Lippincott's Review for NCLEX-PN

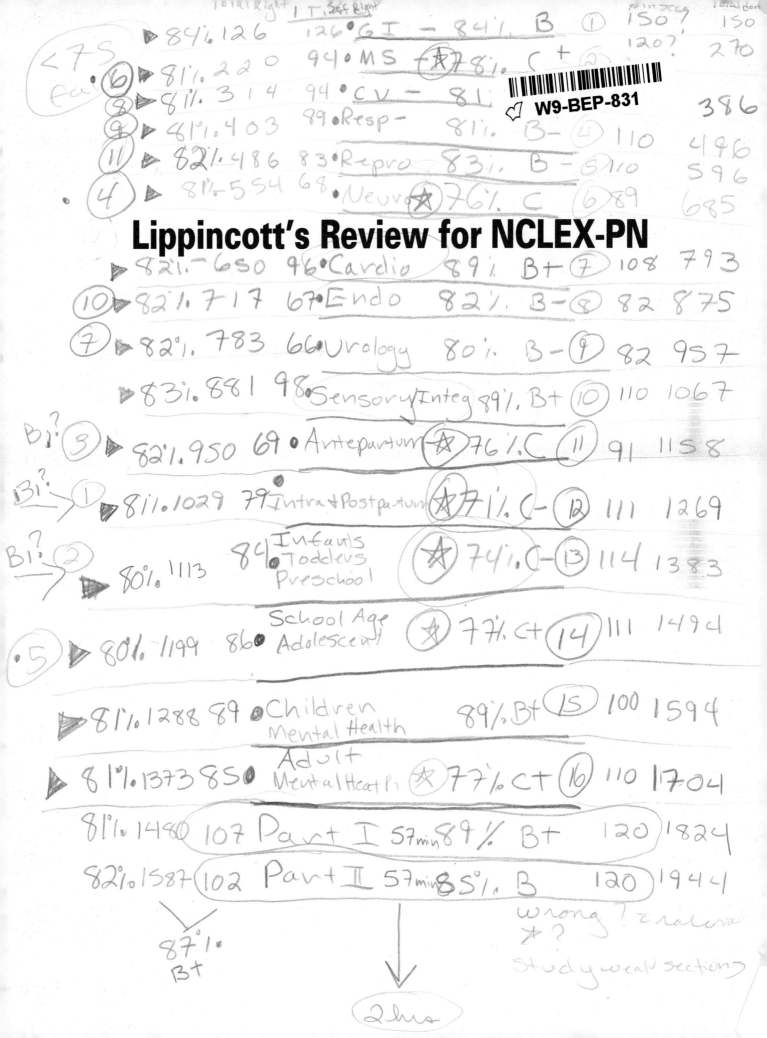

Lippincott's Review for NCLEX-PN

5th Edition

Barbara Kuhn Timby, RNC, BSN, MS

Nursing Professor
Glen Oaks Community College
Centreville, Michigan

Acquisitions Editor: **Susan M. Glover, RN, MSN**
Developmental Editor: **Bridget Blatteau**
Production Editor: **Virginia Barishek**
Production Manager: **Helen Ewan**
Production Service: **Textbook Writers Associates, Inc.**
Compositor: **Bi-Comp**
Printer/Binder: **Courier/Kendallville**
Cover Designer: **William T. Donnelly**
Cover Printer: **Lehigh Press**

5th Edition

9 8 7 6 5 4 3 2 1

Library of Congress Cataloging-in-Publication Data

Timby, Barbara Kuhn.
  Lippincott's review for NCLEX-PN. — 5th ed. / Barbara Kuhn Timby.
    p. cm.
  Includes bibliographical references.
  ISBN 0-397-55471-0
  1. Practical nursing—Examinations, questions, etc.
  [DNLM: 1. Nursing, Practical—examination questions.   WY 18.2
T583L 1998]
RT62.T56   1998
610.73′06′93076—dc21
DNLM/DLC
for Library of Congress   97-36376
                                                       CIP

Care has been taken to confirm the accuracy of the information presented and to describe generally accepted practices. However, the authors, editors, and publisher are not responsible for errors or omissions or for any consequences from application of the information in this book and make no warranty, express or implied, with respect to the contents of the publication.

The authors, editors and publisher have exerted every effort to ensure that drug selection and dosage set forth in this text are in accordance with current recommendations and practice at the time of publication. However, in view of ongoing research, changes in government regulations, and the constant flow of information relating to drug therapy and drug reactions, the reader is urged to check the package insert for each drug for any change in indications and dosage and for added warnings and precautions. This is particularly important when the recommended agent is a new or infrequently employed drug.

Some drugs and medical devices presented in this publication have Food and Drug Administration (FDA) clearance for limited use in restricted research settings. It is the responsibility of the health care provider to ascertain the FDA status of each drug or device planned for use in their clinical practice.

Contributor

Bennita W. Vaughans, RN, MSN

Instructor
Practical Nursing Program
Councill Trenholm State Technical College
Montgomery, Alabama

Coauthor of the Previous Edition

Jeanne C. Scherer, RN, BSN, MS

Formerly Assistant Director and Medical-Surgical Coordinator
Sisters School of Nursing
Buffalo, New York

Contents

Preface

Lippincott's Review for NCLEX-PN, 5th Edition, has been written to help you prepare for the national practical nurse licensing examination. Several features make this review book especially helpful.

First and foremost, the most recent NCLEX-PN Test Plan[1] approved by the National Council of State Boards of Nursing (effective October 1996) was used as a guide for preparing this book. Consequently, the review questions presented here reflect the components in the Test Plan as well as current nursing practice. In addition, the substance of the questions is based entirely on information contained in textbooks that are widely used in practical nursing programs throughout the United States.[2]

An effort also has been made to divide the review book content into comprehensive yet manageable sections. To accomplish this goal, the topics for review are organized into four major units according to specialty areas of nursing practice:

- Unit I: The Nursing Care of Adults with Medical-Surgical Disorders
- Unit II: The Nursing Care of the Childbearing Family
- Unit III: The Nursing Care of Children
- Unit IV: The Nursing Care of Clients with Mental Health Needs

The decision to arrange the content according to specific subject areas was made for several reasons. First, it helps you correlate your review with courses commonly taught in most practical nursing programs. Second, it allows you to focus your energy on reviewing a limited amount of information at any one time.

The four major units are further subdivided into a total of 16 separate review tests. The first unit, which pertains to the nursing care of clients with medical-surgical disorders, contains ten review tests. The remaining three units each contain two review tests. This distribution is appropriate because medical-surgical nursing is the most common clinical area where new practical nurses are employed. And, since the Test Plan is based on a job survey of newly employed practical nurses, it is logical to assume that a majority of the licensing examination questions will reflect items of a medical-surgical nature.

All the questions in the review tests are integrated in the same manner as the licensing examination. This means that underlying each test question—whether it is one that concerns a medical-surgical, maternity, pediatric, or mental health situation—reflects one of the steps in the nursing process and a specific category of client need. Both of these test components are elaborated further in the section on *Frequently Asked Questions* that begins on page xv.

Another helpful feature of this review book is the two-part comprehensive examination that follows the 16 review tests. The examination, beginning on page 453, is as much like the national licensing examination as possible. Like the NCLEX-PN test, the questions in the comprehensive examination are a mix of all nursing content areas and the Test Plan components.

Each part of the comprehensive examination contains 120 items, for a total of 240 items. This is slightly more than the 205 maximum number of questions asked on NCLEX-PN, but it offers you a rough estimate of how long it might take to answer all of the potential NCLEX-PN test items, should that possibility occur.

---

[1] The NCLEX-PN Test Plan is described in detail in the *Frequently Asked Questions* section, which begins on page xv.
[2] References are listed on page 512.

In addition to the two-part comprehensive examination, a similar examination of 115 test items is provided on an accompanying computer diskette. You can use the diskette to realistically simulate the computerized method for taking the NCLEX-PN.

The number of items on the disk is comparable to the average number of questions that most candidates answer when taking the NCLEX-PN examination. Furthermore, because most people taking NCLEX-PN complete it within 2 hours, you can use the disk version to estimate how you compare to the average of those who have taken the national licensing examination.

Other advantages to using this book include use of the sections containing the *Correct Answers and Rationale,* which follow each review test and comprehensive examination. These sections provide the best answer to each test question, the rationale for the correct answer, and reasons why incorrect answers are wrong. Reading the rationales is an excellent technique for reviewing the domain of practical nursing. The cited references and page numbers that correlate with the test questions and answers provide another authoritative resource for review.

Finally, the sections on the *Classification of Test Items* (see page 36, for example) can be used as a diagnostic readiness tool. By following the directions for calculating a percentage test score and competence in each of the test plan components, you can identify the subject areas, steps in the nursing process, or areas of client need where additional review may be beneficial.

In summary, there are 1704 items in the 16 review tests, 240 items in the two-part comprehensive examination, and 115 questions on the computer disk, for a total of 2059 items. Although it is unreasonable to believe that any item in this book will be identical to one in the national examination, it *is* reasonable to expect that NCLEX-PN will test the same kinds of content, knowledge, and skills. Although no review book or licensing examination can cover all aspects of nursing, this book serves as a resource for a comprehensive review and realistic simulation of the NCLEX-PN process.

As a candidate for NCLEX-PN, you are further urged to read the section titled *Frequently Asked Questions,* which begins on page xv. This section provides information about the NCLEX-PN testing process, how the test is designed, and suggestions on how to prepare for the examination.

The *How To Use This Book* section, which begins on page xxix, introduces you to the testing format used in the review book. There also is an overview of how to mark the answer sheets and how to use the answer grids for calculating test results.

Although this book's primary purpose is to help practical nurses prepare for the national licensing examination, it can serve other purposes as well. For example, it can be used to study for various types of achievement tests in nursing. Inactive practical nurses who wish to return to nursing also will find the book useful for review and self-appraisal, as will others who seek course credit by taking challenge examinations for advanced placement. And finally, faculty may find the book helpful for developing expertise in test construction. Regardless of the purpose for which this book is used, however, the ultimate goal is to help prepare practicing nurses for providing safe, effective nursing care.

ACKNOWLEDGMENTS

The author expresses sincere thanks for the contribution of Bennita Vaughans, RN, MSN, who helped revise various categories of test items as well as construct new ones that fit the current test plan. Appreciation is further extended to Jeanne C. Scherer, RN, BSN, MS, the coauthor of the 4th edition, whose previous work made this revision easier.

Finally, recognition is due for the conscientious assistance from the editors and staff who have helped develop this book through its various stages of production. Among that legion, the author wishes to thank Senior Editor Sue Glover and Coordinating Editorial Assistant Bridget Blatteau.

Barbara Kuhn Timby, RNC, BSN, MA

Frequently Asked Questions (FAQ)

The following are frequently asked questions concerning NCLEX-PN and the most current information that is available about the testing process.

WHAT IS NCLEX-PN?

The abbreviation *NCLEX-PN* stands for the *N*ational *C*ouncil *L*icensure *E*xamination for *P*ractical *N*urses. In short, NCLEX-PN is a computerized test developed by the National Council of State Boards of Nursing. The test is used to regulate the licensing of practical and vocational nurses in each of its member states.

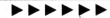

Members of the National Council of State Boards of Nursing

Representatives from:

- All 50 United States
- District of Columbia
- Puerto Rico
- Guam

- American Samoa
- Virgin Islands
- Mariana Islands

WHAT IS THE PURPOSE OF NCLEX-PN?

All National Council member states and territories currently use NCLEX-PN as the standard for licensing practical nurses and vocational nurses. *Practical nurses* and *vocational nurses* are regional terms; they differ in name only. Whether referred to as practical or vocational, each nurse completes similar educational programs, and graduates from both take NCLEX-PN. The terms *practical nurse* and *practical nursing* are used in this book to refer to both.

Licensing serves to assure the public that a graduate practical nurse is a competent practitioner. Passing NCLEX-PN demonstrates that a graduate of a practical nursing program can perform entry-level[1] nursing skills

- that meet the needs of clients with commonly occurring health problems,
- that have predictable outcomes, and
- that demonstrate at least a minimum level of competency.

CAN FOREIGN-EDUCATED NURSES TAKE NCLEX-PN?

Foreign-educated nurses can take NCLEX-PN. Before they can take it, however, they first must meet eligibility requirements in the states where they wish to practice. In most states, foreign-educated nurses are asked to present credentials describing their course of study in the country where they were schooled.

---

[1] *Entry level* is defined as that which is comparable to practical nurses who have been employed for six months or less.

HOW IS NCLEX-PN DEVELOPED?

Before the examination is administered, it goes through several stages of development.

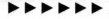

Steps in NCLEX-PN Test Development

- Survey newly licensed practical nurses every 3 years
- Analyze practical nurse job responsibilities
- Formulate a test plan based on the data
- Select and approve item writers
- Submit questions to item reviewers

- Implement trial testing of items
- Give state boards of nursing an opportunity to review items
- Obtain approval of NCLEX-PN items
- Maintain two alternating NCLEX-PN test pools

WHAT IS THE NCLEX-PN TEST PLAN?

The Test Plan, which changes from time to time, serves as the framework for the content that is included in the current NCLEX-PN test. The current Test Plan, which was implemented in October 1996, is based on the results of a study called the *Job Analysis of Newly Licensed Practical Nurses* (1994).

In that study, data were sampled from 3600 newly licensed practical nurses. The participants in the survey were asked to indicate how often they performed each of 238 nursing activities, and whether they could sometimes or never omit the activity without having a major impact on their clients' well-being.

The tabulated results of the job analysis study influence the subject matter tested and the percentage of questions asked in particular NCLEX-PN test categories. The test categories on the current NCLEX-PN Test Plan consist of two broad content areas: *phases of the nursing process*, and *client needs*.

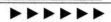

NCLEX-PN Test Plan Categories

Phases of Nursing Process
Data collection
Planning
Implementation
Evaluation

Client Needs
Safe, effective care environment
Physiological integrity
Psychosocial integrity
Health promotion and maintenance

The distribution of questions varies in each of the two test plan categories (Fig. 1). The current NCLEX-PN test includes the following percentages of nursing process items:

- Data collection, 27% to 33%
- Planning, 17% to 23%
- Implementation, 27% to 33%
- Evaluation, 17% to 23%

The distribution of NCLEX-PN test items in the client need categories is as follows:

- Safe, effective care environment, 16% to 22%
- Physiological integrity, 49% to 55%
- Psychosocial integrity, 8% to 14%
- Health promotion and health maintenance, 15% to 21%

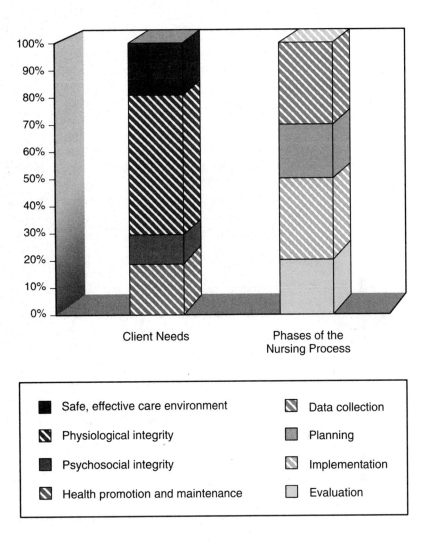

Figure 1. Structure of the Test Plan.

Phases of the Nursing Process

Not all phases of the nursing process are tested equally because some activities are shared between registered nurses and practical nurses in the clinical setting. Therefore those phases that practical nurses perform more often independently, specifically data collection and implementation, are tested in higher proportion.

Data Collection
The *data collection* category of the Test Plan involves questions that are concerned with

- gathering information about clients,
- recording and reporting acquired information, and
- helping to formulate nursing diagnoses.

Planning
The *planning* step of the nursing process is tested in situational questions involving

- formulating goals of care, and
- assisting with the development of a care plan.

Implementation

Implementation items are those questions that relate to

- assisting with the organization and management of client care,
- providing nursing care that leads to goal accomplishment, and
- communicating the outcomes of the care.

Evaluation

Evaluation questions are those whose situations concern

- participating in nursing activities that determine the effectiveness of nursing care,
- documenting the responses that have been identified,
- determining if goals have been achieved, partially achieved, or remain unachieved, and
- assisting with making appropriate changes in the plan of care.

Client Needs

Of the four client need categories, the emphasis is on physiological integrity. The remaining categories, in descending order, are a safe and effective care environment, health promotion and health maintenance, and psychosocial integrity.

Physiological Integrity

Physiological integrity is a category of knowledge tested in questions about

- providing care during acute and chronic phases of health disorders, including emergency situations,
- reducing the potential for developing complications or additional health problems, including the administration of medications, and
- assisting clients with basic care.

Safe, Effective Care Environment

The *safe, effective care environment* category involves questions about

- collaborating with health team members to coordinate client care, including legal and ethical issues,
- protecting clients and personnel from injury, and
- preparing and caring for clients undergoing therapeutic or diagnostic procedures.

Health Promotion and Health Maintenance

The category of *health promotion and health maintenance* tests the examinee's ability to answer questions about

- assisting clients through normal stages of growth and development,
- promoting self-care among clients and support to their significant others, and
- helping clients in the prevention and early detection of health problems and disease.

Psychosocial Integrity

The questions in the *psychosocial integrity* category relate to

- providing care for clients with cognitive and mental health disorders, and
- promoting clients' abilities to cope, adapt, or problem-solve situations involving stressful life events.

WHAT IS THE STYLE OF QUESTIONS ASKED ON NCLEX-PN?

NCLEX-PN uses only multiple-choice questions. A multiple-choice question, also called an *item*, has two main parts: the *stem* and the *options*.

The Stem

The *stem* presents the problem or situation that requires a solution. The stem of an NCLEX-PN multiple-choice question may be stated as an incomplete sentence or as a question.

If all the essential information for answering the question is contained in the stem, it is called a *stand-alone item*. Sometimes the stem is preceded by a *case scenario*, which gives background information that is pertinent to the item.

The Options

The *options* are the choices from which an answer is selected. There are always four options in each multiple-choice question. Options are worded to either end the incomplete sentence or supply an answer to the question in the stem.

The options on NCLEX-PN are labeled *1, 2, 3, 4.* There are no multiple-multiple or compound choices. In other words, there are no combinations like "1 and 2," "all," or "none."

In all cases, there is one and only one *correct* answer. The three incorrect options are called *distractors*. Distractors are intended to appear as good answers; they may even be partially correct. But an option is incorrect if it is not the *best answer* to the question.

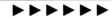

Examples of Stems and Options

Stem as an Incomplete Sentence
Immediately after a pregnant client's membranes rupture, the *most appropriate* nursing action is to

1. monitor the fetal heart rate.*
2. begin the client on antibiotics.
3. put a waterproof pad beneath the client.
4. place the client in the Trendelenberg position.

Stem as a Question
Which assessment finding *best* justifies withholding the continued intramuscular administration of penicillin (Bicillin) until consulting with the prescribing physician?

1. The client states that the injection sites are painful.
2. The client shows the nurse a red, itchy skin rash.*
3. The client's oral body temperature is 100°F.
4. The client has been having two stools a day.

* Correct answer

HOW IS NCLEX-PN ADMINISTERED?

As of April 1994, the former pencil-and-paper method for taking NCLEX-PN was replaced with computerized adaptive testing (CAT). This means that a computer is used to administer the test. The term *adaptive* refers to the fact that the computer creates a unique test for each candidate. (See *How Does the Computer Select Test Questions?* later in the FAQ.)

The computerized method of testing offers several advantages compared to the earlier way of taking NCLEX-PN. For example, it

- facilitates year-round testing,
- offers convenient scheduling choices,
- personalizes the test for each examinee,
- shortens the length of the examination, and
- expedites notification of test results.

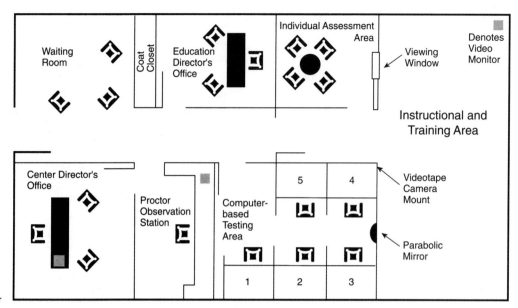

Figure 2. Sample NCLEX test site floor plan. (Redrawn with permission of the National Council of State Boards of Nursing, Inc., Chicago, IL.)

A candidate may request any testing site regardless of the state in which he or she wishes to be licensed. Since the test is adapted to each candidate, it can be completed in 5 hours or less; the average time is less than 2 hours (National Council of State Boards of Nursing, 1995). And because scoring is computerized, examination results are available move rapidly than in the past.

WHAT IS THE TESTING SITE LIKE?

Each of more than 200 testing sites is able to accommodate up to 10 candidates at the same time. A sample of the basic floor plan of a test site is shown in Figure 2. Each examinee is assigned to a separate testing cubicle that contains a table with computer equipment, a desk lamp, and scratch paper. Personal articles can be placed in secured storage or lockers outside the test room.

Persons with special physical needs, or those requesting modifications in the testing process or environment, must make that information known to the board of nursing at the time of application. A letter from a professional confirming the candidate's disability also is required. If the board of nursing approves the applicant's request, special accommodations are made if they do not jeopardize the security of the test or give the candidate an unfair advantage.

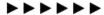 **Test Site Security Policies**

Before the test, each person must

- possess an *Authorization to Test* (ATT) affidavit.*
- present two forms of signature identification.
  - One must contain a recent photograph.
  - The name on the photograph identification must match exactly the name on the ATT.
- be photographed and thumbprinted.

* See *How Do I Register for NCLEX-PN?* on page xxiv.

Precautions are taken to ensure that the candidate who is registered for NCLEX-PN and the person at the test site are one and the same.

Once the examination commences, test security is maintained in three ways. All candidates are observed directly and continuously by a proctor who can view the testing cubicles without entering the room. In addition, candidates are monitored by video and audio equipment that has taping capability.

WILL I BE GIVEN A CHANCE TO PRACTICE USING THE COMPUTER?

Regardless of the candidates' computer skills, each is given an opportunity to practice before the actual test begins. If necessary, computer help also is available during the examination. Candidates with computer experience so far have not demonstrated any advantage in test performance.

HOW DOES THE COMPUTER SELECT TEST QUESTIONS?

The NCLEX-PN questions vary in their level of difficulty. When the test begins, the first questions generally are of moderate difficulty. If a candidate answers such a question incorrectly, the computer selects an easy question next. If the moderately difficult item is answered correctly, the next question is more difficult. Passing the examination depends both on the number of correct answers and on their level of difficulty.

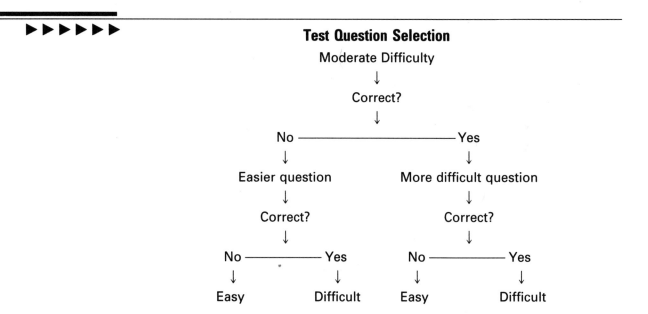

▶ ▶ ▶ ▶ ▶ ▶

Test Question Selection

Moderate Difficulty
↓
Correct?
↓
No ——————————— Yes
↓   ↓
Easier question   More difficult question
↓   ↓
Correct?   Correct?
↓   ↓
No ———— Yes   No ———— Yes
↓   ↓   ↓   ↓
Easy   Difficult   Easy   Difficult

HOW ARE THE TEST QUESTIONS DISPLAYED?

The manner in which stand-alone items and case scenario items are displayed on the computer screen along with the accompanying options is illustrated in Figure 3.

HOW DO I INDICATE MY ANSWERS TO NCLEX-PN QUESTIONS?

Answers are selected by using one of two keys on the keyboard. The only two working keys are the *Space Bar* and the *Enter Key* (Fig. 4). The space bar moves the cursor to highlight a choice. The enter key is pressed to record the highlighted choice. At each computer there is a description of the two keys and a written explanation on how to use them.

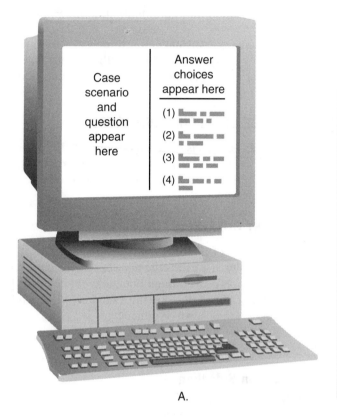 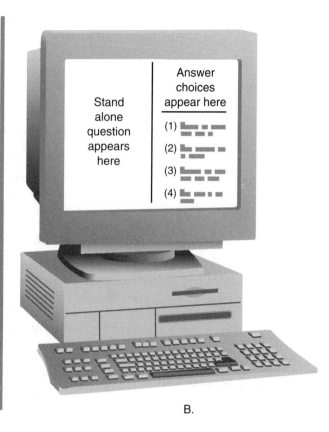

A.
B.

Figure 3. NCLEX questions and answer choices are displayed in either of two ways: (A) Case scenario and question on half of the screen and the numbered answer choices on the other half or (B) stand alone question and answer choices on the screen. (Redrawn with permission of the National Council of State Boards of Nursing, Inc., Chicago, IL.)

HOW LONG DO THE QUESTIONS REMAIN ON THE SCREEN?

Each question remains on the screen until an answer is recorded. Candidates are *not* able to

- skip a question,
- review previous questions, or
- change answers.

The underlying reason is that the difficulty of each test question is based on the examinee's answer to preceding test questions.

HOW MANY QUESTIONS ARE ASKED IN NCLEX-PN?

Each examinee's test is unique. It is made up of a comparatively small number of items from among the vast quantity stored in the memory of the computerized test pool.

To be specific, however, the minimum number of questions that a candidate must answer is 85. Sixty of these are scored questions and 25 are tryout items.[2] The tryout items may be used in subsequent test pools. The maximum number of questions is 205 questions, 180 of which are scored; the remainder are tryout items.

There is no way for the examinee to determine which questions are tryout items. The tryout items are *not* calculated in the final NCLEX-PN score, regardless of whether the examinee answers the questions correctly or not.

On the average, approximately 50% of NCLEX-PN examinees answer the minimum number of test items. Fewer than one-third, or 33% of NCLEX-PN examinees, answer the maximum number of questions. The latter group are usually those whose test performance is on the borderline between pass or fail. The remaining test candidates answer between 85 and 205 items. The average number of items answered by examinees in 1994–1995 was 113 (National Council of State Boards of Nursing, 1995).

---

[2] The number of tryout items on the NCLEX-PN test may vary as the test pool of items accumulates.

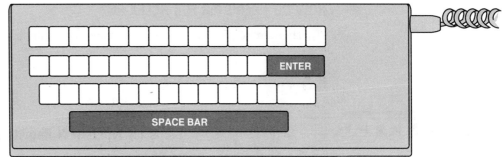

Figure 4. Only the enter key and space bar, which are darkened in the illustration, are used when taking NCLEX-PN. (Redrawn with permission of the National Council of State Boards of Nursing, Inc., Chicago, IL.)

HOW LONG DOES NCLEX-PN TAKE?

Since each test is tailor-made for the examinee, there is no minimum amount of time for the test. The maximum length of time allowed for NCLEX-PN is 5 hours. Most finish much sooner. The examination time varies depending on how speedily the examinee reads and answers each test item *and* on how well or poorly the questions are answered.

▶ ▶ ▶ ▶ ▶ ▶

NCLEX-PN Testing Parameters

Minimum Number of Questions	85
Maximum Number of Questions	205
Minimum Testing Time	None
Maximum Testing Time	5 hours
Mandatory Break	After 2½ hours
Optional Break	After 4 hours

The test is terminated when the computer has sufficient data to determine with 95% confidence whether the candidate has demonstrated sufficient knowledge to pass the examination, or not. The test ends automatically when the examinee

- answers at least a minimum number of 85 questions correctly.
- answers 85 to 205 questions at or below the passing standard.
- answers 205 questions without enough assurity to determine a passing or failing score.
- is still testing when the 5-hour time limit expires.

WHO DECIDES THE PASS/FAIL SCORE FOR NCLEX-PN?

The National Council's Board of Directors ultimately establishes the official minimum passing standard for NCLEX-PN. The Board of Directors' decision is made after receiving recommendations from a panel of nine judges. The panel, who represent diverse geographic regions and areas of clinical practice, determine what portion of minimally competent practical nurses would correctly answer each test question in a sample NCLEX-PN examination.

The passing standard for NCLEX-PN is re-evaluated whenever the test plan changes or at 3-year intervals, whichever comes first. Each state has the authority to set the minimum passing score in its own jurisdiction. Most states, however, use the same minimum passing score proposed by the National Council of State Boards of Nursing.

HOW DO I REGISTER FOR NCLEX-PN?

There are several basic steps that all candidates must complete before taking NCLEX-PN.

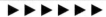

Steps for NCLEX-PN Registration

1. Apply to the board of nursing in the state from which licensure is sought.
2. Request that the nursing program provide the board with proof of eligibility to take NCLEX-PN.
3. Register with the Educational Testing Service.
4. Pay a fee of $88 (as of 1996).

NCLEX-PN applications may be obtained on request from the state board of nursing, or they may be available from the candidate's school of nursing. After receiving an application, the state board of nursing determines if the applicant meets licensure eligibility requirements.

Once the candidate's eligibility is confirmed, NCLEX-PN registration with the Educational Testing Service (ETS) can go forward. ETS registration may be done in either of two ways: directly by mail or phone; or electronically for candidates requesting licensure in Florida, Illinois, Massachusetts, and New York. Forms and information on registering for NCLEX-PN can be obtained by requesting the *NCLEX Candidate Bulletin* from the National Council of State Boards of Nursing.

Fee payment is required at the time of direct registration. Mailed registrations must be accompanied by a certified check, cashier's check, or money order made out to the National Council of State Boards of Nursing. *Personal checks are unacceptable.* Phone registration can be paid by using a valid VISA, MasterCard, or American Express credit card, and requires an additional small service fee. There is no fee payment to the ETS when using electronic registration; information on fee arrangements can be obtained from the boards of nursing in those states using electronic transfer registration.

After the ETS registration is processed, the candidate is sent a publication titled *Scheduling and Taking Your NCLEX*, along with a printed form called an Authorization to Test (ATT). There are three pieces of important information on the ATT. They include a candidate examination number, an authorization number, and an expiration date.

WHEN AND HOW DO I ARRANGE TO TAKE NCLEX-PN?

After receiving an ATT, candidates can schedule a test date by phone with the test site of their choice before the expiration date that appears on the ATT. The locations and phone numbers of all available test sites are provided in the scheduling brochure.

After contacting the test site, first-time candidates are offered a test date within 30 days; repeating candidates may be scheduled within a 45-day period. Either type of candidate can request a date beyond the 30 or 45 days as long as the date occurs prior to the expiration date on the ATT.

If the candidate wishes to cancel or reschedule a testing date, it must be done within 3 business days of the original appointment; otherwise all fees are forfeited and the ATT is revoked. The same policy applies if a candidate is more than 30 minutes late on the date of the test.

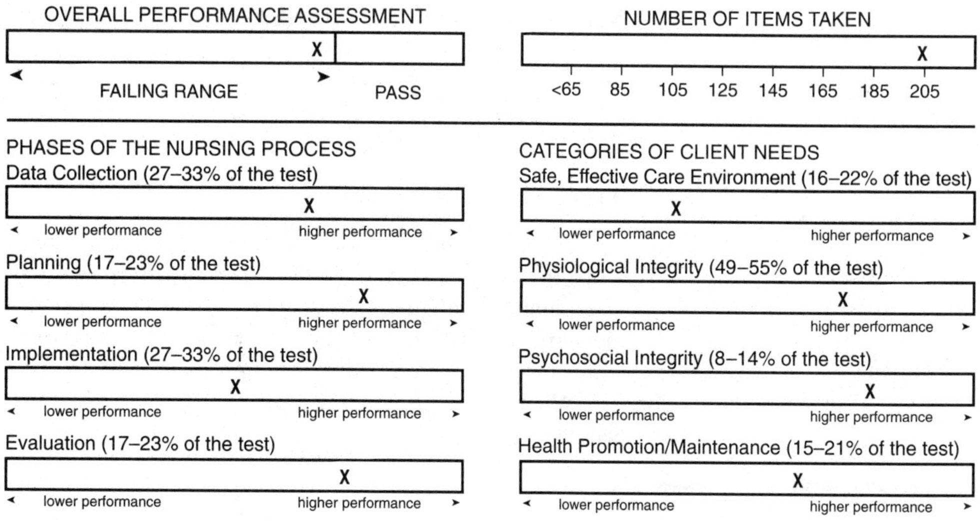

OVERALL PERFORMANCE ASSESSMENT

	X	

◄   FAILING RANGE   ►   PASS

NUMBER OF ITEMS TAKEN

	X

<65   85   105   125   145   165   185   205

Figure 5. The scale titled "Overall Performance Assessment" shows how well you did on NCLEX-PN. The "X" shows how far below passing your performance fell. Passing is indicated by the vertical bar shown in the box. The "X" in each of the eight other boxes shows how well you did in the test plan content areas. (Redrawn with permission of the National Council of State Boards of Nursing, Inc., Chicago, IL.)

PHASES OF THE NURSING PROCESS

Data Collection (27–33% of the test)

	X	

◄ lower performance   higher performance ►

Planning (17–23% of the test)

	X

◄ lower performance   higher performance ►

Implementation (27–33% of the test)

X	

◄ lower performance   higher performance ►

Evaluation (17–23% of the test)

	X

◄ lower performance   higher performance ►

CATEGORIES OF CLIENT NEEDS

Safe, Effective Care Environment (16–22% of the test)

X

◄ lower performance   higher performance ►

Physiological Integrity (49–55% of the test)

	X

◄ lower performance   higher performance ►

Psychosocial Integrity (8–14% of the test)

	X

◄ lower performance   higher performance ►

Health Promotion/Maintenance (15–21% of the test)

X

◄ lower performance   higher performance ►

HOW WILL I BE INFORMED OF MY NCLEX-PN RESULTS?

Test results, either Pass or Fail, are reported by mail from the state board of nursing where the candidate desires licensure. Although each examinee's score is electronically transmitted from the testing service to the respective board of nursing within 48 hours following an examination, the interim for informing the candidate varies from state to state. On the whole, most candidates receive their test results 1 month after taking the examination.

A candidate who fails NCLEX-PN is provided with a testing analysis in the form of a printed diagnostic profile (Fig. 5). The profile gives data on how close the candidate came to the minimum passing score, how many items were answered, and how good or poor a performance was achieved in each of the eight test plan categories. The statistical data is offered to assist failing candidates to improve their potential for success when retaking NCLEX-PN. Weak areas suggest where an unsuccessful candidate might concentrate his or her review.

WHAT IF I FEEL MY TEST RESULT IS INCORRECT?

Some (but not all) states provide a process for reviewing and challenging NCLEX-PN test results. If a failed candidate feels that his or her test performance measurement is invalid, or wants the opportunity to dispute the answer to missed items, arrangements can be made to examine the questions that were answered in error. The review and challenge involves a fee and is limited to no more than 2½ hours.

WHEN CAN I RETAKE NCLEX-PN IF I FAIL?

At present, a repeating candidate may retake the examination up to four times a year, but no more frequently than every 91 days. This allows for a variation in items within the existing test pool. When and if the test pool of items increases, the frequency for retesting may be amended.

WHAT ARE SOME STRATEGIES FOR NCLEX-PN SUCCESS?

There are certain strategies that promote success on the NCLEX-PN examination. Some are more appropriate for long-term planning, while others are more pertinent as the test date for NCLEX-PN nears.

Long-Term Strategies

Long-term strategies are best implemented as early as possible after completion of a nursing program. In fact, some nursing programs include standardized comprehensive examinations for graduating nurses to help predict how well the potential graduate will perform on NCLEX-PN. But most new graduates are left to their own initiative when it comes to preparing for the licensing examination.

Whatever approaches are used, it is best to begin preparing for NCLEX-PN well in advance.

▶ ▶ ▶ ▶ ▶ ▶   **Strategic Plan for NCLEX-PN Preparation**

- Develop a time schedule for a comprehensive review.
- Divide the review topics into manageable amounts.
- Refresh your knowledge of topics in nursing courses.
- Reread sections in nursing textbooks, classroom notes, and written assignments.
- Re-examine tests from previous nursing courses.
- Concentrate on information that is necessary for safe care.
- Use this review book to assess your areas of competence.
- Identify weak areas and restudy or clarify information.

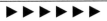

A systematic and comprehensive review is more effective than last-minute cramming. Cramming contributes to disorganized thinking; facts and concepts are likely to be confused. With cramming there is always an underlying fear of being unprepared, which only heightens test anxiety.

One method of continued learning and retention of learned material is to focus on the review of subjects recently covered in the classroom. For example, after a focused review of the nursing care of clients with disorders of the cardiovascular system it is advantageous to take the corresponding review test in this book. This is considered a practical approach because, although NCLEX-PN basically tests the eight categories in the two components of the test plan, the test questions are asked from a medical, surgical, obstetric, pediatric, or mental health perspective.

Above all, it is best to include review strategies that have been successful in the past.

▶ ▶ ▶ ▶ ▶ ▶   **Review Strategies**

- Give priority attention to your weaker subjects first.
- Review key concepts in nursing textbooks.
- Summarize information identified in chapter objectives.
- Process critical-thinking questions in nursing books.
- Concentrate on how each step of the nursing process and client needs apply to the specific review topic.
- Organize or join a study group preparing for NCLEX-PN.
- Select an environment that is conducive to concentration.
- Choose to review when you are most energetic and focused.
- Keep review periods short, regular, and on task.
- Take an NCLEX-PN review course if your motivation weakens.
- Invest in NCLEX-PN computerized testing programs.

Short-Term Strategies

Some strategies are more appropriate as the testing date draws near.

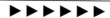

Strategies for Ensuring Success

- Correct vision or hearing problems prior to the test date.
- Make a trial run to the test site location.
- Obtain motel or hotel reservations if the test site is distant.
- Plan some leisure activity the day before the test.
- Get an adequate amount of sleep the night before the test.
- Awaken early.
- Eat sensibly.
- Avoid taking any mind- or mood-altering drugs.
- Take required admission papers and identification.
- Bring a snack or beverage for scheduled breaks.
- Distance yourself from anyone who looks frantic; anxiety is contagious.
- Locate the restroom and use it shortly before the test.
- Utilize relaxation techniques.
- Make positive statements to yourself about your ability.

If you utilize several of the suggested long- and short-term strategies, you can approach the NCLEX-PN examination with a feeling of confidence and a positive mental attitude. You will be off to a good start by continuing to work your way through this review book.

How to Use This Book

This review book, which is a series of tests that cover a wide variety of health-related problems, can be used as one of the strategies for preparing for NCLEX-PN. Answering the majority of questions correctly indicates a solid foundation for taking the national licensing examination and preparation for managing situations in clinical practice. Although one of its objectives is to simulate NCLEX-PN as much as possible, this book's primary goal is to provide graduate nurses with an effective resource for reviewing nursing content.

After reading the *Preface* and the section entitled *Frequently Asked Questions,* you are ready to begin. The topics in this section with which you should become familiar include the *Organization of the Review Book,* the *Testing Format,* the *Correct Answers and Rationale,* the *Classification of Test Items,* and the *Comprehensive Examinations.*

ORGANIZATION OF THE REVIEW BOOK

This review book is divided into four units. Each unit is devoted to a particular specialty area of clinical practice.

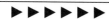

Divisions for Review

- Unit I: The Nursing Care of Adults with Medical-Surgical Disorders
- Unit II: The Nursing Care of the Childbearing Family
- Unit III: The Nursing Care of Children
- Unit IV: The Nursing Care of Clients with Mental Health Needs

The units are subdivided into two or more review tests that concentrate on particular types of clients, health problems, and nursing care. A two-part printed comprehensive examination and a comprehensive examination on a computer disk are provided as a final resource for your NCLEX-PN review.

REVIEW STRATEGIES

There are many strategies for preparing for NCLEX-PN. Whatever plan you use, give yourself sufficient time. One suggestion that may be worth considering is to review one subject area or topic at a time and then analyze your competency by taking the related review test.

TESTING FORMAT

The NCLEX-PN examination and this review book use only multiple-choice questions consisting of a stem and four options. When a case scenario accompanies a question, it is italicized and precedes the stem. Examples of multiple-choice questions and their respective components follow.

Case Scenario

A 49-year-old male is short of breath, has a heart rate of 110 beats per minute, and has moist lung sounds.

Stem in the form of an incomplete sentence

1. The best position for promoting ventilation for this client is

Options

1. supine.   < *distractor*
2. Fowler's.   < *correct answer*
3. prone.   < *distractor*
4. Sims.   < *distractor*

Stem in the form of a question without an accompanying case scenario

2. Which drug can the nurse expect to administer if a client receiving warfarin sodium (Coumadin) begins to hemorrhage?

Options

1. Protamine sulfate   < *distractor*
2. Sodium citrate   < *distractor*
3. Vitamin K   < *correct answer*
4. Vitamin E   < *distractor*

When developing the stems and options for the multiple-choice items in this book, certain editorial policies have been adopted, consistent with those that are found on NCLEX-PN.

EDITORIAL POLICIES

In this review book the word *client* is used when referring to the person receiving nursing services. Although the word *patient* is more familiar to some, *client* is the term that is used throughout NCLEX-PN.

Clients are identified generically by age, gender, and medical information. No personal names are given, as you might have experienced on other examinations. The same principle is followed on NCLEX-PN.

An effort also has been made to avoid using feminine pronouns when referring to the nurse because more and more men are joining their female colleagues in nursing practice. A similar decision was made regarding the use of only masculine pronouns when referring to physicians. In most cases they are identified as *the nurse* or *the physician*. You can assume that the nurse to which the question refers is a practical nurse; if not, that information is identified.

Last, in multiple-choice questions involving drugs, both the generic and a brand name are provided wherever possible. The generic name is given first; a common brand or trade name follows in parentheses.

CHOOSING ANSWERS

There are several necessary steps in choosing an answer. They include analyzing the information, looking for key words or terms, selecting an option, and marking your choice.

Analyzing the Information

It is always best to read each case scenario and stem carefully. Focus on the information that makes the situation unique. Arriving at a correct answer involves integrating the pertinent facts within the context of the question. For example, if you are informed that a client is 3 years old, the answer to the question might be different than if the client is 65 years old, based on variations in the life cycle.

Looking for Key Terms

Key terms are words and their modifiers that help call attention to the critical information in the question. Identifying key terms, which are italicized wherever they appear in the stem of a question, can help you select the answer that fits the intent of the question.

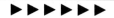

Examples of Key Words and Modifiers

Key Words	Key Words and Modifiers
best	best response
most	best evidence
next	best measure
at this time	best answer
immediately	best explanation
least	most important
except	most appropriate
earliest	most accurate
essential	most indicative
initially	most suggestive

Marking Your Choice

Once you have decided which option is best, you can record your answer by blackening the circle in front of that option in the review test. Alternately, you can follow a similar procedure by removing the perforated answer sheets for the appropriate test in the back of the book (see page 513 for the series of answer sheets).

A word of warning: The correct answers are *randomized,* that is, they do not follow a pattern. It is therefore foolhardy to choose an answer by trying to predict some planned sequence in the numbered choices.

Once you have completed a review test, you can begin to compare your answers with those in the sections titled *Correct Answers and Rationale.* These sections follow each review test and each part of the two-part comprehensive examination.

CORRECT ANSWERS AND RATIONALE

Refer to the sections on correct answers and rationale *after* completing each test and the comprehensive examination. Compare your answers with those identified as the correct answers. Make a check mark next to the items that you answered incorrectly.

Study the rationale for each item regardless of whether it was answered correctly or incorrectly. The rationales often contain additional information that will enhance your NCLEX-PN review.

Next, analyze the reason you chose an incorrect answer. If you answered incorrectly because you did not read the item carefully or because you blackened in the wrong circle, plan to concentrate more on reading and marking the answers more accurately. If you made an error because you lacked the knowledge required to answer the question correctly, it indicates that you should restudy that specific health-related problem. One resource you may wish to use for further review is the cited reference that accompanies each answer and rationale. (In some cases two or more references are given.)

REFERENCES

All of the test questions in this book are based on information found in current nursing textbooks. The references, which appear on page 512, were chosen from among those that are most widely used among programs in practical nursing.

After each answer and rationale, the first number indicates the corresponding numbered reference in which the information in the answer is based. The second number identifies the pertinent page numbers on the subject of the test question in that respective reference.

It is helpful to have as many of these references available as possible. The learning resources library in a school for practical nursing may have some in their collection, or they may be obtained temporarily through an interlibrary loan agreement.

After checking your answers, you can identify your strenghts and weaknesses by tabulating your test results in the section titled *Classification of Test Items*.

CLASSIFICATION OF TEST ITEMS

The *Classification of Test Items* (see page 36, for example) is a collection of grids. The grids code each question in each review test and the comprehensive examination according to the components used in the Test Plan for the NCLEX-PN examination. In other words, the respective step in the nursing process and the specific client need underlying each question are identified. In fact, the items in the two-part comprehensive examination are distributed in exactly the same percentages as those on NCLEX-PN.[1]

Follow the directions at the beginning of the grid and you can calculate your overall percentage on the review test. More important, however, you will be able to determine how well or poorly you performed in any of the Test Plan components. This information can be extremely beneficial in identifying where you need to improve before taking NCLEX-PN.

Although the outcomes are not foolproof, a score of 75% or better overall and the same in each category of the Test Plan indicate a reasonable readiness for passing NCLEX-PN. Scores lower than 75% indicate areas of weakness that may result in failing the licensing examination unless they are strengthened.

COMPREHENSIVE EXAMINATIONS

After taking all of the review tests and completing your review, you are ready to take a comprehensive examination. You may wish to take the two-part examination in the book or the examination on computer disk, or both. Whatever your decision, take these examinations as seriously as if you were taking the actual licensing examination.

Both of these practice examinations are intended to simulate the NCLEX-PN test. The printed version contains a few more items than the maximum number asked on NCLEX-PN. Because of its length, it provides the greatest opportunity for practice in answering a mix of questions from all of the review test material.

The computerized version contains 115 items, which is the approximate number answered by most candidates who pass the NCLEX-PN examination. It, too, contains a mix of questions that relate to topics in each of the four review test units. In addition, the computerized version simulates the same testing process candidates are required to use when taking NCLEX-PN.

When all of the components of this book are utilized along with recommended areas for further review, most candidates can acquire the self-confidence that will make passing the NCLEX-PN examination that much easier.

---

[1] For further information, see page xvi in the section *Frequently Asked Questions*.

The Nursing Care of Adults with Medical-Surgical Disorders

Directions: With a pencil, blacken the circle in front of the option you have chosen for your correct answer.

NURSING CARE OF CLIENTS WITH DISORDERS OF THE MOUTH

A client develops mucositis of the oral cavity while receiving chemotherapy for cancer.

1 Which one of the following items is it *best* for the nurse to withhold from his dietary tray?
- ● 1. Tomato soup
- ○ 2. Lime gelatin
- ○ 3. Canned peaches
- ○ 4. Rice pudding

2 If the client with mucositis needs supplies for performing oral hygiene, it is *best* for the nurse to provide
- ○ 1. pediatric toothbrush.
- ○ 2. waxed dental floss.
- ● 3. sponge-tipped swabs.
- ○ 4. mint-flavored mouthwash.

A nurse is assigned to care for several clients, all of whom will receive oral hygiene.

3 For which one of the following clients should the nurse plan specialized rather than routine oral hygiene measures that are performed by brushing the teeth twice a day?
- ○ 1. Patient A who has full dentures
- ○ 2. Patient B who is on fluid restrictions
- ○ 3. Patient C who is on a low-residue diet
- ● 4. Patient D who sucks on ice chips

4 When the nurse cares for a client's dentures, which one of the following techniques is *most* appropriate?
- ○ 1. The nurse uses hot water while brushing and rinsing the dentures.
- ○ 2. The nurse holds the dentures over a basin of water or soft towel.
- ● 3. The nurse applies solvent to remove the oral adhesive from the dentures.
- ○ 4. The nurse places the dentures in a clean, dry container after brushing.

5 In which position is it *best* for the nurse to place an unconscious client while brushing the client's teeth?
- ○ 1. Supine with head elevated
- ● 2. Side-lying with head lowered
- ○ 3. Prone with head lowered
- ○ 4. Recumbent with head elevated

A client has been taking a tetracycline antibiotic for the past 2 weeks. A candidiasis infection is suspected at this time.

6 If the client has candidiasis, also known as moniliasis or thrush, which one of the following is the nurse *most likely* to observe when inspecting the oral cavity?
- ○ 1. Clear, shiny, domed vesicles on the tongue
- ○ 2. Red, ulcerated patches at the gum margin
- ● 3. White, curd-like patches throughout the mouth
- ○ 4. Dark, brown, flat lesions in the oropharynx

7 The client with candidiasis asks the nurse how he may have acquired this oral infection. The *most accurate* explanation is that most individuals acquire candidiasis by
○ 1. transferring bacteria from unclean dental instruments.
◉ 2. having an unchecked growth of normal mouth organisms.
○ 3. inhaling moist droplets when someone sneezed.
○ 4. consuming contaminated water or tainted food.

The physician prescribes nystatin (Mycostatin) oral suspension for the client with candidiasis.

8 Which one of the following steps should the nurse plan to teach the client when administering nystatin oral suspension?
○ 1. Drink the medication through a straw.
○ 2. Dilute the medication with cold water.
◉ 3. Retain the drug as long as possible in the mouth.
○ 4. Swish the drug in the mouth, but avoid swallowing it.

An older client is referred for suspected cancer of the mouth following a routine dental examination.

9 If the client with cancer of the mouth is typical of others with this diagnosis, which one of the following etiologic factors is the nurse *most likely* to find when reading his medical history?
○ 1. The client drinks decaffeinated coffee on a daily basis.
◉ 2. The client has used smokeless tobacco most of his life.
○ 3. The client has had a partial dental plate for five years.
○ 4. The client chews gum sweetened with aspartame (NutraSweet).

The client's oral cancer is treated with needles containing radioactive cesium that are implanted inside his cheek.

10 Which addition to the care plan is *essential* in the event that the client with the radioactive implant should vomit?
○ 1. Inspect emesis for solid objects before disposing.
○ 2. Rinse emesis basin with diluted household bleach.
◉ 3. Provide plastic emesis basin rather than metal.
○ 4. Cut threads to implanted cesium if vomiting occurs.

11 Assuming the client with mouth cancer enjoys all of the following, which diversional activity is *best* while he is receiving radiation therapy?
○ 1. Allow family to visit as long as they like.
○ 2. Spend an hour playing cards with the client.
◉ 3. Provide kits for building miniature airplanes.
○ 4. Have other clients join in playing board games.

While being prepared for a gynecologic examination, a female client discusses the herpes simplex type I lesion on her mouth which she refers to as a "cold sore."

12 If the client makes all of the following statements about the lesion, which one indicates that she is *misinformed?* She says that
○ 1. the lesion is a result of a viral infection.
○ 2. the infection is spread by direct contact.
○ 3. emotional stress can trigger a recurrence.
◉ 4. the lesions only form on or within the mouth.

The client with the herpes lesion has been taking acyclovir (Zovirax), which was prescribed by her physician.

13 Which statement indicates that the client understands the purpose for her drug therapy? She says that acyclovir
○ 1. kills all of the virus causing the lesion.
◉ 2. shortens the duration of an acute episode.
○ 3. prevents future outbreaks from occurring.
○ 4. must be taken daily for her lifetime.

NURSING CARE OF CLIENTS WITH DISORDERS OF THE ESOPHAGUS

A 60-year-old male client has been experiencing difficulty swallowing. The nurse in the ambulatory surgery department schedules him for an esophagoscopy.

14 Which statement indicates that the client understands how he is to prepare himself for an esophagoscopy? The client says it is essential that he
○ 1. eat a light breakfast before the examination.
○ 2. consume a low-residue diet until the test is done.
◉ 3. avoid food and fluids after midnight before the test.
○ 4. drink a quart of liquid before arriving for the test.

The esophagoscopy reveals that the client has a stricture near the end of his esophagus.

15 To help improve the client's ability to swallow, the *best recommendation* the nurse can make is to tell him to
 ○ 1. eat a variety of baby foods from now on.
 ◉ 2. chew everything that is eaten very thoroughly.
 ○ 3. avoid drinking beverages while eating a meal.
 ○ 4. refrain from consuming milk and dairy products.

A 38-year-old male is admitted with bleeding esophageal varices.

16 As the nurse reviews the client's medical record, which of the following factors is *most likely* related to his present condition? The client
 ○ 1. works at an oil refinery.
 ○ 2. is a lacto-ovovegetarian.
 ○ 3. is extremely underweight.
 ◉ 4. drinks alcohol heavily.

The registered nurse starts an infusion of whole blood and asks the practical nurse to continue monitoring the client with the bleeding esophageal varices during the blood transfusion.

17 If the practical nurse observes all of the following, which one is the *best indication* that a transfusion reaction is occurring?
 ○ 1. The client's urine is very dark yellow.
 ◉ 2. The client becomes dyspneic suddenly.
 ○ 3. The client's skin is pale and cool.
 ○ 4. The client says he is extremely thirsty.

During a postpartum home visit, a client describes what the nurse believes may be symptoms of a hiatal hernia.

18 Which one of the following is *most likely* to be this client's chief complaint?
 ○ 1. Vomiting
 ○ 2. Nausea
 ○ 3. Anorexia
 ◉ 4. Heartburn

19 Until the postpartum client can be seen by a physician, which suggestion can the nurse offer to provide some relief from her symptoms?
 ○ 1. Eat three well-balanced meals a day.
 ○ 2. Eat foods that are easy to swallow.
 ◉ 3. Avoid lying down after eating food.
 ○ 4. Avoid skipping meals when hungry.

20 Which modification in the client's bed is *most appropriate* to recommend at this time?
 ○ 1. Place a bed board between the mattress and springs.
 ○ 2. Consider sleeping in a water bed temporarily.
 ○ 3. Elevate the legs on pillows when retiring at night.
 ◉ 4. Raise the head of the bed on 4-inch blocks.

An older adult with metastatic cancer of the esophagus is undergoing palliative treatment that includes total parenteral nutrition (TPN) through a central subclavian catheter.

21 Which nursing assessment is *essential* for evaluating the client's response to the TPN?
 ○ 1. Test the urine's specific gravity.
 ◉ 2. Monitor the capillary blood glucose.
 ○ 3. Measure the arterial pulse pressure.
 ○ 4. Obtain an apical-radial pulse rate.

22 Which is the *best evidence* that the client is responding favorably to the administration of TPN?
 ○ 1. He remains alert.
 ◉ 2. He gains weight.
 ○ 3. He feels hungry.
 ○ 4. He is pain-free.

In anticipation of transferring the client with cancer of the esophagus to a nursing home or home care, the physician inserts a gastrostomy tube for nourishment.

23 *Immediately* after the gastrostomy tube is inserted, which finding should the nurse consider *normal* when assessing the gastrostomy site?
 ○ 1. Milky-appearing drainage
 ◉ 2. Serosanguineous drainage
 ○ 3. Green-tinged drainage
 ○ 4. Bright bloody drainage

24 Which technique is *best* to use to determine if the tube has migrated after being inserted?
 ○ 1. Test the pH of aspirated secretions.
 ◉ 2. Monitor the results of stomach x-rays.
 ○ 3. Measure the length of external tube.
 ○ 4. Palpate the abdomen for distention.

The nurse fills a tube feeding bag with two (2) 8-ounce cans of commercially prepared formula that will instill continuously through the client's gastrostomy tube via a feeding pump.

25 If the client with the gastrostomy is to receive 120 mL of formula per hour, the nurse can expect that the entire bag of formula will instill in
 ○ 1. 2 hours.
 ◉ 2. 4 hours.
 ○ 3. 6 hours.
 ○ 4. 8 hours.

While the tube-feeding formula is being instilled, the client with the gastrostomy says he feels full and nauseated.

26   The *best* nursing action to take at this time is to
- ○ 1. measure the stomach residual.
- ○ 2. raise the height of the formula.
- ● 3. stop the infusion temporarily.
- ○ 4. add water to dilute the formula.

27   When the tube-feeding formula has instilled, the *next* action the nurse should take is to
- ○ 1. place the client on his left side.
- ○ 2. lower the head of the client's bed.
- ● 3. clamp the opening of the gastrostomy tube.
- ○ 4. instill several ounces of plain tap water.

The client with the gastrostomy is silent and withdrawn as the nurse cares for the insertion site.

28   Which of the nurse's statements is *best* for encouraging him to express his feelings?
- ○ 1. "Are you feeling angry?"
- ● 2. "It must be tough for you."
- ○ 3. "This may get better soon."
- ○ 4. "Lots of people eat this way."

NURSING CARE OF CLIENTS WITH DISORDERS OF THE STOMACH

A 46-year-old male is hospitalized to determine the cause of the intermittent gnawing epigastric pain he has been experiencing.

29   When the admitting nurse obtains the client's health history, if the pain is due to a peptic ulcer, he will most likely report that his discomfort goes away or is less intense when he
- ○ 1. skips a meal.
- ○ 2. goes to bed.
- ● 3. eats food.
- ○ 4. bends over.

30   Which test, if positive, could the nurse perform to further support that the client's symptoms are due to a peptic ulcer?
- ○ 1. The nurse could assess his urine for albumin.
- ○ 2. The nurse could assess his blood for glucose.
- ● 3. The nurse could assess his stool for blood.
- ○ 4. The nurse could assess his emesis for pepsin.

The client with epigastric pain is scheduled for an x-ray of the upper gastrointestinal tract.

31   After the nurse explains the procedure for performing an upper gastrointestinal (GI) x-ray, which statement indicates that the client understands what this test involves?

- ○ 1. "A flexible tube will be inserted into my stomach."
- ○ 2. "Dye will be infused into my vein before the test."
- ○ 3. "My body will be placed within an imaging chamber."
- ● 4. "I will have to swallow a large volume of barium."

Diagnostic tests reveal that the client with epigastric pain has a duodenal ulcer. The physician writes an order for a tetracycline antibiotic and for one ounce of bismuth subsalicylate (Pepto-Bismol) to be administered every six hours.

32   When preparing the bismuth subsalicylate, the nurse is *most correct* in administering which equivalent volume?
- ● 1. 30 mL
- ○ 2. 15 mL
- ○ 3. 10 mL
- ○ 4. 5 mL

The client with the duodenal ulcer questions the nurse as to why an antibiotic has been prescribed for him.

33   The *best* explanation is that antibiotics are used in ulcer therapy to
- ○ 1. heal the irritated mucous membrane of the stomach.
- ● 2. eliminate a microorganism that depletes gastric mucus.
- ○ 3. add a protective coating over the ulcerated mucosa.
- ○ 4. prevent secondary gastrointestinal infections.

The nurse assists the team leader in planning the discharge teaching for the client with a duodenal ulcer. Their goal is to provide him with information that will help prevent further gastrointestinal irritation.

34   For occasional pain and discomfort, it is *best* to tell this client to follow the label directions for taking
- ● 1. acetaminophen (Tylenol).
- ○ 2. aspirin (Anacin).
- ○ 3. ibuprofen (Advil).
- ○ 4. naproxen (Naprosyn).

The nurse is preparing a client with a history of recurrent peptic ulcer disease for abdominal surgery.

35   As the nurse performs a head-to-toe physical assessment, which sign is *most* indicative that the client's ulcer has perforated?
- ○ 1. The client's skin appears ecchymotic.
- ● 2. The client's abdomen feels board-like.
- ○ 3. The client's pupils are widely dilated.
- ○ 4. The client's respirations are rapid.

The registered nurse inserts a gastric sump tube in the client with the perforated ulcer and asks the practical nurse to check its placement.

36 The *most appropriate* technique for determining if the distal end of the tube is in the stomach is to
○ 1. request a portable x-ray of the stomach.
◉ 2. listen over the stomach as air is instilled.
○ 3. instill 100 mL of tap water into the tube.
○ 4. feel for air at the proximal end of the tube.

When the client with the perforated ulcer senses the critical nature of his condition, he says, "Nurse, am I going to make it?"

37 The *best response* from the nurse is,
◉ 1. "We are doing everything we can to do just that."
○ 2. "That's something you'll have to ask your doctor."
○ 3. "Now what kind of a silly question is that?"
○ 4. "I've seen people in a whole lot worse shape."

A gastrojejunostomy, also called a Billroth II, is performed on the client with a perforated ulcer. He is returned to his room after recovering from the anesthesia.

38 When the client does not adequately cough and deep-breathe postoperatively due to incisional pain, which nursing action is most appropriate *at this time*?
○ 1. Explain that he is at high risk for developing pneumonia.
◉ 2. Have him press a pillow against his incision when coughing.
○ 3. Ask the physician to order some form of oxygen for him.
○ 4. Keep the head of the bed elevated at all times of the day.

The nasogastric tube of the postoperative client recovering after gastrojejunostomy stops draining.

39 Which of the following actions is *most appropriate* when the nurse irrigates the nasogastric tube?
○ 1. The nurse instills 30 mL of sterile distilled water.
○ 2. The nurse administers oxygen before the irrigation.
◉ 3. The nurse records the volume instilled and removed.
○ 4. The nurse asks the client to swallow frequently.

The nurse implements the teaching plan on dumping syndrome for the post-gastrojejunostomy client that was developed by the registered nurse.

40 After providing the client with diet instructions for preventing dumping syndrome, the *best evidence* that the client understands what has been taught is his statement that
○ 1. "I should drink a large volume of liquid at meals."
◉ 2. "I should restrict eating sugary and starchy food."
○ 3. "It would be best to eat large meals during the day."
○ 4. "It would be best to reduce my intake of red meat."

41 What other information should the nurse plan to teach the post-gastrojejunostomy client to help reduce the potential for experiencing the symptoms of dumping syndrome?
◉ 1. Lie down for a short time after eating.
○ 2. Sleep with the head of the bed elevated.
○ 3. Walk several times a day between meals.
○ 4. Meditate or relax just prior to eating.

A 74-year-old client is experiencing persistent indigestion, feeling of gastric fullness, and unexplained weight loss.

42 When the nurse reviews the results of several diagnostic tests the client has undergone, which finding is *most suggestive* that the client's symptoms are due to cancer of the stomach?
○ 1. Gastric analysis showed absence of hydrochloric acid.
◉ 2. An elevated level of gastrin was found in the blood.
○ 3. Gastric irritation was noted during a gastroscopy.
○ 4. A urinalysis showed the presence of red blood cells.

The client with stomach cancer is scheduled for a total gastrectomy.

43 When the practical nurse assists the registered nurse insert a single lumen nasogastric tube preoperatively, which one of the following instructions is correct when the tube is in the client's oropharynx?
○ 1. "Breathe deeply as the tube is advanced."
◉ 2. "Hold your head in a sniffing position."
○ 3. "Press your chin to your upper chest."
○ 4. "Avoid coughing until the tube is down."

44 Which setting is be most appropriate to use when connecting the preoperative gastrectomy client's single lumen nasogastric tube to suction?
- ○ 1. Low, intermittent suction
- ◉ 2. Low, continuous suction
- ○ 3. High, intermittent suction
- ○ 4. High, continuous suction

During the postoperative care of the client with the single lumen nasogastric tube, the client indicates that he is very thirsty.

45 In response to the client's statement, which nursing intervention is *most appropriate* to add to the plan of care?
- ○ 1. Offer fluids at least every 2 hours.
- ◉ 2. Provide crushed ice in sparse amounts.
- ○ 3. Increase oral liquids on dietary tray.
- ○ 4. Refill water carafe twice each shift.

The gastrectomy client develops pernicious anemia a year later. A home health nurse administers 1000 mcg of vitamin B₁₂ intramuscularly every month.

46 If the label on the vial of vitamin B₁₂ indicates that there is 1 mg per mL, the nurse is *accurate* in withdrawing which one of the following volumes?
- ○ 1. 0.1 mL
- ◉ 2. 1 mL
- ○ 3. 10 mL
- ○ 4. 0.01 mL

The nurse chooses to use the vastus lateralis muscle as the site for the intramuscular injection of vitamin B₁₂.

47 If the correct technique for administering the injection is followed, the nurse will give the injection in the
- ○ 1. upper arm at a 45-degree angle.
- ◉ 2. outer thigh at a 90-degree angle.
- ○ 3. anterior thigh at a 90-degree angle.
- ○ 4. outer buttock at a 45-degree angle.

NURSING CARE OF CLIENTS WITH DISORDERS OF THE SMALL INTESTINE

A 19-year-old female has been having up to five loose stools per day. She is undergoing diagnostic testing and symptomatic treatment.

48 When the nurse collects a stool specimen for ova and parasites, which action is correct?
- ○ 1. The nurse holds a specimen container under the client's rectum.
- ○ 2. The nurse places the collected specimen in a sterile container.

- ○ 3. The nurse refrigerates the covered specimen after collection.
- ◉ 4. The nurse takes the specimen to the laboratory immediately.

The physician has prescribed diphenoxylate hydrochloride (Lomotil) 5 mg orally q.i.d. for the client with diarrhea.

49 When the nurse checks the medication administration record (MAR), which schedule for administering this drug is correct if military time is used?
- ○ 1. 0730, 1130, 0430
- ◉ 2. 0600, 1200, 1800, 0000
- ○ 3. 0900, 1300, 1700
- ○ 4. 0400, 0800, 1200, 1600, 2000

The physician restricts the diet of the client with diarrhea to clear liquids only.

50 When the client asks for some nourishment, which one of the following is appropriate for the nurse to provide?
- ○ 1. Milk
- ○ 2. Pudding
- ◉ 3. Gelatin
- ○ 4. Custard

The nurse assesses the client with diarrhea for signs of fluid volume deficit.

51 Which assessment finding best indicates that the client is becoming dehydrated?
- ○ 1. The client's blood pressure is elevated.
- ○ 2. The client's heart rate is irregular.
- ○ 3. The client's mucous membranes are pink.
- ◉ 4. The client's urine is dark yellow.

A colonoscopy is scheduled for the client with persistent diarrhea. According to protocol, the nurse administers an electrolyte solution called GoLYTELY orally in amounts of 250 mL every 15 minutes over a 2-hour period.

52 The best evidence that the solution the nurse administers is achieving its *primary* purpose is
- ○ 1. the client's serum electrolytes are normal.
- ○ 2. the client's intake approximates her output.
- ◉ 3. the client's stools become clear liquid.
- ○ 4. the client's bladder fills with urine.

Before the colonoscopy, the client is given conscious sedation using the drug midazolam hydrochloride (Versed).

53 During the colonoscopy and in the immediate recovery period, it is *essential* that the nurse assess the client closely for which potential undesirable effect of midazolam?

○ 1. Unstable blood pressure
○ 2. Cardiac rhythm disturbance
● 3. Respiratory depression
○ 4. Altered consciousness

The colonoscopy reveals that the client with diarrhea has Crohn's disease, also referred to as regional ileitis or regional enteritis. The physician progresses the client to a fiber-controlled diet.

54 After talking with the dietitian, the client demonstrates an understanding of the therapeutic diet by indicating that fiber refers to
○ 1. foods that require chewing.
○ 2. the muscle found in red meat.
○ 3. the semisolid mass in the stomach.
● 4. the indigestible part of plants.

The client with Crohn's disease eventually develops a draining fistula between a loop of the ileum and the skin. The nursing team gathers to revise the client's plan for care.

55 Based on the new complication, which problem is the *highest priority* for planning at this time?
○ 1. Family coping
● 2. Impaired skin
○ 3. Body image
○ 4. Depression

NURSING CARE OF CLIENTS WITH DISORDERS OF THE LARGE INTESTINE

A 52-year-old male client is admitted to the ambulatory surgery department for repair of an inguinal hernia. The nurse takes the operative consent form to the client to obtain his signature.

56 If the operative consent form states that the surgical procedure will be a right inguinal herniorrhaphy and the client says "I hope I can get along without that section of my bowel," which action should the nurse take *next*?
○ 1. Cancel the surgery.
● 2. Notify the physician.
○ 3. Witness his signature.
○ 4. Shave his right groin.

The client returns from surgery which was performed under spinal anesthesia.

57 If all of the following postoperative orders are written on the client's medical record, which one should the nurse question before carrying it out?
○ 1. Diet as tolerated
○ 2. Fluids as desired
○ 3. Vitals until stable
● 4. Fowler's position

58 One of the most important postoperative assessments the nurse should make on this client is his
● 1. ability to urinate.
○ 2. effort at coughing.
○ 3. level of consciousness.
○ 4. tolerance for pain.

59 When the postoperative client asks why the nurse has brought a suspensory (a sling-like support) for him to apply, the *best* explanation is that a suspensory is used to prevent
○ 1. sexual impotence.
● 2. scrotal edema.
○ 3. strain on the incision.
○ 4. wound contamination.

The client who has had an inguinal herniorrhaphy has meperidine hydrochloride (Demerol) 50 mg ordered intramuscularly for pain every 4 hours as needed.

60 If the meperidine hydrochloride is supplied in 100 mg per mL ampules, the nurse is accurate in administering a volume of
○ 1. 1 mL
● 2. 0.5 mL
○ 3. 2 mL
○ 4. 0.2 mL

61 Besides being documented on the medication administration record (MAR), the administration of meperidine hydrochloride (Demerol) also is documented on a(n)
○ 1. computer database.
● 2. narcotic control log.
○ 3. drug enforcement form.
○ 4. agency prescription pad.

A 31-year-old female with a long history of ulcerative colitis is admitted to the hospital for a colectomy.

62 In addition to having severe diarrhea, which other characteristic information is the nurse likely to obtain when admitting this client?
● 1. Mucus and blood are present in the stool.
○ 2. Her bowel sounds are hypoactive.
○ 3. The skin of her abdomen has striae.
○ 4. Shallow ulcerations are found in her mouth.

*The team leader identifies the nursing diagnosis of **Bowel Incontinence Related to Sudden Urgency for Defecation** on the care plan.*

63 If all of the following nursing measures for managing this nursing diagnosis are considered, which one is *least* appropriate?
● 1. Keeping the bedside commode nearby.
○ 2. Answering her signal for help promptly.
○ 3. Putting a disposable diaper on her.
○ 4. Helping her to the bathroom frequently.

The client tells the nurse of the many hospitalizations she has had without much improvement. She says in a discouraged way, "I am sure this surgery won't help either."

64   The *best* nursing response in this situation is
   ○ 1. "You are saying that you doubt that you will get better."
   ◉ 2. "Do you want to talk to your doctor again before surgery?"
   ○ 3. "I'd recommend a more positive attitude this time around."
   ○ 4. "Of course it will. Others wish they'd had it done sooner."

65   After giving the preoperative medication, which consists of meperidine hydrochloride (Demerol), hydroxyzine (Vistaril), and atropine sulfate, the *most important* nursing action is to
   ◉ 1. raise the side rails.
   ○ 2. help her to the toilet.
   ○ 3. provide oral hygiene.
   ○ 4. teach her leg exercises.

The client who had a colectomy performed is transferred to the nursing unit after recovering from anesthesia.

66   When the nurse assesses the client postoperatively, which assessment is *most indicative* of shock?
   ○ 1. Bounding pulse
   ○ 2. Slow respirations
   ◉ 3. Low blood pressure
   ○ 4. High body temperature

The postoperative client with the colectomy is receiving oxygen by nasal cannula at 2 liters per minute (28%).

67   If the client is adequately oxygenated, the pulse oximeter that is attached to her finger should measure oxygen saturation in the range of
   ○ 1. 25% to 30%.
   ○ 2. 35% to 50%.
   ○ 3. 60% to 80%.
   ◉ 4. 95% to 100%.

The care plan for the client with the colectomy includes measures for caring for the ileostomy that also was created at the time of surgery.

68   When implementing the plan of care, the *best* time of day to perform stomal care and change the appliance is after the client
   ◉ 1. awakens in the morning.
   ○ 2. has eaten breakfast.
   ○ 3. has been up and ambulated.
   ○ 4. finishes her last meal.

69   The nurse assesses the stoma of the ileostomy which, if *normal*, appears
   ○ 1. pale pink.
   ◉ 2. bright red.
   ○ 3. dark tan.
   ○ 4. dusky blue.

70   When cleaning the skin around the client's stoma, the *most appropriate* nursing technique is to
   ○ 1. pat it with cotton balls.
   ○ 2. swab it with 70% alcohol.
   ◉ 3. use water and mild soap.
   ○ 4. scrub it with peroxide.

71   The *best* technique for attaching the ileostomy appliance is so that
   ○ 1. the faceplate occludes the opening of the stoma.
   ◉ 2. the appliance opening is ⅛ inch larger than the stoma.
   ○ 3. a ⅛-inch margin of the faceplate adheres to skin.
   ○ 4. the bag is directly at the waist or belt line.

72   While the nurse changes the ostomy appliance, if the client says she would like to do all of the following, which one should the nurse tactfully inform her is *unrealistic* for a client with a conventional ileostomy?
   ○ 1. Go swimming
   ○ 2. Play tennis
   ○ 3. Get pregnant again
   ◉ 4. Control defecation

A 20-year-old female is admitted with pain that is localized on the lower right side of the abdomen, halfway between the umbilicus and the crest of the ileum. Her physician suspects appendicitis.

73   Of the laboratory tests ordered on admission, which one is *most* important for the nurse to monitor at this time?
   ○ 1. Bilirubin level
   ○ 2. Serum potassium
   ○ 3. Prothrombin time
   ◉ 4. Leukocyte count

74   If the client is typical of others with appendicitis, the nurse can expect that when the client's abdomen is palpated midway between the umbilicus and right iliac crest, the client will
   ◉ 1. experience more pain when pressure is released.
   ○ 2. lack any sensation of pain or pressure on palpation.
   ○ 3. have extreme discomfort with the slightest pressure.
   ○ 4. will feel referred pain in the opposite quadrant.

The physician considers removing the client's appendix with laporoscopic surgery.

75 If the client asks the nurse about this type of procedure, which statement is *most accurate*?
   ● 1. The recovery period is shorter.
   ○ 2. No anesthesia is necessary.
   ○ 3. There will be no surgical scar.
   ○ 4. Exercise can be resumed immediately.

The condition of the client with appendicitis worsens. It is feared that her appendix has ruptured. She is prepared for an emergency appendectomy. The laporoscopic approach for removing the appendix is no longer an option.

76 Which one of the client's actions prior to admission is most likely to have contributed to the rupturing of her appendix?
   ○ 1. The client stopped eating and drinking.
   ○ 2. The client continued her usual activities.
   ● 3. The client applied a hot water bottle to her lower abdomen.
   ○ 4. The client took acetaminophen (Tylenol) for her discomfort.

The client returns from surgery with an open drain (Penrose) extending from her incision. The drain is covered by a sterile dressing.

77 Which one of the following body positions is best for the nurse to use for promoting drainage from the wound?
   ○ 1. Lithotomy
   ● 2. Fowler's
   ○ 3. Recumbent
   ○ 4. Trendelenburg

78 When the nurse changes the client's dressing, which nursing action is *correct*?
   ○ 1. The nurse removes the soiled dressing with sterile gloves.
   ○ 2. The nurse frees the tape by pulling it away from the incision.
   ● 3. The nurse encloses the soiled dressing within the latex glove.
   ○ 4. The nurse cleans the wound in circles toward the incision.

A 68-year-old male has noted blood in his stool for the past 6 months. One of the possible diagnoses is colorectal cancer.

79 Besides rectal bleeding, what information in the client's medical history strongly suggests that he may have colorectal cancer?
   ● 1. His bowel habits have changed.
   ○ 2. He has difficulty swallowing.

   ○ 3. He experiences chronic indigestion.
   ○ 4. Some foods give him intestinal gas.

The nurse teaches the client about his scheduled sigmoidoscopy for which he will prepare himself at home.

80 Which one of the following indicates that the client needs more teaching before the sigmoidoscopy?
   ○ 1. The client says he should sit on the toilet to give himself an enema.
   ● 2. The client says he can eat a light meal the evening before the examination.
   ○ 3. The client says a flexible scope will be inserted into his rectum.
   ○ 4. The client says he may take his prescribed medications in the morning.

81 The nurse who assists with the sigmoidoscopy is most correct in placing the client in a
   ○ 1. lithotomy position.
   ● 2. Sim's position.
   ○ 3. orthopneic position.
   ○ 4. Fowler's position.

The client with colorectal cancer will undergo a bowel resection to remove the cancerous tumor.

82 If a low-residue diet is prescribed prior to surgery, which of the following foods is *contraindicated* for him?
   ● 1. Ground meat
   ○ 2. Bran cereal
   ○ 3. Orange juice
   ○ 4. Baked fish

Before colorectal surgery, the client will receive 1 g of neomycin sulfate (Mycifradin) orally every hour for four doses and then 1 g orally every 4 hours for the balance of the 24 hours.

83 If the neomycin sulfate tablets come in a dosage strength of 500 mg per tablet, how many tablets should the nurse administer each time?
   ○ 1. ½ tablet
   ○ 2. 1 tablet
   ● 3. 2 tablets
   ○ 4. 4 tablets

84 When the client asks the nurse why he must take the neomycin sulfate, the *most accurate* explanation *in this case* is that it is given to
   ○ 1. treat any current infection he may have.
   ● 2. suppress the growth of intestinal bacteria.
   ○ 3. prevent the onset of postoperative diarrhea.
   ○ 4. reduce the number of bacteria near the incision.

During the postoperative period, the client's abdominal incision separates and his bowel protrudes through the opening.

85 The *first* action the nurse should take at this time is to
○ 1. check the client's vital signs.
○ 2. call the client's physician.
● 3. cover the bowel with moist gauze.
○ 4. reinsert the bowel internally.

A home health nurse visits a 71-year-old female client and observes that her abdomen is quite distended. She is quite nauseated and has been experiencing persistent vomiting for the last 48 hours.

86 Which one of the following questions is important for the nurse to ask to determine if the client has a bowel obstruction?
○ 1. "When did you last eat a full meal?"
○ 2. "How much fluid are you vomiting?"
● 3. "Does the emesis appear to contain feces?"
○ 4. "Has your appetite changed appreciably?"

The physician admits the client with the bowel obstruction to the hospital and inserts a Miller-Abbott intestinal tube.

87 Immediately after the tube is inserted by the physician, the *next* action the nurse should take is to
○ 1. request an abdominal x-ray.
○ 2. secure the tube to the nose.
○ 3. instill mercury into the tube.
● 4. ambulate the client if possible.

The obstruction is not relieved. The client is scheduled for a laparotomy and possible colon resection and temporary colostomy. The client's preoperative orders include giving her meperidine hydrochloride and atropine sulfate intramuscularly.

88 If the written order for the atropine sulfate says to administer 5 mg intramuscularly and the usual adult preoperative dose is 0.4 to 0.6 mg, which nursing action is best for the nurse to take *next*?
○ 1. Give the usual preoperative dose of atropine.
○ 2. Administer just the meperidine at this time.
● 3. Hold all the medication and notify the physician.
○ 4. Consult the pharmacist on the action to take.

A few days after surgery, the physician orders the nurse to begin daily colostomy irrigations.

89 If all of the following are possible, which position is best to place the client in when irrigating the colostomy?

○ 1. Lying on the left side
● 2. Sitting on the toilet
○ 3. Standing at the sink
○ 4. Kneeling in the bathtub

During a conversation concerning her feelings about the colostomy, the client becomes suddenly silent.

90 At this time it is *best* for the nurse to
○ 1. change the subject to something more pleasant.
○ 2. refrain from interjecting comments or questions.
● 3. provide information about care of the colostomy.
○ 4. offer a referral for psychologic counseling.

The client says to the nurse, "How will I ever adjust to this colostomy."

91 The *best* nursing response at this time is to
○ 1. encourage the client to express her concerns.
● 2. reassure her that adjustment will come with time.
○ 3. recommend she investigate care in a nursing home.
○ 4. say nothing, but quote her statement in the chart.

NURSING CARE OF CLIENTS WITH DISORDERS OF THE RECTUM AND ANUS

When a nurse is invited to assess blood pressures at a senior citizens' community meal site, an older adult discreetly asks if there are any nonprescription laxatives that he should avoid taking.

92 In response to the question, it is appropriate to explain that to avoid interfering with the absorption of fat-soluble vitamins it is best to avoid frequent use of
○ 1. milk of magnesia.
○ 2. cascara sagrada.
○ 3. mineral oil.
● 4. castor oil.

A nurse who works at a nursing home cares for several clients with bowel elimination problems.

93 When an older client tells the nurse that he cannot have a bowel movement without taking a daily laxative, what information is *essential* for the nurse to explain?
● 1. Chronic use of laxatives impairs natural bowel tone.
○ 2. Stool softeners are likely to be less harsh for him.
○ 3. Daily enemas are more preferable than laxatives.
○ 4. Dilating the anal sphincter may aid bowel elimination.

94 Which one of the following is the *best indication* that a client has a fecal impaction?
- ● 1. The client passes liquid stool frequently.
- ○ 2. The client has extremely offending bad breath.
- ○ 3. The client requests medication for a headache.
- ○ 4. The client has not been eating well lately.

95 The *best* technique for confirming that a client has a fecal impaction is to
- ○ 1. administer an oil-retention enema.
- ● 2. insert a gloved finger into the rectum.
- ○ 3. review the results of a lower GI x-ray.
- ○ 4. monitor the client's bowel elimination.

96 Before inserting a rectal tube, which one of the following nursing measures is *most helpful* for eliminating intestinal gas?
- ● 1. Ambulate the client in the hall.
- ○ 2. Provide a carbonated beverage.
- ○ 3. Restrict the intake of solid food.
- ○ 4. Administer a narcotic analgesic.

97 If a rectal tube becomes necessary to relieve a client's distention and discomfort, what is the maximum length of time to leave the tube in place each time it is used?
- ○ 1. 5 minutes
- ○ 2. 20 minutes
- ○ 3. 45 minutes
- ● 4. 1 hour

98 During the administration of a cleansing soapsuds enema, when a client experiences cramping and has the urge to defecate, which is the *best* nursing action at this time?
- ○ 1. Quickly finish instilling the remaining solution.
- ○ 2. Tell the client to hold his or her breath and bear down.
- ● 3. Briefly stop the administration of the enema solution.
- ○ 4. Withdraw the tip of the enema tubing from the rectum.

99 Which one of the following nursing actions is *inappropriate* when inserting a rectal suppository for relieving constipation?
- ● 1. The nurse dons a clean glove on the dominant hand.
- ○ 2. The nurse positions the client on the left side.
- ○ 3. The nurse inserts the suppository approximately ½ inch.
- ○ 4. The nurse tells the client to retain it for 15 minutes.

100 Which one of the following should be planned *first* before beginning bowel retraining on a client who is experiencing bowel incontinence?
- ○ 1. Limit the client's daytime physical activity.
- ● 2. Record the time of day when incontinence occurs.
- ○ 3. Decrease the amount of food eaten at each meal.
- ○ 4. Empty the client's bowel with a soapsuds enema.

A home health nurse reviews the health history of a client who has hemorrhoids.

101 In the information that is documented, which of the following *most probably* contributed to his developing hemorrhoids?
- ○ 1. The client is on a low-sodium diet.
- ○ 2. The client does not tolerate milk well.
- ● 3. The client is frequently constipated.
- ○ 4. The client works as an accountant.

102 Besides increasing his consumption of bulk-forming foods, such as whole grains, fresh fruits, and vegetables, the best diet instruction the nurse can give the client with hemorrhoids is to
- ○ 1. eat small meals frequently.
- ● 2. drink eight glasses of fluid per day.
- ○ 3. avoid snacking between meals.
- ○ 4. reduce the intake of refined sugar.

The client with hemorrhoids eventually has them surgically removed.

103 After assisting the postoperative hemorrhoidectomy client with a Sitz bath, the best indication of its effectiveness is
- ● 1. the client says his rectum is less painful.
- ○ 2. the client has no evidence of body odor.
- ○ 3. the client indicates that he feels refreshed.
- ○ 4. the client's body is pink, warm, and clean.

The physician prescribes docusate sodium (Colace) for the client who has had a hemorrhoidectomy.

104 The nurse is most correct in explaining that the purpose for this medication in the client's case is to
- ○ 1. ease bowel evacuation and its related discomfort.
- ○ 2. irritate the bowel and promote stool elimination.
- ● 3. stimulate peristalsis to move wastes after digestion.
- ○ 4. reduce intestinal activity and decrease stool size.

A client is admitted for the surgical treatment of a pilonidal cyst.

105   When the admitting nurse obtains the client's health history, which of the following is *common* among individuals with this condition?
- ○ 1. There is a history of intermittent rectal bleeding.
- ○ 2. There is an open draining area near the coccyx.
- ○ 3. The client has experienced frequent bouts of diarrhea.
- ● 4. The client has very little or baby fine anorectal hair.

Before discharging the client who had the pilonidal cyst removed, the nurse teaches the client how to apply a non-prescription anesthetic ointment.

106   Which one of the following drug application instructions is *essential* for promoting the drug's local effect?
- ○ 1. Use gloves when applying the ointment.
- ○ 2. Store the ointment in the refrigerator.
- ○ 3. Apply the ointment just before defecating.
- ● 4. Clean the area before applying the drug.

NURSING CARE OF CLIENTS WITH DISORDERS OF THE GALLBLADDER

A 45-year-old female is suspected of having cholecystitis.

107   When the client describes her discomfort to the nurse, she is *most likely* to indicate that the pain she experiences becomes worse
- ● 1. shortly after eating food.
- ○ 2. especially on an empty stomach.
- ○ 3. following periods of activity
- ○ 4. before arising in the morning.

108   If this client is typical of others with cholecystitis, besides localized pain, she may describe feeling pain that is referred to the
- ○ 1. right shoulder.
- ● 2. midepigastrium.
- ○ 3. neck or jaw.
- ○ 4. left upper arm.

109   If the cause of the client's inflamed gallbladder is due to gallstones, laboratory data are most likely to show a(n)
- ○ 1. low red blood cell count.
- ○ 2. low level of hemoglobin.
- ● 3. elevated cholesterol level.
- ○ 4. elevated serum albumin.

110   If gallstones obstruct the flow of bile, the nurse can expect that the client's stools are
- ○ 1. black and tarry.
- ● 2. light clay-colored.
- ○ 3. very dark brown.
- ○ 4. greenish-yellow.

111   If the dietitian explains a low-fat diet, which statement indicates that the client needs *more* teaching?
- ○ 1. The client says she can eat broiled chicken.
- ○ 2. The client says she can eat baked meat loaf.
- ● 3. The client says she can eat fried fish.
- ○ 4. The client says she can eat roast turkey.

The client with possible cholecystitis is scheduled for an oral cholecystography, an x-ray of the gallbladder. The night before the test, the client is to receive several oral tablets that will facilitate a sharp x-ray image.

112   What information is *essential* for the nurse to know before administering the contrast substance to a client undergoing an x-ray of the gallbladder?
- ○ 1. Can the client tolerate holding still?
- ○ 2. How many x-rays has the client had?
- ● 3. Is the client allergic to iodine?
- ○ 4. Does the client want any anesthesia?

The gallbladder is not visualized by cholecystography. An ultrasound of the gallbladder is scheduled for the client with possible cholecystitis.

113   Which one of the client's comments indicates that she has an *accurate* understanding of the nurse's explanation of the preparation for an ultrasound of the gallbladder?
- ● 1. Preparation involves withholding food for approximately 8 to 12 hours.
- ○ 2. Preparation involves drinking a container of barium just before the x-ray.
- ○ 3. Preparation involves eating a large test meal the night before the x-ray.
- ○ 4. Preparation involves inserting a large needle within one of the arm veins.

The physician recommends that the client with gallstones have an open abdominal cholecystectomy. An intramuscular injection of menadiol sodium diphosphate (Synkayvite), a water-soluble derivative of vitamin K, is ordered on the day before surgery.

114   When the client asks the nurse to explain the purpose for the injection of vitamin K, it is most accurate to say it is used to promote
- ○ 1. wound healing.
- ○ 2. liver function.
- ○ 3. general health.
- ● 4. blood clotting.

The prescribed dose of menadiol sodium diphosphate is 10 mg. The drug is supplied in a dosage strength of 5 mg/mL. The nurse prepares 2 mL of the drug.

115 When selecting an intramuscular injection site, which site is *least preferred* when administering this medication?
- ○ 1. Dorsogluteal site
- ○ 2. Ventrogluteal site
- ○ 3. Vastus lateralis site
- ◉ 4. Deltoid site

The client returns from surgery with a nasogastric tube, a T-tube for bile drainage, and a Jackson-Pratt tube for wound drainage.

116 Which of the following best indicates that the T-tube drainage is the color that is expected?
- ○ 1. The drainage is dark red or pale pink.
- ○ 2. The drainage is clear or transparent.
- ○ 3. The drainage is bright red or orange.
- ◉ 4. The drainage is greenish yellow or brown.

117 When the nurse makes all the following T-tube assessments in the early postoperative period, which one requires *immediate* action?
- ○ 1. The drainage bag is hanging below the abdomen.
- ○ 2. The drainage tubing is currently clamped.
- ○ 3. The drainage tube is supported with a roll of gauze.
- ◉ 4. The drainage volume was 100 mL in the last 6 hours.

118 When the client begins to consume food again, which routine for clamping and unclamping the T-tube can the nurse expect to follow?
- ○ 1. Unclamp the tube during the day.
- ○ 2. Unclamp the tube during the night.
- ◉ 3. Unclamp the tube for 2 hours after eating.
- ○ 4. Unclamp the tube for 2 hours before eating.

119 When the nurse empties the drainage in the Jackson-Pratt bulb reservoir, which nursing action is *essential* for re-establishing the negative pressure within this drainage device?
- ◉ 1. The nurse compresses the bulb reservoir, and closes the drainage valve.
- ○ 2. The nurse opens the drainage valve, allowing the bulb to fill with air.
- ○ 3. The nurse fills the bulb reservoir with sterile normal saline.
- ○ 4. The nurse secures the bulb reservoir to the skin near the wound.

NURSING CARE OF CLIENTS WITH DISORDERS OF THE LIVER

A 20-year-old female college student goes to the university health service because she has developed a sudden onset of flu-like symptoms.

120 When the health nurse monitors the client's laboratory test results, which one, if elevated, is *most indicative* that the client's symptoms are related to a liver disorder?
- ○ 1. Serum potassium
- ○ 2. Serum creatinine
- ○ 3. Blood urea nitrogen
- ◉ 4. Amino transferase

The physician determines that the college student with flu symptoms has hepatitis A.

121 When the client asks the nurse how she acquired hepatitis A, the *best answer* is that a common route of hepatitis A transmission is from
- ◉ 1. fecal contamination.
- ○ 2. insect carriers.
- ○ 3. infected blood.
- ○ 4. wound drainage.

An infection control nurse is consulted on measures for reducing the potential transmission of the hepatitis A virus to others.

122 Based on the routes of transmission for this disease, which one of the following infection control measures is *essential* to include in the plan for care?
- ○ 1. Wear gloves whenever entering the client's room.
- ○ 2. Don a mask and gown when providing direct care.
- ◉ 3. Maintain the client in a private room at all times.
- ○ 4. Perform vigorous handwashing after leaving the room.

Several of the college student's friends call the health service because they are concerned about their own risks for acquiring hepatitis A.

123 To prevent the spread of hepatitis A, the nurse is *most correct* in recommending that close contacts receive
- ○ 1. antibiotic therapy.
- ◉ 2. serum immunoglobulin.
- ○ 3. hepatitis vaccination.
- ○ 4. anti-inflammatory drugs.

A 23-year-old male develops jaundice and refers himself to the public health department. He tells the nurse that his skin itches terribly.

124 Which one of the following suggestions is *most appropriate* for helping the client manage his discomfort?
○ 1. Discontinue all bathing temporarily.
● 2. Use only lanolin soap for bathing.
○ 3. Apply rubbing alcohol to your skin.
○ 4. Take showers rather than tub baths.

The cause of the young adult's jaundice is hepatitis B.

125 If the nurse obtains all of the following information in the client's social history, which one strongly predisposes this client to hepatitis B?
○ 1. The client moved here from Alaska.
● 2. The client is an active homosexual.
○ 3. The client abuses alcohol.
○ 4. The client is a carpenter.

126 Which measure is most appropriate if an unvaccinated nurse experienced a needlestick injury while caring for this client?
○ 1. Obtain immediate immunization with hepatitis B vaccine.
● 2. Receive hepatitis B immunoglobulin within one week.
○ 3. Take penicillin (Pentam) for a minimum of 10 days.
○ 4. Scrub the puncture with diluted household bleach.

127 It is essential that the nurse inform the client with hepatitis B that for the remainder of his lifetime he must avoid
○ 1. sexual activity.
● 2. donating blood.
○ 3. active exercise.
○ 4. foreign travel.

A 60-year-old male seeks medical attention because he has been vomiting blood and passing bloody stools. The tentative diagnosis is cirrhosis of the liver.

128 If the client's wife contributes all of the following information, which is *most likely* related to the client's development of cirrhosis?
● 1. He is a heavy user of alcohol.
○ 2. He is a Vietnam veteran.
○ 3. He has osteoarthritis.
○ 4. He has hypertension.

129 If the client's cirrhosis is advanced, which one of the following signs will the nurse *most likely* find during the physical assessment?
○ 1. There is excessive body hair on the shoulders.
● 2. There are spider-like blood vessels on the skin.
○ 3. The scrotum is unusually large.
○ 4. The finger nails appear clubbed.

130 Which one of the following assessments indicate that the client with cirrhosis is bleeding from somewhere in his upper gastrointestinal tract?
○ 1. He has midepigastric pain.
○ 2. He feels very nauseated.
● 3. His stools are black.
○ 4. His abdomen is distended.

The nursing care plan indicates that the nurse should monitor the ascites on the client with cirrhosis each day.

131 To carry out this nursing order, which one of the following nursing actions is *most appropriate*?
○ 1. The apical and radial pulse rate are counted.
○ 2. The lying and sitting blood pressure are taken.
○ 3. The specific gravity of the urine is checked.
● 4. The circumference of the abdomen is measured.

The physician considers performing a liver biopsy on the client with cirrhosis.

132 If a liver biopsy is performed, *immediately afterward* it is *most important* for the nurse to assess the client for signs of
● 1. hemorrhage.
○ 2. infection.
○ 3. blood clots.
○ 4. collapsed lung.

133 After a liver biopsy, which nursing order is *most appropriate* to add to the plan of care?
○ 1. Ambulate the client twice each shift.
○ 2. Keep the client in high Fowler's position.
○ 3. Position the client on his right side.
● 4. Elevate the client's legs on two pillows.

Instead of a liver biopsy, a magnetic resonance imaging (MRI) test is ordered.

134 Before the MRI is performed, which nursing action is *essential*?
○ 1. The nurse administers a pretest sedative.
● 2. The nurse removes the client's dental bridge.
○ 3. The nurse records the client's body weight.
○ 4. The nurse inserts a Foley retention catheter.

The MRI confirms the diagnosis of hepatic cirrhosis and reveals a large amount of fluid in the peritoneal cavity. A paracentesis is planned.

135 Which one of the following nursing actions is *most appropriate* prior to assisting with the paracentesis?
- ● 1. The nurse asks the client to void.
- ○ 2. The nurse withholds food and water.
- ○ 3. The nurse washes the client's abdomen.
- ○ 4. The nurse obtains a suction machine.

136 After the paracentesis has been performed, which of the following is an *essential* nursing responsibility?
- ○ 1. Increasing the client's oral fluid intake
- ● 2. Recording the volume of withdrawn fluid
- ○ 3. Administering a prescribed analgesic
- ○ 4. Encouraging the client to deep-breathe

137 When administering an intramuscular injection to the client with cirrhosis of the liver and others with a similar diagnosis, which nursing action is *essential* to perform?
- ○ 1. Cleansing the site with povidone-iodine (Betadine)
- ○ 2. Injecting volumes of 1 mL or less in any one site
- ○ 3. Using glass syringes rather than disposable plastic
- ● 4. Applying prolonged pressure to the injection site

138 If all the following laboratory test results on the client with cirrhosis are elevated, which one is *most indicative* that the client may develop hepatic encephalopathy?
- ○ 1. Serum creatinine
- ○ 2. Serum bilirubin
- ● 3. Blood ammonia
- ○ 4. Blood urea nitrogen

139 Which one of the following assessment findings is *most indicative* that the cirrhotic client's condition is worsening?
- ● 1. He is difficult to arouse.
- ○ 2. His urine output is 100 mL/h.
- ○ 3. He snores when he is asleep.
- ○ 4. His blood pressure is 122/60

The seriousness of the client's condition is explained to his wife. She is prepared for the possibility of her husband's death.

140 When the client's wife cries as she recalls various significant events she and her husband shared together, which nursing action is *most therapeutic* at this time?

- ○ 1. Tell her to call a close family member.
- ● 2. Listen to her express her thoughts.
- ○ 3. Suggest that she write in a diary.
- ○ 4. Ask about her future plans in life.

NURSING CARE OF CLIENTS WITH DISORDERS OF THE PANCREAS

A 48-year-old male is brought to the emergency department because he has severe upper abdominal pain. It came on suddenly a few hours ago, and nothing thus far has relieved it. The nurse observes that the client is curled in a fetal position and is rocking back and forth.

141 Which one of the following actions would help the nurse *most* to further assess the client's pain?
- ○ 1. Determine if the client can stop moving about.
- ● 2. Ask the client to rate his pain from 0 to 10.
- ○ 3. Observe if the client is perspiring heavily.
- ○ 4. Give the client a prescribed pain-relieving drug.

142 If all of the following initial laboratory tests are ordered, which one, if elevated, is the *best indication* that the client's pain is caused by pancreatitis?
- ○ 1. Serum bilirubin
- ● 2. Serum amylase
- ○ 3. Lactose tolerance
- ○ 4. Glucose tolerance

The physician orders a nasogastric sump tube inserted.

143 To determine the length for inserting the tube, the nurse is *most correct* in placing the tip of the tube at the client's nose and measuring the distance from there to the
- ○ 1. jaw and then midway to the sternum.
- ○ 2. mouth and then between the nipples.
- ○ 3. midsternum and then to the umbilicus.
- ● 4. ear and then to the xiphoid process.

144 If the client turns blue and coughs as the nasogastric tube is inserted, which *additional sign* indicates that the tube has entered the respiratory tract?
- ● 1. The client cannot speak.
- ○ 2. The client cannot swallow.
- ○ 3. The client begins to sneeze.
- ○ 4. The client begins to vomit.

The client's fluid and nutritional needs are temporarily being met by administering intravenous fluid.

145 While assessing the infusion, what finding should be reported to the charge nurse *immediately*?
- ○ 1. The tubing is coiled on the top of the mattress.
- ○ 2. The container has approximately 250 mL of fluid left.
- ○ 3. The fluid is infusing in the client's nondominant hand.
- ◉ 4. Less fluid than ordered has infused at this time.

After being kept NPO (nothing by mouth) for several days, the nasogastric tube is removed and the client is placed on a bland, low-fat diet.

146 If all of the following foods are on the client's breakfast tray, which one should the nurse remove?
- ○ 1. Stewed prunes
- ○ 2. Skim milk
- ◉ 3. Scrambled eggs
- ○ 4. Whole wheat toast

147 Before discharging the client who is recovering from pancreatitis, what information is essential for him to receive?
- ○ 1. He must never donate blood again.
- ○ 2. He must avoid lifting heavy objects.
- ◉ 3. He must not drink alcohol in any form.
- ○ 4. He must forgo taking strong laxatives.

A 69-year-old female is admitted with the diagnosis of cancer of the pancreas.

148 If this client is typical of most others who develop cancer of the pancreas, the nurse can expect that one of the earliest problems for which the client sought treatment is
- ○ 1. sharp pain.
- ◉ 2. weight loss.
- ○ 3. bleeding.
- ○ 4. fainting.

The client with cancer of the pancreas has metastatic disease that makes aggressive treatment unrealistic. She is in a terminal state.

149 When the client says to the nurse, "Am I dying?" The best response from the nurse is
- ○ 1. "Yes, you have little time left."
- ○ 2. "No, you are not going to die."
- ◉ 3. "Tell me about how you are feeling."
- ○ 4. "Who would you like me to call?"

The client with metastatic cancer of the pancreas has an advance directive that requests no aggressive treatment. She is referred for hospice care.

150 If the client has pain medication ordered every 3 to 4 hours as necessary, which of the following is the best action for the hospice nurse to take to provide her with maximum comfort at this time?
- ◉ 1. Give the medication immediately at her request.
- ○ 2. Administer the medication every 3 hours.
- ○ 3. Ask the physician to prescribe a high dose.
- ○ 4. Give the medication when the pain is severe.

Correct Answers and Rationale

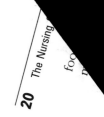

Directions: Two numbers appear in parentheses following each rationale. The first number identifies the textbook listed in the references, page 512, and the second number identifies the page(s) in that textbook on which the correct answer can be verified. Occasionally two or more textbooks are given for verifying the correct answer.

NURSING CARE OF CLIENTS WITH DISORDERS OF THE MOUTH

1 1. When the mucous membrane of the oral cavity is inflamed, it is best to eliminate foods that are acidic, salty, spicy, dry, or very hot. Other than tomato soup, none of the other foods have any of these characteristics. (6:616)
 Nursing Process—Implementation
 Client Need—Physiological integrity

2 3. Oral swabs may clean plaque from the teeth, promote more comfort, and produce less irritation than a toothbrush—regardless of its size. Even a soft-bristled toothbrush may cause too much trauma. Dental floss alone is not the best choice for mouth care. Normal saline mouth rinse is preferable to one that is flavored. Flavoring may only refresh the breath and may irritate the mouth as well. (18:1153; 21:157; 25:319)
 Nursing Process—Implementation
 Client Need—Physiological integrity

3 2. Clients who are limited in the amount of fluid they may consume need frequent mouth care. Limited hydration can reduce the volume of saliva. Saliva helps keep the teeth clean and inhibits bacterial growth. A client with full dentures has the same oral hygiene needs as a person with natural teeth. A low-residue diet is one that reduces the volume of undigested substances in the bowel; in and of itself, it is not a criteria for specialized oral hygiene. Eating raw fruits or vegetables, like apples and celery, can act as a dental cleanser. Sucking on ice chips is not an indication for modifying routine measures for oral hygiene. (18:510; 25:321)
 Nursing Process—Planning
 Client Need—Physiological integrity

4 2. Holding dentures over a basin of water or soft towel prevents breaking them if they slip from the hands. Hot water may warp the plastic from which some dentures are made. Oral adhesives do not require a special solvent for removal. Dentures are kept moist when not being used to retain their fit and color. (18:511; 25:320)
 Nursing Process—Implementation
 Client Need—Physiological integrity

5 2. The potential for aspiration is best prevented by placing unconscious clients on their side with the head slightly lowered when administering oral hygiene. It is difficult to provide mouth care with a client in the prone or face-down position. Elevating the head regardless of whether the client is supine or recumbent increases the potential for aspiration. (18:512; 25:318)
 Nursing Process—Implementation
 Client Need—Safe, effective care environment

6 3. Candidiasis appears as small white patches on the mucous membrane of the mouth and tongue. Their appearance has been described as resembling milk curds. Red ulcerated patches near the margin of the teeth and gums are characteristic of gingivitis. Herpes simplex lesions are vesicles that become transformed to shallow ulcers. Herpes simplex is not restricted to the tongue. The last option does not describe any particular oral disease. (4:660)
 Nursing Process—Data collection
 Client Need—Physiological integrity

7 2. An infection with the yeast organism, *Candida albicans*, is usually acquired from an overgrowth of normal flora found in and on the skin and mucous membranes of the gastrointestinal tract. Candidiasis is considered an opportunistic infection because the source of the infection is usually the client. Antibiotic therapy can upset the ecologic balance of organisms in the body, allowing some natural microbes to grow unchecked. It may be possible to acquire organisms from soiled dental instruments, but since most dentists follow guidelines for sterilizing their equipment between uses, this is not the most reasonable explanation. Candidiasis is not transmitted from vectors, contaminated water, or

d. Because the organisms are present in the mouth, it is possible, but highly improbable, that the infection could be acquired by inhaling respiratory droplets from another individual. (4:660)

Nursing Process—Implementation
Client Need—Health promotion/maintenance

8 3. Because nystatin is poorly absorbed from the gastrointestinal tract, holding the liquid suspension in the mouth as long as possible facilitates contact of the drug with the organism. The client is allowed to swallow the medication after swishing it around. There is no reason to use a straw or dilute the medication. (20:108)

Nursing Process—Planning
Client Need—Health promotion/maintenance

9 2. Factors that predispose to cancer of the mouth include any source of chronic irritation, such as holding a pipe in the mouth, holding chewing or smokeless tobacco in the mouth, consumption of alcohol, prolonged contact with rough dental appliances or jagged teeth. Having a partial plate, as long as it fits well, is not as likely to cause cancerous changes as the chronic use of smokeless tobacco. Certain processes for extracting caffeine have been linked with some forms of cancer but not cancer of the mouth. No hazards for cancer have been reported from chewing gum sweetened with aspartame (NutraSweet) at this time. (21:667; 3:160)

Nursing Process—Data collection
Client Need—Safe, effective care environment

10 1. All emesis is inspected to detect the presence of radioactive needles that may have been displaced. If one or more becomes dislodged, it is never touched with the hands. It is retrieved with long forceps and placed in a lead container. Bleach is not required for cleaning or disinfecting the emesis basin. There is no reason for using a plastic rather than metal emesis basin. The threads are never cut; they are counted each shift to make sure that the original number inserted are still present. (18:1154)

Nursing Process—Planning
Client Need—Safe, effective care environment

11 3. Whenever implanted radiation is used, others are protected by limiting time and distance from the patient and by using other physical methods of shielding them from absorbing the radiation. Therefore, a solitary activity is more appropriate than those involving one or more people. (18:1154; 21:151)

Nursing Process—Implementation
Client Need—Safe, effective care environment

12 4. Herpes simplex type 1 lesions appear on the face, cheeks, and nose as well as in the perioral (mouth) area. Handwashing and good personal hygiene are used during the time the virus is replicating and being shed. All the other statements about herpes simplex 1 are true. (18:1243)

Nursing Process—Evaluation
Client Need—Health promotion/maintenance

13 2. Acyclovir does not cure the infection or prevent future outbreaks. It only shortens the time during which the virus is replicating and being shed. Some of the virus retreats within nerve fibers and escapes detection by the body's immune system where it remains dormant until stimulated. The drug is taken when the client first becomes aware of symptoms, such as an area of itching and tingling on the mucous membrane. Oral doses are generally taken for 10 days. (17:135)

Nursing Process—Evaluation
Client Need—Health promotion/maintenance

NURSING CARE OF CLIENTS WITH DISORDERS OF THE ESOPHAGUS

14 3. Food and fluid are avoided to reduce the potential for aspiration. All other choices are incorrect because they involve eating or drinking. (7:715; 18:1230; 21:656)

Nursing Process—Evaluation
Client Need—Safe, effective care environment

15 2. Chewing food thoroughly helps the bolus slip through the narrowed stricture. Switching to baby food is too drastic at this time. Drinking liquids throughout a meal is beneficial in thinning the bolus of food. Eliminating dairy products will not promote the ability to swallow food. (6:418; 21:677)

Nursing Process—Implementation
Client Need—Health promotion/maintenance

16 4. Chronic consumption of alcohol can damage the liver and interfere with blood flow from the esophagus and other abdominal organs. The hypertension created by the stagnation of blood causes esophageal veins to distend and bleed. None of the other facts in the client's social and medical history relate to his current condition. (4:705; 21:676)

Nursing Process—Data collection
Client Need—Physiological integrity

17 2. Dyspnea, hypotension, chest constriction, and back pain are some of the symptoms associated with an incompatibility transfusion reaction. An incompatibility reaction is life-threatening. The other assessments in this item are signs associated with hypovolemia. In this client's case, the remaining signs and symptoms are probably due to blood loss. (18:1133; 25:293)

> Nursing Process—Data collection
> Client Need—Physiological integrity

18 4. A hiatal hernia results when a weakened area of the diaphragm allows a portion of the stomach to protrude into the esophagus. The acid contents of the stomach reflux into the esophagus causing irritation and inflammation which the client describes as "heartburn." The remaining signs and symptoms are unrelated to the medical diagnosis. (4:695; 21:675)

> Nursing Process—Data collection
> Client Need—Physiological integrity

19 3. An upright position for at least two hours after eating keeps swallowed food and gastric contents within the stomach by gravity. A person with a hiatal hernia is also encouraged to sleep with the head of his bed elevated. A client with this condition should eat small, frequent meals to avoid overdistending the stomach. Eating soft foods or eating when hungry have no effect on relieving the discomfort associated with this condition. (18:1247; 25:676)

> Nursing Process—Implementation
> Client Need—Health promotion/maintenance

20 4. Elevating the head of the bed helps to prevent gastric reflux. The other suggestions may provide comfort, but they are not therapeutic for relieving the client's symptoms. (18:1247; 25:676)

> Nursing Process—Implementation
> Client Need—Health promotion/maintenance

21 2. It is essential to monitor the blood glucose levels frequently because TPN solutions contain high concentrations of glucose. Insulin coverage may be needed to maintain the blood sugar within an acceptable range. The specific gravity may become lower if the client begins to excrete large volumes of urine, but it is not generally monitored. Pulse pressure is the difference between the systolic and diastolic arterial pressure measurements. Pulse pressure is usually unaffected by hyperalimentation. There is nothing specifically related to TPN that necessitates taking the apical and radial pulse. (18:746; 21:221; 25:295)

> Nursing Process—Data collection
> Client Need—Safe, effective care environment

22 2. One of the best criteria that a client is responding favorably to TPN is a gradual and steady gain in weight. The client could remain alert despite improvement in his nutritional state. Hunger is both an emotional and physical phenomenon. Well-nourished, satiated people can feel hungry when they see, smell, or even think about food. The client's tolerance of pain may increase with improved nutrition, but it is not be the best criterion for determining the effectiveness of TPN. (18:747; 25:294)

> Nursing Process—Evaluation
> Client Need—Physiological integrity

23 2. Slight bleeding or clear serum drainage at the site of the gastrostomy is a normal finding that can be expected immediately after a gastrostomy has been performed. Milky drainage suggests an infection, or, if it occurs after feedings have been initiated, it may indicate leakage of formula. Intestinal secretions cause green-tinged drainage, but the gastrostomy is located in a client's stomach. Bright bloody drainage indicates arterial bleeding which is not a normal finding. (25:611)

> Nursing Process—Data collection
> Client Need—Physiological integrity

24 3. Comparing the measured length of tubing extending from the gastrostomy site is an easy and appropriate technique for determining tube migration. A change in pH from acid to alkaline indicates intestinal migration, but most gastrostomy tubes are too short to reach the small intestine. X-rays are expensive and expose clients to unnecessary radiation. A distended abdomen may indicate many complications, but tube migration is not one of them. (18:314)

> Nursing Process—Implementation
> Client Need—Safe, effective care environment

25 2. Since each ounce equals 30 mL, it will take a total of four hours to instill 480 mL (2 × 8 ounces) at a rate of 120 mL/hr. (25:254)

> Nursing Process—Implementation
> Client Need—Safe, effective care environment

26 3. It is important that the stomach not become overdistended. The stomach residual is checked prior to administering an intermittent feeding. As a rule of thumb, the gastric residual should be no more than 100 to 150 mL of the previous intermittent feeding or, if continuous, no more than half of the previous hour's infusion volume. Raising the formula causes the liquid nourishment to run in at a faster rate. Adding water to formula adds more volume. (21:671; 25:614)

> Nursing Process—Implementation
> Client Need—Physiological integrity

27 4. It is important to rinse the feeding tube after each use to maintain its patency and to meet the client's needs for water. A tube-fed client should always have the head of the bed elevated during and for at least a half hour after a tube feeding to prevent aspiration. Gastrostomy tubes may be clamped intermittently, but only after they have been rinsed with water. (25:616)

> Nursing Process—Implementation
> Client Need—Physiological integrity

28 2. Sharing perceptions or what some refer to as validation is the best therapeutic communication technique in this case for encouraging the client to discuss his feelings. Most clients tend to deny feeling angry if asked a direct question. Telling clients their situation may get better is false reassurance. When clients know the situation will not get better, they lose trust in the nurse's ability to be supportive. Just because "lots of people" are nourished by tube feedings doesn't necessarily make it easier for the client to cope. (9:152; 25:79)

> Nursing Process—Implementation
> Client Need—Psychosocial integrity

NURSING CARE OF CLIENTS WITH DISORDERS OF THE STOMACH

29 3. Individuals with peptic ulcers generally find that eating relieves their discomfort. The pain is caused by irritation of the eroded mucosa with hydrochloric acid and pepsin. Food tends to dilute the acid, thereby raising the pH of the secretions. This reduces irritation of the ulcerated tissue. Skipping a meal increases the pain because the acid secretions become very concentrated. Many ulcer clients report awakening at night with pain. Bending over does not cause or relieve the discomfort associated with an ulcer. (18:1249; 21:679)

> Nursing Process—Data collection
> Client Need—Physiologic integrity

30 3. Blood in the stool is a significant finding. Its presence indicates that bleeding is occurring within the gastrointestinal tract. If the bleeding is occurring in the upper gastrointestinal tract, the stool appears black. This finding is called *melana*. However, blood may be present without an obvious change in the normal color of stool. This finding is referred to as *occult blood*. Identifying blood in the stool is not proof that the client has an ulcer, but it aids the differential diagnosis. Albumin in the urine is a finding associated with kidney disease. Elevated glucose levels in the blood could be due to diabetes mellitus. Emesis is not tested for the presence of pepsin. (3:666: 7:263–264, 21:679)

> Nursing Process—Data collection
> Client Need—Physiological integrity

31 4. An upper gastrointestinal x-ray uses barium as a contrast medium. The client must drink the barium during the x-ray procedure. This opaque substance fills the hollow structures of the esophagus and stomach, improving their image. A gastroscopy involves inserting a flexible tube in the stomach. Intravenous dye is used in some x-rays of the gallbladder. A client is placed within a chamber when a computerized axial tomography scan is performed. (7:705; 18:1228)

> Nursing Process—Evaluation
> Client Need—Safe, effective care environment

32 1. There is approximately 30 mL per ounce. None of the other volumes are approximate equivalents. (20:33; 18:575)

> Nursing Process—Implementation
> Client Need—Physiological integrity

33 2. Antibiotics, like tetracyclines, eliminate *Helicobactor pylori*, a bacteria that has been found to deplete gastric mucus, which causes the majority of peptic ulcers. This therapeutic treatment may ultimately heal the irritated mucous membrane of the stomach, but that is not the most specific answer to the question. Tetracyclines do not coat the stomach, nor are they prescribed in this case to prevent secondary infections. (17:280; 18:1248; 25:678)

> Nursing Process—Implementation
> Client Need—Health promotion/maintenance

34 1. Acetaminophen is not associated with gastritis or ulcer formation. However, the link between salicylates, like aspirin, and the nonsteroidal anti-inflammatory drugs, like ibuprofen and naproxen, with gastric irritation and ulcer formation is well documented. (18:1249; 25:678)

> Nursing Process—Implementation
> Client Need—Health promotion/maintenance

35 2. When the stomach or other gastrointestinal structure perforates, the abdomen becomes very hard, rigid, and tender. The skin becomes pale due to vasoconstriction associated with shock. Dilated pupils are due to a variety of causes, such as mydriatic eye medication, eye surgery, cerebral anoxia, and so on. Rapid respirations are not as significant as a tense abdomen. (18:1251; 25:701)

> Nursing Process—Data collection
> Client Need—Physiological integrity

36 2. Hearing a whooshing sound over the stomach as a bolus of air is instilled through the proximal end of the gastric tube is one method for determining placement. If the tube is in the esophagus, the client will belch. Another technique is to aspirate secretions from the tube and test the pH. If the secretions are coming from the stomach, the pH will be very acid. A portable x-ray is an accurate method, but the cost and unnecessary radiation exposure make this method inappropriate. Liquids are never instilled through a nasogastric tube until placement has been verified. If the tip is not in the stomach, aspiration could occur. Feeling for air is an unacceptable technique for determining placement. (18:1238; 25:598)

Nursing Process—Implementation
Client Need—Safe, effective care environment

37 1. The nurse offers the client a basis for hope by validating the conscientious efforts that are being made. The response is objective without giving false reassurance. The client may interpret the nurse's unwillingness to answer, in the second example, as an indication that his worst fear is confirmed. By implying that his serious question is frivolous, as in the third example, the client may be discouraged from attempting further communication about his fears and feelings. The last example shows a disregard for the client's unique perception and fears. (25:79–80)

Nursing Process—Implementation
Client Need—Psychosocial integrity

38 2. Splinting or supporting the incision promotes deeper inhalation and more forceful coughing. An explanation of his risks is not as likely to result in efforts to clear the airway as relieving the client's discomfort. Oxygen is not necessary unless ventilation is compromised. A high Fowler's position facilitates the potential for a larger volume of air, but unless the client actively uses his respiratory muscles, that will not happen. (21:239; 25:551)

Nursing Process—Implementation
Client Need—Physiological integrity

39 3. Any fluid instilled or removed is recorded to maintain an accurate intake and output record. A nasogastric tube is irrigated with normal saline, which does not have to be sterile. Oxygen is administered prior to tracheobronchial suctioning. Swallowing does not affect a gastric tube irrigation. (4:675; 25:607)

Nursing Process—Implementation
Client Need—Safe, effective care environment

40 2. Consuming carbohydrates triggers the release of insulin, causing postprandial hypoglycemia. Therefore, to prevent this component of the dumping syndrome, postgastrectomy clients are taught to follow a low-carbohydrate diet. Fluids are not con-

sumed with meals because this increases the rapidity with which consumed food is dumped into the small intestine. Eating small meals is recommended for limiting the bolus of food present in the stomach. Reducing the consumption of red meat is a healthy dietary change, but it does not prevent dumping syndrome. (4:374; 21:680–681)

Nursing Process—Evaluation
Client Need—Health promotion/maintenance

41 1. Lying down delays the movement of food from the stomach into the small intestine. People with a hiatal hernia should sleep with the head of the bed elevated. Walking, meditation, and relaxation are healthy behaviors, but they are unrelated to preventing dumping syndrome. (3:671; 26:364)

Nursing Process—Planning
Client Need—Health promotion/maintenance

42 1. Absence of free hydrochloric acid in the stomach is associated with stomach cancer. This finding distinguishes the etiology of the symptoms from other causes, such as peptic ulcer, esophageal stricture, and so on. Gastrin is a hormone secreted by the mucosa of the pylorus and stomach. Gastrin causes hypersecretion of gastric acid. Gastritis is a common finding that has multiple etiologies. The presence of a few red blood cells in the urine indicates blood loss within the urinary tract from conditions such as cystitis, glomerulonephritis, and others. (7:973; 18:1252; 21:681)

Nursing Process—Data collection
Client Need—Physiological integrity

43 3. Placing the chin to the chest helps to direct the tube into the esophagus rather than the lower airway. The client is given water to sip which would make it difficult to breathe deeply. A sniffing position is appropriate when first inserting the tube into a client's nose. Coughing occurs as a reflex if the tube enters the airway; it is a helpful sign that the tube must be raised from its present location. (4:673; 25:601)

Nursing Process—Implementation
Client Need—Safe, effective care environment

44 1. Low intermittent suction is the best setting for a single lumen nasogastric tube. This setting reduces trauma to the gastric mucosa and reduces the volume of electrolytes that are withdrawn from the client's gastric secretions. Low continuous suction is used for vented, or double lumen, nasogastric tubes. (26:369)

Nursing Process—Implementation
Client Need—Safe, effective care environment

45 2. Clients with nasogastric tubes that are connected to suction are generally NPO (nothing by mouth). Giving water or other fluids, which are subsequently removed from the stomach, is likely to dilute and deplete electrolyte levels. (25:604)
  Nursing Process—Planning
  Client Need—Physiological integrity

46 2. There are 1000 mcg in 1 mg. Therefore the correct volume in this case is 1 mL. (17:70)
  Nursing Process—Implementation
  Client Need—Physiological integrity

47 2. Intramuscular injections are given at a 90° angle. The vastus lateralis muscle is located at the outer thigh. The deltoid site is in the upper arm. The rectus femoris site is on the anterior thigh and the dorsogluteal site is in the upper outer quadrant of the buttock. (25:740)
  Nursing Process—Implementation
  Client Need—Physiological integrity

NURSING CARE OF CLIENTS WITH DISORDERS OF THE SMALL INTESTINE

48 4. Stool specimens that may contain ova and parasites should be examined when the feces is fresh. Ova and parasites will not survive long below body temperature. Drying and cooling destroy the organisms and result in invalid findings. The client can use a bedpan or toilet for bowel elimination. The nurse can transfer a portion of stool to a waxed, covered container using a tongue blade. The specimen container need not be sterile. (7:256; 18:559)
  Nursing Process—Implementation
  Client Need—Safe, effective care environment

49 2. The abbreviation *q.i.d.* means that the drug is to be administered four times a day. Scheduled hours may differ depending on the predetermined timetable set by the health agency. However, in following the order as it is written, administration can be no less or no more than four times during a 24-hour period. Military time is based on a 24-hour clock. Each hour is numbered in continuous sequence. (25:98)
  Nursing Process—Evaluation
  Client Need—Safe, effective care environment

50 3. A clear liquid diet includes fat-free bouillon, tea or coffee, flavored gelatin, fruit ices, carbonated beverages like ginger ale, some clear fruit juices like apple and grape. Honey and sugar also may be used. No milk or milk products are permitted. (6:53; 25:242)

  Nursing Process—Implementation
  Client Need—Physiological integrity

51 4. Dark yellow urine indicates a concentration of urinary pigment in a small volume of water. Pink mucous membranes is a normal finding. An elevated blood pressure and irregular heart rate are abnormal findings, but these signs are not associated with fluid volume deficit. (25:254)
  Nursing Process—Data collection
  Client Need—Physiological integrity

52 3. GoLYTELY is given as a colonic lavage. Within 30 minutes of ingesting the first volume of the solution, the client should experience the first of many bowel movements. This solution is preferable to other forms of bowel cleansing because it is less likely to deplete electrolytes or cause water intoxication. The other choices are expected outcomes of administering the colonic lavage solution, but they are not the main reasons for its administration. (3:654; 7:808)
  Nursing Process—Evaluation
  Client Need—Physiological integrity

53 3. Respiratory depression is a potential effect when midazolam hydrochloride is administered. It is *expected* that the client will be able to communicate and cooperate during the procedure, but have no memory of doing so afterward. Many drugs can cause instability in blood pressure and cardiac dysrhythmias, but these effects are not commonly manifested by those who receive midazolam. (28:1155)
  Nursing Process—Data collection
  Client Need—Physiological integrity

54 4. Fiber is the portion of fruits, vegetables, grains, and nuts that is not broken down and absorbed during the digestive process. Animal products are not a source of dietary fiber. Food that requires chewing is too limited a definition for fiber. The semisolid mass of food in the stomach is called chyme. (6:133; 18:281)
  Nursing Process—Evaluation
  Client Need—Health promotion/maintenance

55 2. Ileal drainage contains enzymes and bile salts that are very damaging to the skin. Family coping, body image, and depression are likely to occur whenever an individual develops a complication. However, standards for care are not met if nursing measures for maintaining or restoring skin integrity are omitted from the nursing plan for care. (25:22)
  Nursing Process—Planning
  Client Need—Physiological integrity

NURSING CARE OF CLIENTS WITH DISORDERS OF THE LARGE INTESTINE

56 2. The client's statement contradicts the procedure that has been scheduled. For the consent to be valid, a person must understand that to which he is giving his consent. The physician is responsible for providing the explanation. The nurse is responsible for witnessing the client's signature and ensuring that the legal aspects of the contract are upheld. If the nurse determines that the client does not understand the information provided by the physician, the physician is notified. If the client's misinformation is clarified, the surgery need not be canceled. The nurse never allows a client to sign a contract he does not fully understand. The nurse does not proceed with skin preparation until the discrepancy is settled. (4:21; 25:197)

    Nursing Process—Implementation
    Client Need—Safe, effective care environment

57 4. To help prevent headaches after spinal anesthesia, it is customary to keep the client's head flat for 6 to 12 hours postoperatively. The remaining orders in this item are appropriate. (21:238)

    Nursing Process—Implementation
    Client Need—Safe, effective care environment

58 1. Although pain is important to assess, the safety and welfare of the client is jeopardized if the client experiences urinary retention which is undetected. Coughing is contraindicated following this type of surgery. The client is alert if spinal anesthesia is administered. (4:694; 21:243)

    Nursing Process—Data collection
    Client Need—Physiological integrity

59 2. A suspensory is used following a herniorrhaphy on a male patient to help prevent scrotal swelling. A suspensory does not prevent impotence, strain on the incision, or wound contamination. (4:694; 21:710)

    Nursing Process—Implementation
    Client Need—Health promotion/maintenance

60 2. The client should receive half of the total volume in the ampule. Dosages are calculated by dividing the desired dose by the dose supplied and then multiplying it times the volume. (20:36; 25:699)

    Nursing Process—Implementation
    Client Need—Physiological integrity

61 2. The federal government mandates that the manufacturing, distributing, and dispensing of addictive drugs like meperidine hydrochloride be controlled. Therefore, an accurate accounting of its administration is kept on a narcotic control log. (18:660)

    Nursing Process—Implementation
    Client Need—Safe, effective care environment

62 1. Clients with ulcerative colitis may have 12 or more diarrheal stools per day that contain blood and mucus along with fecal material. Bowel sounds are likely to be hyperactive. Striae are red or white streaks on the skin due to stretching. Because the client with ulcerative colitis suffers from weight loss and emaciation, striae are not a common finding. Ulcerated lesions in this disease are confined to the colon. (18:1257; 21:697)

    Nursing Process—Data collection
    Client Need—Physiological integrity

63 3. Using a diaper on a person with fecal incontinence is usually emotionally devastating. It is done only as a last resort, preferably with the client's permission. Keeping the bedside commode nearby, answering her signal promptly, and helping her to the bathroom frequently are acceptable methods for dealing with the urgency that results in incontinence. (26:28)

    Nursing Process—Planning
    Client Need—Psychosocial integrity

64 1. Reflecting is a response that lets the client know that both the content and the feelings are understood. The nurse avoids any emotional support or involvement by offering to arrange contact with the physician. Giving advice and disagreeing with a client are blocks to therapeutic communication. (9:150; 25:79)

    Nursing Process—Implementation
    Client Need—Psychosocial integrity

65 1. Once the preoperative medication is given, the side rails are raised and the client instructed to remain in bed. Elimination and oral hygiene are accomplished prior to giving the preanesthetic drugs. Meperidine and hydroxyzine depress the central nervous system, making it difficult for the client to remain alert during attempts at teaching leg exercises. (18:623)

    Nursing Process—Implementation
    Client Need—Safe, effective care environment

66 3. A dropping blood pressure frequently suggests that the client is going into shock. A systolic pressure of 90 to 100 mm Hg indicates shock is approaching. Below 80 mm Hg, shock is present. Other signs of shock include a rapid, thready pulse; pale, cold, and clammy skin; rapid respirations; a falling body temperature; restlessness; and a decreased level of consciousness. (4:453; 25:235)

    Nursing Process—Data collection
    Client Need—Physiological integrity

67 4. Normal oxygen saturation is between 95% and 100%. The measurements in the other options indicate hypoxemia. (25:402)

Nursing Process—Evaluation
Client Need—Physiological integrity

68 1. The best time for changing an appliance and providing stomal care is when the bowel is somewhat inactive. This is usually in the morning before any food has been eaten. Exercise and eating tend to increase bowel activity, making it likely that intestinal contents will spill onto the skin if the procedure is done at that time. (21:723; 25:684)

Nursing Process—Implementation
Client Need—Physiological integrity

69 2. A normal healthy stoma appears bright red or pink because of its rich blood supply. If the stoma is light pink or dusky blue, the blood supply to the tissue is compromised. A tan stoma is atypical even in non-Caucasians and further assessments are necessary to determine the cause. (21:722)

Nursing Process—Data collection
Client Need—Physiological integrity

70 3. A mild soap and tepid water are most often recommended for cleaning the skin around the stoma. Patting the skin with cotton is ineffective for cleansing. Alcohol is drying and irritating to the skin. Scrubbing is avoided because friction is likely to irritate the skin. (21:724; 25:685)

Nursing Process—Implementation
Client Need—Physiological integrity

71 2. The appliance opening must be large enough to avoid impairing circulation to the stoma, but small enough that ileal drainage will not damage the skin. There should be only a ¹⁄₁₆- to ⅛-in margin of skin exposed around the stoma. This allows room to attach the faceplate to the skin rather than to the stoma itself. However, it covers an adequate amount of skin to prevent excoriation due to contact with enzymes and bile salts in ileal drainage. The stomal opening must not be obstructed or stool will not be passed. The appliance will not adhere to the skin if only a ⅛-in. margin is in contact with skin. The appliance must cover the stoma; the bag may or may not be directly at the waist or belt line. (21:723; 25:686)

Nursing Process—Implementation
Client Need—Physiological integrity

72 4. Because there is no sphincter to control the watery discharge from a conventional ileostomy, it is difficult for most to gain control of bowel elimination. It is realistic for people with an ileostomy to play tennis, swim, have sexual relations, get pregnant, and in general pursue careers and enjoy all manner of social activities. (4:686; 18:1241)

Nursing Process—Implementation
Client Need—Health promotion/maintenance

73 4. Appendicitis is an inflammation of the appendix. Infection often accompanies the inflammation. The white blood cells, also called leukocytes, increase when these conditions are present to wall off, destroy, or remove damaged tissue and pathogens. The bilirubin level is usually monitored on an adult with liver or gallbladder disease. The serum potassium is important if the client had anorexia, vomiting, or diarrhea. The prothrombin time is generally monitored when the client is receiving the anticoagulant warfarin sodium (Coumadin). (18:1259; 21:700)

Nursing Process—Data collection
Client Need—Physiological integrity

74 1. Appendicitis is often accompanied by *rebound tenderness* which is characterized as more pain after pressure is released than when applied. There may be pain with palpation, but the hallmark of appendicitis is the rebound phenomenon. The other options are inconsistent with appendicitis. (4:689; 18:1259; 21:700)

Nursing Process—Data collection
Client Need—Physiological integrity

75 1. A shorter recovery period is only one of the many advantages of laporoscopic surgery. However, some form of anesthesia is used. There is a smaller than usual surgical scar. And there are still restrictions in activity, which include lifting, for a minimum of 10 to 15 days postoperatively. (18:1259)

Nursing Process—Implementation
Client Need—Health promotion/maintenance

76 3. Applications of heat are avoided whenever there is a possibility that abdominal discomfort is due to appendicitis. The heat dilates blood vessels, increases swelling, and promotes rupture of the vermiform appendix. Withholding oral nourishment is advantageous if the symptoms are due to gastroenteritis or if emergency surgery is necessary. Pain generally limits activity. Because it did not in this case, the activity probably would not affect the course of the appendicitis. Acetaminophen is a nonsalicylate. It lowers a fever and relieve discomfort but does not predispose to rupturing the appendix. (18:1259)

Nursing Process—Data collection
Client Need—Physiological integrity

77 2. An open drain relies on gravity to remove secretions that are then absorbed by the dressing. Neither a lithotomy, recumbent, or Trendelenberg position promotes the collection of wound drainage near the drain. (4:482; 25:571)
Nursing Process—Implementation
Client Need—Physiological integrity

78 3. Soiled dressings are enclosed in a receptacle or container, like the nurse's glove, to prevent the transmission of infectious microorganisms. A clean glove is used to remove soiled dressings. Tape is pulled toward the wound to prevent separating the healing edges. Wounds are always cleansed so as to carry microorganisms and debris away from the incision. (25:571–574)
Nursing Process—Implementation
Client Need—Physiological integrity

79 1. A change in bowel habits is one of the seven danger signals for cancer identified by the American Cancer Society. Difficulty swallowing and indigestion also are warning signs of cancer. However, these symptoms are more likely associated with cancer of upper gastrointestinal structures, such as the esophagus and stomach. Most individuals experience an increased production of flatus from eating common gas-forming foods. (21:147)
Nursing Process—Data collection
Client Need—Physiological integrity

80 1. An enema solution cannot be distributed very well in a sitting position. Overall there will be a less than desirable cleansing effect. Also, the person usually experiences a need to defecate sooner because of the pooling of solution within the rectum. Clients can eat lightly the evening before a sigmoidoscopy. A flexible scope is more common than one that is rigid. Medications are taken before the test and do not interfere with the test findings. (7:807; 25:209, 682)
Nursing Process—Evaluation
Client Need—Safe, effective care environment

81 2. A Sim's position, which is a left lateral side-lying position, is commonly preferred when a flexible sigmoidoscope is used. A knee-chest position is used if the sigmoidoscope is of the rigid type. A lithotomy position is used for cystoscopy and vaginal examinations. An orthopneic position is helpful for promoting rest for dyspneic individuals. Fowler's position is used for many reasons, one of which is improving ventilation. (7:806; 25:210)
Nursing Process—Implementation
Client Need—Safe, effective care environment

82 2. A low-residue diet contains no fruits, vegetables, or whole grain breads and cereals. Fruit and vegetable juices, with the exception of prune juice, are allowed in minimal amounts. Tender or ground meat can be eaten, as can refined carbohydrates, such as pasta. (6:575)
Nursing Process—Implementation
Client Need—Safe, effective care environment

83 3. There are 1000 mg in 1 g. To administer 1 g of neomycin the nurse gives the client two 500 mg tablets. A common formula to compute proper dosage is as follows (20:34; 25:699):

$$\frac{\text{dosage desired}}{\text{dosage on hand}} \times \text{quantity} = \text{amount to administer}$$

$$\frac{1000 \text{ mg}}{500 \text{ mg}} \times 1 \text{ tablet} = \frac{1000}{500} = 2 \text{ tablets to administer}$$

Nursing Process—Implementation
Client Need—Physiological integrity

84 2. During the operative procedure the bowel is opened, and some contents can leak within the peritoneum. The neomycin destroys intestinal bacteria and reduces the risk of a postoperative infection. (17:141; 20:73)
Nursing Process—Implementation
Client Need—Health promotion/maintenance

85 3. The first action to take in the case of evisceration is to cover the bowel with preferably sterile gauze moistened with sterile normal saline. The physician is notified and vital signs are taken after taking emergency action. The bowel is not manipulated except by the physician. (4:473; 18:637; 21:242)
Nursing Process—Implementation
Client Need—Physiological integrity

86 3. When an obstruction interferes with the movement of intestinal contents toward the rectum for elimination, the client begins to experience distention and vomiting. At first the emesis contains gastric contents. As time passes the vomitus may contain fecal matter and have a foul odor. The other questions are appropriate to ask, but they do not necessarily provide information associated with an intestinal obstruction. (21:703)
Nursing Process—Data collection
Client Need—Physiological integrity

87 4. Clients are ambulated immediately after the insertion of an intestinal tube to promote its passage through the pyloric valve. An x-ray is ordered several hours after the intestinal tube is inserted. The tube is not secured until it has reached the intestine, although it is supported in a taped sling. The physician instills the mercury in a Miller-Abbott tube once it passes the pyloric valve. Other types of intestinal tubes, like the Cantor and Harris tubes, have a pre-filled mercury chamber. (21:705)

Nursing Process—Implementation
Client Need—Safe, effective care environment

88 3. Any written order that is unclear or unsafe is questioned. This includes a drug dose that is higher or lower than the dosages given in approved references. The nurse never administers a different dose until consulting with a physician. Written orders for combined preoperative medication indicate they are given together. The pharmacist is a reliable source for obtaining drug information; however, the only person who can revise the order is the physician. (25:697)

Nursing Process—Implementation
Client Need—Physiological integrity

89 2. The best position for performing a colostomy irrigation is sitting on the toilet. This position and the environment simulate normal bowel elimination. The toilet also is convenient for hanging the distal end of the irrigating sleeve. The stool is easily flushed away along with the drained irrigating solution. Because it takes some time for the bowel evacuation to be complete, clients often appreciate the privacy that the bathroom provides. If sitting on the toilet is not possible, provide privacy while the client sits on or in bed with the end of the sleeve placed within a bedpan. (21:731; 25:689)

Nursing Process—Implementation
Client Need—Physiological integrity

90 2. Silence, when used appropriately, is a powerful means of communicating without verbalizing. Among other things, silence conveys acceptance, provides the client time to collect his thoughts, allows relief from emotionally charged content, and gives the client the opportunity to proceed when ready. Changing the subject is nontherapeutic. It indicates that the nurse cannot handle the topic of conversation. Switching the discussion to physical care is a form of changing the subject. Active listening, rather than psychologic counseling, is sufficient based on the data in the situation. (10:92; 25:79)

Nursing Process—Implementation
Client Need—Psychosocial integrity

91 1. Encouraging the expression of concerns provides the client an opportunity to ventilate feelings without fear of retaliation. An open discussion can effectively lower a client's frustration level. Reassurance, in this case, is somewhat premature. The client needs to verbalize and clarify the specific problems she perceives. With the assistance of the nurse and

other health care professionals, the client ought to achieve the ability to accomplish self-care. Maintaining the client's independence is more preferable than institutionalized care. Saying nothing indicates to the client that the nurse prefers not to become involved with emotional problems. Quoting a client, however, is always appropriate when documenting information. (9:159; 25:812)

Nursing Process—Implementation
Client Need—Psychosocial integrity

NURSING CARE OF CLIENTS WITH DISORDERS OF THE RECTUM AND ANUS

92 3. Mineral oil is a petroleum product that has lubricating properties. Humans lack the ability to digest and absorb mineral oil. It passes through the digestive system unchanged. Any fat-soluble vitamins present when food is consumed with mineral oil are not absorbed. Occasional use of mineral oil, if taken at bedtime, is not harmful, but frequent use should be avoided. None of the other laxatives interfere with the absorption of fat-soluble vitamins. (3:292; 6:628)

Nursing Process—Implementation
Client Need—Health promotion/maintenance

93 1. Long-term use of laxatives causes the bowel to become sluggish because it is repeatedly subjected to artificial stimulation. Stool softeners are less harsh than laxatives. However, it is best to determine the cause of the constipation and treat the etiology with life-style changes rather than continue to rely on pharmaceutical interventions. Daily enemas are just as habituating as laxative abuse. Dilating the anal sphincter is not usually a technique for promoting bowel elimination. (1:389–390; 20:397)

Nursing Process—Implementation
Client Need—Health promotion/maintenance

94 1. A client with a fecal impaction tends to expel liquid stool around the hardened mass. Bad breath is not usually a sign of constipation or fecal impaction. If halitosis is chronic, the nurse should suspect dental disease, ineffective oral hygiene, or esophageal diverticula. Headaches have been anecdotally associated with constipation, but a relationship has not been proven scientifically. Loss of appetite may be either the cause or the effect of impaired bowel elimination. Its presence is not necessarily an indication of a fecal impaction. (18:544; 25:670)

Nursing Process—Data collection
Client Need—Physiological integrity

95 2. By inserting a lubricated gloved finger within the rectum, it is possible to confirm the presence of a hard mass of stool. An x-ray may confirm the presence of a mass in the rectum, but is expensive and relatively unnecessary. An oil-retention enema is a method for relieving the impaction after its presence is confirmed. Monitoring bowel elimination patterns causes unnecessary delay in treating the problem. (25:670)

Nursing Process—Data collection
Client Need—Physiological integrity

96 1. Activity promotes the movement of gas toward the anal sphincter where it can be released. Carbonated beverages can increase gas accumulation. Restricting food is inappropriate. It may prevent additional gas from forming, but it does not help eliminate what is already present. Narcotic analgesics tend to slow peristalsis and contribute to the retention of stool and intestinal gas. (25:671)

Nursing Process—Implementation
Client Need—Physiological integrity

97 2. A rectal tube remains in place only approximately 20 to 30 minutes at one time to help relieve distention from accumulating gas. Placement for only 5 minutes is not likely to achieve an optimal effect, yet longer than 30 minutes is unnecessary. The tube is removed and replaced again in 1 to 2 hours if gas continues to accumulate. (18:548; 25:672)

Nursing Process—Planning
Client Need—Physiological integrity

98 3. Interrupting the instillation of enema solution allows time for the bowel to adjust to the distention. Rapidly instilling the remaining solution may cause the client to lose control of his elimination. Taking deep breaths or panting rather than holding the breath relieves some discomfort. To finish administering the remaining enema solution, the withdrawn tip needs to be reinserted. (18:546; 25:680)

Nursing Process—Implementation
Client Need—Physiological integrity

99 3. A rectal suppository is inserted approximately 2 to 4 in. For the best effect, the suppository must be beyond the internal sphincter. A glove is used to avoid contact with organisms in the rectum, stool, or blood. A left lateral position provides anatomic access to the rectal area. Retaining the suppository until feeling an urge to defecate ensures its effectiveness. (18:722; 25:674–676)

Nursing Process—Implementation
Client Need—Physiological integrity

100 2. Bowel elimination tends to occur in a cyclic pattern. Assessing the bowel elimination pattern precedes

selecting interventions. Limiting activity impairs rather than promotes bowel elimination. The diet should have adequate amounts of water and bulk-forming foods to help the client form soft, rather than constipated, stool. The regular administration of enemas eventually may help to regulate bowel elimination, but it is not the first step in a bowel retraining program. (1:364; 18:547; 21:591)

Nursing Process—Planning
Client Need—Physiological integrity

101 3. Chronic constipation, hereditary factors, and conditions that increase venous pressure in the abdomen and pelvic area, such as pregnancy, ascites, and liver disease, foster the development of hemorrhoids. A low-sodium diet tends to keep venous fluid volume within a low to normal level. Lactose intolerance causes bloating, gassiness, cramping, and diarrhea. An occupation that interferes with the use of the toilet when feeling the urge to defecate can predispose to constipation and the development of hemorrhoids. However, generally the work of an accountant does not fit that category. (21:713)

Nursing Process—Data collection
Client Need—Physiological integrity

102 2. The cellulose that remains after eating high-fiber foods absorbs water in the bowel. Lack of adequate fluid makes constipation more severe. None of the other recommendations aid in preventing or eliminating constipation. (3:298; 6:415–416)

Nursing Process—Implementation
Client Need—Health promotion/maintenance

103 1. A sitz bath is primarily a comfort measure. The warmth of the water soothes the discomfort in the surgical area. Secondarily, a sitz bath keeps the incisional area clean and promotes healing. Because only the buttocks are submerged in water, evidence of personal hygiene is not an appropriate criterion for effectiveness. (25:304, 590)

Nursing Process—Evaluation
Client Need—Physiological integrity

104 1. Docusate sodium is a stool softener. Retaining water in the stool softens the mass and makes the stool easier and less painful to pass. Some categories of laxatives, like castor oil, stimulate bowel evacuation by irritating the intestinal mucosa. Bulk-forming laxatives, like psyllium (Metamucil), stimulate peristalsis by adding bulk and water to the stool. A drug that reduces intestinal activity promotes constipation rather than stool elimination. (17:276–277; 20:391)

Nursing Process—Implementation
Client Need—Health promotion/maintenance

105　2. A pilonidal cyst is actually a sinus with one or more openings onto the skin. Once the integrity of the skin is impaired, microorganisms enter and cause subsequent infection evidenced by purulent drainage. Neither rectal bleeding nor diarrhea are associated with a pilonidal cyst. The word pilonidal means a "nest of hair." The growth of stiff body hair in the anorectal area at puberty often precipitates irritation within the sinus tract. (18:1263; 21:714–715)

> Nursing Process—Data collection
> Client Need—Physiological integrity

106　4. Cleaning the area where a topical medication is applied ensures that it is maximally absorbed. The client may wish to wear gloves for aesthetic and aseptic reasons, but their use does not affect the local effect of the medication. For comfort an ointment that is applied to a sensitive area is kept at room temperature unless otherwise directed by the manufacturer. It is more appropriate to apply this type of medication immediately following a bowel movement, because pain is greater at that time. In addition this drug can be routinely applied in the morning and evening. (20:21; 25:714)

> Nursing Process—Implementation
> Client Need—Health promotion/maintenance

NURSING CARE OF CLIENTS WITH DISORDERS OF THE GALLBLADDER

107　1. The characteristic pain of cholecystitis comes on after eating. It is especially aggravated when the meal has a high fat content. Besides pain, the fat intolerance due to impaired flow of bile causes nausea, vomiting, distention, and flatulence. Ulcers are more likely to cause pain when the stomach is empty. Activity ought not to influence the discomfort of cholecystitis. The volume and type of food are more of a factor in the symptoms of gallbladder disease than the time of day. (18:1268; 21:749)

> Nursing Process—Data collection
> Client Need—Physiological integrity

108　1. The referred pain of cholecystitis is felt either in the right shoulder or, as some describe it, in the back at the level of the shoulder blades. Ulcers and esophageal reflux cause pain in the midepigastric region. Angina pectoris may be experienced as pain in the neck, jaw, or down the left arm. (18:1268; 21:749)

> Nursing Process—Data collection
> Client Need—Physiological integrity

109　3. Evidence suggests that an elevated cholesterol level predisposes to developing gallstones. The majority of gallstones are thought to form when bile in the gallbladder is thick, high in cholesterol, and low in bile acids. A low red cell count and hemoglobin commonly are found in people with bleeding, nutritional deficiency, or bone marrow disorders. Elevated serum albumin is not generally a common laboratory finding with any pathologic condition. (7:411; 18:1268; 21:749)

> Nursing Process—Data collection
> Client Need—Physiological integrity

110　2. Bile pigments cause the normal brown appearance of stool. If bile is prevented from entering the small intestine, the stool that forms is likely to appear clay colored. Black, tarry stools indicate bleeding high in the gastrointestinal tract or the administration of oral iron therapy. Dark brown stool is normal; the shade may vary depending on the food that has been eaten. Greenish yellow stool is more often associated with diarrhea. (4:711; 18:1268)

> Nursing Process—Data collection
> Client Need—Physiological integrity

111　3. Greasy fried foods and fatty meats are not allowed on a low-fat diet. Baked fish, poultry, and lean meat are allowed. Leaner cuts of beef, such as round steak, could be ground and used in recipes that call for hamburger. Hard cheese, cream, gravies, salad oil, rich desserts, and nuts are restricted. Whole milk, butter or margarine, and sometimes eggs can be used in limited amounts. (6:521; 18:1268)

> Nursing Process—Evaluation
> Client Need—Health promotion/maintenance

112　3. Radiography of the gallbladder involves the use of an oral iodine contrast medium. If a client is allergic to iodine, he is at risk for experiencing an allergic reaction to the radiopaque substance. Allergic reactions can be life-threatening. Most clients can cooperate by holding still for the brief amount of time required during the gallbladder x-ray. Determining the number of previous x-rays is appropriate in terms of teaching and preparing a client. However, all individuals receive an explanation before any procedure is performed. No anesthesia is given prior to or during an x-ray of the gallbladder. (6:686; 25:206)

> Nursing Process—Data collection
> Client Need—Physiological integrity

113　1. The person undergoing an ultrasound of the gallbladder must not eat food for approximately 8 to 12 hours before the test. Restricting food helps to eliminate the presence of gas. Intestinal gas interferes with the transmission of sound waves toward the gallbladder and the scan of the structure's image. Water is permitted. Barium is used as a contrast medium for upper and lower gastrointestinal x-rays. During ultrasonography, the gallbladder is imaged by applying a water-soluble lubricant to a hand-held transducer and passing it across the abdomen. (6:846; 18:1233)

Nursing Process—Evaluation
Client Need—Health promotion/maintenance

114 4. Biliary obstruction often is accompanied by hypo-prothrombinemia. The preoperative administration of vitamin K reduces the risk of hemorrhage. A single dose usually restores the normal prothrombin time within 8 to 24 hours. Vitamins A and C promote wound healing. Adequate intake of all water- and fat-soluble vitamins is necessary for general health. No specific vitamin promotes liver function. (4:1269; 20:465)

Nursing Process—Implementation
Client Need—Health promotion/maintenance

115 4. The deltoid muscle is not capable of absorbing large amounts of solution. Intramuscular injections into the deltoid muscle of an adult are limited to 1 mL of solution. The deltoid is not used as a site for injecting medication in an infant or child because it is not sufficiently developed to absorb medication adequately. The dorsogluteal, ventrogluteal, and vastus lateralis are large muscle sites that can absorb greater volumes of injected drugs. (18:736; 20:740)

Nursing Process—Planning
Client Need—Physiological integrity

116 4. The pigment found in bile is derived from hemoglobin. Depending on the concentration of pigment, the normal appearance of bile drainage is described as being greenish yellow to orange brown. Bile is generally clear, but clear is not a color. Dark red drainage indicates that venous blood is mixed with the biliary drainage. Bright red drainage is a sign of fresh or arterial bleeding. (4:484, 648)

Nursing Process—Data collection
Client Need—Physiological integrity

117 2. A T-tube remains unclamped until the client begins to resume oral feedings. Clamping the tube results in reflux of bile toward the liver. It is appropriate to support the tubing so it is not kinked or dislodged. Placing the drainage bag in a dependent position facilitates gravity drainage. A volume of up to 500 mL in 24 hours is not unusual. (4:713)

Nursing Process—Data collection
Client Need—Physiological integrity

118 3. Since bile is essential to digestion, the T-tube generally is unclamped for up to 2 hours after a meal is consumed. As healing takes place and edema is reduced, some bile begins draining into the small intestine even when the tubing is clamped. (4:713)

Nursing Process—Planning
Client Need—Physiological integrity

119 1. To establish negative pressure, air and drainage are eliminated from the bulb reservoir and the opening capped before releasing the squeezed bulb. A Jackson-Pratt drain is an example of a closed drainage device. The Jackson-Pratt device could drain by gravity, not negative pressure, if the drainage valve were left open. The bulb reservoir is never filled with normal saline. The reservoir is secured to the skin with tape. However, this is to prevent tension on the tubing and possibly pulling it from its insertion site. (4:482, 484; 25:571, 576)

Nursing Process—Implementation
Client Need—Safe, effective care environment

NURSING CARE OF CLIENTS WITH DISORDERS OF THE LIVER

120 4. Alanine and aspartate amino transferase, previously called transaminase, are blood tests performed to assess liver function. Liver and other organ disease and damage result in elevated levels of these particular enzymes. The tests are repeated periodically to evaluate the client's response to treatment. Serum potassium is performed to monitor electrolyte balance when a client's nutritional or fluid balance has been altered. Serum creatinine and blood urea nitrogen tests are performed to monitor kidney function. (4:708; 7:381; 21:742)

Nursing Process—Data collection
Client Need—Physiological integrity

121 1. Infectious hepatitis A is generally spread by the oral-fecal route. In other words, the stool contains the virus, and the pathogen is spread to the mouth of a susceptible individual. Transmission is direct following contact with the excrement of an infected person or indirect by ingesting fecally contaminated food or water or food handled by an individual with the virus. This virus also is present in the blood and saliva of infected individuals. However, transmission through these routes is more rare. (18:1265; 21:743)

Nursing Process—Implementation
Client Need—Health promotion/maintenance

122 4. Conscientious handwashing is the best defense against the transmission of disease. Gloves are worn when nursing care involves direct contact with the client, his excrement, or other body fluids. Wearing gloves does not eliminate the need for handwashing. A gown is used if soiling is possible, but a mask is not necessary. Only individuals who cannot be relied on to practice good handwashing are placed in a private room. (4:709; 21:744)

Nursing Process—Planning
Client Need—Health promotion/maintenance

123 2. Immunoglobulin, formerly known as gamma globulin, is recommended for postexposure to an infected person with hepatitis A. It is most effective if administered within 48 hours to 2 weeks following exposure. Antibiotic therapy is ineffective in preventing or eliminating a viral infection. The current vaccine that is available is used to prevent hepatitis B infection. Anti-inflammatory drugs, such as salicylates, nonsalicylates, and steroids, are not effective therapy in preventing the spread of hepatitis A. (21:744)

Nursing Process—Implementation
Client Need—Health promotion/maintenance

124 2. Lanolin is an emollient. It softens skin and prevents moisture loss. Dry skin adds to the itching sensation caused by the release of bile salts onto the skin. Bathing is not discontinued altogether. Even in the worst situations, the skin is bathed with tepid water. Alcohol is drying to the skin. Its use contributes to itching. There is no advantage to substituting a shower for a tub bath. (21:746)

Nursing Process—Implementation
Client Need—Health promotion/maintenance

125 2. Homosexual men are at particularly high risk for acquiring blood-borne infections. The source of the hepatitis B virus is the blood of infected people or carriers. The virus is present in semen, saliva, and blood. It is transmitted by sexual contact, contaminated blood products, or accidental puncture with objects that contain traces of infected blood. There is no more connection between having lived in Alaska than in any other state. Abusing alcohol compounds the liver damage concurrent with hepatitis, but it is not a cause of it. Being a carpenter is not a known risk factor in acquiring hepatitis B. (21:496)

Nursing Process—Data collection
Client Need—Health promotion/maintenance

126 2. For anyone who is previously unvaccinated, the best action to prevent acquiring hepatitis B infection following exposure to the blood of someone with the disease is to receive hepatitis B immunoglobulin within 24 hours, but no later than 7 days. Vaccination immediately after exposure does not provide sufficient antibody protection. Viruses are unaffected by antibiotics like penicillin. Bleach is an effective antiseptic, but it is not the best prophylaxis when there is exposure to the hepatitis B virus. (21:744)

Nursing Process—Implementation
Client Need—Health promotion/maintenance

127 2. Donating blood is not recommended for people who have had hepatitis. The virus remains in the blood, even years after the person has had the acute illness, and can be passed on to others. Blood collection personnel are taught to screen and reject any potential donor who indicates that he has had jaundice in the past. Safe sex may be practiced, which would include using a latex condom. Convalescence is prolonged following the acute phase of hepatitis, but eventually there are no permanent physical restrictions. Individuals with hepatitis antibodies are not barred from foreign travel. (21:747)

Nursing Process—Implementation
Client Need—Health promotion/maintenance

128 1. The etiology for Laënnec's portal cirrhosis, the most common form in the United States, is chronic malnutrition and alcoholism. Malnutrition is often a consequence of alcoholism. Vietnam veterans were exposed to toxic chemicals during their military service, but their medical problems have not resulted in a predominant incidence of cirrhosis. If the client uses salicylates or nonsteroidal anti-inflammatory drugs, it may be a factor in his gastrointestinal bleeding, but not the cirrhosis. The hypertension could be secondary to his alcohol abuse. (4:703; 21:737)

Nursing Process—Data collection
Client Need—Health promotion/maintenance

129 2. The skin of a person with cirrhosis usually manifests multiple vascular lesions with a central red body and radiating branches. These are known as spider angiomas. They also are referred to as telangiectasias, spider nevi, or vascular spiders. There is usually scant body hair on someone with cirrhosis. The testes atrophy due to the liver's inability to fully metabolize estrogen. Clubbed finger nails are a common finding in clients who have had longstanding cardiac or pulmonary disorders. (4:704; 21:738)

Nursing Process—Data collection
Client Need—Physiological integrity

130 3. In the absence of taking an oral iron supplement, stool that appears black or tarry is an indication that a significant amount of blood is being lost from the stomach or somewhere in the proximal end of the intestine. Gastric hemorrhage is not usually accompanied by pain, nausea, or abdominal distention. (18:535)

Nursing Process—Data collection
Client Need—Physiological integrity

131 4. Ascites is the collection of fluid within the peritoneal cavity. An appropriate technique for monitoring the increase or decrease in this condition is measuring the abdominal girth. Either the apical or radial pulse measurement are appropriate for a general assessment. The position in which the blood pressure is measured must be consistent, but it may be taken either while the client is lying down or sitting. The specific gravity usually is monitored when there is a problem with intravascular fluid volume or renal disease. (7:480; 14:875)

Nursing Process—Implementation
Client Need—Safe, effective care environment

132 1. After a liver biopsy, the client is monitored closely for signs of hemorrhage. The nurse positions the client so that body weight puts pressure on the needle site. A person with cirrhosis is at especially high risk for bleeding because liver disease results in diminished prothrombin. Prothrombinemia causes a prolonged delay in the time it takes for blood to clot. (4:313; 18:1232; 21:653)

Nursing Process—Data collection
Client Need—Physiological integrity

133 3. By positioning the client on the right side, the weight of the body tends to put pressure on the puncture that was created. The compression is used to reduce or prevent bleeding. Ambulation is contraindicated since it promotes bleeding. Neither high Fowler's nor elevating the legs is appropriate for controlling bleeding. (4:313; 18:1232; 21:653)

Nursing Process—Planning
Client Need—Physiological integrity

134 2. Metallic objects present a safety hazard during an MRI. Consequently, internal metal objects are a contraindication for performing an MRI. Any external metal devices are removed. Sedation is not usually required except for clients who are severely claustrophobic. There is no relationship between body weight and urinary elimination, although giving the client an opportunity to void is a conscientious comfort measure. (7:969–970; 25:206)

Nursing Process—Implementation
Client Need—Safe, effective care environment

135 1. The bladder is emptied just prior to a paracentesis. A full bladder may be punctured as the needle is inserted through the abdominal wall. The client can eat and drink before the test. There is no need for

additional skin hygiene other than what already has been routinely provided; the physician prepares the skin with an antiseptic. There is no need for a suction machine. (25:212)

Nursing Process—Implementation
Client Need—Safe, effective care environment

136 2. Documentation of the total volume of aspirated fluid is essential. Fluid replacement is determined more by the client's urinary output and vital signs rather than on the volume of aspirated fluid. As a rule, clients do not require pain relief after a paracentesis. Ventilation is improved after ascitic fluid has been removed; clients generally do not need additional encouragement to deep breathe. (25:212)

Nursing Process—Implementation
Client Need—Safe, effective care environment

137 4. Due to the tendency to bleed, the nurse applies sustained pressure for a longer period to prevent hematoma formation and bruising. There is no scientific rationale for performing any of the other actions. (18:1264)

Nursing Process—Implementation
Client Need—Physiological integrity

138 3. Rising levels of ammonia in the blood are toxic to the central nervous system. Serum bilirubin is monitored to assess the ability of the liver to form bile and send it to the gallbladder for concentration. Serum creatinine and blood urea nitrogen are tests used to monitor renal function. (4:706; 7:347; 21:741–742)

Nursing Process—Data collection
Client Need—Physiological integrity

139 1. Difficulty in arousing the cirrhotic client indicates a significant neurologic change. It is a sign that the client is progressing into hepatic coma. The client's physiologic and safety needs become even more important at this time. Convulsions may occur. The urine output and blood pressure are within normal limits. The fact that he snores is unrelated to his mental status. (4:706; 18:1265; 21:742)

Nursing Process—Data collection
Client Need—Physiological integrity

140 2. Grief work involves dealing with the loss. Reviewing one's life is often a task that takes place in anticipatory grieving. This is therapeutic and is not suppressed. Suggesting that a close family member be called is an example of changing the subject. Writing in a diary is therapeutic. However, this action is more appropriate at a later time. At the moment, spontaneous verbalization is most therapeutic. It is unrealistic to expect that the client's wife is able to think about future plans before she has dealt with the reality of the loss. (9:359; 10:101)

> Nursing Process—Implementation
> Client Need—Psychosocial integrity

NURSING CARE OF CLIENTS WITH DISORDERS OF THE PANCREAS

141 2. Pain is a subjective experience. Asking the client to rate pain numerically helps to assess its intensity. The rating scale is used later to evaluate the effectiveness of pain-relief techniques that are used. Noting if a client can stop moving about is not a valid assessment technique. A cooperative client may make an effort to stop moving despite the continuation of severe pain. Perspiration is a physiologic sign that may accompany pain. However, because many factors can cause perspiration, its presence or absence is not the best assessment technique. Administering an analgesic is an intervention, not a form of assessment. (25:366–367)

> Nursing Process—Data collection
> Client Need—Physiological integrity

142 2. Elevated serum amylase is the most reliable evidence of pancreatitis. The bilirubin level becomes elevated if the cause of the pancreatitis is due to an obstruction of the common bile duct or pancreatic duct. Glucose tolerance test abnormalities indicate dysfunction of the endocrine functions of the pancreas, which are secondary to pancreatitis. Elevated bilirubin and abnormal glucose tolerance tests, in and of themselves, are not the best indication of pancreatitis. Lactose tolerance test results have no relationship to pancreatitis. (4:715; 21:754)

> Nursing Process—Data collection
> Client Need—Physiological integrity

143 4. The distance from the nose (N) to the earlobe (E) to the xiphoid (X) is called the NEX measurement. It is used to determine the approximate distance to the stomach. None of the other landmarks are correct for approximating the length for nasogastric tube insertion. (4:672; 25:597)

> Nursing Process—Implementation
> Client Need—Safe, effective care environment

144 1. The presence of the tube between the folds of the vocal cords interferes with vibration and the ability to speak. The tube is withdrawn to the level of the oropharynx while the client reestablishes his ability to breathe. Swallowing is not affected. Sneezing and vomiting are not appropriate signs to evaluate

if a gastric tube is in the wrong location. (4:673; 25:601)

> Nursing Process—Data collection
> Client Need—Physiological integrity

145 4. The nurse assigned to care for a client with an intravenous infusion has a responsibility to monitor the infusion to ensure that it is instilling the prescribed volume at the correct rate. If the volume is more or less than prescribed, it is reported to the nurse in charge. The infusion can flow by gravity with the tubing coiled on the bed. The nondominant hand is preferred for an intravenous infusion. There is ample time, with 250 mL left, to postpone reporting the information temporarily. (4:461; 25:272)

> Nursing Process—Implementation
> Client Need—Physiological integrity

146 3. The nurse is most correct in removing the scrambled eggs from the dietary tray of a client on a bland, low-fat diet. One scrambled egg made with milk and butter has approximately 8 g of fat. One cup of cooked unsweetened prunes has only a trace of fat. One cup of nonfat skim milk has a trace of fat. One slice of unbuttered whole-wheat toast has 1 g of fat. (7:161–162, 644, 646, 652, 656)

> Nursing Process—Implementation
> Client Need—Safe, effective care environment

147 3. There is an established relationship between the chronic consumption of alcohol and the incidence of pancreatitis. Once an acute attack of pancreatitis has occurred, the client is at risk for chronic pancreatitis. Use of alcohol leads to continued inflammation of this organ. It is essential to protect the pancreas from further irritation because complications include destruction of the organ itself, peritonitis, shock, and even death. Having had pancreatitis does not disqualify someone from donating blood, doing heavy lifting, or taking laxatives. (4:716; 21:758)

> Nursing Process—Implementation
> Client Need—Health promotion/maintenance

148 2. Anorexia and weight loss are signs and symptoms that appear early in the onset of cancer of the pancreas. Pancreatic cancer, like most other forms of cancer, does not usually cause acute pain in the early stages. If the client with pancreatic cancer experiences pain early on, it is usually dull and more apparent at night. Bleeding is not usually a problem unless the cancer also has affected the liver. Fainting, unless from weight and fluid loss, is not a common sign of cancer of the pancreas. (4:716; 21:758)

Nursing Process—Data collection
Client Need—Physiological integrity

149 3. The most therapeutic response in this situation is to encourage the client to talk about thoughts and feelings. People who are dying often know they are terminal without being told. It is more important to support a client's hope than to bluntly confirm suspicions. It is unethical to deny that the terminal client will improve. It is appropriate to act as a liaison in contacting someone who will help the client take care of unfinished business. However, this is not the first or best nursing response in this case. (9:355–357; 25:158)

Nursing Process—Implementation
Client Need—Psychosocial integrity

150 2. It is better to control pain before it escalates. When pain is intense, relief is more difficult to achieve. Peaks and valleys of pain are reduced by administering pain-relieving drugs on a routine schedule throughout the 24-hour period rather than just when it becomes absolutely necessary to do so. The goal is to keep the client free from pain yet not dull his or her consciousness or ability to communicate. Asking the physician to order a high dose initially is premature. Tolerance is likely to develop later. It is appropriate at that time for the nurse to consult the physician about changing the medication order. (9:363–364; 21:156; 25:815)

Nursing Process—Implementation
Client Need—Physiological integrity

Classification of Test Items

Unit I Review Test 1

The Nursing Care of Clients with Disorders of the Gastrointestinal System and Accessory Organs of Digestion

Directions: After each question, the correct answer is given, as well as a classification of each test question. Compare the correct answer with your answer. If a question has been answered *incorrectly*, draw a line to the end of all the columns. When finished, add up the number of your correct answers in each column and place that number in the respective box at the end in the area identified as *Number Correct*.

To determine the percentage of questions you answered correctly and your performance in each of the test plan categories, divide the *Number Correct* in each column by the *Number Possible* in each column. Then multiply the decimal by 100 to get the percentage. For example:

$$\frac{\text{Number Correct: } 78}{\text{Number Possible: } 94} = 0.83 \times 100 = 83\%$$

Any score that is less than 75% indicates an area where further review would be beneficial.

KEY TO ITEM CLASSIFICATION:

NURSING PROCESS	CLIENT NEEDS
D = Data collection	S = Safe, effective care environment
P = Planning	P = Physiological integrity
I = Implementation	M = Psychosocial integrity
E = Evaluation	H = Health promotion/maintenance

Question #	Answer #	Nursing Process				Client Needs			
		D	P	I	E	S	P	M	H
1	1			I			P		
2	3			I			P		
3	2		P				P		
4	2			I			P		
5	2			I		S			
6	3	D					P		
7	2			I					H
8	3		P						H
9	2	D				S			
10	1		P			S			
11	3			I		S			
12	4				E				H
13	2				E				H
14	3				E	S			
15	2			I					H

1D 4I
35
2P

		Nursing Process				Client Needs			
Question #	Answer #	D	P	I	E	S	P	M	H
16	4	D					P		
17	2	D					P		
18	4	D					P		
19	3			I					H
20	4			I					H
21	2	D				S			
22	2				E		P		
23	2	D					P		
24	3			I		S			
25	2			I		S			
26	3			I			P		
27	4			I			P		
28	2			I				M	
29	3	D					P		
30	3	D					P		
31	4				E	S			
32	1			I			P		
33	2			I					H
34	1			I					H
35	2	D					P		
36	2			I		S			
37	1			I				M	
38	2			I			P		
39	3			I		S			
40	2				E				H
41	1		P						H
42	1	D					P		
43	3			I		S			
44	1			I		S			
45	2		P				P		
46	2			I			P		
47	2			I			P		

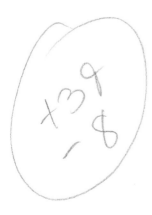

Question #	Answer #	Nursing Process				Client Needs			
		D	P	I	E	S	P	M	H
48	4			I		S			
49	2				E	S			
50	3			I			P		
51	4	D					P		
52	3				E		P		
53	3	D					P		
54	4				E				H
55	2		P				P		
56	2			I		S			
57	4			I		S			
58	1	D					P		
59	2			I					H
60	2			I			P		
61	2			I		S			
62	1	D					P		
63	3		P					M	
64	1			I				M	
65	1			I		S			
66	3	D					P		
67	4				E		P		
68	1			I			P		
69	2	D					P		
70	3			I			P		
71	2			I			P		
72	4			I					H
73	4	D					P		
74	1	D					P		
75	1			I					H
76	3	D					P		
77	2			I			P		
78	3			I			P		
79	1	D					P		

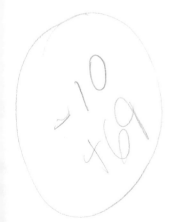

2DSI1P   2S 4P 2M 1H

Question #	Answer #	Nursing Process				Client Needs			
		D	P	I	E	S	P	M	H
80	1				E	S			
81	2			I		S			
82	2			I		S			
83	3			I			P		
84	2			I					H
85	3			I			P		
86	3	D					P		
87	4			I		S			
88	3			I			P		
89	2			I			P		
90	2			I				M	
91	1			I				M	
92	3			I					H
93	1			I					H
94	1	D					P		
95	2	D					P		
96	1			I			P		
97	2		P				P		
98	3			I			P		
99	3			I			P		
100	2		P				P		
101	3	D					P		
102	2			I					H
103	1				E		P		
104	1			I					H
105	2	D					P		
106	4			I					H
107	1	D					P		
108	1	D					P		
109	3	D					P		
110	2	D					P		
111	3				E				H

Question #	Answer #	Nursing Process				Client Needs			
		D	P	I	E	S	P	M	H
112	3	D					P		
113	1				E				H
114	4			I					H
115	4		P				P		
116	4	D					P		
117	2	D					P		
118	3		P				P		
119	1			I		S			
120	4	D					P		
121	1			I					H
122	4		P						H
123	2			I					H
124	2			I					H
125	2	D							H
126	2			I					H
127	2			I					H
128	1	D							H
129	2	D					P		
130	3	D					P		
131	4			I		S			
132	1	D					P		
133	3		P				P		
134	2			I		S			
135	1			I		S			
136	2			I		S			
137	4			I			P		
138	3	D					P		
139	1	D					P		
140	2			I				M	
141	2	D					P		
142	2	D					P		
143	4			I		S			

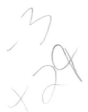

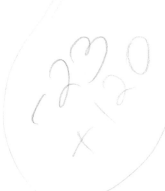

		Nursing Process				Client Needs			
Question #	Answer #	D	P	I	E	S	P	M	H
144	1	D					P		
145	4			I			P		
146	3			I		S			
147	3			I					H
148	2	D					P		
149	3			I				M	
150	2			I			P		
Number Correct	126	41	7	66	14	25	69	4	31
Number Possible	150	45	13	78	14	30	79	8	33
Percentage Correct	84%	91	53	84	100	83	87	50	93

Handwritten annotations:

Top: 1 I   1 P

Left margin: +1 +6   −24 +126 (circled)   +126

Within table (handwritten): 4D, 6P, 12 I, 0 E, 5 S, 10 P; +126 +41 +7 +66 +14

Bottom row: B (circled)   A   ↑   B   A   B   B   ↑   A
4D

wrong ?s
slows
weak areas

Review Test 2

The Nursing Care of Clients with Musculoskeletal Disorders

Directions: With a pencil, blacken the circle in front of the option you have chosen for your correct answer.

NURSING CARE OF CLIENTS WITH TRAUMATIC INJURIES

A male client who golfs at least three times a week has been experiencing wrist pain aggravated by movement. The physician diagnosed his condition as tenosynovitis and recommends temporarily avoiding repetitive wrist motion.

1 If the client made all of the following statements to the nurse, which one is the *best evidence* that the client understands the therapeutic plan?
- ○ 1. The client says that he should keep his hand as still as possible.
- ◑ 2. The client says that he should stop playing golf for the time being.
- ○ 3. The client says that he can substitute playing miniature golf.
- ○ 4. The client says that he can wear a tight leather glove when golfing.

The nurse examines a female client who slipped and fell while climbing stairs and now has swelling of her ankle and pain on movement.

2 If the nurse documents that the client's ankle is *ecchymotic*, it indicates that the skin appears
- ○ 1. freckled.
- ○ 2. mottled.
- ◑ 3. bruised.
- ○ 4. blanched.

3 While the client who slipped and fell awaits an ankle x-ray, which nursing measure is *most helpful* for relieving the soft tissue swelling?
- ○ 1. Dangle the client's foot.
- ◑ 2. Apply ice to the ankle.
- ○ 3. Exercise the client's foot.
- ○ 4. Immobilize the client's foot.

The ankle x-ray reveals that the bones of the client who slipped and fell are intact. The physician tells the client that she has a severely sprained ankle.

4 When the physician directs the nurse to wrap the client's lower extremity with an elastic roller bandage, where should the nurse *begin* applying the bandage?
- ○ 1. Below the knee
- ○ 2. Above the ankle
- ◉ 3. Across the phalanges
- ○ 4. At the metatarsals

5 In the case of the client with the sprained ankle, which application technique is *best* for the nurse to use when wrapping the roller bandage?
- ◑ 1. Making figure-of-eight turns with the bandage
- ○ 2. Making spiral-reverse turns with the bandage
- ○ 3. Making recurrent turns with the bandage
- ○ 4. Making spica turns with the bandage

Before the client with the sprained ankle is released from the emergency department, the nurse provides home care instructions.

6 Besides routinely removing and reapplying the roller bandage, it is *essential* that the nurse tell the client with the sprained ankle to *rewrap* the roller bandage anytime that
- ○ 1. she sits for a long time.
- ○ 2. her ankle feels painful.
- ◉ 3. her toes appear swollen.
- ○ 4. she wears a cotton sock.

A client presents in the emergency room with a shoulder injury after falling from a short stepladder.

7 When the nurse assesses the client's injuries, which finding is *most suggestive* that the client has *dislocated* his shoulder?

○ 1. The client is experiencing intense pain.
○ 2. There is obvious swelling about the joint.
○ 3. The client is hesitant to move his arm.
● 4. The arm appears displaced from the shoulder.

The physician tells the client that he plans to correct the client's shoulder dislocation by manipulation.

8 When the client asks the nurse what is meant by the term "manipulation," the *best explanation* is that this procedure involves
○ 1. making an incision to realign the bones.
○ 2. inserting a pin or wire into the joint.
● 3. repositioning the bone ends manually.
○ 4. strengthening the joint with exercise.

The client with the dislocated shoulder cannot afford a commercial canvas sling. As an alternative, the nurse teaches a family member how to apply a triangular sling made from muslin.

9 If the person who will apply the triangular sling makes all of the following statements, which one indicates a need for *more teaching?*
● 1. The person says the client's hand should be elevated higher than the elbow.
○ 2. The person says the knot should be tied at the back of the neck.
○ 3. The person says the client's elbow should be flexed within the sling.
○ 4. The person says the sling is used to elevate and support the arm.

While backpacking with a church youth group, a 17-year-old sustains an injury to the lower leg. A nurse who is accompanying the group suspects a fracture of the tibia.

10 To immobilize the suspected fracture of the tibia, it is *best* to apply a splint from
○ 1. below the knee to above the hip.
○ 2. above the knee to below the hip.
○ 3. above the ankle to below the knee.
● 4. below the ankle to above the knee.

An x-ray of the injured adolescent reveals a comminuted fracture of the distal tibia.

11 The nurse is *most correct* in explaining that a comminuted fracture is one in which
● 1. one bone end is driven into the other.
○ 2. the bone is splintered into pieces.
○ 3. there is no open break in the skin.
○ 4. a portion of the bone is split away.

The adolescent with the fractured tibia will require surgery to realign the bone.

12 In this case, from whom is it *most appropriate* to obtain consent to perform the surgical procedure?
○ 1. The client himself
○ 2. The client's physician
○ 3. The client's minister
● 4. The client's parent

13 If the adolescent who will undergo surgery is wearing a class ring, which nursing action is *most correct?*
○ 1. Put the ring in the bedside stand.
○ 2. Leave the ring on the client's finger.
○ 3. Give the ring to a security guard.
● 4. Lock the ring with his valuables.

14 After surgery, one of the *first signs* of a fat embolism is
● 1. respiratory distress.
○ 2. abdominal distention.
○ 3. difficulty swallowing.
○ 4. absent bowel sounds.

An adult female has several fractured ribs as a result of being thrown against the steering wheel during a motor vehicle accident.

15 If the nurse collects all of the following data, which is *most indicative* that the client is experiencing a secondary complication from the primary injury?
○ 1. Pulse rate is irregular.
● 2. Chest expands asymmetrically.
○ 3. Bowel sounds are hyperactive.
○ 4. Bladder is slightly distended.

A nurse stops to assist an adult female involved in a motor vehicle accident. The nurse assumes the victim was not wearing a seat belt and was thrown from the car.

16 Of the following emergency measures, which one should the nurse perform *first?*
● 1. Check the victim's breathing.
○ 2. Cover the victim with a blanket.
○ 3. Move the victim to the curb.
○ 4. Look for signs of injuries.

The nurse sees that a bone fragment is protruding from the thigh of the motor vehicle accident victim and there is profuse bleeding from the wound.

17 The *best technique* the nurse could use in this situation to control the bleeding is to
○ 1. place a tourniquet around the leg.
● 2. apply direct pressure at the wound.
○ 3. compress the femoral artery.
○ 4. elevate the injured extremity.

The nurse suspects that the motor vehicle accident victim also might have a broken back.

18 When emergency medical personnel arrive, the *preferred position* in which the victim with a back injury is transported is
○ 1. side-lying position.
○ 2. face-lying position.
◉ 3. back-lying position.
○ 4. semi-sitting position.

An adult female is hospitalized with a fracture between the trochanters of her right femur.

19 During the nurse's admission assessment, the *most typical sign* of an intertrochanteric fracture of the hip is
○ 1. paralysis of the affected leg.
○ 2. bruising of the affected leg.
◉ 3. lengthening of the affected leg.
○ 4. external rotation of the leg.

20 If the nurse finds all of the following information in the medical record of the client with the fractured hip, which one is the *most significant risk factor* for sustaining a fracture?
◉ 1. The client is postmenopausal.
○ 2. The client is somewhat obese.
○ 3. The client likes to do gardening.
○ 4. The client was born in England.

After the client's fractured hip is stabilized with an open reduction and internal fixation, the nurse teaches her to perform isometric quadriceps setting exercises with her unaffected leg.

21 If the client performs this exercise correctly, the nurse will observe her
○ 1. move her toes toward and away from her head.
○ 2. contract and relax the muscles of her thigh.
○ 3. lift her lower leg up and down from the bed.
◉ 4. bend her knee and pull her lower leg upward.

The client who has had her fractured hip repaired wears knee-high antiembolism stockings.

22 When the client asks how antiembolism stockings prevent blood clots, the nurse is *most accurate* in explaining that the stockings
◉ 1. prevent blood from pooling in the legs.
○ 2. reduce blood flow to the extremities.
○ 3. keep the blood pressure lower in the legs.
○ 4. decrease the volume of red blood cells.

23 Which of the following indicates that the nursing assistant caring for the client with the repaired fractured hip has applied the elastic stockings *correctly*?
○ 1. The nursing assistant applies the stockings before getting the client out of bed.
○ 2. The nursing assistant applies the stockings just before helping the client do leg exercises.
○ 3. The nursing assistant applies the stockings when noting that the client's legs are cool or swollen.
◉ 4. The nursing assistant applies the stockings at night prior to the client's bedtime.

An Austin-Moore prosthesis is used to repair a subcapital fracture of the hip sustained by an older adult male.

24 Postoperatively, before turning the client with the hip prosthesis onto his unoperative side, the nurse would *first*
◉ 1. place pillows between his legs.
○ 2. have him point his toes downward.
○ 3. flex his knee on the affected side.
○ 4. elevate the head of his hospital bed.

25 When the client with the hip prosthesis is allowed to get up in a chair, it is best for the nurse to place the chair
○ 1. at the end of the bed.
○ 2. perpendicular to the bed.
◉ 3. parallel with the bed.
○ 4. against a side wall.

The client with the hip prosthesis is allowed to ambulate with a walker using a three-point partial weight-bearing gait.

26 The *best evidence* that the client is performing this gait correctly is that the client advances the walker and his operative leg while putting most of his weight on
○ 1. the hand grips of the walker.
○ 2. the back legs of the walker.
○ 3. the toes of his operative leg.
◉ 4. the heel of his unoperative leg.

NURSING CARE OF CLIENTS WITH CASTS

A plaster arm cast will be applied to an adult male client with a fracture of his radius.

27 When preparing the client for the cast application, the nurse is *accurate* in explaining that
○ 1. the cast will feel very tight as it is applied.
◉ 2. his arm will feel warm as the wet plaster sets.
○ 3. there will be a foul odor until the cast is dry.
○ 4. he may experience itching while the cast is wet.

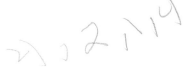

28 While the physician wraps the arm with rolls of wet plaster, it is *most appropriate* for the nurse to support the wet cast
- ○ 1. on a soft mattress.
- ○ 2. on a firm surface.
- ○ 3. with the tips of the fingers.
- ● 4. with the palms of the hand.

The client with the plaster arm cast asks the nurse about casts made of synthetic materials, like fiberglass.

29 The nurse is *accurate* in stating that an advantage of fiberglass casts is that they are generally
- ○ 1. less expensive.
- ● 2. more lightweight.
- ○ 3. more flexible.
- ○ 4. less restrictive.

30 After the arm cast has been applied, which of the following observations is *most indicative* that the client is developing compartment syndrome?
- ● 1. The client experiences severe pain.
- ○ 2. The client's hand becomes reddened.
- ○ 3. The fingers develop muscle spasms.
- ○ 4. The radial pulse feels bounding.

A long leg plaster cast is applied following an open reduction of a fractured femur.

31 When the client returns to the nursing unit after surgery, what is *best* to place under the wet cast?
- ○ 1. Synthetic sheepskin
- ● 2. A vinyl sheet
- ○ 3. An absorbent pad
- ○ 4. Several pillows

32 Which of the following nursing actions is *best* for drying the wet plaster cast?
- ● 1. Leave the leg in the cast uncovered.
- ○ 2. Apply a heating blanket to the cast.
- ○ 3. Use a hair dryer to blow hot air.
- ○ 4. Place a heat lamp above the cast.

The nurse observes bloody drainage on the long leg plaster cast.

33 What is the *next action* that the nurse should take?
- ○ 1. Document the finding in the medical record.
- ○ 2. Call the physician and report the finding.
- ● 3. Circle it with ink and write down the time.
- ○ 4. Apply an ice bag over the spot of drainage.

34 Which of the following techniques is *best* for assessing the circulation in the casted extremity of the client with the long leg plaster cast?
- ○ 1. Ask the client if the cast feels exceptionally heavy.
- ○ 2. Feel the cast to determine if it is unusually cold.
- ● 3. Depress the nailbed and time the return of color.
- ○ 4. See if there is room to insert a finger in the cast.

After a young adult sustains a fracture of the shaft of the femur in a motorcycle accident, a hip spica cast that covers the trunk, the full length of the fractured leg, and the upper circumference of the uninjured leg is applied.

35 When the client says, "My father is furious with me. He doesn't want me to ride a motorcycle," which of the following nursing responses is *best?*
- ○ 1. "As they say, 'Father knows best.' "
- ● 2. "All parents want their children to be safe."
- ○ 3. "It can be frustrating when a father and son disagree."
- ○ 4. "You are old enough to make your own decisions now."

36 When the nurse analyzes the communicated information from the client involved in the motorcycle accident, it suggests that he, like most young adults, is struggling with the developmental task that involves
- ○ 1. Searching for his sexual identity.
- ○ 2. Testing his physical abilities.
- ● 3. Acquiring his own independence.
- ○ 4. Learning to control his emotions.

37 While planning nursing care for the client in the hip spica cast, what equipment is *best* for facilitating the client's bowel elimination?
- ○ 1. bedside commode
- ● 2. fracture bedpan
- ○ 3. mechanical lift
- ○ 4. raised toilet seat

The client in the hip spica cast asks the nurse to explain the purpose of the bar that runs from the plaster on one thigh to the other.

38 The *most accurate answer* is that the bar is used for
- ○ 1. Lifting and turning clients.
- ○ 2. Performing physical exercise.
- ● 3. Strengthening the cast.
- ○ 4. Hanging personal items.

The client in the hip spica cast tells the nurse that his skin itches terribly beneath the cast.

39 What is the *best nursing action* at this time?
- 1. Collaborate with the physician on prescribing an antipruritic medication.
- 2. Encourage the client to think about something else for the time being.
- 3. Bend a wire coat hanger so the client can scratch inside the cast.
- 4. Drop an ice cube inside the client's cast and let it melt.

After the client has had the hip spica cast for nearly 3 weeks, the nurse detects a foul odor coming from the cast.

40 The *best reason* for reporting this finding promptly is that an unpleasant smell is usually a sign that
- 1. the plaster has dried improperly.
- 2. there is bleeding under the cast.
- 3. the cast is disintegrating.
- 4. there is an infected wound.

The physician cuts a small window in the hip spica cast to inspect the underlying tissue.

41 What is the *best nursing action* after the piece of plaster is removed to create a window in the cast?
- 1. Dispose of the piece of plaster in a plastic bag.
- 2. Replace the piece of plaster in the cast hole with tape.
- 3. Save the piece of plaster in the dirty utility room.
- 4. Send the piece of plaster to the laboratory for a culture.

42 When the rough edges on the client's hip spica cast edges begin to threaten the integrity of the skin, the *best nursing action* is to
- 1. line the cast edge with adhesive petals of moleskin.
- 2. apply a fresh strip of plaster to the cast edge.
- 3. trim the rough cast edge with a cast cutter.
- 4. cover the cast edge with a gauze dressing.

43 Which of the following suggests that the client in the hip spica cast may be developing "cast syndrome"?
- 1. The client becomes nauseated and vomits.
- 2. The client becomes disoriented and confused.
- 3. The client becomes feverish and delirious.
- 4. The client becomes dyspneic and hyperventilates.

NURSING CARE OF CLIENTS WITH TRACTION

Before undergoing surgery for a fractured hip, an older adult female is placed in Buck's traction.

44 When changing the linen on the bed of the client in Buck's traction, it is *best* for the nurse to
- 1. roll the client from one side of the bed to the other.
- 2. apply the linen from the foot to the top of the bed.
- 3. leave the bottom sheets in place until after surgery.
- 4. raise the client from the bed with a mechanical lift.

45 While providing nursing care for the client in Buck's traction, which one of the following indicates a need for *immediate action*?
- 1. The traction weights are hanging above the floor.
- 2. The leg is in line with the pull of the traction.
- 3. The client's foot is touching the end of the bed.
- 4. The rope is in the groove of the traction pulley.

46 Which one of the following techniques is the *best* strategy for assessing the circulation in the leg in Buck's traction?
- 1. Observe if the client can wiggle or move her toes.
- 2. Palpate for pulsation of the dorsalis pedis artery.
- 3. Take the blood pressure on the leg with a thigh cuff.
- 4. See if the client can feel sharp and dull sensations.

An older adult male is placed in Russell's traction while awaiting surgery to repair his fractured hip.

47 Where is it *essential* to inspect the skin while the client is in Russell's traction?
- 1. Over the ischial spines
- 2. In the popliteal space
- 3. Near the iliac crests
- 4. At the zygomatic arch

On the day of surgery, the client in Russell's traction will be transported to the operating room in his bed.

48 When the client is transported, which of the following nursing actions is *correct*?

● 1. The nurse leaves the traction just as it is.
○ 2. The nurse removes the weights during his transport.
○ 3. The nurse rests the weights on the end of the bed.
○ 4. The nurse takes the client's leg out of the traction.

A client with a fractured femur is in skeletal traction with a pin through the distal femur. The leg in traction is supported by balanced suspension.

49 Which substance is *best* for covering the tips of the pin to prevent injuries while caring for the client in skeletal leg traction?
○ 1. Gauze squares
○ 2. Cotton balls
○ 3. Cork blocks
● 4. Rubber tubes

50 Which finding is *most suggestive* that the client has an infection at the pin site?
○ 1. The nurse observes that there is serous drainage at the pin site.
○ 2. The nurse observes that there is bloody drainage at the pin site.
○ 3. The nurse observes that there is mucoid drainage at the pin site.
● 4. The nurse observes that there is purulent drainage at the pin site.

The physician orders antibiotic therapy for the client with a pin site infection.

51 If the client is allergic to penicillin, it is *essential* that the nurse question the medical order for which one of the following types of antibiotics?
○ 1. Aminoglycosides, like gentamicin sulfate (Garamycin)
○ 2. Cephalosporins, like cefaclor (Ceclor)
● 3. Tetracyclines, like doxycycline (Vibramycin)
○ 4. Sulfonamides, like trimethoprim-sulfamethoxazole (Bactrim)

52 If the nurse makes all of the following observations of the traction apparatus applied to the client in Russell's traction, which is *interfering* with its effectiveness?
○ 1. The rope is strung tautly from pulley to pulley.
○ 2. The trapeze is hanging above the client's chest.

● 3. The rope is knotted at the location of a pulley.
○ 4. The weight is hanging about 24 inches from the floor.

A cervical halter type of skin traction is applied to a client who has experienced a whiplash injury in a motor vehicle accident.

53 When the nurse makes rounds at the beginning of the shift, which observation requires *immediate* attention?
○ 1. The halter rests under the client's chin and occiput.
○ 2. The client's ears are clear of the traction ropes.
○ 3. The weight hangs between the headboard and wall.
● 4. There is a soft pillow beneath the client's head.

An adult male client with a fracture of a cervical vertebra is put in halo skeletal traction consisting of pins inserted into the skull that are incorporated into a vest of plaster.

54 When the nurse is asked the purpose of this type of traction, the *best response* is,
○ 1. "It restricts neck movement, but enables physical activity."
○ 2. "It allows head movement, while immobilizing the spine."
○ 3. "It accelerates healing by facilitating physical therapy."
● 4. "It promotes faster bone repair in a short span of time."

55 Which of the following is the *best indication* that the halo traction device is applied appropriately?
○ 1. The client has full range of motion in the neck.
○ 2. The client's neck pain is within a tolerable level.
○ 3. The client can speak and hear at preinjury levels.
● 4. The client reports the ability to see straight ahead.

56 If the nurse gathers all of the following data, which one is *most indicative* that the halo traction needs to be readjusted by the physician?
○ 1. The client experiences postural hypotension.
○ 2. The client needs assistance with shaving.
● 3. The client cannot open his mouth widely.
○ 4. The client eats about 75% of served food.

An adult female has acute low back pain for which pelvic-belt traction has been ordered intermittently throughout the day.

57 When the nurse helps the client apply the pelvic-belt traction, it is *most correct* to place the *top* of the belt
  ○ 1. just below the rib cage.
  ○ 2. even with her waistline.
  ◉ 3. level with the iliac crest.
  ○ 4. where it is most comfortable.

NURSING CARE OF CLIENTS WITH INFLAMMATORY JOINT DISORDERS

An adult female consults a physician about persistent joint pain and stiffness.

58 If the client with joint pain has all of the following laboratory tests, which one, if elevated, is *most diagnostic* for rheumatoid arthritis?
  ◉ 1. Erythrocyte sedimentation rate (ESR)
  ○ 2. Partial thromboplastin time (PTT)
  ○ 3. Fasting blood sugar (FBS)
  ○ 4. Blood urea nitrogen (BUN)

A client with rheumatoid arthritis takes a total of 5 g of acetylsalicylic acid (Bayer aspirin) per day.

59 If each tablet contains 5 grains, how many tablets should the nurse make sure are stocked in the medicine cart for the client in each 24-hour period?
  ○ 1. 5 tablets
  ○ 2. 10 tablets
  ◉ 3. 15 tablets
  ○ 4. 20 tablets

The client with rheumatoid arthritis says she is surprised the physician prescribed such a common drug as aspirin.

60 The nurse is *most correct* in explaining that aspirin is one of the best drugs used in the treatment of arthritis because it relieves discomfort and
  ○ 1. stimulates the immune system.
  ○ 2. relaxes skeletal muscles.
  ◉ 3. reduces joint inflammation.
  ○ 4. interrupts nerve synapses.

The client with rheumatoid arthritis tells the nurse that she gets an upset stomach when she takes the aspirin.

61 Which of the following changes is *most appropriate* to add to the client's plan of care to relieve the discomfort she experiences when taking the aspirin?
  ○ 1. Give aspirin before meals only.
  ○ 2. Give aspirin with cold water.
  ○ 3. Give aspirin with hot tea.
  ◉ 4. Give aspirin with food or meals.

The client with rheumatoid arthritis says that when she watches television, her discomfort is decreased.

62 Which of the following nursing conclusions is *most likely* the correct one?
  ○ 1. The client is improving due to electronic signals.
  ○ 2. The client is having less pain than she thinks.
  ○ 3. The client is experiencing a slight case of arthritis.
  ◉ 4. The client is being distracted from her pain.

63 When planning the care of the client with rheumatoid arthritis, the nurse can expect that the time when the client will need *more time and assistance* with activities of daily living is
  ◉ 1. early morning.
  ○ 2. noontime.
  ○ 3. late afternoon.
  ○ 4. bedtime.

64 Which nursing recommendation has the *greatest potential* for helping the client with rheumatoid arthritis to sustain her ability to care for herself?
  ○ 1. Learn to play a musical instrument.
  ◉ 2. Buy clothes that can be slipped on.
  ○ 3. Enroll in an aerobic exercise class.
  ○ 4. Eat food without chemical additives.

During an acute episode, the physician asks the nurse to apply a splint to each of the hands of the client with rheumatoid arthritis.

65 The nurse is most accurate in explaining to the client that the *primary purpose* of the splints is to
  ◉ 1. rest the affected joints.
  ○ 2. cure her joint disease.
  ○ 3. improve her hand strength.
  ○ 4. increase her range of motion.

A friend of the client with rheumatoid arthritis told her that her arthritis was cured by wearing copper bracelets. The client is thinking of doing the same.

66 What is the *best information* the nurse can provide the client about wearing copper bracelets?
  ○ 1. The relief of symptoms can be attributed to restoring electrolyte balance.
  ◉ 2. The relief of symptoms can be attributed to spontaneous remission.
  ○ 3. The relief of symptoms can be attributed to metallic attraction.
  ○ 4. The relief of symptoms can be attributed to chemical restoration.

An older adult female has been a long-term client at the Rheumatology Clinic. Her hands and wrists are affected by rheumatoid arthritis.

67 When the nurse examines the hands of the client with rheumatoid arthritis, which finger joints are *most often affected*?
○ 1. Proximal finger joints
○ 2. Medial finger joints
○ 3. Distal finger joints
◉ 4. Lateral finger joints

68 If the older client is typical of most people with rheumatoid arthritis, the nurse can expect that she *first developed symptoms*
○ 1. in very early childhood.
○ 2. at the onset of puberty.
○ 3. during young adulthood.
◉ 4. as she neared retirement.

The older female with rheumatoid arthritis has not responded to the usual drug therapy. She now takes prednisone (Meticorten) daily.

69 While the client with rheumatoid arthritis takes prednisone, a corticosteroid, which one of the following assessments is *most essential* for the nurse to monitor?
◉ 1. Daily weight
○ 2. Pulse rate
○ 3. Bowel sounds
○ 4. Skin integrity

70 If the client with rheumatoid arthritis makes all of the following statements about corticosteroid therapy, which one is *incorrect*?
○ 1. The client says she is susceptible to acquiring infections.
○ 2. The client says she should never stop taking her medication abruptly.
○ 3. The client says she may become very depressed and perhaps suicidal.
◉ 4. The client says she may develop low blood sugar and need glucose.

In addition to prednisone (Meticorten), the client with rheumatoid arthritis also takes methotrexate (Rheumatrex), a drug usually used to treat clients with cancer.

71 Which assessment finding is *most likely* a sign of an adverse effect from methotrexate therapy?
○ 1. Constipation
○ 2. Polyuria
◉ 3. Mouth sores
○ 4. Chest pain

The physician recommends that the nurse apply heat to the hands of the older client with rheumatoid arthritis to relieve some of her discomfort.

72 If all of the following are available, which one is *best* for the nurse to use?
○ 1. Hot water bottle
○ 2. Warm moist compresses
◉ 3. Electric heating pad
○ 4. Infrared heat lamp

An older adult male with osteoarthritis in his left hip has been told by his physician to apply a heating pad to his hip periodically.

73 It is *essential* for the nurse to tell the client with osteoarthritis that when he uses the heating pad
◉ 1. it should be kept on the low setting.
○ 2. he should secure it with safety pins.
○ 3. it should be covered with plastic.
○ 4. he should apply it for two hours.

The client with osteoarthritis asks the nurse if there are special foods that help treat arthritis.

74 The *most accurate information* the nurse can provide is that there is no specific diet, but the stress on painful joints can be minimized by
◉ 1. maintaining normal weight.
○ 2. eating green leafy vegetables.
○ 3. increasing the intake of fruit.
○ 4. becoming more physically active.

The client with osteoarthritis uses a cane when ambulating.

75 When the nurse observes him walk, which observation indicates that the client *needs more instruction* about using a cane?
○ 1. The tip of the cane is covered with a rubber cap.
○ 2. The client wears athletic shoes with nonskid soles.
◉ 3. The client uses the cane on his painful side.
○ 4. He holds his head up and looks straight ahead.

The client with osteoarthritis takes 400 mg of ibuprofen (Motrin) four times a day.

76 Which one of the following questions is *most appropriate* to ask a client who takes a nonsteroidal anti-inflammatory drug (NSAID) to determine if a common side effect is occurring?
○ 1. Have you noticed any hand tremors?
○ 2. Are you urinating more frequently?
○ 3. Has your interest in sex changed?
◉ 4. What is the color of your stools?

A total hip replacement (hip arthroplasty) is planned for a 70-year-old male with osteoarthritis. The physician instructs the client to stop taking his enteric coated aspirin (Ecotrin) 1 week prior to surgery.

77 The *most accurate* explanation for the physician's instruction is that aspirin
- ○ 1. increases the risk of wound infection.
- ◉ 2. impairs the ability to control bleeding.
- ○ 3. makes it difficult to assess his pain.
- ○ 4. interferes with the ability to heal.

Before the total hip replacement, the nurse teaches the client how to use an incentive spirometer.

78 Which statement indicates that the client has a *correct understanding* of its use?
- ◉ 1. The client says that he should position the mouthpiece and inhale deeply.
- ○ 2. The client says that he should position the mouthpiece and exhale forcefully.
- ○ 3. The client says that he should position the mouthpiece and cough effectively.
- ○ 4. The client says that he should position the mouthpiece and breathe naturally.

Just before the total hip replacement surgery, a wide area of the client's skin in the operative area is prepared.

79 Which of the following describes the *best technique* for the nurse to use when shaving the operative area?
- ○ 1. Avoid using soap to see the hair better.
- ○ 2. Press the razor deeply into the skin while shaving.
- ○ 3. Use long strokes in a medial to lateral direction.
- ◉ 4. Pull the razor in the direction of hair growth.

80 After the client undergoes a total hip replacement, it is *essential* for the nurse to maintain the operative hip in a position of
- ○ 1. adduction.
- ◉ 2. abduction.
- ○ 3. flexion.
- ○ 4. rotation.

81 Which of the following is *most helpful* for facilitating the postoperative nursing care of the client who underwent a total hip replacement?
- ○ 1. A bed cradle
- ○ 2. A bed board
- ◉ 3. An overhead trapeze
- ○ 4. Lower side rails

82 Which of the following items is *best* for preventing external rotation of the operative leg when caring for the client with the total hip replacement?

- ○ 1. A foot board
- ◉ 2. A trochanter roll
- ○ 3. A turning sheet
- ○ 4. A foam mattress

The nurse caring for the client after the total hip replacement implements a portion of the discharge teaching by instructing him on positions he must temporarily avoid.

83 Which of the following statements indicates that the client has a *correct understanding* of the restrictions he must follow?
- ◉ 1. The client says he cannot cross his legs.
- ○ 2. The client says he cannot point his toes.
- ○ 3. The client says he cannot lay flat in bed.
- ○ 4. The client says he cannot stand upright.

84 Before the client with the total hip replacement is discharged, it is *essential* that the nurse help him obtain which of the following items for his home care?
- ○ 1. A wheelchair
- ○ 2. A hospital bed
- ◉ 3. A raised toilet seat
- ○ 4. A mechanical lift

85 Which area of health teaching is *essential* to include in the discharge instructions of a client who has undergone a total hip replacement?
- ◉ 1. Modifying ways of donning clothing
- ○ 2. Using special equipment for eating
- ○ 3. Taking daily supplemental vitamins
- ○ 4. Avoiding bowel elimination problems

A 36-year-old male client undergoes an arthroscopy of his right knee for purposes of diagnosing and treating the joint, which has been chronically painful.

86 Which one of the following is *most appropriate* to teach the client before the arthroscopy procedure is performed?
- ○ 1. The signs and symptoms of arthritis
- ◉ 2. The technique for using crutches
- ○ 3. The side effects of drug therapy
- ○ 4. The need to balance rest and exercise

A middle-aged male with osteoarthritis will have a knee arthroplasty during which an artificial joint will replace his natural knee joint. A continuous passive motion (CPM) machine will be used postoperatively.

87 The nursing explanation that *best describes* the *primary* purpose of the CPM machine is that it is used to
- ○ 1. strengthen leg muscles.
- ○ 2. relieve foot swelling.
- ○ 3. reduce surgical pain.
- ◉ 4. restore joint function.

88 When documenting the client's progress while using a CPM machine, it is *essential* that the charting indicate the degree of joint flexion, the number of cycles per minute, and the
- ● 1. condition of the sutures around the incision.
- ○ 2. amount of time the client used the machine.
- ○ 3. characteristics of drainage from the wound.
- ○ 4. presence and quality of arterial pulses.

89 Which activity is the *best evidence* that the client who had a knee arthroplasty can discontinue wearing the resting knee extension splint (immobilizer)?
- ○ 1. The client has minimal pain when ambulating.
- ● 2. The client can flex the operative knee 90 degrees.
- ○ 3. The client can perform straight leg raising.
- ○ 4. The client's surgical wound is approximated.

A 54-year-old male is being treated for gout.

90 When the nurse examines the client with gout, if he is typical of others with this condition, which structure is *most likely affected*?
- ● 1. Great toe
- ○ 2. Index finger
- ○ 3. Sacrococcygeal vertebrae
- ○ 4. Temporomandibular joint

91 If the physician orders the following laboratory tests on the client who has gout, the elevation of which one *correlates most* with the client's diagnosis?
- ○ 1. Creatinine clearance
- ○ 2. Blood urea nitrogen
- ● 3. Serum uric acid
- ○ 4. Serum calcium

92 While the client with gout is experiencing an acute attack, which one of the following items is *best* for promoting his comfort?
- ● 1. A bed cradle
- ○ 2. An electric fan
- ○ 3. A foam mattress
- ○ 4. A fracture bedpan

The client with gout is on a low purine diet.

93 It is *most appropriate* for the nurse to consult the dietitian if the client is served
- ○ 1. beets.
- ○ 2. milk.
- ○ 3. eggs.
- ● 4. liver.

During an acute attack of gout, the physician prescribes colchicine to be given every hour until the client's pain is relieved.

94 Which of the following is an indication that the administration of colchicine needs to be discontinued even if the client's pain is unrelieved?
- ○ 1. The client develops vomiting.
- ○ 2. The client develops dizziness.
- ○ 3. The client develops drowsiness.
- ● 4. The client develops a headache.

To reduce the potential for forming urinary stones, the nursing care plan indicates that the client with gout is to have 3000 mL of fluid daily.

95 When implementing the plan of care, the *best time* to offer proportionately greater amounts of fluid to the client is
- ○ 1. before bedtime.
- ○ 2. early evening.
- ● 3. in the morning.
- ○ 4. midafternoon.

The nurse advises the client with gout to continue consuming a high intake of fluid following discharge.

96 The nurse is correct in telling the client that fluid which is *contraindicated*, even in small amounts, for those with gout is
- ○ 1. Coffee
- ● 2. Alcohol
- ○ 3. Cranberry juice
- ○ 4. Carbonated drinks

NURSING CARE OF CLIENTS WITH DEGENERATIVE BONE DISORDERS

A middle-aged female asks the nurse about methods for preventing or delaying the onset of osteoporosis.

97 The nurse is *most accurate* in telling the client that prophylaxis is often achieved by
- ○ 1. having a pregnancy just before menopause.
- ○ 2. breast feeding infants more than one year.
- ○ 3. limiting pregnancies to no more than two.
- ● 4. taking estrogen hormones postmenopausally.

98 When managing the nursing care of clients, the nurse is *correct* in planning measures to reduce skeletal degeneration for clients with
- ○ 1. chronic indigestion.
- ● 2. prolonged immobility.
- ○ 3. inadequate sleep.
- ○ 4. insufficient fluid.

99 When examining clients, which finding is *most suggestive* that a client has osteoporosis?
- ○ 1. The client's joints are swollen.
- ○ 2. The client has discomfort sitting.
- ● 3. The client has a spinal deformity.
- ○ 4. The client's energy is diminished.

100 When planning instructions for teaching a client with osteoporosis on methods for reducing the progression of the disorder, the nurse is correct in recommending that the client *avoid*
- ○ 1. aspirin and carbonated beverages.
- ● 2. nicotine and sources of caffeine.
- ○ 3. sodium and substances with alcohol.
- ○ 4. calcium and dairy products.

A middle-aged client has developed bone necrosis as a result of chronic osteomyelitis in the tibia of his left leg.

101 All of the following nursing measures are appropriate when caring for the client with osteomyelitis; which one is *best* for preventing a pathological fracture?
- ○ 1. Encourage a high fluid intake.
- ○ 2. Provide a nutritional diet.
- ● 3. Support the limb during movement.
- ○ 4. Relieve pressure on bony prominences.

An older adult immigrant to the United States has a pronounced spinal curve and recent vertebral collapse. His condition is diagnosed as Pott's disease.

102 When the client asks the nurse to clarify the physician's explanation of the cause of his condition, the *best answer* is that Pott's disease is caused by
- ● 1. bacteria that cause tuberculosis.
- ○ 2. pollutants that exist in the environment.
- ○ 3. chemical toxins like those in lead paint.
- ○ 4. food additives to which he is sensitive.

A person with osteomalacia, weakening of the bones, has been told that his condition may improve with more vitamin D.

103 In addition to recommending the consumption of foods like milk and margarine that are fortified with vitamin D, it is *correct* for the nurse to suggest that the client
- ● 1. get more direct exposure to sunlight.
- ○ 2. eat meat from growth-stimulated cattle.
- ○ 3. consume bright orange vegetables.
- ○ 4. purchase organically grown produce.

NURSING CARE OF CLIENTS HAVING AMPUTATIONS

During a farming accident, a middle aged male's arm is caught in a corn auger. His lower left arm and hand are crushed.

104 If the farm accident victim is in shock, what position is *best* while the nurse continues to assess and care for him?
- ○ 1. Prone
- ○ 2. Supine
- ● 3. On his back with his legs elevated
- ○ 4. On his side with his neck extended

The victim of the farm accident is rushed to surgery where his arm is amputated above the elbow.

105 Postoperatively, when the client screams obscenities with the realization that his forearm is missing, the *best action* for the nurse is to
- ○ 1. leave the room until he has worked through his anger.
- ● 2. stay quietly with him at his bedside.
- ○ 3. tell him to get control of himself.
- ○ 4. call the hospital chaplain for him.

The client with the amputated arm says, "I know my arm is not there, but I feel it throbbing."

106 The *most accurate* explanation the nurse can give is that the client is experiencing
- ○ 1. referred pain.
- ● 2. phantom pain.
- ○ 3. psychogenic pain.
- ○ 4. intractable pain.

The physician orders transcutaneous electric nerve stimulation (TENS) in the location of the discomfort on the arm opposite the amputation.

107 When the client asks the nurse how the TENS unit is supposed to help, one of the *most widely held* theories is that the sensation created by the TENS machine
- ○ 1. blocks the brain's perception of pain impulses.
- ● 2. travels to the nerve root of the amputated arm.
- ○ 3. destroys the brain's pain center.
- ○ 4. weakens the arm's sensory nerves.

An older adult diabetic female is admitted with vascular problems. Some toes on her left foot are black. She is scheduled for a below-the-knee (BK) amputation.

108 When planning the postoperative care of the diabetic client who has had a BK amputation, which position is *least desirable* for this client?
- ○ 1. Lying prone
- ○ 2. Lying supine
- ○ 3. Sitting in a chair
- ● 4. Standing to shower

The nursing team gathers to develop a plan to strengthen the muscles of the client with the BK amputation to prepare her for ambulating with crutches.

109 If all of the following activities are suggested, which one is *best* to begin implementing *immediately* after surgery?
- ○ 1. Stand at the side of the bed.
- ○ 2. Balance between parallel bars.
- ● 3. Lift herself with the trapeze.
- ○ 4. Transfer from bed to chair.

The client with the BK amputation asks the nurse why the stump is wrapped with elastic roller bandages several times a day.

110 The *best explanation* for stump bandaging is that it is done to
- ○ 1. lengthen and tone muscles.
- ● 2. shrink and shape the stump.
- ○ 3. maintain joint flexibility.
- ○ 4. absorb blood and drainage.

NURSING CARE OF CLIENTS WITH SKELETAL TUMORS

Just before his 18th birthday, a male client is diagnosed as having a cancerous bone tumor (osteogenic sarcoma) in his femur. An above-the-knee (AK) amputation is performed.

111 Which of the following items is *best* to keep at the bedside during the *immediate* postoperative care?
- ○ 1. Gauze dressings
- ● 2. Rubber tourniquet
- ○ 3. Oropharyngeal airway
- ○ 4. Oxygen equipment

A rigid plaster shell surrounds the stump of the client who has undergone an AK amputation. A pylon, or temporary prosthesis, allows the client to ambulate with crutches soon after surgery.

112 Which of the following observations is *most indicative* that the crutches the client is using need further adjustment?
- ○ 1. The client stands straight without bending forward.
- ○ 2. The elbows are slightly flexed when standing in place.
- ○ 3. The top bars of the crutches fit snugly into the axillae.
- ● 4. The wrists are hyperextended when grasping the handgrips.

113 Due to the *location* of a malignant bone tumor like osteogenic sarcoma, it is *most appropriate* for the nurse to assess for which accompanying complication?
- ○ 1. Bowel obstruction
- ○ 2. Liver dysfunction
- ○ 3. Anorexia
- ● 4. Anemia

114 If all of the following are ordered on a client with osteogenic sarcoma, the findings of which diagnostic test is the nurse *most correct* in checking for evidence of metastasis?
- ● 1. Lung scan
- ○ 2. Urinalysis
- ○ 3. Spinal tap
- ○ 4. Blood glucose

NURSING CARE OF CLIENTS WITH A HERNIATED INTERVERTEBRAL DISK

A middle-aged male construction worker has an acute onset of severe low back pain. The physician suspects that the client has a herniated intervertebral disk in the lumbar spine.

115 While assessing the characteristics of the client's pain, the nurse can expect that a person with a herniated disk will have an increase in the *intensity* of pain when
- ○ 1. eating.
- ○ 2. sneezing.
- ● 3. resting.
- ○ 4. urinating.

116 If the client with a herniated lumbar disk is typical of others with this same condition, he also will report to the nurse that he has
- ● 1. radiating pain into the buttocks and leg.
- ○ 2. tenderness over one or both iliac crests.
- ○ 3. diminished sensation in one or both knees.
- ○ 4. brief periods when his toes feel quite cold.

The physician prescribes 10 mg of diazepam (Valium) orally t.i.d. for the client with the tentative diagnosis of herniated intervertebral disk.

117 Besides diminishing anxiety, the nurse is *correct* in explaining to the client with symptoms of a herniated intervertebral disk that this medication is used *in his case* to
- ○ 1. reduce emotional depression.
- ● 2. relax skeletal muscles.
- ○ 3. promote restful sleep.
- ○ 4. relieve inflammation.

A myelogram with a water-soluble contrast dye is ordered to confirm the diagnosis of a herniated intervertebral disk.

118 After the client returns from the myelogram, it is *most appropriate* for the nurse to keep the client quiet and to
- ○ 1. reduce glare from bright lights.
- ● 2. withhold food and fluids for 12 hours.
- ○ 3. administer sedatives every 6 hours.
- ○ 4. encourage a high fluid intake.

Conservative treatment does not relieve the client's symptoms and physical disability. The client with the herniated intervertebral disk consents to have a laminectomy and spinal fusion in the lumbar area of the spine.

119 Before turning the client postoperatively, which nursing instruction is *most important* for preventing postoperative complications?
- ○ 1. "Hold your breath as you are turning."
- ○ 2. "Move your upper body first then legs."
- ○ 3. "Curl up in a ball before I help you turn."
- ● 4. "Let me roll you as if you were a log."

The nurse plans to include principles of good body mechanics in the discharge teaching of the client who has undergone spinal surgery.

120 The nurse is *correct* in telling the client that when he picks something up, he should
- ● 1. flex both his knees.
- ○ 2. keep his feet together.
- ○ 3. lift with arms extended.
- ○ 4. bend from the waist.

Directions: Two numbers appear in parentheses following each rationale. The first number identifies the textbook listed in the references, page 512, and the second number identifies the page(s) in that textbook on which the correct answer can be verified. Occasionally, two or more textbooks are given to verify the correct answer.

NURSING CARE OF CLIENTS WITH TRAUMATIC INJURIES

1 2. Temporarily eliminating the activity that has injured the tendons, in this case playing golf, is the best action to take at this time. It is unnecessary to keep the hand and wrist immobile. Playing miniature golf would continue to injure the tendon. Golfers wear gloves to prevent their skin from becoming blistered. Wearing a tight glove does not protect the joint from injury. (18:1007)
> Nursing Process—Evaluation
> Client Need—Health promotion/maintenance

2 3. Ecchymosis refers to a black and blue skin discoloration caused by the rupture of small blood vessels with bleeding into the skin. Freckled skin is evidenced as scattered small brown pigmented spots on the skin. Mottled skin contains patchy, light-colored or blue skin color. Mottled skin is seen primarily in hypothermic infants and dying clients. Blanched skin appears pale. (21:1065)
> Nursing Process—Data collection
> Client Need—Physiological integrity

3 2. Applying ice and elevating a swollen extremity relieves swelling. Dangling the foot puts the foot in a dependent position and increases the amount of swelling. Exercise causes pain and further swelling in the early stage of the injury. Immobilization is used to relieve pain and promote healing. (18:1007; 21:969)
> Nursing Process—Implementation
> Client Need—Physiological integrity

4 4. When wrapping the lower extremity with a roller bandage, bandaging starts at the metatarsals. The metatarsal bones form the ball of the foot and instep. The toes, or phalanges, are left uncovered to assess circulation. To relieve swelling the injured area is wrapped distally to proximally. If wrapped from below the knee toward the foot, swelling would not be relieved. (18:563)
> Nursing Process—Implementation
> Client Need—Physiological integrity

5 1. The figure-of-eight turn is made by overlapping the roller bandage in an alternately ascending and descending oblique pattern around a joint. Each turn crosses the one preceding it so that it resembles the number eight. A spiral reverse turn is used to bandage a cone-shaped body part, such as the thigh or leg. The recurrent turn is used to cover the tip of a body part, such as the stump of an amputated limb. A spica turn is an adaptation of the figure-of-eight wrap. It is used when the wrap goes around an adjacent body part, such as the thumb and hand, thigh and hip, and so on. (25:577)
> Nursing Process—Implementation
> Client Need—Physiological integrity

6 3. If the roller bandage is applied too tightly, venous blood and lymph are trapped in the toes, producing a swollen appearance. The toes also may feel numb. Rewrapping the extremity may restore or improve circulation. Sitting is not likely to disturb the application of the bandage. The injured area will not be pain free until the swelling subsides and injured tissue heals. Wearing a cotton sock is not an indication for rewrapping the elastic bandage. (18:563)
> Nursing Process—Implementation
> Client Need—Health promotion/maintenance

7 4. A dislocation results in the temporary displacement of a bone from its normal position within a joint. It is caused by the tearing of the ligaments that connect two bone ends within a joint. Most traumatic musculoskeletal injuries, including sprains, strains, and fractures, are accompanied by pain, swelling, and compromised mobility. (18:1007; 21:969)
> Nursing Process—Data collection
> Client Need—Physiological integrity

8 3. Restoring function for a dislocation involves repositioning two adjacent bones so that they are again in contact with one another. The repositioning is done manually with or without anesthesia. A surgical incision is necessary when doing a procedure called an open reduction. Inserting a pin or wire is a type of internal fixation. Exercise is prescribed only after a period of stabilization to allow time for healing. (18:1007; 21:970)

Nursing Process—Implementation
Client Need—Health promotion/maintenance

9 2. When a triangular sling is used, the knot is tied at the side of the neck to avoid pressure on the cervical vertebrae. All the other statements indicate correct information concerning the application and use of a triangular sling. (18:351; 25:519)

Nursing Process—Evaluation
Client Need—Health promotion/maintenance

10 4. To immobilize a broken bone, a splint is applied so that it prevents movement of the joints above and below the injury. The tibia is between the knee and the ankle. Therefore it is correct to apply the splint from below the ankle to above the knee. (4:1562; 25:515)

Nursing Process—Implementation
Client Need—Physiological integrity

11 2. A comminuted fracture means that there are pieces or fragments of bone in the area where the bone was broken. An impacted fracture is one in which the bone ends are driven together. A simple, or closed, fracture is one in which there is no break in the skin. A greenstick fracture is the name given to a fracture in which there is a longitudinal split that extends partially through one side of the bone. (4:607; 21:972)

Nursing Process—Implementation
Client Need—Health promotion/maintenance

12 4. The hospital first attempts to obtain permission from a minor's parent or guardian. Minors cannot give permission under most circumstances. If permission is obtained over the telephone, at least two people must hear the verbal consent and co-sign as witnesses to what they heard. (14:441; 25:32)

Nursing Process—Implementation
Client Need—Safe, effective care environment

13 4. Jewelry is removed preoperatively, itemized, identified, and locked in a secure area. Another alternative is to give the client's valuables to a member of the family. The nurse has a responsibility to document in the client's record the items that were taken and how they are being kept secure. In some agencies the client is given a receipt for his property. If a client asks that a wedding ring be left on, the nurse can secure it to the finger or hand with tape or a strip of gauze. Class rings generally contain multiple grooves or crevices that trap and hold microorganisms. Therefore, to reduce the potential for infection, it is best to remove and safeguard the ring. The ring is subject to theft if left in the bedside

stand. Security guards usually are not responsible for the safekeeping of personal valuables. (4:450; 25:557)

Nursing Process—Implementation
Client Need—Safe, effective care environment

14 1. Most fat emboli travel to the pulmonary circulation. Once the emboli partially or totally occlude blood flow through a pulmonary vessel, the client experiences dyspnea, rapid breathing and heart rate, cyanosis, chest pain, cough, blood-streaked sputum, and a feeling of doom. Emboli also may travel to the brain, causing confusion, agitation, and coma. (18:997; 21:310)

Nursing Process—Data collection
Client Need—Physiological integrity

15 2. The ribs enclose the lungs. This makes injuries to the pulmonary system the prime complication associated with fractured ribs. The broken ribs may puncture the pleura and collapse a lung. One of the classic signs of a flail chest injury is asymmetrical or paradoxical chest expansion. The heart also is in the thorax but somewhat better protected in the center of the chest. Tachycardia and a weak or thready pulse is more likely to indicate damage to major blood vessels than an irregular pulse rate. Hyperactive bowel sounds are characteristic of hyperperistalsis as occurs in diarrhea. A distended bladder indicates a need for urinary elimination, rather than secondary trauma. (26:308)

Nursing Process—Data collection
Client Need—Physiological integrity

16 1. All of the measures described in this item are necessary in an emergency, but the first step a rescuer takes is to see that the victim is breathing. Maintaining ventilation is a priority for sustaining life. (4:1550; 21:249)

Nursing Process—Implementation
Client Need—Physiological integrity

17 3. The best method for controlling bleeding in the case of a compound fracture is compressing the major artery above the site of the injury. Direct pressure on the wound itself may cause additional injuries to the soft tissue surrounding the fracture. A tourniquet is used only if all other efforts to control bleeding are unsuccessful. If used, a tourniquet is periodically released to allow oxygenated blood to the distal tissue. Elevation of the extremity is helpful after applying pressure on the artery. (4:1553; 21:250)

Nursing Process—Implementation
Client Need—Physiological integrity

18 3. The neck and back of an accident victim with a suspected spinal injury are immobilized before transport. The victim is positioned flat on his or her back and secured to a rigid stretcher before being moved and transported. Rescuers need to keep the spine extended. Flexion may cause more injury to the vertebrae or the spinal cord. (4:1564; 21:576)
   Nursing Process—Implementation
   Client Need—Physiological integrity

19 4. Typical signs of a fractured hip include external rotation and shortening of the affected leg. Bruising may or may not be present depending on the circumstances of the fracture. Sensation is intact. Movement results in increased pain. (4:610; 21:986)
   Nursing Process—Data collection
   Client Need—Physiological integrity

20 1. Estrogen deficiency, which occurs postmenopausally, is linked to loss of calcium from the bones. Decreased bone mass weakens the skeletal system increasing a person's susceptibility for fractures. Being overweight exerts more stress on the skeletal system, but as long as the integrity of the bones is intact, the risk for fractures is the same as for the general population. Doing gardening and being born in England do not potentiate the client's risk for a fracture. (4:597; 21:986, 1000)
   Nursing Process—Data collection
   Client Need—Physiological integrity

21 2. Isometric exercises are performed by tensing and releasing muscles. They do not involve any appreciable movement of a joint. The quadriceps muscles are on the anterior of the thigh. All of the other options in this item describe isotonic exercises that involve joint movement. (4:580; 25:531)
   Nursing Process—Evaluation
   Client Need—Health promotion/maintenance

22 1. Elastic stockings, known as antiembolism or thromboembolic disease (TED) hose, support the valves within veins. The supported valves prevent blood from falling back into the lower legs and feet. When blood moves, rather than stands still, it is less likely to clot. When properly fitted, antiembolism stockings do not restrict arterial blood from flowing into the extremities or affect arterial blood pressure. Red blood cells, or erythrocytes, do not play a role in forming blood clots. Platelets, or thrombocytes, are the type of blood cells that clump together, especially when there has been an injury. (4:774; 25:551)
   Nursing Process—Implementation
   Client Need—Health promotion/maintenance

23 1. To prevent trapping venous blood in the lower extremities, elastic stockings are applied while in a nondependent position. The best time to apply these stockings is in the morning before getting out of bed or after elevating the legs a short time. Elastic stockings are worn almost continuously. They are removed once per shift or once per day to assess the skin. (18:565; 25:553)
   Nursing Process—Evaluation
   Client Need—Safe, effective care environment

24 1. A client who has a prosthesis inserted to repair a fractured hip is turned using sufficient pillows so that the operative leg remains slightly abducted. Hip abduction prevents displacement of the fixation device. Pointing the toes, flexing the knee, or elevating the head will not promote hip abduction. (4:613; 25:987)
   Nursing Process—Implementation
   Client Need—Physiological integrity

25 3. When helping a client transfer from the bed to a chair, it is best to place the chair parallel to and near the head of the bed on the client's stronger side. The nurse makes the distance as short as possible to promote safety when the client is weak or may lose his balance. Transferring to a chair at the end of the bed or against a side wall requires much more physical effort and involves safety hazards. Placing the chair perpendicularly interferes with assisting the client. (4:248; 25:483)
   Nursing Process—Planning
   Client Need—Safe, effective care environment

26 1. In a three-point partial weight-bearing gait, the weaker leg and walker are advanced together. The majority of the weight is supported by the hands while the stronger leg is lifted and advanced. (4:629; 25:541)
   Nursing Process—Evaluation
   Client Need—Health promotion/maintenance

NURSING CARE OF CLIENTS WITH CASTS

27 2. When plaster combines with water a chemical reaction takes place. Energy is given off in the form of heat. The client is warned that his arm may feel quite warm temporarily. Steam or heat waves may even be seen rising from the surface of the wet cast. The cast supports the broken bone, but it should not constrict the underlying tissue. Wet plaster does not produce a disagreeable odor. Itching is not a common experience at the time a cast is applied. (21:975–976; 25:522)
   Nursing Process—Implementation
   Client Need—Health promotion/maintenance

28 4. A wet cast is held and supported with the palms of the hands. Using the fingers is likely to cause indentations in the cast. The inward dents create pressure areas on the underlying tissue. After the cast is applied, it is dried while supported on a soft surface. If the wet cast is on a hard surface is can become flattened. (18:986; 25:523)

> **Nursing Process—Implementation**
> **Client Need—Physiological integrity**

29 2. Casts made of fiberglass or other synthetic materials have several advantages, one of which is that they tend to weigh less than plaster casts. A synthetic cast dries more quickly. It is more durable and not likely to soften if the cast becomes wet. They are no less flexible or less restrictive than plaster casts. The major disadvantage is that they are more expensive than traditional plaster casts. (18:987; 25:520)

> **Nursing Process—Implementation**
> **Client Need—Health promotion/maintenance**

30 1. Sharp pain is the first symptom of compartment syndrome. The pain is due to ischemia, the impairment of arterial blood flow, caused by swelling of the surrounding muscle within the inelastic fascia. Paralysis and sensory loss follow as nerves become damaged by compression and lack of blood supply. The hand appears pale or white and cold from inadequate arterial blood. If the radial artery is assessed, the nurse finds that it is weak or absent. (4:619; 18:998)

> **Nursing Process—Data collection**
> **Client Need—Physiological integrity**

31 4. A wet cast is supported along its entire length with soft pillows as it dries. The soft support distributes the weight of the cast over a greater surface and prevents flattening of the underlying portion. Use of pillows helps in elevating the extremity to relieve temporary swelling. A synthetic sheepskin or vinyl sheet interferes with evaporation of water from the wet plaster. An absorbent pad does not cushion the weight of the cast sufficiently. (4:625; 25:523–524)

> **Nursing Process—Implementation**
> **Client Need—Physiological integrity**

32 1. Natural evaporation is the best way to dry a plaster cast. This process takes 24 to 48 hours. It involves turning the client at frequent intervals so that the entire cast circumference is exposed to the air. Intense heat such as with a heating blanket, hot air

drying, or heat lamp, may burn the client or just dry the superficial surface of the cast. (18:986; 25:523)

> **Nursing Process—Implementation**
> **Client Need—Physiological integrity**

33 3. Circling the outer margin of the drainage on the cast helps the nurse evaluate the status of the bleeding. The nurse needs to return soon for another assessment. By comparing the subsequent size of the bloody spot, the nurse evaluates the seriousness of the bleeding. It is important to monitor the vital signs each time the drainage is assessed. All information is documented. If the bleeding is not controlled, and the vital signs indicate that the client's condition is changing, the physician is notified immediately. An ice bag is generally used to control swelling postoperatively. In some small way it also may decrease bleeding. (25:524)

> **Nursing Process—Implementation**
> **Client Need—Physiological integrity**

34 3. The nurse assesses circulation in an extremity by performing the blanching test to determine capillary refill time. After releasing pressure on the nailbed, the color normally returns within 2 to 3 seconds. The assessment also is performed on the opposite extremity. If the capillary refill time is similar in both extremities, the cast or tissue swelling is not a factor. Asking if the cast feels heavy or palpating it to feel the cast temperature are not appropriate techniques for assessing circulation. Determining that there is space between the cast and the skin is not a totally reliable assessment technique. If the circulation is impaired due to compartment syndrome, there may still be room to insert a finger at the margins of the cast. (4:627; 25:523)

> **Nursing Process—Data collection**
> **Client Need—Physiological integrity**

35 3. When a client expresses a concern, it is best for the nurse to verbalize the feeling or message that the sender conveyed. This response shows understanding and a willingness to listen. Using clichés, agreeing with the client, or stereotyping the family interaction are all nontherapeutic. They are of little help to a client who is struggling with a personal problem. (23:85–89; 25:79–80)

> **Nursing Process—Implementation**
> **Client Need—Psychosocial integrity**

36 3. Most young adults seek to become independent of their parents and develop an intimate relationship with a nonrelative. Developmental tasks concerned with self-identity, sexuality, testing the body's abilities, and learning to control emotional behavior

occur more commonly before young adulthood. (2:310–313; 21:44)
  Nursing Process—Evaluation
  Client Need—Health promotion/maintenance

37 2. A hip spica cast interferes with hip flexion and assuming a sitting position. A fracture bedpan elevates the buttocks just slightly enough for bowel elimination. Because this client cannot sit, a bedside commode, mechanical lift, and raised toilet seat are inappropriate. (18:994; 25:521)
  Nursing Process—Planning
  Client Need—Physiological integrity

38 3. One of the weakest areas of a hip spica cast is at the groin areas. This area tends to crack because it is stressed when turning and repositioning the client. The bar is *never* used for lifting or turning, performing physical exercise, or hanging personal items. (25:521)
  Nursing Process—Implementation
  Client Need—Health promotion/maintenance

39 1. Obtaining a medical order for administering an antihistamine/antipruritic drug like cyproheptadine (Periactin) chemically relieves the client's itching. Distraction may also be an alternative technique for relieving discomfort, but it takes commitment and repeated practice to be effective. The client is cautioned against using any method that scratches the skin. If the integrity of the skin is impaired, organisms may begin to grow in the warm, dark, moist environment. Administering an analgesic for itching is inappropriate. Moisture from melting ice cubes could soften a plaster cast. (17:377; 14:645)
  Nursing Process—Implementation
  Client Need—Physiological integrity

40 4. The most frequent cause of an odor from a cast is an infected wound. Infected wounds produce purulent drainage. There is often an unpleasant odor as pus accumulates. To confirm the suspicion that an infection exists, the nurse monitors the client for a cluster of additional signs and symptoms such as an elevated temperature, tachycardia, anorexia, and malaise. (21:979)
  Nursing Process—Data collection
  Client Need—Physiological integrity

41 2. The piece of plaster that is removed to make a window is replaced in the opening and secured with tape or a roller bandage. If the window remains open, tissue tends to bulge into the opening. The uneven pressure on the skin can cause it to break down. (21:976; 25:524)
  Nursing Process—Implementation
  Client Need—Physiological integrity

42 1. Rough or crumbling edges of a plaster cast are smoothed or repaired by applying petals made from moleskin or adhesive tape. Petals, formed in rectangular or oval pieces, are inserted on the inside of the cast edge and then folded over the outside edge of the cast. The strips are made to overlap, resembling the appearance of flower petals. The physician usually applies more plaster strips or uses a cast cutter if it is needed. Trimming a cast does not usually stop it from crumbling. Fragments of plaster are likely to continue breaking off if the nurse uses gauze to cover the cast edge. (18:986; 25:524; 26:639)
  Nursing Process—Implementation
  Client Need—Physiological integrity

43 1. Cast syndrome, also known as superior mesenteric syndrome, causes gastrointestinal symptoms such as abdominal distention, bloating, nausea, vomiting, and abdominal pain. The symptoms are caused by a partial or total intestinal obstruction. The other symptoms, if they develop, are more likely to be caused by complications other than cast syndrome. (4:625; 18:994)
  Nursing Process—Data collection
  Client Need—Physiological integrity

NURSING CARE OF CLIENTS WITH TRACTION

44 2. The leg of the client in Buck's traction must remain in alignment with the pull of the traction. This means that rather than making the bed as usual from side to side, the nurse removes and applies linen at the top or bottom of the bed and pulls it underneath the client. A person in Buck's traction is not turned from side to side or raised with a mechanical lift. A client in traction, as any other hospitalized client, has bed linen changed whenever it is soiled, wet, or needs replacement. (4:628; 25:527)
  Nursing Process—Implementation
  Client Need—Physiological integrity

45 3. To maintain countertraction, the client's foot must never press against the foot of the bed. If this is observed, the nurse helps pull the client back up toward the head of the bed. The weights must always hang free rather than rest on the floor or the bed. The body must be in alignment with the pull of the traction. The traction rope must move freely within the groove of the pulley. (18:996; 21:978; 25:527)
  Nursing Process—Implementation
  Client Need—Physiological integrity

46 2. The best technique for assessing circulation among the options provided is to palpate the distal peripheral pulse. The dorsalis pedis artery is on the top of the foot. Other pertinent circulatory assessments include observing the color and temperature of the skin, capillary refill time, and subjective complaints concerning pain. Checking movement and sensation are neurologic assessment techniques. Taking the blood pressure on the thigh rather than the arm is unnecessary. (4:628; 21:971)
    Nursing Process—Planning
    Client Need—Physiological integrity

47 2. The popliteal space behind the knee is especially prone to pressure and irritation when Russell's traction is used. This area is suspended in a sling, which can become wrinkled. A piece of thick felt is sometimes used to line the sling to keep the surface smooth. The ischial spines are part of the inferior portion of the pelvic bones. The iliac crests are the upper flared portion of the bony pelvis. The zygomatic arches are in the cheek. (4:628; 25:526)
    Nursing Process—Data collection
    Client Need—Physiological integrity

48 1. Preoperatively the traction remains applied to the client at all times, even during transport to the operating room. Its purpose is to relieve muscle spasm and immobilize the fractured bone. If the traction is removed or the weights released, muscle spasms recur. Any realignment that may have been achieved with the use of traction is jeopardized. (18:996; 26:540)
    Nursing Process—Implementation
    Client Need—Physiological integrity

49 3. The tips of the pin used for skeletal traction are skewered into a block of cork or a rubber ball like those used for playing jacks. Gauze and cotton are inadequate for preventing punctures and abrasions. Rubber tubes may also be pierced by the pin, thus exposing the sharp tip. (25:527; 26:541)
    Nursing Process—Implementation
    Client Need—Safe, effective care environment

50 4. Purulent drainage is sometimes referred to as pus. Purulent drainage is a collection of fluid containing white blood cells and pathogens. The presence of white blood cells indicates that the body is attempting to destroy and remove infecting organisms. Serous drainage is clear; it is made up of plasma or serum. Bloody drainage indicates trauma. Mucoid drainage is sticky and transparent. It is released from mucous membranes. (18:422; 21:120)
    Nursing Process—Data collection
    Client Need—Physiological integrity

51 2. There is a high probability that individuals who are allergic to penicillin also will exhibit a cross-sensitivity to cephalosporins. Both of these drugs are very similar in their structure. Although everyone with a drug sensitivity is observed closely when a new medication, especially an antibiotic, is administered, individuals with a penicillin allergy seem to react more often to the cephalosporins than to others. (20:60)
    Nursing Process—Implementation
    Client Need—Physiological integrity

52 3. Two pieces of rope are sometimes spliced together with a knot to provide sufficient length for traction. However, if the knot prevents free movement over and within a pulley, it interferes with the effectiveness of the traction. Traction ropes are taut. Locating the trapeze above the client's chest facilitates its use. Traction weights must hang freely above the floor for effective use. (21:974; 26:540)
    Nursing Process—Data collection
    Client Need—Physiological integrity

53 4. A pillow is usually contraindicated when a client is in cervical skin traction because it alters the direction of pull. If any kind of head support is necessary, it is usually provided with a cervical or neck pillow that fits under the nape of the neck. (25:527; 26:541)
    Nursing Process—Data collection
    Client Need—Physiological integrity

54 1. Halo skeletal traction immobilizes the vertebrae in the neck while allowing clients to assume erect posture, to sit, and ambulate. Halo skeletal traction restricts head movement. Veterbral fractures proceed to heal at a standard rate regardless of whether halo traction or some other medical or surgical management is instituted. Physical therapy is not prescribed until the vertebral fracture is stabilized and the halo traction is removed. (4:618)
    Nursing Process—Implementation
    Client Need—Health promotion/maintenance

55 4. A client's ability to see straight ahead is the best sign that halo traction is keeping the neck immobilized in a neutral position. Clients should not be able to move the neck at will while in halo traction. Clients may experience mild neck discomfort even though halo traction is applied appropriately. The ability to speak and hear are unrelated to the use of halo traction. (18:994)
    Nursing Process—Data collection
    Client Need—Physiological integrity

56 3. Signs that the metal rods in halo traction require readjustment include an inability to fully open the mouth and difficulty swallowing. Postural hypotension, if it occurs, is not due to the malfunction of the halo traction. Adult males need help with shaving because they are unable to change their head position to see areas of the face while shaving. Reduced appetite or appetite changes require nursing interventions, but they are not related to the effectiveness of the halo traction. (18:994)

> Nursing Process—Data collection
> Client Need—Physiological integrity

57 3. The uppermost edge of a pelvic belt hugs the client's hips. The pelvic belt helps to relieve spasms and pain in the muscles in the lumbar area. Placing the belt below the rib cage or at midabdomen does not promote the maximum effectiveness from its use. Though using pelvic belt traction will promote comfort, the location for its application is not arbitrarily determined on that basis. (26:541)

> Nursing Process—Implementation
> Client Need—Physiological integrity

NURSING CARE OF CLIENTS WITH INFLAMMATORY JOINT DISORDERS

58 1. The erythrocyte sedimentation rate is a nonspecific test that indicates the presence and progress of an inflammatory disease. It is elevated in a number of inflammatory conditions including rheumatoid arthritis. A PTT time is ordered to determine a person's ability to clot blood. It is commonly ordered when a person is on heparin therapy. A fasting blood sugar is performed to diagnose and evaluate the treatment of diabetes mellitus. The BUN is a common test for assessing renal function. (4:592; 7:74)

> Nursing Process—Data collection
> Client Need—Physiological integrity

59 3. Five grams of drug supplied in a dosage strength of 5 grains per tablet requires 15 tablets in a 24-hour period.

> 1 g contains approximately 15 grains
> 5 g contains 75 grains (5 × 15 = 75)

To solve the problem using a ratio and proportion method, use the following steps (20:33; 25:699):

> 5 grains:1 tablet = 75 grains:X tablets
> 5X = 75
> X = 15 tablets

> Nursing Process—Implementation
> Client Need—Physiological integrity

60 3. Aspirin has the ability to produce analgesic, anti-inflammatory, and antipyretic effects. Its analgesic and anti-inflammatory effects are probably

achieved by inhibiting chemicals called prostaglandins, not by interrupting nerve synapses. Prostaglandins increase sensitivity of peripheral pain receptors. Aspirin does not relax skeletal muscles or stimulate the immune system. (17:227; 20:401)

> Nursing Process—Implementation
> Client Need—Health promotion/maintenance

61 4. Taking irritating drugs with food or at mealtime helps decrease gastric distress. Aspirin, especially in large doses, tends to irritate the stomach mucosa. Giving aspirin on an empty stomach increases discomfort. Cold water or hot tea are not substances that protect the stomach or alter the acidity of the aspirin. The caffeine in tea actually stimulates an increase in the production of stomach acid. (17:227; 20:5)

> Nursing Process—Planning
> Client Need—Physiological integrity

62 4. Distraction is a legitimate and often very effective method for the relief of discomfort. Watching television is one method of distraction. There are no reports that electronic television signals are an effective treatment for arthritis. If the client had only a slight case of arthritis, she would be likely to feel pain relief at times other than when watching television. (18:611; 25:169)

> Nursing Process—Evaluation
> Client Need—Physiological integrity

63 1. People with rheumatoid arthritis are more stiff and uncomfortable in the early morning hours after being inactive during the hours of sleep. Therefore, it is best to allow extra time and distribute self-care activities over later hours of the day. (4:592; 21:990)

> Nursing Process—Planning
> Client Need—Physiological integrity

64 2. Hand deformity and muscle atrophy make it difficult to perform fine motor movement with the fingers. Purchasing clothes that are pulled on or slipped on enables the client with rheumatoid arthritis to maintain a degree of independence. It is important for the person with arthritis to maintain joint mobility through exercise. However, it is unlikely that the client would be able to perform the finger coordination required to play a musical instrument. Aerobic exercise is unrealistic because it is likely to be too strenuous. Clients with rheumatoid arthritis are often anemic and tire easily. There is no known connection between chemical additives and the symptoms of arthritis. (4:594; 21:998)

> Nursing Process—Planning
> Client Need—Health promotion/maintenance

65 1. During an acute attack, splints are used primarily to keep the inflamed joints somewhat inactive. Resting the part suppresses additional stress on the diseased joints. The acute inflammation subsides with a combination of drug therapy and the body's natural healing processes. Secondarily, a certain amount of strength and joint flexibility are preserved by limiting the damage during the acute attack. (21:993; 26:841)
Nursing Process—Implementation
Client Need—Health promotion/maintenance

66 2. The symptoms of rheumatoid arthritis can spontaneously go away. Many give credit for their remission to some unrelated activity or unorthodox treatment. The use of copper bracelets in the treatment of arthritis is a common folk medicine myth. Because people who suffer from chronic and incurable diseases, like arthritis, are desperate for something that will cure their illness, they are extremely vulnerable to fraudulent treatment. Through health teaching, the nurse helps individuals with incurable or terminal diseases avoid becoming victims of quackery. (4:592; 25:990–991)
Nursing Process—Implementation
Client Need—Health promotion/maintenance

67 1. The proximal finger joints are affected the most in rheumatoid arthritis. There may be so much involvement that the fingers actually turn laterally. In osteoarthritis the distal finger joints are more often deformed. Traumatic arthritis, which is associated with a specific injury, affects any joint. (21:990)
Nursing Process—Data collection
Client Need—Physiological integrity

68 3. Although some acquire juvenile arthritis, most experience the onset of rheumatoid arthritis early in their adult life. The disease profoundly affects the ability to maintain employment during the productive years of life. (4:592; 18:1005)
Nursing Process—Data collection
Client Need—Physiological integrity

69 1. Corticosteroid therapy causes sodium and water retention. The consequence of hypernatremia is evidenced by weight gain. With an excess of fluid, blood pressure also becomes elevated and is closely monitored. The pulse rate is not likely to change appreciably. However, the pulse may feel bounding with an increase of fluid in the blood volume. Peristalsis is unaffected by corticosteroids. The skin of a person taking steroids undergoes various changes. However, the skin generally remains intact. The nurse may observe that the skin becomes thin and bruises easily. There may be increased hair growth,

petechiae, redistribution of body fat, and striae. If the skin does become impaired as a result of injury or surgery, wound healing is prolonged. (20:353; 21:992)
Nursing Process—Data collection
Client Need—Physiological integrity

70 4. Individuals receiving corticosteroids tend to have elevated blood sugar. Diabetics may need to increase their dosage of insulin or oral hypoglycemic agents. Nondiabetics also are monitored for hyperglycemia and glucosuria. Because steroids depress the inflammatory response, they place the client at high risk for acquiring infections. Steroids are withdrawn gradually if therapy is discontinued to prevent acute adrenal insufficiency. Depression is common among individuals receiving corticosteroids. (17:241; 21:992)
Nursing Process—Evaluation
Client Need—Health promotion/maintenance

71 3. The mucosa of the mouth and entire gastrointestinal tract may become ulcerated as a consequence of taking methotrexate. Therefore, it is especially important to inspect the oral cavity. This drug also causes diarrhea and renal failure. Chest pain is not a usual side effect of methotrexate. (20:407; 28:715)
Nursing Process—Data collection
Client Need—Physiological integrity

72 2. Moist heat is more effective than forms of dry heat like a hot water bottle, electric heating pad, or infrared heat lamp. This phenomenon is attributed to the fact that water is a better conductor of heat than air. Whenever any form of heat is used, the nurse takes care that the client is not accidentally burned. (18:569; 25:584)
Nursing Process—Implementation
Client Need—Physiological integrity

73 1. To avoid burning the skin, a heating pad is always kept on a low setting. The client is cautioned not to turn the heat setting higher when becoming adapted to the sensation of warmth. It is hazardous to use safety pins. There is a potential for electric shock if metal pins puncture a heating wire. A heating pad is covered with fabric, such as flannel. Heat is not applied for longer than 20 to 30 minutes at a time. (18:575)
Nursing Process—Implementation
Client Need—Safe, effective care environment

74 1. Obesity puts additional stress on weight-bearing joints and contributes to discomfort. Eating green leafy vegetables and fruit are healthy behaviors, but they do not directly relieve the effects of arthritis.

Physical activity is likely to cause more discomfort to a person whose hips are affected by osteoarthritis. (4:594; 21:991, 998)

> Nursing Process—Implementation
> Client Need—Health promotion/maintenance

75 3. A cane is always held on the uninvolved side. By doing so the client can transfer or redistribute body weight from the painful joint to the hand with the cane when taking a step. Covering the tip with a rubber cap, wearing supportive shoes, and maintaining good posture are all appropriate techniques for using a cane. (4:630; 25:534)

> Nursing Process—Evaluation
> Client Need—Health promotion/maintenance

76 4. Gastrointestinal side effects and the potential for bleeding are common among clients who take nonsteroidal anti-inflammatory drugs. This category of drugs is used cautiously in individuals with a history of peptic ulcer disease. By asking the client to identify the color of his stools, the nurse is assessing if the drug is causing gastrointestinal bleeding. NSAIDS are not known to cause changes in libido, increased urination, or hand tremors. (20:401,4; 28:577)

> Nursing Process—Planning
> Client Need—Physiological integrity

77 2. Aspirin increases the possibility of postoperative bleeding. It interferes with the ability of platelets to clump together, one of the first mechanisms in clot formation. Aspirin does not increase the risk of wound infection or the ability to heal. Aspirin is not discontinued to facilitate the assessment of the client's pain. (21:994)

> Nursing Process—Implementation
> Client Need—Health promotion/maintenance

78 1. An incentive spirometer helps a client measure the effectiveness of deep inhalation. It is important postoperatively for the client to breathe deeply to open the airways and alveoli. This helps to improve the oxygenation of blood, eliminate carbon dioxide, and prevent atelectasis and pneumonia. None of the other three options indicates a correct use of an incentive spirometer. (4:454; 26:328)

> Nursing Process—Evaluation
> Client Need—Health promotion/maintenance

79 4. The strokes with the razor are made with the grain of the hair shaft. This technique avoids nicking or scraping the skin. Impairing the integrity of the skin and bleeding increase the risk of postoperative wound infections. Soap is used to decrease the numbers of transient skin organisms. The razor is held so that it glides across the surface of the skin.

The direction of the razor strokes is determined by the direction of the hair growth. (4:444; 18:626)

> Nursing Process—Implementation
> Client Need—Safe, effective care environment

80 2. The hip of a client who has undergone a total hip replacement (arthroplasty) is maintained in a position of abduction. If the client flexes his hip more than 90° or adducts the hip, the prosthetic femoral head may become dislocated. A triangular foam wedge is generally kept between the client's legs while in bed. (4:633; 21:994)

> Nursing Process—Implementation
> Client Need—Physiological integrity

81 3. A trapeze is an item that allows the client to help move and lift himself or herself. Encouraging the client to participate actively helps maintain muscular strength and reduces the effort the nurse provides when moving and positioning a client. A bed cradle is used to keep bed linen off of lower extremities. A bed board is used to support the client's spine. Lower side rails are appropriate when maintaining the safety of a confused client or one with a perceptual disorder. (18:507; 25:471–472)

> Nursing Process—Planning
> Client Need—Physiological integrity

82 2. A trochanter roll is used to maintain the hip in a position of extension. Placing this positioning device at the trochanter helps keep the hip from rotating outward. A foot board is used to prevent plantar flexion and foot drop deformity. A turning sheet is used to reposition a client. A foam mattress helps to relieve pressure from bony prominences. (18:995; 25:470)

> Nursing Process—Implementation
> Client Need—Physiological integrity

83 1. A client with a total hip replacement is instructed to avoid crossing the legs. Crossing the legs places the hip in a position of adduction and flexion. These two positions can displace the prosthetic device. Pointing the toes as in plantar flexion or dorsiflexion will not impair the surgical procedure. Laying flat and standing upright are not harmful. (25:994; 26:524)

> Nursing Process—Evaluation
> Client Need—Health promotion/maintenance

84 3. Postoperatively and for an extended time afterward, a client with a total hip replacement must avoid flexing the hip more than 90°. This necessitates using a raised toilet seat. The client does not need a wheelchair. He or she ambulates using a walker. The client can continue to use his or her own bed at home. The client is taught techniques for transferring from bed to a chair. Therefore, a mechanical lift is unnecessary. (4:634; 25:994)

Nursing Process—Planning
Client Need—Health promotion/maintenance

85 1. The client with a total hip replacement must avoid bending over to put on or take off socks, pants, and shoes. Someone helps with these items of clothing or assistive devices are obtained. Another approach is to modify the clothing so that the client can slip them on without flexing the hip more than 90 degrees. No special equipment is needed for eating. Taking supplemental vitamins is not necessary as long as the client consumes an adequate diet. It is helpful to discuss how to avoid bowel elimination problems with any client who is prone to constipation or diarrhea. However, this is not unique to the care of the client with a total hip replacement. (4:634; 25:994)

Nursing Process—Planning
Client Need—Health promotion/maintenance

86 2. Most who undergo an arthroscopy use crutches for a period of time following the procedure. Since postprocedural discomfort and recovery from local anesthesia or light conscious sedation interferes with learning and practice, it is best to teach clients how to use crutches during their preoperative preparation. Most clients who undergo arthroscopy have already personally experienced the signs and symptoms of arthritis. Drug teaching is postponed until the physician writes postoperative orders. Balancing rest with exercise is important, but specific orders are indicated by the physician following the procedure. (7:822; 26:527)

Nursing Process—Implementation
Client Need—Health promotion/maintenance

87 4. A CPM machine is used primarily to restore full range of joint motion. Clients with knee joint replacement often are reluctant to exercise the operative knee actively because of pain. Exercise tones and strengthens muscles and relieves dependent swelling by promoting venous circulation; however, these are considered secondary benefits. Discomfort usually accompanies use of the CPM machine. It is appropriate for the nurse to administer a prescribed analgesic before the client uses a CPM machine. (18:493, 495; 25:510)

Nursing Process—Implementation
Client Need—Health promotion/maintenance

88 2. The length of time the CPM machine is used provides additional documentation of the client's response to treatment. Inspecting and documenting

the appearance of the wound, the drainage on the dressing, and the presence and quality of arterial pulses are important data to record. However, this information is more pertinent to general physical assessment findings. (25:510)

Nursing Process—Implementation
Client Need—Safe, effective care environment

89 3. A resting knee extension splint (immobilizer) is worn on the operative leg until the client demonstrates enough quadriceps strength to independently perform straight leg raising. A decrease in pain, wound approximation, and increase in knee flexion are positive signs of healing and rehabilitation, but they are not criteria for discontinuing the immobilizer. (4:632)

Nursing Process—Evaluation
Client Need—Physiological Integrity

90 1. Gout can affect any joint, but approximately 80% of the people who have gout experience symptoms in their great toe. (4:596; 18:1002; 21:994)

Nursing Process—Data collection
Client Need—Physiological integrity

91 3. An elevated serum uric acid level is diagnostic among clients with gout. An elevated serum creatinine clearance and blood urea nitrogen are indicative of renal failure. Serum calcium is elevated in hyperparathyroidism; primary cancers, such as Hodgkin's disease or multiple myeloma; and metastasis to the bone. (4:591; 25:995)

Nursing Process—Data collection
Client Need—Physiological integrity

92 1. Of all the items, a bed cradle is best for preventing the affected joints from being touched or bumped. There is no relationship between gout and the need for an electric fan, foam mattress, or fracture bedpan. (4:596; 18:1002)

Nursing Process—Implementation
Client Need—Physiological integrity

93 4. Organ meats, such as liver, kidney, brain, and sweetbreads, are high in purines. Other high sources are fish roe, sardines, and anchovies. Foods that are moderately high in purines are meats, seafood, dried beans, lentils, spinach, and peas. (6:626; 18:1002)

Nursing Process—Implementation
Client Need—Physiological integrity

94 1. The nurse withholds the administration of colchicine when the client manifests adverse gastrointestinal disturbances, such as nausea and vomiting, abdominal pain, or diarrhea. Dizziness, drowsiness,

and headache are not signs of an adverse reaction to colchicine. (17:247; 20:403)
　　Nursing Process—Implementation
　　Client Need—Physiological integrity

95 3. It is best to serve the greater share of fluid in the morning to compensate for the long period without oral fluids during the hours of sleep. Serving a large volume of fluid after a meal contributes to gastrointestinal fullness or upset. Consuming large amounts of fluid during evening hours or before bedtime usually interferes with sleep. The client is likely to be awakened with a full bladder and the need to urinate. (25:260)
　　Nursing Process—Implementation
　　Client Need—Physiological integrity

96 2. There seems to be a relationship between the consumption of alcohol and the recurrence of gout symptoms. Therefore, it is best to teach clients with gout to abstain from drinking alcohol. Coffee, cranberry juice, and carbonated beverages are safe to consume. (18:1002; 21:995)
　　Nursing Process—Implementation
　　Client Need—Health promotion/maintenance

NURSING CARE OF CLIENTS WITH DEGENERATIVE BONE DISORDERS

97 4. Estrogen replacement therapy is one method for reducing the potential for osteoporitic skeletal changes. There is nothing in the literature to substantiate recommending a premenopausal pregnancy, prolonged breast-feeding, or limiting the number of pregnancies to two or less. (18:1347; 21:1000)
　　Nursing Process—Implementation
　　Client Need—Health promotion/maintenance

98 2. Bone density is decreased with prolonged inactivity. The loss of calcium from the bones of inactive clients predisposes to forming renal stones. Brittle, porous bones are not related to indigestion and disturbed sleep patterns. A reduced fluid intake is a remote etiological factor if the client's consumption of food and liquids is deficient in calcium. (4:597; 25:1000)
　　Nursing Process—Planning
　　Client Need—Physiological integrity

99 3. Clients with osteoporosis tend to present with spinal deformities such as kyphosis (dowager's hump) or an inability to assume an erect posture. Although swollen joints, discomfort in sitting, and diminished energy are experienced by clients with osteoporo-

sis, they are not uniquely associated with this disorder. (4:597; 18:1347)
　　Nursing Process—Data collection
　　Client Need—Physiological integrity

100 2. Smoking and consumption of caffeine contribute to the severity of osteoporosis. Although aspirin, carbonated beverages, and sodium are best used in moderation, they are not considered to be pathologically related to osteoporosis. Alcohol is associated with loss of bone density. Currently it is unclear if chronic alcohol ingestion destroys bone-forming cells, interferes with calcium absorption, or contributes to osteoporosis simply because of its correlation with an inadequate nutritional intake. Supplemental calcium and consumption of dairy products are therapeutic measures for individuals who are at risk for or who have acquired osteoporosis. (4:599; 6:214–215)
　　Nursing Process—Planning
　　Client Need—Health promotion/maintenance

101 3. Supporting the limb affected by osteomyelitis and handling it gently help to reduce the risk of a pathological fracture. Meeting the client's needs for nutrition and fluids addresses the metabolic problems that accompany an infection that is often accompanied by a fever. Since the activity of a client with osteomyelitis is often limited, using pressure-relieving devices becomes imperative in maintaining the integrity of the skin. (18:997; 21:1001)
　　Nursing Process—Implementation
　　Client Need—Physiological integrity

102 1. Pott's disease is a form of tuberculosis in which the infectious bacteria localize in the spine. Although the condition is rare in the United States, its occurrence is found in foreign visitors or those who have immigrated to this country. There is no etiological relationship between Pott's disease and toxins, pollutants, or food additives. (4:997, 1196)
　　Nursing Process—Implementation
　　Client Need—Health promotion/maintenance

103 1. Vitamin D is necessary for the absorption of calcium. Exposure to sunlight helps to convert dehydrocholesterol in the skin and ergosterol, a plant precursor, to provitamins that eventually become vitamin D. The beneficial and harmful effects of eating cattle that have been injected with bovine growth hormone have not been conclusively determined. Orange vegetables are good sources of beta carotene, a precursor of vitamin A. Organically grown produce is not any more nutritious than others; however, there may be beneficial effects from coincidentally eliminating the ingestion of chemical fertilizers, herbicides, and pesticides. (6:225; 20:467)

> Nursing Process—Implementation
> Client Need—Health promotion/maintenance

NURSING CARE OF CLIENTS HAVING AMPUTATIONS

104   3. With very few exceptions, a person in shock is kept flat with the lower extremities slightly elevated. Gravity helps to maintain blood in the area of the vital organs. Supine position is a back-lying position but does not provide the added benefit of elevating the legs. Prone is a face-lying position. Keeping the client on his side interferes with the emergency assessment and care. (18:631)

> Nursing Process—Implementation
> Client Need—Physiological integrity

105   2. Staying with a grief-stricken client indicates that the nurse is there for his emotional support. The client is more likely to feel that he can depend on the nurse to be available and respond to his future needs. Leaving an uncomfortable situation is one method health professionals use to cope with their own feelings of inadequacy. The client will likely interpret the desertion as a sign that the nurse is not a caring individual. It is therapeutic for a person to release his rage as long as it does not endanger himself or others. Feeling angry is one of the early steps in the grieving process. The hospital chaplain may be helpful later, but the nurse should not leave the client alone at this time. (9:357; 18:1000)

> Nursing Process—Implementation
> Client Need—Psychosocial integrity

106   2. Phantom pain or sensation is a phenomenon experienced by some people who have a limb amputated. The person feels a physical sensation in the missing limb. The feeling ranges from a sense that the amputated part is still there or other sensations that cause discomfort, such as pain, cramping, burning, and itching. Referred pain is discomfort that is experienced in a location that is distant from the actual area of pathology. Psychogenic pain is discomfort that is emotional in origin. Intractable pain is severe and unrelenting. (18:998; 25:1008)

> Nursing Process—Implementation
> Client Need—Health promotion/maintenance

107   1. Most believe that the TENS unit generates sensations that the brain perceives in place of the pain from the missing limb. This phenomenon is referred to as the *gate-control theory*. The process is compared to a car waiting while a train crosses the highway. The impulses from the TENS unit are like the train. As long as the TENS impulses flood the brain, the pain impulses are blocked. (4:1109–1110; 25:378)

> Nursing Process—Implementation
> Client Need—Health promotion/maintenance

108   3. Sitting in a chair, especially if it is done frequently or for long periods of time, is undesirable because below-the-knee amputees are prone to developing knee flexion contractures. A knee flexion contracture interferes with wearing a prosthesis and being able to walk again. For this reason, the stump is kept in an extended or neutral position as much as possible. The prone, supine, and standing positions provide extension of the stump. (4:635; 21:1011)

> Nursing Process—Planning
> Client Need—Physiological integrity

109   3. Almost immediately after surgery, the nurse encourages the client to lift up using the trapeze, since the muscles that most need strengthening prior to ambulating with crutches are those in the arms, neck, shoulders, chest, and back. The client also may squeeze rubber balls and perform arm push-ups. Doing arm push-ups involves placing the palms flat on the bed and raising the buttocks. Some provide the client with sawed-off crutches to use in bed to condition the same muscles that are needed during ambulation. (18:1000; 21:530–531)

> Nursing Process—Planning
> Client Need—Physiological integrity

110   2. Wrapping the stump decreases stump edema. A permanent prosthesis is not constructed until the stump is cone shaped and no longer undergoing changes in size. An equal amount of compression is applied with each turn of the roller bandage. Isotonic and isometric exercises are used to tone muscles. Range of motion exercises maintain joint flexibility. Gauze dressings absorb blood and drainage. (4:635; 21:1009)

> Nursing Process—Implementation
> Client Need—Health promotion/maintenance

NURSING CARE OF CLIENTS WITH SKELETAL TUMORS

111   2. A tourniquet is kept at the bedside in the event that hemorrhage, if it should occur, cannot be controlled with elevation of the stump and direct pressure. There ought not to be an urgent need for gauze dressings. If the airway becomes compromised, the nurse maintains temporary patency by using the chin-lift/head tilt maneuver. Most clients are transferred to the nursing unit from the recovery room with oxygen already being administered. (18:999; 26:526)

Nursing Process—Planning
Client Need—Physiological integrity

112 3. If crutches are measured and fitted appropriately, there is room for at least two fingers between the axilla and the axillary bar of the crutch. Prolonged pressure under the arm affects circulation or impairs nerve function, resulting in permanent paralysis. All of the other observations are indications that the crutch length and the position of the handgrips are correct. (18:481; 25:535)

Nursing Process—Evaluation
Client Need—Physiological integrity

113 4. Malignant bone tumors cause secondary anemia if bone marrow function is disrupted. Although primary bone tumors can spread to any organ, the bowel and liver are not common metastatic sites. Anorexia may be present, but it is not due to the location of a bone tumor. (4:601)

Nursing Process—Data collection
Client Need—Physiological integrity

114 1. The most common site for bone tumor metastasis is the lungs. If tests such as a urinalysis, spinal tap, or blood glucose are done, it is for reasons other than determining if the primary tumor has metastasized. (4:601; 26:866)

Nursing Process—Data collection
Client Need—Physiological integrity

NURSING CARE OF CLIENTS WITH A HERNIATED INTERVERTEBRAL DISK

115 2. Any activity that increases intraspinal pressure, such as sneezing, causes the lower back pain to intensify. Other activities that make the pain more severe include coughing, lifting an object, and straining to have a bowel movement. Neither eating nor urinating tend to affect the intensity of pain. Resting and inactivity help relieve the pain caused by a herniated intravertebral disk. (21:579)

Nursing Process—Data collection
Client Need—Physiological integrity

116 1. Many clients feel pain radiate into their buttocks and down the leg where the herniating disk protrudes on the spinal nerve root. The sciatic nerve is commonly affected when the herniated disk occurs between lumbar vertebrae. The iliac crests, knees,

and toes are not generally symptomatic. (4:1531; 21:579)

Nursing Process—Data collection
Client Need—Physiological integrity

117 2. Diazepam relieves skeletal muscle spasm. By doing so, the client experiences a certain amount of relief from pain. Drugs, other than minor tranquilizers, are used to reduce depression, promote sleep, and relieve inflammation. (17:338, 340–341; 20:400)

Nursing Process—Implementation
Client Need—Health promotion/maintenance

118 4. Encouraging extra fluids and keeping clients quiet following a myelogram helps to prevent post-procedural headaches. Drinking fluid dilutes and hastens the excretion of the contrast medium used during a myelogram. Increasing oral fluid intake aids in replacing cerebrospinal fluid that has been withdrawn prior to or after the procedure. Keeping the room dim relieves a spinal headache once it is manifested, but it is not generally done as a standard of care following a myelogram. Food is withheld if the client becomes nauseous, but it is not routinely done. Administering sedatives at scheduled intervals following a myelogram masks early assessment of central nervous system complications. (7:738–739; 21:517)

Nursing Process—Implementation
Client Need—Physiological integrity

119 4. The client with a herniated disk rolls from side to side without twisting the spine. This type of movement prevents displacing bone grafts until they have become solidly fused. Holding one's breath increases discomfort if it is accompanied by bearing down. It is difficult to turn a patient who is curled up in a ball. (18:1001; 26:512)

Nursing Process—Planning
Client Need—Physiological integrity

120 1. Bending both knees and keeping the back straight makes best use of the longest and strongest muscles in the body. The feet are spread apart for a broad base of support. Extending the arms puts strain on weaker muscles by placing the weight of the lifted object outside the body's center of gravity. (4:235; 25:467)

Nursing Process—Implementation
Client Need—Health promotion/maintenance

Classification of Test Items

Unit **I** Review Test **2**

The Nursing Care of Clients with Musculoskeletal Disorders

Directions: After each question, the correct answer is given as well as a classification of each test question. Compare the correct answer with your answer. If a question has been answered *incorrectly*, draw a line to the end of all the columns. When finished, add up the number of your correct answers in each column and place that number in the respective box at the end in the area identified as *Number Correct*.

To determine the percentage of questions you answered correctly and your performance in each of the test plan categories, divide the *Number Correct* in each column by the *Number Possible* in each column. Then multiply the decimal by 100. For example:

$$\frac{\text{Number Correct: 95}}{\text{Number Possible: 120}} = 0.791 \times 100 = 79\%$$

Any score that is less than 75% indicates an area where further review would be beneficial.

KEY TO ITEM CLASSIFICATION:

NURSING PROCESS	CLIENT NEEDS
D = Data collection	S = Safe, effective care environment
P = Planning	P = Physiological integrity
I = Implementation	M = Psychosocial integrity
E = Evaluation	H = Health promotion/maintenance

2 I   2 I I E   1 P   2 H

	Question #	Answer #	Nursing Process				Client Needs			
			D	P	I	E	S	P	M	H
	1	2				E				H
	2	3	D					P		
	3	2			I			P		
	4	4			I			P		
	5	1			I			P		
	6	3			I					H
	7	4	D					P		
	8	3			I					H
	9	2				E				H
	10	4			I			P		
	11	2			I					H
	12	4			I		S			
	13	4			I		S			
	14	1	D					P		
	15	2	D					P		

-3
+12

3D   4I 3E 1S 6P 1M

Question #	Answer #	Nursing Process				Client Needs			
		D	P	I	E	S	P	M	H
16	1			I			P		
17	3			I			P		
18	3			I			P		
19	4	D					P		
20	1	D					P		
21	2				E				H
22	1			I					H
23	1				E	S			
24	1			I			P		
25	3		P			S			
26	1				E				H
27	2			I					H
28	4			I			P		
29	2			I					H
30	1	D					P		
31	4			I			P		
32	1			I			P		
33	3			I			P		
34	3	D					P		
35	3			I				M	
36	3				E				H
37	2		P				P		
38	3			I					H
39	1			I			P		
40	4	D					P		
41	2			I			P		
42	1			I			P		
43	1	D					P		
44	2			I			P		
45	3			I			P		
46	2		P				P		
47	2	D					P		

-10
+22

-13
+34
74%

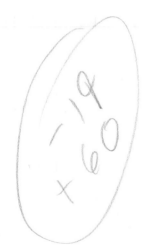

Question #	Answer #	Nursing Process				Client Needs			
		D	P	I	E	S	P	M	H
48	1			I			P		
49	3			I		S			
50	4	D					P		
51	2			I			P		
52	3	D					P		
53	4	D					P		
54	1			I					H
55	4	D					P		
56	3	D					P		
57	3			I			P		
58	1	D					P		
59	3			I			P		
60	3			I					H
61	4		P				P		
62	4				E		P		
63	1		P				P		
64	2		P						H
65	1			I					H
66	2			I					H
67	1	D					P		
68	3	D					P		
69	1	D					P		
70	4				E				H
71	3	D					P		
72	2			I			P		
73	1			I		S			
74	1			I					H
75	3				E				H
76	4		P				P		
77	2			I					H
78	1				E				H
79	4			I		S			

	Question #	Answer #	Nursing Process				Client Needs			
			D	P	I	E	S	P	M	H
	80	2			I			P		
	81	3		P				P		
	82	2			I			P		
	83	1				E				H
	84	3		P						H
	85	1		P						H
	86	2			I					H
	87	4			I					H
	88	2			I		S			
	89	3				E		P		
	90	1	D					P		
	91	3	D					P		
	92	1			I			P		
	93	4			I			P		
	94	1			I			P		
	95	3			I			P		
	96	2			I					H
	97	4			I					H
	98	2		P				P		
	99	3	D					P		
	100	2		P						H
	101	3			I			P		
	102	1			I					H
	103	1			I					H
	104	3			I			P		
	105	2			I				M	
	106	2			I					H
	107	1			I					H
	108	3		P				P		
	109	3		P				P		
	110	2			I					H
	111	2		P				P		

-24
+87

Question #	Answer #	Nursing Process				Client Needs			
		D	P	I	E	S	P	M	H
112	3				E		P		
113	4	D					P		
114	1	D					P		
115	2	D					P		
116	1	D					P		
117	2			I					H
118	4			I			P		
119	4		P				P		
120	1			I					H
Number Correct	94	22	15	49	7	5	56	1	31
Number Possible	120	28	16	63	13	8	73	2	37
Percentage Correct	78%	79%	94	78	54	63	77	50	84

Nursing Care of Clients with Venous Disorders
Nursing Care of Clients with Arterial Disorders
Nursing Care of Clients with Red Blood Cell Disorders
Nursing Care of Clients with White Blood Cell Disorders
Nursing Care of Clients with Bone Marrow Disorders

Nursing Care of Clients with Coagulation Disorders
Nursing Care of Clients with Inflammatory and Obstructive Lymphatic Disorders
Correct Answers and Rationale
Classification of Test Items

Directions: With a pencil, blacken the circle in front of the option you have chosen for your correct answer.

NURSING CARE OF CLIENTS WITH VENOUS DISORDERS

While helping a female client into stirrups for a pelvic examination, The nurse notes that the client has some large protruding leg veins.

1 Which one of the client's statements is *most suggestive* that the client has varicosed leg veins?
○ 1. "My legs feel heavy and tired by evening."
○ 2. "My feet perspire heavily during the day."
● 3. "I wake up at night with leg cramps."
○ 4. "I have pain in my shins when I jog."

2 Which nursing suggestion is *most beneficial* in helping to relieve the client's symptoms caused by varicose veins?
● 1. Elevate your legs frequently during the day.
○ 2. Wear two pair of thick cotton socks.
○ 3. Walk about when experiencing leg cramps.
○ 4. Take up something less active, like knitting.

3 Which of the following is *most important* for the nurse to tell the client with varicose veins to *avoid*?
○ 1. Walking in high heeled shoes
○ 2. Wearing nylon pantyhose
● 3. Sitting with crossed knees
○ 4. Shaving her lower legs

A 67-year-old client has developed venous stasis ulcers on her lower leg.

4 When the nurse assesses the skin lesions, the *most characteristic* finding is that the areas appear
○ 1. to contain purulent drainage.
● 2. blanched around the open area.
○ 3. dark brown, dry, and crusty.
○ 4. as a fluid-filled blister.

A physician writes a medical order for the application of wet-to-dry dressings over the venous stasis ulcers.

5 When the client asks the nurse why the dressings are being applied, the *best explanation* is that these dressings help to
○ 1. prevent wound infections.
● 2. remove dead cells and tissue.
○ 3. absorb blood and drainage.
○ 4. protect the skin from injury.

6 The *best evidence* that a stasis ulcer is healing is the size becomes smaller and
○ 1. there is more drainage.
○ 2. there is less discomfort.
● 3. the cavity appears pink.
○ 4. the wound margins are white.

Eventually the wet-to-dry dressings are discontinued and the nurse is asked to cover the client's leg ulcer with Duo-DERM, a type of air-occlusive dressing.

7 The nurse is most correct in telling the client that the main advantage in using this type of dressing is that it
○ 1. reduces the formation of scar tissue.
○ 2. relieves pain from skin irritation.
○ 3. is less expensive than gauze dressings.
● 4. speeds healing by keeping the wound moist.

A 55-year-old male truck driver is scheduled for a vein stripping procedure as treatment for his varicose veins.

8 If the nurse reads all of the following information in the truck driver's health history, which one is most related to his development of varicose veins?
   ⬤ 1. His mother also has varicose veins.
   ○ 2. He has smoked cigarettes for 20 years.
   ○ 3. He was a track athlete in high school.
   ○ 4. He tries to follow a vegetarian diet.

After the surgeon explains the vein stripping procedure to the client with varicose veins, the client asks the nurse how his blood will circulate in his legs after surgery.

9 The *best explanation* the nurse can provide is that
   ○ 1. some of the arteries begin to function as veins.
   ⬤ 2. new veins grow to replace the ones that were removed.
   ○ 3. other veins take over the work of those removed.
   ○ 4. the healthy vein ends are attached to other veins.

10 Although all of the following nursing actions are important when planning the postoperative care of a client following a vein stripping, which one is of *highest priority*?
   ○ 1. Providing the client with nutritious food
   ○ 2. Orienting the client to his surroundings
   ⬤ 3. Ambulating the client frequently
   ○ 4. Offering regular oral hygiene

Postoperatively, the client who has had the vein stripping procedure asks the nurse for medication for his pain. The physician has ordered propoxyphene hydrochloride (Darvon), 65 mg, orally every 4 hours as needed for pain.

11 When offered the propoxyphene, the client says to the nurse, "If that's Darvon, I don't want it. It makes me sick to my stomach." The *best action* the nurse can take *at this time* is to
   ○ 1. tell the client that the drug is propoxyphene.
   ○ 2. explain that this is what the physician ordered.
   ○ 3. advise him to take the drug with lots of water.
   ⬤ 4. report the information to the nurse in charge.

A 57-year-old female is recovering after having an abdominal hysterectomy two days earlier.

12 If the nurse makes all of the following observations, which one is *most likely* to predispose this client to developing venous thrombosis in a lower extremity?

   ⬤ 1. The client resists ambulation.
   ○ 2. The client breathes shallowly.
   ○ 3. The client requests analgesics frequently.
   ○ 4. The client drinks coffee excessively.

The care plan for the client who has had an abdominal hysterectomy indicates that the client should wear antiembolism stockings.

13 The *best evidence* that the antiembolism stockings are a correct size and fit for the client is that
   ○ 1. the stockings extend to mid-calf.
   ⬤ 2. the toes feel warm when touched.
   ○ 3. the stockings are easily donned.
   ○ 4. the heels do not appear reddened.

14 When the nurse assesses the client who had a hysterectomy for Homans' sign, the *most correct* technique is to
   ○ 1. have the client push each foot against the mattress.
   ⬤ 2. extend the legs and flex each foot toward the knee.
   ○ 3. sit up in bed and point all the toes forward.
   ○ 4. ask the client to contract the thigh muscles.

15 If the client who had a hysterectomy has developed a thrombus in one of her leg veins, when the nurse assesses for Homans' sign, the client will
   ⬤ 1. experience sharp calf pain immediately.
   ○ 2. complain of sudden numbness in her foot.
   ○ 3. be unable to bend her knee when asked.
   ○ 4. feel tingling throughout her affected leg.

16 Besides a positive Homans' sign, which *additional assessment finding* best supports the assumption that the client who had a hysterectomy has a thrombus in a leg vein?
   ○ 1. The foot on the affected leg appears blue.
   ○ 2. The affected leg is warmer than the other.
   ○ 3. The capillary refill takes 2 seconds.
   ⬤ 4. The lower affected leg is swollen.

17 Based on the assessments that indicate the client with the hysterectomy has a thrombus in a leg vein, which one of the following changes is *most appropriate* to add to the nursing care plan?
   ○ 1. Ambulate twice each shift
   ⬤ 2. Refrain from massaging legs
   ○ 3. Caution to avoid leg elevation
   ○ 4. Encourage active leg exercises

The physician prescribes warm moist compresses to the affected leg in which the thrombus is located.

18 Which of the following nursing actions is *correct* when applying the warm moist compress?

○ 1. The nurse heats the water to 120°F.

● 3. The nurse inspects the skin every 4 hours.

○ 4. The nurse covers the wet gauze with a towel.

The physician orders heparin calcium (Calciparine) 7500 U subcutaneously.

19 When the client asks why she is receiving the medication, the *best explanation* the nurse can give is that heparin

○ 1. helps shrink blood clots.

○ 2. helps dissolve blood clots.

● 3. prevents more clots from forming.

○ 4. prevents the clot from dislodging.

20 Before giving any and all subsequent injections of heparin calcium (Calciparine), it is *essential* for the nurse to report the results of the patient's

● 1. partial thromboplastin time (PTT).

○ 2. complete blood count (CBC).

○ 3. packed cell volume (PCV).

○ 4. prothrombin time (PT).

21 When the nurse withdraws the heparin calcium from the multidose vial, which of the following is *correct?*

○ 1. The nurse removes the rubber stopper in the top of the vial.

● 2. The nurse instills an equal volume of air as liquid to be withdrawn.

○ 3. The nurse mixes the drug by rolling it in the palms of the hands.

○ 4. The nurse shakes the drug vigorously to distribute the drug evenly.

22 When the nurse administers the heparin subcutaneously to the client who is of average weight for her height, which of the following actions is *correct?*

○ 1. The nurse selects the dorsogluteal site.

○ 2. The nurse uses a 22-gauge, 1½-inch needle.

● 3. The nurse inserts the needle at a 45-degree angle.

○ 4. The nurse massages the site immediately afterward.

23 After assessing the client who has been receiving daily injections of heparin, which finding should the nurse report *immediately?*

○ 1. The client says bathing makes her very tired.

○ 2. The client never eats all the food on her tray.

● 3. The client's gums bleed after brushing her teeth.

○ 4. The client's bowel movements occur twice a day.

24 The drug the nurse should plan to have available in case it becomes necessary to overcome the effects of heparin therapy is

○ 1. calcium lactate.

○ 2. sodium benzoate.

● 3. protamine sulfate.

○ 4. aluminum phosphate.

A nurse applies prolonged pressure to an injection site of a client who is on anticoagulant therapy.

25 The nurse's action is

○ 1. inappropriate because it promotes hematoma formation.

○ 2. inappropriate because it delays drug absorption.

○ 3. appropriate because it distributes the drug evenly.

● 4. appropriate because it diminishes blood loss.

A client will be discharged and continue taking warfarin sodium (Coumadin) on a daily basis.

26 The best evidence that this client understands his risk for bleeding is that he indicates he must report having

○ 1. dark amber urine.

● 2. tar-colored stools.

○ 3. green-tinged emesis.

○ 4. yellow skin color.

A postoperative client has been receiving intravenous fluids through the same site for several days.

27 If the client is developing phlebitis at the intravenous site, the nurse *most likely* observes that the vein

● 1. appears red and feels warm.

○ 2. looks dark and feels cool.

○ 3. seems pale and feels hard.

○ 4. is purplish and feels spongy.

28 The *most appropriate* action the nurse can take if a phlebitis is suspected at an intravenous site is to

○ 1. elevate the extremity where the fluid is infusing.

○ 2. apply pressure to the current intravenous site.

○ 3. administer the intravenous solution at a faster rate.

● 4. remove the needle or catheter from the current site.

NURSING CARE OF CLIENTS WITH ARTERIAL DISORDERS

An older adult who is a resident in a nursing home has arteriosclerosis.

29 Which of the following physical assessments is *common* among individuals with arterial insufficiency secondary to peripheral arteriosclerosis?
- ● 1. The toenails are thick and tough.
- ○ 2. Hair growth on the legs is extensive.
- ○ 3. Knee jerk reflexes are hyperactive.
- ○ 4. Peripheral pulses are bounding.

30 When a client with peripheral arterial insufficiency actively exercises, which is most likely to occur?
- ○ 1. Cyanosis of the feet
- ○ 2. Burning of the toes
- ● 3. Pain in both legs
- ○ 4. Sensitivity to the sun

31 If the client with peripheral arterial insufficiency tells the nurse her feet are cold, which of the following nursing actions is *best*?
- ○ 1. Apply a hot water bottle
- ○ 2. Use an electric heating pad
- ● 3. Wrap them in a warm blanket
- ○ 4. Elevate her feet on a stool

The nurse prepares to use a Doppler ultrasound device to assess blood flow through the dorsalis pedis artery.

32 Which of the following actions is *correct* when using the Doppler device?
- ○ 1. The nurse places the probe beside the ankle.
- ● 2. The nurse applies acoustic gel to the skin.
- ○ 3. The nurse records the time of capillary refill.
- ○ 4. The nurse measures the temperature of the skin.

A 36-year-old woman who has had Raynaud's disease for several years comes to donate a unit of blood during a blood drive.

33 In which part of the body can the nurse expect the client's symptoms to be *chiefly located*?
- ○ 1. In her legs
- ● 2. In her hands
- ○ 3. In her chest
- ○ 4. In her neck

34 Which one of the following would the client with Raynaud's disease *most likely* correlate with the onset of her discomfort?
- ○ 1. Exposure to heat
- ● 2. Exposure to cold
- ○ 3. Exposure to sun
- ○ 4. Exposure to wind

35 The teaching plan for clients with Raynaud's disease includes explaining that it is important to *avoid*
- ● 1. wearing gloves.
- ○ 2. emotional stress.
- ○ 3. drinking alcoholic beverages.
- ○ 4. bathing with perfumed soap.

A 32-year-old male has been diagnosed as having thromboangiitis obliterans, also known as Buerger's disease.

36 When the client describes his earliest symptoms, he is *most likely* to tell the nurse that he experienced
- ○ 1. a heavy feeling in his lower extremities.
- ○ 2. frequent problems with ingrown toenails.
- ● 3. leg pain accompanying walking or exercise.
- ○ 4. swollen feet at the end of the day.

37 When the nurse palpates the peripheral pulses in the lower extremities of the client with thromboangiitis obliterans (Buerger's disease), the *most common finding* is that they feel
- ○ 1. strong.
- ○ 2. normal.
- ○ 3. full.
- ● 4. weak.

38 If the client with thromboangiitis obliterans (Buerger's disease) understands the potential complications from his disease process, he will tell the nurse that it is *most important* for him to regularly see a(n)
- ● 1. podiatrist for foot care.
- ○ 2. dietitian for weight control.
- ○ 3. ophthalmologist for eye care.
- ○ 4. counselor for emotional therapy.

The physician discusses the possibility of treating the client with thromboangiitis obliterans (Buerger's disease) by performing a sympathectomy.

39 The *best evidence* that the client understood the physician's explanation of the purpose for this surgical procedure is when he says that a sympathectomy will
- ● 1. promote vasodilation.
- ○ 2. aid muscle relaxation.
- ○ 3. relieve mental stress.
- ○ 4. slow his heart rate.

The client with thromboangiitis obliterans (Buerger's disease) is taught to perform Buerger-Allen exercises.

40 When the client returns the nurse's demonstration, he is performing these exercises *correctly* if he lies flat with his legs elevated for several minutes and then
- ○ 1. sits on the edge of the bed.
- ● 2. stands and touches his toes.
- ○ 3. jogs in place at the bedside
- ○ 4. pretends to climb stairs.

41 When preparing the client with thromboangiitis obliterans (Buerger's disease) to manage his disorder, it is essential that the nurse plan to inform him that
○ 1. heavy lifting is contraindicated.
○ 2. use of tobacco must be avoided.
◉ 3. airplane travel is restricted.
○ 4. sexual activity is prohibited.

In addition to evidence of an intestinal disorder, an older client who is undergoing an abdominal x-ray is found to have an arterial aneurysm in his abdominal aorta.

42 When the nurse collects assessment data, which information in the client's history is the *most predisposing factor* to the formation of an aortic aneurysm?
○ 1. The client is lactose-intolerant.
◉ 2. The client has chronic hypertension.
○ 3. The client has a sedentary lifestyle.
○ 4. The client takes digoxin (Lanoxin).

43 When conducting a physical assessment of the client with an abdominal aortic aneurysm, which of the following is the nurse most likely to find?
○ 1. The client's feet show signs of edema.
○ 2. The client's bowel sounds are hypoactive.
○ 3. There are multiple abdominal petichiae.
◉ 4. There is a pulsating abdominal mass.

44 If the client has a correct understanding of the physician's explanation of his condition, he will tell the nurse that an aneurysm is
○ 1. a weakened valve in a major blood vessel.
○ 2. a stationary blood clot in a large vein.
○ 3. a fatty deposit in the wall of an artery.
◉ 4. an outpouching in the wall of an artery.

A 78-year-old client who resides in a long-term care facility also has an abdominal aortic aneurysm for which she has refused surgical treatment.

45 Which one of the following symptoms is the client *most likely* to manifest if the aneurysm becomes *larger* or begins to *dissect*?
○ 1. Hematuria
○ 2. Indigestion
○ 3. Rectal bleeding
◉ 4. Low back pain

Several years ago the client with the abdominal aortic aneurysm prepared an advance directive indicating that she did not want heroic measures performed to sustain her life. The physician wrote a "do not resuscitate" order on her medical record.

46 If the client loses consciousness and remains unresponsive, the *next action* the nurse should take is to

○ 1. have her transferred to the hospital.
○ 2. call the local ambulance service.
◉ 3. notify her attending physician.
○ 4. call her immediate next of kin.

NURSING CARE OF CLIENTS WITH RED BLOOD CELL DISORDERS

The complete blood count of a 71-year-old client indicates that his erythrocytes are below normal.

47 If the client has all of the following conditions, which one is the *most likely explanation* for the client's red blood cell loss?
○ 1. Mitral valve regurgitation
○ 2. Arteriosclerotic heart disease
◉ 3. Peptic ulcer disease
○ 4. Prostatic hypertrophy

48 Once the cause of the client's low red blood cell count is being treated, which nursing instruction is most appropriate for reducing his lethargy?
○ 1. Get at least 8 hours of sleep.
○ 2. Breathe deeply whenever possible.
○ 3. Eat more simple carbohydrates.
◉ 4. Take frequent rest periods.

An 18-year-old female college student has been feeling extremely tired and makes an appointment at the university's health office.

49 Which one of the following laboratory tests can the nurse expect to be *lower than normal* if the cause of the client's fatigue is due to iron-deficiency anemia?
○ 1. Prothrombin time
○ 2. Bleeding time
○ 3. Fibrinogen level
◉ 4. Hemoglobin level

50 If the college student with anemia provides the health service nurse with all of the following information, which one is *most related* to her anemia?
○ 1. She has chronic constipation.
○ 2. She experiences menstrual cramps.
◉ 3. She feels chilled most of the time.
○ 4. She had rheumatic fever as a child.

The nurse takes a diet history from the client with iron-deficiency anemia.

51 If the client says she consumes *very little* of the following foods, which one *most likely* contributes to her iron-deficiency anemia?
○ 1. Milk
◉ 2. Meat
○ 3. Fruit
○ 4. Candy

The physician prescribes ferrous sulfate (Feosol) 1 tablet orally t.i.d. for the college student with iron deficiency anemia.

52   For the *best absorption* of oral iron preparations the nurse is *most accurate* in telling the client to take ferrous sulfate
   ○ 1. between meals.
   ◉ 2. with each meal.
   ○ 3. just before eating.
   ○ 4. just before bedtime.

53   To *potentiate* the *maximum absorption* of the oral iron supplement, the nurse is *most accurate* in advising the college student to take the tablet with
   ○ 1. milk.
   ○ 2. tea.
   ○ 3. a soft drink.
   ◉ 4. orange juice.

54   If the college student understands the nurse's explanation concerning the effects from taking iron, she will say that this drug will cause her stools to become
   ○ 1. medium brown.
   ◉ 2. quite black.
   ○ 3. clay-colored.
   ○ 4. light green.

An 80-year-old client who resides in a nursing home has difficulty swallowing the capsule of iron that the physician has prescribed. The physician changes the medical order to a liquid preparation.

55   When the nurse plans the administration of the liquid iron preparation, it is *essential* to give it
   ◉ 1. through a straw.
   ○ 2. in a paper cup.
   ○ 3. with a metal spoon.
   ○ 4. without any water.

A 42-year-old female develops anemia due to heavy menstrual blood loss.

56   When the office nurse interviews the client, which of the following information is *most likely related* to her anemia?
   ◉ 1. She fainted last week at work.
   ○ 2. She has occasional insomnia.
   ○ 3. Her gallbladder has been removed.
   ○ 4. Her abdomen is somewhat tender.

57   During the physical assessment of the anemic client, the nurse is *most likely* to observe that her skin appears
   ○ 1. mottled.
   ○ 2. flushed.
   ◉ 3. pale.
   ○ 4. blue.

The physician instructs the office nurse to administer iron dextran (InFeD) intramuscularly to the client with anemia due to blood loss. The nurse will administer the injection by Z-track (zig-zag) technique.

58   Which one of the following muscles is *best* for the nurse to plan on using when giving the injection by Z-track technique?
   ○ 1. Deltoid
   ○ 2. Trapezius
   ◉ 3. Gluteus medius
   ○ 4. Latissimus dorsi

59   The *best reason* the nurse can give the client for administering the injection by Z-track technique is that iron dextran stains superficial tissue and therefore, is
   ○ 1. absorbed slowly.
   ◉ 2. sealed deeply.
   ○ 3. instilled quickly.
   ○ 4. massaged vigorously.

60   When administering an injection using the Z-track technique, just before inserting the needle into the muscle, the nurse is *correct* to pull the tissue at the injection site
   ◉ 1. laterally.
   ○ 2. diagonally.
   ○ 3. downward.
   ○ 4. upward.

A 50-year-old female is suspected of having pernicious anemia. She is hospitalized for diagnostic purposes.

61   If the nurse writes all of the following information on a traditional, source-oriented record using narrative charting, which one contains *inappropriate information* in the nurses' notes?
   ○ 1. States, "I get nauseated when I eat."
   ◉ 2. Has Medicare insurance for health care.
   ○ 3. Skin over back and buttocks is flushed.
   ○ 4. Has asked to see a Presbyterian minister.

62   If the client with pernicious anemia has developed neurologic symptoms, she is *most likely* to describe to the nurse that she has
   ◉ 1. numbness and tingling in the extremities.
   ○ 2. morning headaches and sudden dizziness.
   ○ 3. restlessness and sleep pattern disturbances.
   ○ 4. periods of temporary amnesia and fainting.

The physician orders a Schilling test.

63   The nurse is *accurate* in telling the client with possible pernicious anemia that a Schilling test involves collecting

○ 1. urine.
● 2. blood.
○ 3. stool.
○ 4. sputum.

The Schilling test confirms that the client has pernicious anemia.

64 When the client with pernicious anemia asks the nurse how her disorder will be treated, the *best answer* is that the physician will probably prescribe
 ○ 1. blood transfusions.
 ○ 2. iron medication.
 ● 3. vitamin B₁₂ injections.
 ○ 4. vitamin K injections.

65 The nurse is correct in stating that pernicious anemia is also *common* among people who have had
 ○ 1. their stomach removed.
 ● 2. any type of hepatitis.
 ○ 3. exposure to toxic wastes.
 ○ 4. severe allergic reactions.

The nursing unit is informed to expect a 30-year-old male who is experiencing a sickle cell crisis.

66 If this new admission fits the profile of individuals in the United States with sickle cell anemia, the nurse can expect that his ethnic background is
 ○ 1. Mexican American
 ○ 2. Asian American
 ○ 3. Native American
 ● 4. African American

67 During the admission assessment, which one of the following can the nurse attribute to the client's blood disease?
 ○ 1. His tongue is white.
 ○ 2. His urine is cloudy.
 ● 3. He is jaundiced.
 ○ 4. He is nauseated.

68 During a sickle cell crisis, which problem is most likely the *priority* for nursing care?
 ○ 1. Improving nutrition
 ○ 2. Controlling pain
 ● 3. Assisting ventilation
 ○ 4. Relieving anxiety

69 When the nurse observes that the knee of the client with sickle cell anemia is swollen, which nursing measures is *most appropriate* to add to the plan of care?
 ○ 1. Perform passive range of motion during each shift.
 ● 2. Help to change positions to achieve comfort.
 ○ 3. Ambulate the client at frequent intervals.
 ○ 4. Encourage quadriceps setting exercises.

70 Which one of the following nursing interventions is the *best approach* for maintaining tissue perfusion during a sickle cell crisis?
 ○ 1. Provide a large intake of fluids.
 ○ 2. Apply thigh-high elastic stockings.
 ○ 3. Elevate the lower extremities.
 ● 4. Dangle on the side of the bed.

71 The *best evidence* that the client understands a factor that precipitates a sickle cell crisis is when he identifies
 ○ 1. obesity.
 ○ 2. fatigue.
 ● 3. overexertion.
 ○ 4. overhydration.

72 When a client asks the significance of having sickle cell trait, the *best answer* from the nurse is that people with sickle cell trait
 ○ 1. manifest the disease later in life.
 ● 2. have a milder form of disease symptoms.
 ○ 3. do not develop symptoms of the disease.
 ○ 4. have a much shorter life expectancy.

NURSING CARE OF CLIENTS WITH WHITE BLOOD CELL DISORDERS

A nurse cares for a 70-year-old male with chronic myelogenous leukemia.

73 All of the following assessment information is reported; which one *most indicates* a possible infection?
 ○ 1. Blood in the stool
 ○ 2. Prolonged vomiting
 ● 3. Cloudy urine
 ○ 4. Extreme fatigue

The nurse notes that the leukemia client's mouth bleeds after he brushes his teeth.

74 Which of the following is the *best alternative* for mouth care at this time?
 ● 1. Use foam mouth swabs.
 ○ 2. Use only dental floss.
 ○ 3. Discontinue oral hygiene.
 ○ 4. Eliminate the use of toothpaste.

75 When the nurse helps the leukemia patient who has an ulcerated mouth select foods from his menu, which one of the following foods is *best*?
 ○ 1. Spaghetti with meatballs
 ○ 2. Grilled cheese sandwich
 ○ 3. Salad with French dressing
 ● 4. Creamed potato soup

A leukemic client is receiving antineoplastic drugs to treat his disease.

76   The nurse should plan to prepare the client for which one of the following *common side effects?*
   ◉ 1. Hair loss
   ○ 2. Body rash
   ○ 3. Constipation
   ○ 4. Headaches

Laboratory test results indicate that the client with leukemia has a low platelet count.

77   Which one of the following nursing interventions is *most appropriate* at this time?
   ○ 1. Limit the client's visitors to family.
   ○ 2. Place the client in protective isolation.
   ◉ 3. Use small-gauge needles for injections.
   ○ 4. Provide rest periods between activities.

The physician tells a client who has been receiving drug therapy for his leukemia that his condition is in remission.

78   The client understands what this term means if he tells the nurse that
   ○ 1. he will never need cancer treatment again.
   ○ 2. he will need drugs again in a few months.
   ○ 3. his disease has responded to treatment.
   ◉ 4. his disease is cured at the present time.

A client with terminal leukemia will be discharged in a few days. Although the client's condition is stable, the physician has discussed with the client and his family that he will probably not survive more than 6 more months.

79   To which one of the following organizations is it *best* to refer this client and his family?
   ○ 1. Public health department
   ○ 2. Centers for Disease Control and Prevention
   ◉ 3. The local hospice organization
   ○ 4. The local United Way

A young college student contracts infectious mononucleosis.

80   When the student asks the health service nurse how she acquired this condition, the *best answer* is that the virus causing this disease is transmitted by
   ○ 1. contact with microorganisms in blood.
   ◉ 2. direct contact with an infected person.
   ○ 3. consuming contaminated food or water.
   ○ 4. the bite of an insect, such as a mosquito.

81   Which one of the following is likely to have been one of the *first symptoms* experienced by a client with infectious mononucleosis?

   ○ 1. Abdominal discomfort
   ◉ 2. Aching joints
   ○ 3. Sore throat
   ○ 4. Intestinal upset

82   Which one of the following is *essential* for the nurse to stress when discussing self-care with the client with infectious mononucleosis?
   ○ 1. Complying with antibiotic therapy
   ◉ 2. Restricting physical activity
   ○ 3. Taking supplemental vitamins
   ○ 4. Returning for blood transfusions

A 32 year-old male with Hodgkin's disease, is being admitted to the hospital.

83   If this client is typical of most people who develop Hodgkin's disease, one of the *chief manifestations* is
   ◉ 1. severe itching.
   ○ 2. unsteady gait.
   ○ 3. frequent headaches.
   ○ 4. chronic diarrhea.

84   When performing a physical assessment of the client in the early stages of Hodgkin's disease, the nurse is *most likely* to find that the client's lymph nodes are
   ◉ 1. enlarged and painless.
   ○ 2. small and firm.
   ○ 3. swollen and tender.
   ○ 4. fixed and hard.

The client with Hodgkin's disease will undergo external radiation of his cervical and axillary lymph nodes.

85   Which of the following instructions should the teaching plan include when preparing a client for radiation therapy?
   ○ 1. "Don't get skin in your axillae and neck wet."
   ◉ 2. "Don't use any deodorants with aluminum hydroxide."
   ○ 3. "Shave the hair from your neck and axillae daily."
   ○ 4. "After each treatment apply zinc oxide ointment."

86   What is the *best response* when the client who is receiving external radiation becomes concerned that his skin is reddened?
   ○ 1. Explain that this is an expected outcome with radiation.
   ◉ 2. Tell him that the heat from radiation causes vasodilation.
   ○ 3. Inform him that the redness indicates superficial bleeding.
   ○ 4. Reassure him that the redness is hardly noticeable.

The client with Hodgkin's disease will continue his radiation treatment as an outpatient following his hospital discharge.

87 Before the client goes home, the *most important* information to include in his discharge instructions is that when he goes outside, he should
- ○ 1. wear several layers of warm clothing.
- ○ 2. avoid becoming chilled or too warm.
- ○ 3. wear a mask to filter dust and pollen.
- ◉ 4. protect his irradiated skin from sunlight.

A client with advanced non-Hodgkin's lymphoma is being treated with antineoplastic drugs to control his condition.

88 Which one of the following should be reported *immediately* because it indicates that the client receiving cancer chemotherapy needs to be placed in reverse (protective) isolation?
- ○ 1. The client has anorexia and loses weight.
- ○ 2. The client experiences frequent diarrhea.
- ◉ 3. The client has a low white blood cell count.
- ○ 4. The client becomes disoriented and confused.

When the client with non-Hodgkin's lymphoma does not respond to medical treatment, the physician asks the nurse to accompany him when he tells the client that his condition is terminal.

89 Which nursing action is *most helpful* in assisting the client with terminal disease deal with his impending death?
- ○ 1. Provide literature on death and dying.
- ○ 2. Allow him privacy to think by himself.
- ◉ 3. Let him talk about how he is feeling.
- ○ 4. Encourage him to get a second opinion.

A 24-year-old male makes an appointment with his physician because he has been losing weight and has noted swollen lymph nodes in his axillae and groin.

90 If the client tells the nurse all of the following, which one places him at *high risk* for acquired immunodeficiency syndrome (AIDS)?
- ○ 1. He had surgery 6 months ago.
- ○ 2. He went to Mexico on his vacation.
- ○ 3. He breeds and sells poodles.
- ◉ 4. He is an intravenous drug user.

The physician orders several laboratory tests on the client who may have acquired immunodeficiency syndrome.

91 Which laboratory test is *most specific* for diagnosing antibodies to the human immunodeficiency virus (HIV)?
- ○ 1. Schick test
- ○ 2. Dick test

- ◉ 3. Enzyme-linked immunosorbent assay (ELISA) test
- ○ 4. Veneral disease research laboratory (VDRL) test

92 Which one of the following nursing practices is *best* to prevent acquiring AIDS from a person of unknown infectious status?
- ○ 1. Wearing a face mask when changing a dressing.
- ◉ 2. Refraining from capping needles after injections.
- ○ 3. Wearing a cover-gown when giving a bed bath.
- ○ 4. Donning gloves before taking a client's vital signs.

A client with AIDS is admitted with an opportunistic respiratory infection. He makes statements to the nurse that imply a sense of hopelessness.

93 Which one of the following nursing approaches is *most therapeutic* to plan at this time?
- ○ 1. Encouraging him to set small, daily goals.
- ◉ 2. Making a referral to the hospital chaplain.
- ○ 3. Planning periodic distractions, such as television.
- ○ 4. Recommending that he contact a lawyer.

NURSING CARE OF CLIENTS WITH BONE MARROW DISORDERS

A client with polycythemia vera has an enlarged spleen.

94 The position that will provide the *most comfort* for the client with an enlarged spleen is
- ○ 1. sitting upright.
- ◉ 2. lying on the back.
- ○ 3. lying on the side.
- ○ 4. elevating the legs.

95 To prevent the formation of blood clots when a person has polycythemia, the *best nursing action* is to
- ○ 1. provide protein foods.
- ◉ 2. increase fluid intake.
- ○ 3. restrict dietary sodium.
- ○ 4. encourage weight loss.

The physician tells the client with polycythemia that a phlebotomy will be performed.

96 The *best evidence* that the client understands the physician's explanation is when he tells the nurse that
- ○ 1. blood will be removed from his vein.
- ○ 2. tourniquets will be applied to his arms.
- ○ 3. some veins will be surgically occluded.
- ◉ 4. he will receive a blood transfusion.

97 Which symptom, if manifested by a client with polycythemia vera, should the nurse recognize as a *consequence* of the disorder?
- ● 1. Angina
- ○ 2. Dyspepsia
- ○ 3. Dysuria
- ○ 4. Anorexia

The physician plans to perform a bone marrow aspiration on a 67-year-old client who has had unexplained low counts of all blood cell components. The physician suspects aplastic anemia.

98 If the nurse has explained the anatomic location for the bone marrow aspiration in terms that the client can understand, to which area will the client point when asked to identify the site where the specimen will be taken?
- ● 1. The posterior hip
- ○ 2. The lower spine
- ○ 3. The upper arm
- ○ 4. The groin area

99 One of the *chief responsibilities* of the nurse during a bone marrow aspiration is helping to
- ● 1. minimize discomfort.
- ○ 2. hold instruments.
- ○ 3. regulate suction.
- ○ 4. administer oxygen.

100 After a bone marrow aspiration has been completed, it is *essential* for the nurse to monitor
- ○ 1. trends in the blood pressure.
- ● 2. bleeding from the puncture site.
- ○ 3. changes in the client's pulse.
- ○ 4. the client's level of consciousness.

The results of the bone marrow aspiration confirm that the client has aplastic anemia.

101 When the client with aplastic anemia is bathing, which one of the following observations is the *best indication* that she is having difficulty tolerating the current level of activity?
- ● 1. She becomes short of breath.
- ○ 2. She feels extremely nauseated.
- ○ 3. Her pulse rate drops below 60.
- ○ 4. Her skin becomes moist and cool.

102 When the nurse performs a physical assessment on the client with aplastic anemia, which finding is *most likely* due to a low number of platelets?
- ● 1. Multiple bruises
- ○ 2. Coarse body hair
- ○ 3. Thick toenails
- ○ 4. Cool extremities

103 Because the client with aplastic anemia has a reduced leukocyte count, it is *most important* for all caregivers to
- ● 1. perform conscientious handwashing.
- ○ 2. relieve pressure over bony prominences.
- ○ 3. provide daily high-protein nourishment.
- ○ 4. monitor heart rate and rhythm each shift.

The physician tells the client with aplastic anemia that she will be receiving 2 units of packed blood cells.

104 When the client asks how packed cells are different from the usual blood transfusion, the nurse is *most correct* in explaining that packed cells
- ○ 1. contain the same blood cells in less fluid volume.
- ● 2. contain more blood cells in the same fluid volume.
- ○ 3. are less likely to cause an allergic reaction.
- ○ 4. will stimulate her own bone marrow to function.

The client with aplastic anemia has type A, Rh positive blood.

105 If all of the following units of packed cells are available for transfusion, which one should the nurse *refuse* to administer because it is *incompatible* for this client?
- ○ 1. A, Rh negative
- ○ 2. O, Rh positive
- ○ 3. O, Rh negative
- ● 4. AB, Rh positive

106 During the first 15 minutes of the infusion, which of the following is *most indicative* that the client is experiencing a transfusion reaction?
- ○ 1. The client feels an urgent need to urinate.
- ● 2. The client's blood pressure becomes low.
- ○ 3. There is localized swelling at the infusion site.
- ○ 4. The skin is pale at the site of the infusing blood.

A 58-year-old female with aplastic anemia tells the nurse that she has been receiving corticosteroid treatment for more than 1 year in an effort to treat her disease.

107 While the nurse examines the client, which assessment finding is *most likely* due to the administration of corticosteroids?
- ○ 1. The client's voice is quite husky.
- ● 2. The client's face is moon-shaped.
- ○ 3. The client's muscles are large.
- ○ 4. The client's skin looks tanned.

108 Which one of the following statements is *most indicative* that the client with aplastic anemia has a complication from the use of corticosteroid administration?
1. The client says, "I've been experiencing such heartburn lately."
2. The client says, "I've been taking long naps during the day."
3. The client says, "I seem to have lost my appetite."
4. The client says, "I've noticed that my urine is light yellow."

Because corticosteroid therapy has not been effective, the client with aplastic anemia has consented to have a bone marrow transplant. She undergoes total body irradiation.

109 Just prior to and for several weeks following the bone marrow transplant, the *highest* priority when planning the nursing care of this client is
1. relieving depression.
2. promoting nutrition.
3. preventing infection.
4. monitoring hydration.

NURSING CARE OF CLIENTS WITH COAGULATION DISORDERS

The physician makes a tentative medical diagnosis of idiopathic thrombocytopenia and notes that the client has purpura.

110 When conducting the physical assessment the nurse looks for
1. small skin hemorrhages.
2. dark areas of cyanosis.
3. flushed red skin.
4. protruding veins.

111 When the nursing team plans the care of the client with thrombocytopenia, one of the *priorities* must include
1. encouraging fluids.
2. promoting activity.
3. restricting visitors.
4. preventing injury.

Before discharging a client with hemophilia who experienced a minor closed head injury, the nurse reviews the signs and symptoms that indicate bleeding.

112 The *best evidence* that the client understands his discharge instructions is if he identifies an *early indication* of intracranial bleeding as

1. convulsions.
2. drowsiness.
3. ringing in the ears.
4. diminished appetite.

A client with hemophilia is concerned about becoming HIV-positive from receiving transfusions of publicly donated blood.

113 Which of the following is the *most accurate response* to the comment made by the client with hemophilia?
1. Blood donors are tested before their blood is accepted.
2. No donated blood contains the virus causing AIDS anymore.
3. Donated blood is tested for AIDS antibodies once collected.
4. There is no way to identify the AIDS virus in blood yet.

NURSING CARE OF CLIENTS WITH INFLAMMATORY AND OBSTRUCTIVE LYMPHATIC DISORDERS

An infection develops where an older female has been scratched on her arm by her cat.

114 A sign that the infection is complicated by lymphangitis is
1. the arm becomes stiff near the joints.
2. red streaks extend up the client's arm.
3. there is progressively ascending numbness.
4. there is serous drainage from the wound.

A nurse reads in the transfer form that an older adult female who has just been admitted to the nursing home has lymphedema of her right arm.

115 If the client's medical history reveals all of the following, which one is *most likely* to have contributed to the development of the lymphedema?
1. The client has a healed fracture of the humerus.
2. The client had a radical mastectomy years ago.
3. The client is being treated for pernicious anemia.
4. The client was immunized for smallpox as a child.

116 Which one of the following is essential when planning the care of the client with lymphedema?
1. Avoid giving injections in her right arm.
2. Avoid turning the client on her right side.
3. Avoid active exercise of her right arm.
4. Avoid use of nail polish on her right hand.

Correct Answers and Rationale

The Nursing Care of Clients with Peripheral Vascular, Hematologic, and Lymphatic Disorders

Directions: Two numbers appear in parentheses following each rationale. The first number identifies the textbook listed in the references, page 512, and the second number identifies the page(s) in that textbook on which the correct answer can be verified. Occasionally two or more textbooks are given to verify the correct answer.

NURSING CARE OF CLIENTS WITH VENOUS DISORDERS

1 1. Most people with varicose veins describe that their legs ache and feel heavy and tired. At night, symptoms are relieved because the impaired circulation is most prominent when the person sits or stands for a long period of time. Leg pain during activity is more likely to be caused by inadequate arterial blood flow or a sport-related injury. (4:774; 21:385)
Nursing Process—Data collection
Client Need—Physiological integrity

2 1. Symptoms associated with varicose veins are relieved by elevating the legs periodically during the day. Other techniques that improve venous circulation, such as isometric or isotonic exercise, also are helpful. Wearing cotton socks does not provide symptomatic relief from varicose veins; wearing elastic support hose, however, is beneficial. Walking helps improve venous circulation, but this should be done frequently throughout the day. Knitting does not promote venous circulation because it generally involves sitting for long periods of time. (4:774; 21:386)
Nursing Process—Implementation
Client Need—Health promotion/maintenance

3 3. Clients with varicose veins must avoid anything that promotes venous stasis like sitting with crossed knees, standing for long periods of time, wearing tight undergarments or knee-high stockings. Walking promotes circulation whether low-heeled or high-heeled shoes are worn. Pantyhose are better than hose that end at the calf. Shaving the legs is not contraindicated. (4:775; 21:386)
Nursing Process—Implementation
Client Need—Health promotion/maintenance

4 3. Stasis ulcers appear darkly pigmented, dry, and scaly. Venous congestion causes edema. The localized swelling interferes with adequate arterial blood flow, causing poor oxygenation and nourishment of skin tissue. This combined with the retention of metabolic wastes leads to inflammation of the skin, sometimes referred to as cellulitis. The inflamed tissue chronically breaks open, forming craters that are difficult to heal. (4:775–776)
Nursing Process—Data collection
Client Need—Physiological integrity

5 2. Wet-to-dry dressings provide a means for debriding the ulcerated areas of necrotic tissue. Although covering impaired skin reduces the entrance of microorganisms, absorbs drainage, and protects the skin, they are not the primary reasons for their use. (4:775; 18:643)
Nursing Process—Implementation
Client Need—Health promotion/maintenance

6 3. The appearance of pink tissue indicates that granulation tissue is being formed. Granulation tissue consists of capillaries and fibrous collagen that seals and nourishes the tissue. An increase in drainage suggests that cellular death is continuing or the wound is infected. Relief of discomfort is a positive sign; however, venous ulcers are not severely painful even in the acute stage. White or black wound margins suggest an extension of cell death. (4:465; 25:566)
Nursing Process—Evaluation
Client Need—Physiological integrity

7 4. A moist wound undergoes accelerated healing. An air occlusive dressing prevents evaporation of wound moisture. The moist environment allows healing by second intention to occur at a more rapid rate. Some feel that the reason healing is faster using an air occlusive dressing is that by preventing oxygen from reaching the wound externally, capillary growth to the wound is stimulated. This type of dressing can remain in place for up to 7 days unless it comes loose or there are signs of an infection. Air occlusive dressings, like DuoDERM, are initially more expensive than traditional gauze dressings. The need for less frequent changing tends to reduce the initial cost for some individuals. (25:570)

Nursing Process—Implementation
Client Need—Health promotion/maintenance

8 1. Heredity is a predisposing factor in developing varicose veins. Other contributing factors include occupations that require prolonged standing or sitting, obesity, and the pressure on veins from an enlarging uterus during the later months of pregnancy. Although smoking is definitely unhealthy, nicotine has a major vasoconstricting effect on arterioles rather than veins. An active lifestyle or athletic exercise is more likely beneficial for the cardiovascular system. Eating a vegetarian diet, as long as it contains all the essential amino acids, generally promotes health rather than endangers it. (18:1121; 21:385)

Nursing Process—Data collection
Client Need—Health promotion/maintenance

9 3. Following a vein-stripping procedure, blood returns to the right side of the heart through other veins that are deeper in the leg. Arteries cannot transport both oxygenated and unoxygenated blood. New veins are not formed as replacements. The ends of the removed veins are sutured closed. They are not reconnected to other blood vessels. (21:386)

Nursing Process—Implementation
Client Need—Health promotion/maintenance

10 3. Early and frequent ambulation is essential following vein stripping and vein ligation surgery. During the immediate postoperative period, walking is ordered hourly while the client is awake. Even during the night, the client is aroused and assisted to walk several times. Walking helps to promote venous circulation that has been temporarily compromised by the removal of some leg veins. Most individuals having surgery can reduce their intake of food for a short period of time without severe consequences. Orienting a confused person is important, but disorientation is not usually a problem among most surgical clients. Oral hygiene is a basic component of good nursing care. However, if ambulation is not performed, the client is at risk for developing postoperative complications. (18:1121)

Nursing Process—Planning
Client Need—Physiological integrity

11 4. When a person states that an unfavorable reaction is experienced when taking a particular medication, the drug is withheld and the information reported to the nurse in charge or the physician. It is unethical to try to deceive a client by giving the generic name for a drug. A medical order is changed by consulting with the physician. Taking phene with a lot of water is not likely prevent gastrointestinal upset. (4:407;

Nursing Process—Implementation
Client Need—Physiological integrity

12 1. Thrombi most often form as a result of venous stasis. A common cause of venous stasis is inactivity. Postoperative clients are encouraged to perform active leg exercises and to ambulate frequently to promote venous circulation. Shallow breathing predisposes to pneumonia. Analgesics may make clients lethargic and less willing to ambulate, but relieving pain is not a direct cause of thrombus formation. Caffeine constricts arteries and arterioles, which can impair blood flow, but thrombi generally form in veins.(21:356; 25:551)

Nursing Process—Data collection
Client Need—Physiological integrity

13 2. Besides premeasuring the circumference of the calf from the heel to the popliteal space, signs of adequate circulation provide evidence that the antiembolism stockings are of correct size and fit. The toes should feel warm. The capillary refill should occur in less than 3 seconds. Antiembolism stockings should cover the entire calf. If antiembolism stockings are easily donned, they are too large for the client. Antiembolism stockings are not intended to prevent redness of the heels. (25:554)

Nursing Process—Evaluation
Client Need—Physiological integrity

14 2. Checking Homans' sign, an assessment used to detect venous thrombosis, is correctly performed by having the client extend each leg separately and dorsiflex the foot. None of the actions and positions in the other options are described correctly. (18:636; 25:553)

Nursing Process—Data collection
Client Need—Physiological integrity

15 1. If the client experiences pain in the calf immediately after dorsiflexing the foot, there is a possibility that the discomfort is due to a thrombus. Numbness, tingling, and impaired function are not classic signs of phlebothrombosis. (21:357)

Nursing Process—Data collection
Client Need—Physiological integrity

16 4. The area distal to the thrombus tends to swell due to the stasis of venous blood and redistribution of plasma to the interstitial space from increased hydrostatic pressure in the capillaries. Below the thrombus, the leg feels cool and looks pale. A normal capillary filling time is less than 3 seconds. (4:773)

Nursing Process—Data collection
Client Need—Physiological integrity

17 2. Whenever a thrombus is suspected, the legs must not be massaged. Activity is generally restricted. Ambulation, exercise, or massage can cause a blood clot, if present, to break away from the vessel wall and circulate possibly to the lung. Although there is some controversy, elevating the legs is recommended by some to relieve local swelling. At no time, however, are pillows placed under the knees or the bed gatched at the knees. (4:773; 18:1119)

Nursing Process—Planning
Client Need—Physiological integrity

18 4. A dry towel and a waterproof cover act as insulators and prevent rapid heat and moisture loss from the compress. To avoid burning the skin, the temperature of the compress solution is between 98°F and 105°F. The skin is inspected at least every 30 minutes to monitor for thermal injury. Sterile technique is not necessary as long as the skin is intact. (25:583)

Nursing Process—Implementation
Client Need—Physiological integrity

19 3. Heparin prevents future clots from forming and those that have formed from becoming larger. Heparin is an anticoagulant that inhibits the conversion of fibrinogen to fibrin. Only thrombolytic agents, such as streptokinase, will shrink and dissolve clots that already have formed. The use of thrombolytic agents is extremely hazardous. The risks usually outweigh the benefits in the case of thrombophlebitis. Drug therapy will not prevent a thrombus from becoming dislodged. (17:471; 20:275)

Nursing Process—Implementation
Client Need—Health promotion/maintenance

20 1. The partial thromboplastin time (PTT) is used to monitor the client's response to heparin therapy. The therapeutic range is 1.5 to 2.5 times the control time. A complete blood count (CBC) reports the number of blood cells, not blood clotting factors. Packed cell volume (PCV) is the same as a hematocrit. It measures the percentage of cells in a volume of blood. The prothrombin time (PT) is a test that is used to monitor the response of a client who is receiving an oral anticoagulant, such as warfarin sodium. Another test that is used when clients are on warfarin sodium therapy is the international normalized ratio (INR). (20:276)

Nursing Process—Implementation
Client Need—Physiological integrity

21 2. When a drug is withdrawn from a vial, the nurse instills a volume of air equal to the amount of fluid that will be withdrawn. Adding air to the contents of a vial facilitates withdrawing the drug. If air is not instilled, a partial vacuum is created making it difficult to remove solution. If too much air is instilled, solution will surge into the syringe and in some cases force the plunger from the barrel of the syringe. If the rubber stopper is removed, the drug will not remain sterile. Modified insulins, not heparin, are rotated gently prior to withdrawal to mix the additive and insulin together. Heparin is not shaken before withdrawing it from the vial. (4:420; 25:729)

Nursing Process—Implementation
Client Need—Physiological integrity

22 3. When the adult client is of average or thin size, it is acceptable practice to insert a needle intended for subcutaneous administration at a 45-degree angle to the skin. For obese adults it is recommended that the nurse use a 90-degree angle to insert the needle. The dorsogluteal site is used for intramuscular injections. The needle size for a subcutaneous injection is between ½ to ⅝ inch and 23 to 26 gauge. The injection site following the administration of heparin is not massaged because this increases the tendency for local bleeding. (4:426, 429)

Nursing Process—Implementation
Client Need—Physiological integrity

23 3. When a client receiving anticoagulant therapy manifests any sign of bleeding, it is reported. Feeling tired, leaving food on the tray require further nursing assessment and care planning, but they are not as potentially dangerous as bleeding. Having a bowel movement more than once a day is a normal pattern for some clients. A change in bowel habits is not a common side effect of heparin therapy. (20:280)

Nursing Process—Implementation
Client Need—Physiological integrity

24 3. Protamine sulfate is the antagonist for heparin. It is given to counteract the anticoagulant effects of heparin and restore more normal clotting mechanisms. Calcium lactate is a mineral supplement. Sodium benzoate is used as a food preservative. Aluminum phosphate is an ingredient in some antacid products. (17:479; 20:277; 28:552)

Nursing Process—Planning
Client Need—Physiological integrity

25 4. When injections cannot be avoided, it is appropriate for the nurse to apply pressure to the injection site for several minutes to prevent oozing of blood or localized bruising. Pressure is not applied to distribute the drug. Hematomas do not form as a result of applying pressure. Drug absorption is not significantly affected by several minutes of local pressure. (17:481)

Nursing Process—Implementation
Client Need—Physiological integrity

26 2. Black or tar-colored stools is a sign of bleeding from the upper gastrointestinal tract. Dark amber urine is more indicative of low fluid volume. Emesis is usually green-tinged or clear. A coffee-grounds appearance to emesis is more suggestive of gastrointestinal bleeding. Jaundiced skin indicates a liver or biliary disorder or rapid hemolysis of red blood cells. (20:275))

Nursing Process—Evaluation
Client Need—Health promotion/maintenance

27 1. Signs of an inflammation include redness, tenderness, warmth, and swelling. An inflamed vein also feels indurated (hard) or cordlike, but its appearance is not purple. A pale or dark appearance is not typical of inflamed tissue, nor is it common that an inflamed vein is cool or spongy. (4:773)

Nursing Process—Data collection
Client Need—Physiological integrity

28 4. The cause of the inflamed vein is either the presence of the foreign infusion device, irritating solution, or trauma to the vein wall. In any case, the infusion is discontinued to prevent further injury to the vein and promote healing. Elevating the extremity is appropriate to relieve swelling after the needle or catheter has been removed. Applying pressure does not diminish the current problem, rather it slows the rate of infusion. Increasing the rate of infusion is contraindicated since it has not been medically approved and places the client at risk for fluid volume excess. (25:281)

Nursing Process—Implementation
Client Need—Physiological integrity

NURSING CARE OF CLIENTS WITH ARTERIAL DISORDERS

29 1. Individuals with peripheral vascular disease develop *trophic changes*, like thick, hard nails. Other signs include thin, shiny skin with little hair growth. Trophic changes are the result of chronic impaired blood flow to the epidermal tissues. The peripheral pulses are often weak and difficult to detect in a client with peripheral vascular disease. Hyperactive knee jerk reflexes are not a characteristic of peripheral vascular disease. (3:153; 1:217)

Nursing Process—Data collection
Client Need—Physiological integrity

30 3. When the muscles of the legs become ischemic, the client with peripheral arterial insufficiency is most likely to report having pain in both legs. The pain goes away with rest, which is the reason the symptom is referred to as *intermittent claudication.* Cyanosis is associated more with venous congestion. Poor distal arterial circulation tends to heighten a person's sensation of being cold. Feeling that the toes are burning and photosensitivity are not common symptoms of peripheral arterial insufficiency. (3:307–308; 27:56)

Nursing Process—Data collection
Client Need—Physiological integrity

31 3. Extra clothing or blankets, rather than applying direct heat, are used whenever possible for individuals with peripheral arterial insufficiency. Because of their disease process, they are often insensitive to warm temperatures and are at high risk for being burned. Layers of loosely woven fibers, especially of natural material like cotton or wool, help hold pockets of warm air close to the body surface. This promotes a feeling of warmth. Elevating the feet relieves edema but does not necessarily make the feet feel warmer. (4:768; 21:384–385)

Nursing Process—Implementation
Client Need—Physiological integrity

32 2. The nurse applies acoustic gel to the skin when using a Doppler ultrasound device. The gel helps beam the ultrasound toward the blood vessel being assessed. Movement of red blood cells through an artery produces an intermittent, pulsating sound. Movement of blood through a vein makes a continuous sound like whistling wind. The dorsalis pedis artery is on the top of the foot. The posterior tibialis artery is beside the ankle. When assessing capillary refill, the nurse releases a compressed nailbed and counts the number of seconds it takes for blood to return. A Doppler ultrasound device does not measure skin temperature. (25:384)

Nursing Process—Implementation
Client Need—Safe, effective care environment

33 2. The symptoms of arterial vasospasm associated with Raynaud's disease are generally confined to an individual's hands or feet. The nose, ears, and chin are less commonly involved. The client experiences periodic episodes during which the affected areas feel cold, painful, numb, and prickly due to poor circulation. As blood flow resumes, the deprived areas become flushed and warm. A throbbing sensation is then experienced. (4:772; 21:382)

> Nursing Process—Data collection
> Client Need—Safe, effective care environment

34 2. Conditions that lead to vasoconstriction, such as exposure to cold or emotional upsets, aggravate or exacerbate the symptoms experienced by individuals with Raynaud's disease. The effect of wind depends on the temperature of the air. (4:772; 21:382)

> Nursing Process—Data collection
> Client Need—Physiologic integrity

35 2 Stress stimulates the sympathetic nervous system, causing vasoconstriction. When the arterioles narrow, blood flow is impaired, and the client experiences an episodic attack of pain, numbness, pallor, and so on. Wearing warm gloves while out of doors in cold weather is beneficial. Drinking alcoholic beverages and bathing with perfumed soap are not necessarily contraindicated for a person with Raynaud's disease. (4:370)

> Nursing Process—Implementation
> Client Need—Health promotion or maintenance

36 3. Individuals with thromboangiitis obliterans (Buerger's disease) report that they experience leg pain or muscle cramps during periods of active movement. This symptom is referred to as *intermittent claudication*. The discomfort is relieved by rest at first; eventually the pain occurs even while inactive. People with varicose veins report feeling a sense of heaviness in their legs. If a client with thromboangiitis obliterans has ingrown toenails, it is a coincidental finding and not related to the disease process. Edema occurs among clients with Buerger's disease, but it is more likely when the disease is far advanced. (4:771; 21:358)

> Nursing Process—Data collection
> Client Need—Physiological integrity

37 4. Thromboangiitis obliterans (Buerger's disease) is an acute inflammation of the arteries and veins in the lower extremities. This disorder results in decreased blood flow in the legs and feet, although the hands are also sometimes affected. The distal peripheral pulses are frequently found to be diminished or absent. A normal peripheral pulse feels strong or full. It is easily felt with only moderate pressure. (7:387)

> Nursing Process—Data collection
> Client Need—Physiological integrity

38 1. Because of impaired arterial and venous circulation, a person with thromboangiitis obliterans (Buerger's disease) can easily develop gangrene. A podiatrist is a professional who cares for feet. The services of a podiatrist are used for nail care, treatment of corns and calluses, or other foot problems. Some individuals with this condition eventually undergo amputation when foot lesions become infected or do not heal. Weight control, visual examination, and seeking counseling for emotional problems are all positive health habits, but they are not directly related to the complications of Buerger's disease. (18:1120; 21:359)

> Nursing Process—Data collection
> Client Need—Health promotion/maintenance

39 1. A sympathectomy is a procedure that promotes vasodilation of peripheral arterioles. It involves cutting sympathetic nerve fibers from the autonomic nervous system. Severing these particular nerve fibers will not produce skeletal muscle relaxation, relieve mental stress, or slow the heart rate. (4:771; 21:358)

> Nursing Process—Evaluation
> Client Need—Health promotion/maintenance

40 1. When Buerger-Allen exercises are performed, the legs are alternately elevated while lying down and then lowered to a dependent position by sitting on the edge of the bed or couch. When the legs flush, the client returns to lying flat in bed again. (18:1120; 21:358)

> Nursing Process—Evaluation
> Client Need—Health promotion/maintenance

41 2. Because nicotine causes vasoconstriction, cigarette smoking is avoided by a person with thromboangiitis obliterans (Buerger's disease). There are no contraindications for heavy lifting, traveling by air, or engaging in sexual activity based on the pathology involved in Buerger's disease. (4:771; 18:1120; 21:358)

> Nursing Process—Planning
> Client Need—Health promotion/maintenance

42 2. There are several predisposing factors for developing an aortic aneurysm, such as hypertension, which may be secondary to arteriosclerosis, trauma, and congenital weakness. Lactose intolerance is more likely to cause digestive problems. A sedentary lifestyle predisposes to many cardiac risks, but it is not as highly correlated with aneurysm formation as hypertension and arteriosclerosis. Digoxin (Lanoxin) is a cardiac glycoside that increases the strength of myocardial contraction and lowers the heart rate. Neither its use, side effects, nor conditions for which it is prescribed are linked to the formation of aneurysms. (18:1120; 21:388)

> Nursing Process—Data collection
> Client Need—Physiological integrity

43 4. When palpating the abdomen of a client with an abdominal aortic aneurysm, it may be possible to feel a pulsating mass. The extremities are more likely to manifest signs of diminished circulation, such as looking pale, feeling cool, and having faint peripheral pulses. Occasionally thrombi may form and occlude blood flow to one or both legs. Occlusion of arterial blood flow causes intense leg or foot pain. A *bruit*, a purring or blowing sound, may be auscultated, but this sound is quite different from bowel sounds. Abdominal petichiae are more often associated with liver or blood disorders. (4:770; 21:388)

> **Nursing Process**—Data collection
> **Client Need**—Physiological integrity

44 4. An aneurysm is a balloon-like outpouching in the wall of an artery. Aneurysms commonly occur in the thoracic or abdominal aorta and in cerebral arteries. Weakened valves in veins cause blood vessels in the legs to appear distended and twisted. A stationary blood clot is referred to as a thrombus. A fatty deposit in the wall of an artery is called plaque. (4:770; 18:1122; 21:387)

> **Nursing Process**—Data collection
> **Client Need**—Health promotion/maintenance

45 4. Pressure from an enlarging or dissecting abdominal aortic aneurysm is most likely to be manifested as low back pain. The client indicates that no position or nursing measure relieves the pain. Because the blood loss from a dissecting aneurysm is internal, the cause of rectal bleeding or blood in the urine is from some other cause. The client may complain of cramping abdominal pain but not indigestion if the intestine's blood supply is inadequate. (21:388)

> **Nursing Process**—Data collection
> **Client Need**—Physiological integrity

46 3. The nurse informs the physician of the change in the client's condition. Pertinent assessments, such as vital signs and skin color, are reported at the same time. If the client is not breathing and pulseless, it is unethical to violate her wishes by performing cardiopulmonary resuscitation. The nurse is not following the physician's written order if resuscitation efforts are initiated. The physician is the one to decide about transferring the client based on the information the nurse communicates. The physician generally notifies next of kin, but the task may be delegated to the nurse. (4:1580–1581; 25:41)

> **Nursing Process**—Implementation
> **Client Need**—Safe, effective care environment

NURSING CARE OF CLIENTS WITH RED BLOOD CELL DISORDERS

47 3. Complications of peptic ulcer disease include chronic bleeding or hemorrhage. Blood loss occurs as the ulcer penetrates one or more blood vessels. If the bleeding is slight, but continuous, it may go unnoticed until the client becomes weak and fatigued. Mitral valve regurgitation, arteriosclerosis, and an enlarged prostate are not usually associated with chronic or severe blood loss. (18:1135, 1250)

> **Nursing Process**—Data collection
> **Client Need**—Physiological integrity

48 4. Balancing rest between activities is one way of maintaining a consistent energy level and avoiding excessive energy expenditures. Adequate sleep, breathing deeply, and eating nutrients that provide energy are all healthy behaviors, but they are not likely to make as significant an improvement as balancing energy use with rest. (4:794)

> **Nursing Process**—Planning
> **Client Need**—Health promotion/maintenance

49 4. Iron is necessary for the formation of hemoglobin. Therefore, a deficiency of iron is reflected by a low hemoglobin level. If the hemoglobin level is below 12 g/dL in an adult female or 14 g/dL in a male, the person is considered anemic. Since there are causes other than iron deficiency for a low hemoglobin level, additional diagnostic tests may be necessary. However, prothrombin time, bleeding time, and fibrinogen level are all tests that are performed if a person is suspected of having a clotting problem or at high risk for bleeding. (18:1130; 21:450)

> **Nursing Process**—Data collection
> **Client Need**—Physiological integrity

50 3. An anemic person is likely to feel colder than usual most of the time. This symptom is most likely due to impaired cellular oxygenation from reduced levels of hemoglobin. Without oxygen, the body's ability to produce calories of heat during metabolism is affected. Constipation, dysmenorrhea, and a history of rheumatic fever are not related to iron-deficiency anemia. (18:1135)

> **Nursing Process**—Data collection
> **Client Need**—Physiological integrity

51 2. Omitting meat from the diet can cause iron-deficiency anemia. Good food sources of iron include meat, fish, certain beans, iron-enriched cereals, whole grain products, and green leafy vegetables. Iron is more poorly absorbed from plant sources. Milk, citrus fruits, and candy are not good sources of iron. Milk is a good source of calcium and protein. Citrus fruits are a good source of potassium and vitamin C and aids in the absorption of iron. Candy is a source of empty calories. That is, it is high in calories without any appreciable contribution to nutrition. The health of a person who does not consume candy would not be harmed. (4:798–799; 6:207)

> Nursing Process—Data collection
> Client Need—Health promotion/maintenance

52 1. Iron is absorbed very poorly from the gastrointestinal tract. Absorption occurs best when the drug is taken on an empty stomach with water. Taking the drug between meals, or at least 1 hour before meals, is the best routine for maximum benefit. Taking the drug just before eating or with the meal causes the drug to be present in the stomach with food. When food and some other drugs, like antacids, are taken at the same time as iron, its absorption is decreased. However, if a client experiences gastrointestinal upset while taking iron, rather than discontinuing the medication, the client may reduce the discomfort by taking the ferrous sulfate with food or milk. If the client only takes the ferrous sulfate before bedtime, she is not following the prescribed daily schedule for taking this drug three times a day. (17:517; 20:473)

> Nursing Process—Implementation
> Client Need—Health promotion/maintenance

53 4. The presence of vitamin C, found in orange or other citrus juices, improves the absorption of iron. For this reason some pharmaceutical companies combine iron and vitamin C in the same capsule or tablet. Iron taken with milk interferes with its absorption. Taking iron with tea or a soft drink is not likely to be any more beneficial than taking it with water. (6:207; 18:1135)

> Nursing Process—Implementation
> Client Need—Health promotion/maintenance

54 2. Most individuals who take iron observe that their stools become jet black or dark green. Stool is normally a medium brown color. Clay-colored stools are associated with liver or biliary disease. The stool becomes light green with diarrhea, or it assumes this color from eating certain foods. (17:517; 20:473)

> Nursing Process—Evaluation
> Client Need—Health promotion/maintenance

55 1. Liquid iron preparations stain the teeth. Drinking the medication through a straw minimizes contact of the drug with the teeth. Using a paper cup or metal spoon does not protect the teeth from unsightly staining. Diluting the liquid iron with at least

2 to 4 oz of water also reduces the potential for staining teeth. (17:517)

> Nursing Process—Planning
> Client Need—Physiological integrity

56 1. People who are anemic from blood loss often experience dizziness and fainting. This is probably due to low blood volume or an inability to maintain adequate oxygenation to the brain. Anemia is also likely to cause an individual to feel tired and require more sleep. Having had the gallbladder removed and having a tender abdomen are unrelated to anemia from blood loss. (4:795; 21:449)

> Nursing Process—Data collection
> Client Need—Physiological integrity

57 3. The skin of someone with anemia is most likely to appear pale. This is generally due to the fact that tissue oxygenation, which causes the skin and mucous membranes to appear pink, is impaired from reduced amounts of hemoglobin or red blood cells. Cyanosis is more likely caused by the buildup of carbon dioxide in the blood. Flushed appearance is due to factors such as vasodilation, increased blood volume, and thermal injury. Mottled skin is a condition characterized by generalized purplish, spotted areas. It is often seen in newborns who are chilled or inactive. (4:795; 21:449)

> Nursing Process—Data collection
> Client Need—Physiological integrity

58 3. The ventrogluteal site, which includes the gluteus medius and gluteus minimus muscles, is the preferred site for administering an injection by Z-track technique. Z-track injections are given deeply into a large muscle. The deltoid muscle is used for intramuscular injections; however, it is a smaller muscle in comparison to other intramuscular injection sites. Neither the trapezius muscle, located in the back and shoulder, nor the latissimus dorsi, the widest muscle in the back, are used for injections. (4:427; 25:741)

> Nursing Process—Planning
> Client Need—Physiological integrity

59 2. Using a Z-track technique helps to deposit a substance that stains tissue or that is irritating deeply within the muscle so that it will not leak into subcutaneous tissues. Absorption occurs at the same rate as any other intramuscular injection. Z-track administration involves injecting the drug with slow, even pressure. The nurse waits approximately 10 seconds before removing the needle after the drug is

instilled. Injections given by Z-track technique are not massaged afterward. (4:425; 18:737)
　　Nursing Process—Implementation
　　Client Need—Health promotion/maintenance

60 1. When administering an injection using the Z-track technique, the tissue is pulled laterally until it is taut. It is held in that position during the injection as well. The position of the tissue is not released until after the needle is withdrawn. (18:737; 25:741)
　　Nursing Process—Implementation
　　Client Need—Physiological integrity

61 2. The company and type of health insurance an individual has is obtained by personnel in the admissions or business office. Nurses document subjective and objective assessment data, nursing care, treatment interventions, and the client's responses in narrative nursing notes. (4:71; 25:93)
　　Nursing Process—Implementation
　　Client Need—Safe, effective care environment

62 1. Pernicious anemia impairs peripheral and spinal cord nerve fibers, causing symptoms such as tingling and numbness in the extremities, loss of position sense, a staggering gait, and partial or total paralysis. Headaches are not a classic complaint among individuals with pernicious anemia nor is restlessness or sleep disturbances. Some experience confusion, depression, personality changes, and memory loss, but not to the point of amnesia. (18:1136; 21:452)
　　Nursing Process—Data collection
　　Client Need—Physiological integrity

63 1. When a Schilling test is performed, all the client's urine is collected for 24 to 48 hours after oral and injected doses of vitamin B_{12}. Subnormal levels of vitamin B_{12} in the urine suggest pernicious anemia. (7:718–720)
　　Nursing Process—Implementation
　　Client Need—Safe, effective care environment

64 3. Pernicious anemia is not curable, but the manifestations of the disease can be treated by lifelong injections of vitamin B_{12}. Blood transfusions are administered to someone who has hemolytic anemia or severe loss of red blood cells and hemoglobin. Iron preparations are given for nutritional anemia and when blood cells or hemoglobin are low, but the condition is not life-threatening. Vitamin K is administered for clotting disorders in which the client's prothrombin level is low. (18:1136; 21:452)
　　Nursing Process—Implementation
　　Client Need—Health promotion/maintenance

65 1. Absorption of vitamin B_{12}, the extrinsic factor, depends upon adequate intrinsic factor in gastric secretions. Those who have had a total gastrectomy eventually develop pernicious anemia unless prophylactically treated with injections of vitamin B_{12}. (6:235)
　　Nursing Process—Implementation
　　Client Need—Health promotion/maintenance

66 4. The gene for sickling hemoglobin is found in 1 out of every 10 African-Americans. In Africa the sickling effect developed as a genetic adaptation protecting Africans from malaria. When African-Americans were forced into slavery in America and other western countries, the genetic characteristic continued in generation after generation. Because malaria in the United States is minimal, the genetic phenomenon is detrimental rather than protective. This disease also occurs in smaller numbers among people from Mediterranean and Middle Eastern countries. (18:1136; 21:450)
　　Nursing Process—Data collection
　　Client Need—Health promotion/maintenance

67 3. Jaundice is commonly present in individuals with sickle cell anemia. It is due to the fact that sickled red blood cells are destroyed more rapidly than normal red blood cells. A white, coated tongue indicates a fungal infection or mouth breathing. Cloudy urine is a sign associated with a urinary tract infection. Nausea has multiple causes, but it is not particularly a common symptom among people with sickle cell anemia. (4:799; 21:450)
　　Nursing Process—Data collection
　　Client Need—Physiological integrity

68 2. Severe pain is the major problem for clients experiencing a sickle cell crisis. The pain is caused by tissue ischemia secondary to blockage of blood vessels by sickled red cells. The pain is likely to trigger anxiety, but if the pain is controlled, anxiety is relieved as well. Adequate nutrition is a concern for all clients, as is ventilation. Usually these physiological functions are not typically affected in a sickle cell crisis unless complications such as a cerebral or pulmonary infarction develop. (4:799–800; 21:450–451)
　　Nursing Process—Planning
　　Client Need—Physiological integrity

69 2. It is important to change positions to avoid complications of immobility, but activity is limited during a sickle cell crisis to reduce the client's discomfort. No specific position is ideal; the goal is to relieve pressure and promote comfort. Exercise and ambulation are contraindicated because they increase the client's need for tissue oxygenation at a time when

the oxygen-carrying capacity of red blood cells is very limited. (4:800)
Nursing Process—Planning
Client Need—Physiological integrity

70 1. Increasing and maintaining a high volume of fluid intake by oral or intravenous routes promotes the circulation of sickled blood cells through blood vessels. Elastic stockings promote venous return of blood; however, the arterial blood contains the oxygen needed by cells and tissue. Elevating the legs relieves swelling associated with thrombus formation. However, in sickle cell crisis there are likely to be many microemboli. Neither elevating the legs nor dangling them helps move red blood cells that accumulate and form thrombi. (4:800; 21:451)
Nursing Process—Implementation
Client Need—Physiological integrity

71 3. Sickle cell crises occur when clients with this disorder become overexerted, dehydrated, acquire an infection, ingest alcohol, smoke, are exposed to cold weather or high altitudes. (4:799)
Nursing Process—Evaluation
Client Need—Health promotion/maintenance

72 3. People with sickle cell trait inherited one defective gene and one normal gene for hemoglobin. Since the defective gene is a recessive trait, the disease is never manifested. However, children born to couples with the recessive trait may each transmit the defective gene to their offspring, who then manifest the disease. Genetically, these same couples could transmit their normal genes so that there is a possibility that some children are free of the sickle cell trait. Or, some children acquire one defective and one normal gene and continue to carry the sickle cell trait. (18:1136)
Nursing Process—Implementation
Client Need—Health promotion/maintenance

NURSING CARE OF CLIENTS WITH WHITE BLOOD CELL DISORDERS

73 3. Cloudy urine is a common sign associated with a urinary tract infection. Other findings that suggest an infection include fever, cough, increased respirations and heart rate, and ulcerated oral mucous membranes. Blood in the stool is associated with altered clotting mechanisms. Prolonged vomiting is a side effect of chemotherapy. Extreme fatigue accompanies reduced numbers of red blood cells, causing anemia. (25:634)
Nursing Process—Data collection
Client Need—Physiological integrity

74 1. Foam mouth swabs are less likely to traumatize the gums and oral mucous membranes. They are substituted for the toothbrush temporarily. Oral hygiene is not discontinued because the mouth contains organisms that are the source of an opportunistic infection. The potential for injury continues to exist if the nurse eliminated toothpaste but not the use of the toothbrush. (4:806; 18:1138)
Nursing Process—Implementation
Client Need—Physiological integrity

75 4. Soft, bland foods, such as creamed soups, cottage cheese, baked fish, macaroni and cheese, custard, and pudding, help to maintain nutrition but relieve oral discomfort from coarse or irritating foods. Spicy foods are avoided. (4:806; 6:616–617; 18:1138)
Nursing Process—Implementation
Client Need—Physiological integrity

76 1. The client who receives antineoplastic drugs is likely to experience hair loss. The hair loss is not permanent; the hair returns when the drug therapy is discontinued. In the meantime the nurse lets the client discuss how he or she feels about the potential hair loss. If the client is troubled by the loss of hair, the nurse offers suggestions for disguising the fact that hair loss is occurring. Some possible alternatives include wearing a turban, baseball cap, scarf, or wig. (17:631; 20:445)
Nursing Process—Planning
Client Need—Physiological integrity

77 3. A low platelet count places clients at risk for bleeding. Using a small-gauge needle for injections reduces the amount of blood loss. Switching to oral medications when possible is even better. It is appropriate to place clients in protective isolation and limit contact with visitors who may be infectious when the number of mature white blood cells is low. Rest periods are appropriate to counteract the effects of a low red blood cell count. (18:1138)
Nursing Process—Implementation
Client Need—Physiological integrity

78 3. The term remission means that the disease is not currently progressing and there may even be an absence of the original signs and symptoms. However, this does not mean the condition is cured. Although a remission is a good sign, the client's prognosis continues to be guarded because it is difficult to predict how long the remission will last. If the disease is manifested again, treatment is reinstituted at that time. For this reason it is very important to stress that the person maintain regular

checkups with his physician. In the meantime, they are encouraged to live as fully and normally as possible. (18:1486; 25:46)
> **Nursing Process—Evaluation**
> **Client Need—Health promotion/maintenance**

79 3. Hospice organizations offer assistance to dying individuals who have less than 6 months to live. They provide services to assist the family in caring for the terminally ill individual's physical and emotional needs. They continue working with the family, even after the client's death, to help them resolve their grief. The public health department provides preventive services in the area of immunizations, care of well babies, diagnosing sexually transmitted and other communicable diseases, inspecting sanitary conditions of buildings and food establishments, and so on. The Centers for Disease Control and Prevention studies the incidence of communicable diseases and recommends practices for controlling their spread. The local United Way is a philanthropic organization that collects and distributes funds to many social welfare organizations in the community. (21:69; 25:126, 813)
> **Nursing Process—Planning**
> **Client Need—Health promotion/maintenance**

80 2. Mononucleosis is transmitted by direct contact with the droplets or oral secretions of another infected person. This disease is referred to as the "kissing disease" because the virus passes from one individual to another by the oral route. Sharing eating utensils and cigarettes also are ways of transmitting this disease. (18:924–925)
> **Nursing Process—Implementation**
> **Client Need—Health promotion/maintenance**

81 3. One of the first signs of infectious mononucleosis is a sore throat. It is accompanied by a fever and headache. In severe cases the lymph nodes, including the spleen, become enlarged. If complications develop, jaundice occurs. Abdominal discomfort, aching joints, and intestinal upset are not common symptoms among people with infectious mononucleosis. (18:925; 21:472)
> **Nursing Process—Data collection**
> **Client Need—Physiological integrity**

82 2. Rest is essential for the recovery from infectious mononucleosis. Physical activity is likely to intensify symptoms, prolong recovery, or contribute to complications involving the liver, spleen, heart, and nervous system. Treatment is usually symptomatic, involving oral fluids, analgesics, and antipyretics. (21:472)
> **Nursing Process—Implementation**
> **Client Need—Health promotion/maintenance**

83 1. Clinical manifestations of Hodgkin's disease include extreme pruritus (itching), anorexia, weight loss, enlarged lymph nodes and lymphatic organs such as the spleen. Bone pain may occur later as the disease progresses. An unsteady gait, headaches, and easy bruising, if they occur, are not necessarily related to the primary disorder. (4:813; 21:473)
> **Nursing Process—Implementation**
> **Client Need—Health promotion/maintenance**

84 1. Hodgkin's disease is characterized by lymph nodes that are enlarged yet painless. The physical change in cervical lymph nodes is generally one of the first abnormal signs of this disease. Later the axillary and inguinal lymph nodes also may become involved. Regardless of the location in the body, cancerous growths are hardly ever painful in the early stages of the disease. This explains why early warning signs of cancer tend to be ignored. (18:1138; 21:473)
> **Nursing Process—Data collection**
> **Client Need—Safe, effective care environment**

85 2. Deodorants or other skin preparations that contain metals are avoided. They absorb the x-rays and increase skin irritation. The skin can be washed with tepid water, mild soap, and a soft wash cloth. The hair in the area is not shaved. In fact, shaving may further impair the integrity of the skin, which is somewhat damaged temporarily by the radiation. Zinc oxide contains a metal and is not applied to the skin. If the skin does become dry, blistered, or peeled, the physician may prescribe a topical application, such as vitamin A and D ointment, lanolin, pure aloe vera gel, or cortisone ointment. (4:1197; 18:1154)
> **Nursing Process—Planning**
> **Client Need—Safe, effective care environment**

86 1. Reddening or bronzing of the skin is expected in the area that is irradiated. It is best to inform clients about skin changes before therapy begins, stressing that the discoloration is only temporary. Although ionizing radiation used in cancer therapy is a form of energy, it does not produce heat or bleeding under the skin. The client's concern is not likely about the cosmetic change, but rather about fear that an adverse reaction is occurring. Therefore, reassuring him that the redness is hardly noticeable is inappropriate. (21:156)
> **Nursing Process—Implementation**
> **Client Need—Health promotion/maintenance**

87 4. The most important information to give the client with irradiated skin is to protect it from direct sunlight. Advising the client to wear several layers of warm clothing is appropriate if there is an accompanying problem of poor circulation. For comfort, any individual should avoid becoming chilled or too warm. Wearing a face mask is only warranted if the client has allergies to inhaled substances, has cardiovascular disease in which vasoconstriction causes ischemia, or needs a barrier to infectious microorganisms or environmental pollutants. (4:1197; 21:161)

    Nursing Process—Planning
    Client Need—Health promotion/maintenance

88 3. If the white blood cell count drops to dangerously low levels, the client becomes susceptible to infection. Chemotherapy drugs can depress bone marrow function. Periodic blood cell counts are monitored to assess for this potential side effect. Anorexia, nausea, vomiting, weight loss, and diarrhea also are side effects of cancer treatment, but they are not indications that the client should be placed in protective isolation. Confusion and disorientation suggest that the client is experiencing neurologic problems and should be observed closely to protect his safety, but the symptoms do not justify implementing protective isolation. (21:474)

    Nursing Process—Implementation
    Client Need—Physiological integrity

89 3. Grieving is facilitated by discussing feelings with another person. The client is not left alone immediately after hearing this information. It is important for the nurse to stay with the client as he processes the information he was just given. The client also benefits from talking with other supportive individuals, such as a spouse, family member, friend, or clergyman. Reading literature on the subject and thinking in private help some people but are not believed to be as effective as verbalizing thoughts. If the client requested a second opinion, the request is not denied. However, it is inappropriate for the nurse to initiate the suggestion. It is considered a form of false reassurance and could prolong denial. (9:356; 23:254)

    Nursing Process—Implementation
    Client Need—Psychosocial integrity

90 4. Intravenous drug users who share needles, male homosexuals, bisexuals, women who have intercourse with these males, and infants of infected mothers are at greatest risk for developing AIDS. Haitians and Africans also have a high incidence of this disease among their native populations. Vacationing in Mexico, breeding dogs, and having had surgery in and of itself does not place the client at

any greater risk for AIDS than other individuals. (21:496; 25:451)

    Nursing Process—Data collection
    Client Need—Health promotion/maintenance

91 3. The ELISA test detects the presence of antibodies to viral antigens. A reactive ELISA test is generally repeated. If it continues to be reactive, more specific tests for the HIV antibodies, such as the Western blot test or Murex SUDS-HIV-1 test, are performed before making a definitive diagnosis of AIDS. A VDRL test is used as a screening test for syphilis. The Schick test is used to determine if a person has antibodies to the bacterial toxins of the organism causing diphtheria. The Dick test is used to assess the immunologic status of a person to the toxins associated with an infection of scarlet fever. (7:536–537; 21:498)

    Nursing Process—Data collection
    Client Need—Physiological integrity

92 2. Standard precautions are used when a person's infectious status is unknown. Standard precautions involve donning one or more protective garments, depending upon the potential for coming into contact with blood or body fluids, and taking precautionary actions to avoid penetrating injuries with objects that are contaminated with blood or body fluid. In *all* situations, it is important to avoid recapping needles to avoid an accidental needlestick injury. A face mask does provide protection from being splashed with blood or body fluid; however, most dressings absorb liquid drainage and wearing gloves is more appropriate. Wearing a cover gown is appropriate if there is the potential that blood and body fluid may penetrate clothing, but this measure is unnecessary when giving most clients a bed bath. Gloves are appropriate when touching areas of the body where there may be contact with blood or body fluids. Wearing gloves while taking vital signs is generally unnecessary. (21:139; 25:452)

    Nursing Process—Implementation
    Client Need—Safe, effective care environment

93 1. Setting and reaching realistic daily goals can help the client experience a sense of hope. Hope is a powerful influence on a dying person's will to live and can do much to lift a depressed person's spirits. A referral to the chaplain is appropriate if the client requests contact with a clergyman. Distraction does not help a client deal with his feelings or promote a sense of hope. Contacting a lawyer helps an individual take care of unfinished business, but it is only arranged if the client indicates that he would

like the nurse's assistance in this matter. (2:121–122; 3:445–448)
>   Nursing Process—Planning
>   Client Need—Psychosocial integrity

NURSING CARE OF CLIENTS WITH BONE MARROW DISORDERS

94 1. Sitting upright allows abdominal organs, like the spleen, liver, and intestines, to fall away from the diaphragm. By reducing crowding of the diaphragm, dyspnea is reduced, and the client feels more comfortable. (25:404, 469)
>   Nursing Process—Planning
>   Client Need—Physiological integrity

95 2. Keeping a person with polycythemia well hydrated reduces the viscosity or thickness of the blood. Thrombi are less likely to form if the excessive numbers of blood cells are kept diluted within the plasma. In that way they move more easily throughout the circulatory system, reducing the possibility of clumping together within a small blood vessel. Providing protein foods, restricting dietary sodium, and encouraging weight loss are healthful interventions, but they do not have a therapeutic effect on preventing the formation of blood clots. (26:239, 242)
>   Nursing Process—Implementation
>   Client Need—Physiological integrity

96 1. Treatment for polycythemia vera include measures that remove blood. As much as 500 to 2000 mL of blood are removed by performing a phlebotomy. This is similar to the technique for donating a unit of blood. Afterward, intravenous fluid is infused to dilute the remaining circulating cells. More aggressive therapy using radiophosphorus and radiation is used in an effort to decrease the bone marrow's production of cells. (4:801; 21:455)
>   Nursing Process—Evaluation
>   Client Need—Health promotion/maintenance

97 1. Angina may result as a consequence of thrombosis in a coronary artery and subsequent myocardial infarction. Clots are more likely to form due to the viscous nature of the circulating blood volume and the fact that there is an increased number of platelets as well as red and white blood cells. Indigestion, burning on urination, and loss of appetite are not ignored, but they are not commonly associated with polycythemia vera. (4:801; 21:455)
>   Nursing Process—Data collection
>   Client Need—Physiological integrity

98 1. Bone marrow is aspirated from the iliac crest, the curved rim along the upper border of the ilium. It is felt in the hip area near the level of the waist. The sternum, or breastbone, located in the center of the chest is an alternate site for aspirating a sample of bone marrow. The iliac crest is generally the first choice as a site for this procedure because it contains more bone marrow than the sternum. The lower spine, upper arm, and groin area are not sites from which bone marrow is aspirated. (4:794; 21:444)
>   Nursing Process—Evaluation
>   Client Need—Health promotion/maintenance

99 1. The client undergoing a bone marrow aspiration needs the help of the nurse in minimizing pain. Despite the use of local anesthesia, a person usually feels pressure as the needle is driven within the bone. Brief but sharp pain is experienced as the needle finally enters the bone and marrow is withdrawn. Premedication is helpful, as well as using distractive techniques and supportive encouragement. The physician generally needs no assistance with instruments during the procedure. A suction machine is not used. Oxygen is not needed under most conditions. (4:309; 18:1131)
>   Nursing Process—Implementation
>   Client Need—Safe, effective care environment

100 2. Bleeding from the puncture site is one of the most common problems following a bone marrow aspiration. If bleeding is not controlled, a painful hematoma forms. Firm pressure or an ice pack is used to limit bleeding. Under usual circumstances, a bone marrow aspiration does not cause shock. Though the blood pressure and pulse may fluctuate somewhat, it is usually due to anxiety and fear rather than from loss of blood volume. The client remains awake and alert throughout and following the procedure. (4:309; 7:133)
>   Nursing Process—Data collection
>   Client Need—Safe, effective care environment

101 1. Rapid or labored breathing indicates that an adequate amount of oxygen is not available for a client's metabolic needs. It is important for the nurse at this time to provide the dyspneic client with a period of rest. Feeling nauseated is not generally associated with hypoxemia. The pulse rate increases with activity and poor oxygenation. Cool, moist skin accompanies a drop in blood pressure or other physical problems. It is not usually a classic sign of fatigue or intolerance of activity. (21:454)
>   Nursing Process—Data collection
>   Client Need—Physiological integrity

102 1. A low number of platelets, also known as thrombocytes, increases the risk for bleeding. Bruises indi-

cate bleeding into the skin. Coarse body hair, thick toenails, and cool extremities are not associated with thrombocytopenia. (4:796–797)
> Nursing Process—Data collection
> Client Need—Physiological integrity

103 1. A client with leukopenia, a low number of white blood cells, is at high risk for infection. Handwashing is the best technique for reducing the spread of microorganisms. Maintaining skin integrity, adequate nourishment, and assessing vital signs are all components of good nursing care. However, these actions are not directly related to the depressed white blood cell count. (4:797; 18:1136)
> Nursing Process—Implementation
> Client Need—Physiological integrity

104 1. Packed cells contain similar numbers of blood cells. A unit of packed blood cells is prepared by removing approximately two-thirds of the plasma from a unit of whole blood. The administration of packed cells is preferred for clients who need a blood transfusion but for whom additional water within the circulatory system is hazardous. Typically the candidate for packed cells is someone who is prone to congestive heart failure or who has poor kidney function. Packed cells pose the same risk for an allergic reaction as whole blood. Packed cells do not stimulate the bone marrow to produce blood cells. (18:1132; 21:215; 25:263)
> Nursing Process—Implementation
> Client Need—Health promotion/maintenance

105 4. A person with blood type A, Rh positive would have a reaction if transfused with AB, Rh positive blood. It is always best to administer the same blood type. However, O type blood is referred to as the universal donor. In an emergency, anyone can receive type O blood. People who are Rh positive can receive compatible blood types that are either Rh positive or Rh negative. The reverse is not true; in other words a person who is Rh negative should never be given Rh positive blood. (13:208; 25:264)
> Nursing Process—Implementation
> Client Need—Physiological integrity

106 2. Hypotension is one of the signs of a serious blood transfusion reaction. In a serious transfusion reaction, urine formation is decreased. Swelling and pale skin at the infusion site are indications that there is a problem with the administration of the blood rather than a reaction to the blood product. (18:1133; 25:293)
> Nursing Process—Data collection
> Client Need—Physiological integrity

107 2. Long-term administration of endogenous corticosteroids cause body changes like a "moon" face and "buffalo" hump on the back of the neck, which resemble signs of Cushing's syndrome caused by a hyperfunctioning adrenal cortex. The voice is not affected. There is apt to be muscle wasting with long-term corticosteroid use. Anabolic steroids cause muscle enlargement. Steroid administration causes the skin to appear thin and transparent. Purple striae are found on the abdomen and hips. Bronzed skin is found in individuals who have Addison's disease due to an inadequately functioning adrenal cortex. (17:241; 20:349)
> Nursing Process—Data collection
> Client Need—Physiological integrity

108 1. Steroids are known to cause peptic ulcers. For this reason the physician also may prescribe drugs to protect the gastric mucosa from erosion. Drowsiness, anorexia, and light-colored urine are not generally experienced by individuals who take corticosteroids. (17:241; 20:351)
> Nursing Process—Data collection
> Client Need—Physiological integrity

109 3. Total body irradiation destroys the client's bone marrow and places the individual at high risk for infection. Medical asepsis is scrupulously followed, prophylactic antibiotics and antifungal medications are administered, and visitors are restricted to prevent the client from acquiring an infection from which he or she may not recover. The nurse never neglects to promote optimum nutrition and hydration and to help the client cope with fear and depression. However, if these problems occur, they are more easily treated than an infection. (4:1203; 18:1134)
> Nursing Process—Planning
> Client Need—Physiological integrity

NURSING CARE OF CLIENTS WITH COAGULATION DISORDERS

110 1. Small hemorrhages in the skin, mucous membranes, or subcutaneous tissues are referred to as purpura. Bleeding also occurs internally when a person has thrombocytopenia. There is no other additional term for dark areas of cyanosis. The term for flushed red skin is *erythema*. Protruding veins are referred to as distended or as being *varicosities*. (18:1139; 21:463)
> Nursing Process—Data collection
> Client Need—Physiological integrity

111 4. Preventing injury is a priority concern when caring for people with thrombocytopenia because they are prone to bleeding. The care plan specifies careful handling of the client, padding the side rails with soft material, avoiding injections, using a soft toothbrush for mouth care, using extended pressure when discontinuing intravenous infusions, and so on. Activity is restricted to reduce the potential for injury. Generally, individuals with thrombocytopenia are not at high risk for infection; therefore, visitors are not restricted. A normal intake of oral fluid is appropriate unless a client experiences a large loss of blood volume. (18:1139; 21:466)

Nursing Process—Implementation
Client Need—Safe, effective care environment

112 2. Drowsiness, or a change in the level of consciousness, is one of the earliest signs of increased pressure from intracranial bleeding. Other signs include headache, visual problems, vomiting, motor weakness or paralysis, and personality changes. Convulsions occur later as the bleeding progresses. Tinnitus, or ringing in the ears, is not commonly associated with active intracranial bleeding. The individual does not lose his appetite but may vomit with or without nausea. (4:1111; 21:570)

Nursing Process—Evaluation
Client Need—Health promotion/maintenance

113 3. Once collected, all donated blood is tested for HIV antibodies. Donated blood is the safest it has ever been since early 1985. However, it is still not 100% safe because some blood donors who have the virus in their blood have not produced sufficient antibodies to cause a positive reaction when the blood is tested. All potential blood donors are asked questions about lifestyle behaviors that indicate a risk for HIV infection, but some do not answer the questions honestly. Blood donors are encouraged to call the blood collection agency later and report an identifying number, but not their name, if they feel someone is at risk if they received a unit of their donated blood. (7:588; 21:496)

Nursing Process—Implementation
Client Need—Health promotion/maintenance

NURSING CARE OF CLIENTS WITH INFLAMMATORY AND OBSTRUCTIVE LYMPHATIC DISORDERS

114 2. Red streaks that follow the course of lymph channels suggest that lymphangitis is present. Lymphangitis is generally a consequence of a bacterial infection. There may be limitation of movement due to tenderness and swelling, but it is not limited to the joints. Most experience tenderness and pain. Drainage may be present from the original wound, but it is most likely purulent rather than serous. (21:471)

Nursing Process—Data collection
Client Need—Physiological integrity

115 2. When the axillary lymph nodes are removed during a radical mastectomy, lymph circulation is impaired. The lymph collects and pools within the arm on the side of the mastectomy. The condition is generally permanent once it develops. Elevation of the affected arm and hand, applying an inflatable pressure sleeve or elasticized bandage, squeezing a rubber ball, and active exercise are immediate postoperative interventions designed to prevent, reduce, or eliminate the development of lymphedema. (21:866)

Nursing Process—Data collection
Client Need—Physiological integrity

116 1. Because circulation in the arm with lymphedema is impaired, certain nursing interventions, such as administering injections, taking a blood pressure, obtaining blood, or starting an intravenous infusion, are avoided. Prolonged pressure during positioning is avoided, but there is no contraindication at this late date to lying on the affected side for brief periods. Active exercise is encouraged. Though nail polish interferes with assessing capillary refill, it is not necessary to totally discourage its use. (14:912; 16:704)

Nursing Process—Planning
Client Need—Physiological integrity

Classification of Test Items

Unit I Review Test **3**

The Nursing Care of Clients with Peripheral Vascular, Hematologic, and Lymphatic Disorders

Directions: After each question, the correct answer is given as well as a classification of each test question. Compare the correct answer with your answer. If a question has been answered *incorrectly*, draw a line to the end of all the columns. When finished, add up the number of your correct answers in each column and place that number in the respective box at the end in the area identified as *Number Correct*.

To determine the percentage of questions you answered correctly and your performance in each of the test plan categories, divide the *Number Correct* in each column by the *Number Possible* in each column. Then multiply the decimal by 100. For example:

$$\frac{\text{Number Correct: 93}}{\text{Number Possible: 116}} = 0.801 \times 100 = 80.$$

Any score that is less than 75% indicates an area where further review would be beneficial.

KEY TO ITEM CLASSIFICATION:

NURSING PROCESS

D = Data collection
P = Planning
I = Implementation
E = Evaluation

CLIENT NEEDS

S = Safe, effective care environment
P = Physiological integrity
M = Psychosocial integrity
H = Health promotion/maintenance

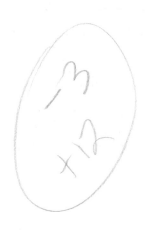

Question #	Answer #	Nursing Process				Client Needs			
		D	P	I	E	S	P	M	H
1	1	D					P		
2	1			I					H
3	3			I					H
4	3	D					P		
5	2			I					H
6	3				E		P		
7	4			I					H
8	1	D							H
9	3			I					H
10	3		P				P		
11	4			I			P		
12	1	D					P		
13	2				E		P		
14	2	D					P		
15	1	D					P		

Question #	Answer #	Nursing Process				Client Needs			
		D	P	I	E	S	P	M	H
16	4	D					P		
17	2		P				P		
18	4			I			P		
19	3			I					H
20	1			I			P		
21	2			I			P		
22	3			I			P		
23	3			I			P		
24	3		P				P		
25	4			I			P		
26	2				E				H
27	1	D					P		
28	4			I			P		
29	1	D					P		
30	3	D					P		
31	3			I			P		
32	2			I		S			
33	2	D				S			
34	2	D					P		
35	2			I					H
36	3	D					P		
37	4	D					P		
38	1	D							H
39	1				E				H
40	1				E				H
41	2		P						H
42	2	D					P		
43	4	D					P		
44	4	D							H
45	4	D					P		
46	3			I		S			
47	3	D					P		

Question #	Answer #	Nursing Process				Client Needs			
		D	P	I	E	S	P	M	H
48	4		P						H
49	4	D					P		
50	3	D					P		
51	2	D							H
51	2	D							H
52	1			I					H
53	4			I					H
54	2				E				H
55	1		P				P		
56	1	D					P		
57	3	D					P		
58	3		P				P		
59	2			I					H
60	1			I			P		
61	2			I		S			
62	1	D					P		
63	1			I		S			
64	3			I					H
65	1			I					H
66	4	D							H
67	3	D					P		
68	2		P				P		
69	2		P				P		
70	1			I			P		
71	3				E				H
72	3			I					H
73	3	D					P		
74	1			I			P		
75	4			I			P		
76	1		P				P		
77	3			I			P		
78	3				E				H

1 2 2 1   2 1 3

Question #	Answer #	Nursing Process				Client Needs			
		D	P	I	E	S	P	M	H
79	3		P						H
80	2			I					H
81	3	D					P		
82	2			I					H
83	1			I					H
84	1	D				S			
85	2		P			S			
86	1			I					H
87	4		P						H
88	3			I			P		
89	3			I				M	
90	4	D							H
91	3	D					P		
92	2			I		S			
93	1		P					M	
94	1		P				P		
95	2			I			P		
96	1				E				H
97	1	D					P		
98	1				E				H
99	1			I		S			
100	2	D				S			
101	1	D					P		
102	1	D					P		
103	1			I			P		
104	1			I					H
105	4			I			P		
106	2	D					P		
107	2	D					P		
108	1	D					P		
109	3		P				P		
110	1	D					P		

3 4 10 3 1 7 1 11

Question #	Answer #	Nursing Process				Client Needs			
		D	P	I	E	S	P	M	H
111	4			I		S			
112	2				E				H
113	3			I					H
114	2	D					P		
115	2	D					P		
116	1		P				P		
Number Correct	94	39	13	35	7	10	58	0	26
Number Possible	116	43	17	45	11	11	66	1	38
Percentage Correct	81%	91%	76	78	64	91	88	0	68

Directions: With a pencil, blacken the circle in front of the option you have chosen for your correct answer.

NURSING CARE OF CLIENTS WITH UPPER RESPIRATORY INFECTIONS

During a visit to the physician's office, a client complains to the nurse that the physician would not prescribe an antibiotic for a head cold.

1 The *best explanation* the nurse can provide is that
- ● 1. antibiotics are ineffective in treating viral infections.
- ○ 2. once cold symptoms develop, antibiotics are ineffective.
- ○ 3. antibiotics only prevent the spread of colds to others.
- ○ 4. they are only used for immunosuppressed individuals.

2 Which symptom, if reported by a person with a common cold, is the *best indication* that complications are developing?
- ○ 1. The client reports having nasal stuffiness.
- ○ 2. The client reports having a dry cough.
- ● 3. The client reports having a high fever.
- ○ 4. The client reports having a scratchy throat.

3 To avoid aggravating a pre-existing medical condition, it is *best* to determine if a client with a cold has which one of the following disorders before recommending the use of a nonprescription decongestant?
- ○ 1. Arthritis
- ● 2. Asthma
- ○ 3. Hypertension
- ○ 4. Diabetes

4 The nurse is *most correct* in warning a client with a common cold that overuse of a topical nasal decongestant is likely to result in

- ● 1. nasal stuffiness.
- ○ 2. physical dependence.
- ○ 3. mucosal ulceration.
- ○ 4. microbial resistance.

5 To prevent a secondary ear infection while experiencing typical symptoms of a head cold, it is *best* for the nurse to recommend
- ● 1. sleeping with the head elevated.
- ○ 2. blowing the nose very gently.
- ○ 3. inserting cotton into the ears.
- ○ 4. covering the ears when outdoors.

An adult female who has a prolonged upper respiratory infection sees the doctor because she continues to have a low-grade fever, poor appetite, and malaise.

6 If the client has sinusitis in the maxillary sinuses, it is *most likely* she will tell the nurse that she feels pain
- ○ 1. over her eyes.
- ○ 2. near her eyebrows.
- ● 3. in her cheeks.
- ○ 4. above her ears.

The physician recommends that the client with sinusitis purchase and use an over-the-counter nasal spray.

7 It is *essential* that the nurse stress that the client follow the directions exactly as they are stated on the container because overuse of nasal decongestants
- ○ 1. leads to physical addiction in a very short time.
- ● 2. offers shorter and shorter periods of symptomatic relief.
- ○ 3. thins the mucous membranes, causing them to bleed.
- ○ 4. lowers a person's resistance to various pathogens.

8 The nurse is correct in instructing clients who use nose drops that to promote accurate application the *best position* for instilling the medication is
○ 1. bending the head forward.
○ 2. pushing the nose laterally.
◉ 3. tilting the head backward.
○ 4. opening the mouth wide.

A client at a clinic tells the nurse that she has an old-fashioned steam vaporizer at home. She plans to use it to help relieve her child's nasal congestion.

9 The *best reason* for the nurse to discourage the client from using a steam vaporizer is that it can cause
○ 1. a fire if the water reservoir boils rapidly.
○ 2. excess moisture saturation in the room.
○ 3. burns from contact with heated water vapor.
◉ 4. rapid growth of environmental pathogens.

NURSING CARE OF CLIENTS WITH INFLAMMATORY AND ALLERGIC DISORDERS OF THE UPPER AIRWAYS

The physician orders a culture on a client with pharyngitis.

10 Which one of the following describes the *best technique* for collecting the specimen?
○ 1. The nurse asks the client to expectorate sputum in a cup.
○ 2. The nurse wipes the inner mouth and tongue with gauze.
◉ 3. The nurse swabs the throat with a sterile cotton applicator.
○ 4. The nurse collects saliva in a sterile culture tube.

Oral potassium penicillin V (V-cillin K) is prescribed for the client with pharyngitis caused by group A streptococci microorganisms.

11 The nurse is correct in stressing that all of the prescribed medication must be taken because if the infection is untreated or undertreated, it may be followed by
◉ 1. glomerulonephritis.
○ 2. chickenpox.
○ 3. shingles.
○ 4. whooping cough.

A singer talks to the nurse at the physician's office and asks what she might do to treat her laryngitis.

12 The *best* nursing advice until the client is examined is to tell the client to
○ 1. take a multivitamin.
◉ 2. rest the voice.
○ 3. maintain bed rest.
○ 4. massage the throat.

The hoarseness the client with laryngitis experiences is still present after 2 weeks of symptomatic treatment. The physician schedules the client for a direct laryngoscopy.

13 Which one of the following statements is the *best indication* that the client understands the reason a direct laryngoscopy is ordered in cases of chronic or prolonged hoarseness?
○ 1. "This test is done because hoarseness is associated with emphysema."
○ 2. "This test is done because hoarseness is associated with bronchitis."
◉ 3. "This test is done because hoarseness is associated with laryngeal cancer."
○ 4. "This test is done because hoarseness is associated with enlarged adenoids."

A 23-year-old female notes that every fall her nasal passages become swollen, she sneezes endlessly, and her eyes become red, itchy, and watery. She makes an appointment with an allergist.

14 When the physician prescribes an antihistamine, terfenadine (Seldane), for symptomatic relief, the *most appropriate* health teaching the nurse can provide is that this drug may cause
○ 1. weight loss.
○ 2. constipation.
◉ 3. drowsiness.
○ 4. depression.

The physician recommends that the client with allergy symptoms undergo skin testing.

15 When the client asks the nurse why skin testing is beneficial, the *best explanation* is that
◉ 1. her symptoms may be due to more than one substance.
○ 2. skin testing helps to build up blocking antibodies.
○ 3. testing is an example of high-quality medical care.
○ 4. insurance generally covers diagnostic skin testing.

16 When the client undergoes scratch skin testing, which of the following signs is *most indicative* that the client has a hypersensitivity to the scratched substance?
○ 1. The skin at the test site feels numb.
○ 2. The skin at the test site feels painful.
○ 3. The skin at the test site looks pale.
◉ 4. The skin at the test site looks red.

Based on the outcome of the skin tests, the client begins desensitization treatment. She comes back every week for injections of diluted antigens to which she is allergic.

17 Each week after the client receives her injection, it is *essential* that the nurse remind her to
  ○ 1. take a couple of aspirin before leaving.
  ◉ 2. wait at least 20 minutes before going home.
  ○ 3. make sure someone else drives the car.
  ○ 4. call the office as soon as she arrives home.

18 When caring for a client with allergies, which one of the following is an *early indication* that the client is developing anaphylaxis?
  ◉ 1. The client has difficulty breathing.
  ○ 2. The client complains of a headache.
  ○ 3. The client develops a sore throat.
  ○ 4. The client loses bladder control.

19 Which one of the following drugs should the nurse plan to have available whenever there is a possibility that a person may develop a *severe* allergic reaction?
  ○ 1. Codeine sulfate
  ○ 2. Morphine sulfate
  ○ 3. Dopamine (Intropin)
  ◉ 4. Epinephrine (adrenalin)

20 The *most important* assessment for the nurse to make while managing the care of a client experiencing a severe allergic reaction is
  ○ 1. urine output.
  ○ 2. skin color.
  ◉ 3. blood pressure.
  ○ 4. pupil response.

21 If a person experiencing a severe allergic reaction becomes unresponsive, which of the following actions should the nurse take *first*?
  ○ 1. Administer a single blow to the sternum.
  ○ 2. Raise the client's head to 90 degrees.
  ◉ 3. Lift the chin and tilt the head back.
  ○ 4. Cover the individual with a blanket.

NURSING CARE OF CLIENTS HAVING A TONSILLECTOMY

22 Besides monitoring the vital signs of a client immediately after a tonsillectomy, the *best indication* that the client is experiencing postoperative bleeding is
  ◉ 1. frequent swallowing.
  ○ 2. periodic belching.
  ○ 3. occasional coughing.
  ○ 4. grinding of teeth.

23 Until the tonsillectomy client regains consciousness, the *best* body position to maintain is

  ○ 1. dorsal recumbent.
  ◉ 2. side-lying.
  ○ 3. high Fowler's.
  ○ 4. horizontal recumbent.

NURSING CARE OF CLIENTS WITH CANCER OF THE LARYNX

A client with cancer of the larynx is undergoing a total laryngectomy. The team gathers to develop a nursing care plan.

24 When the client returns from the post-anesthesia reacting room, which sign is an *early indication* that the client's oxygenation status is compromised?
  ○ 1. The client's dressing is bloody.
  ◉ 2. The client becomes restless.
  ○ 3. The client's heart rate is irregular.
  ○ 4. The client indicates he is thirsty.

25 Which one of the following nursing actions is the *best plan* for dealing with the client's impaired verbal communication?
  ○ 1. Lip-read the client's attempts at communication.
  ○ 2. Inform the client to speak slowly when talking.
  ○ 3. Listen attentively to the client's vocalizations.
  ◉ 4. Provide the client with paper and pencil.

The nursing team discusses a client's angry and depressed reaction to his diagnosis of cancer, the change in his body image, and the loss of speech following a laryngectomy.

26 Which one of the following best indicates that the client who had a laryngectomy is beginning to resolve his grief?
  ○ 1. The client wants only his wife to visit him.
  ○ 2. The client says his doctor made an incorrect diagnosis.
  ○ 3. The client looks at the tracheostomy tube in a mirror.
  ◉ 4. The client asks the nurse to help him bathe and shave.

NURSING CARE OF CLIENTS WITH INFLAMMATORY AND INFECTIOUS DISORDERS OF THE LOWER AIRWAYS

27 Although all of the following information is appropriate to gather when assessing a client with a cough, it is *most important* to document the characteristics of the cough and the
  ○ 1. client's family history of respiratory disease.
  ○ 2. current assessment of the client's vital signs.
  ◉ 3. appearance of respiratory secretions.
  ○ 4. any self-treatment that is being used.

A client who has had a persistent upper respiratory infection develops acute bronchitis and is given a prescription for elixir of terpin hydrate with codeine.

28 Which one of the following drug administration instructions is *most appropriate* for the nurse to provide?
○ 1. "Don't take the drug more frequently than prescribed."
○ 2. "Avoid taking the medication before going to sleep."
○ 3. "Drink extra fluids throughout your waking hours."
○ 4. "Warm the syrup to make the taste more acceptable."

The prescribed dose of a liquid cough syrup is 5 mL.

29 Which household measurement is the equivalent to recommend when teaching a client how to self-administer the prescribed amount of liquid cough syrup?
○ 1. 1 ounce
○ 2. 1 tablespoon
○ 3. 1 teaspoon
○ 4. 1 dram

A client is scheduled to receive liquid cough syrup and several other solid oral tablets at the same scheduled time.

30 Which of the following is *most appropriate* when administering the liquid cough syrup and the solid medications?
○ 1. Administer the cough syrup and then the solid tablets.
○ 2. Wait 15 minutes after the cough syrup before giving the solid tablets.
○ 3. Give the cough syrup in between administering the oral tablets.
○ 4. Administer the solid tablets and then the cough syrup.

A client with acute bronchitis is receiving aerosol therapy.

31 The *best evidence* that the client understands the purpose of his treatment is the statement that aerosol therapy is used to
○ 1. relieve tissue irritation.
○ 2. kill infectious organisms.
○ 3. dry respiratory passages.
○ 4. slow the respiratory rate.

A client with bronchitis asks the nurse why he is receiving guaifenesin (Robitussin AC), an antitussive that contains codeine.

32 The *best explanation* is that the guaifenesin liquefies mucus while the codeine

○ 1. relieves discomfort.
○ 2. dilates the bronchi.
○ 3. suppresses coughing.
○ 4. reduces inflammation.

When an adult male client with a diagnosis of pneumonia arrives, the nurse observes that he has shaking chills and a fever of 104.2°F. A chest x-ray and sputum specimens for culture and sensitivity are ordered.

33 Which of the following nursing actions is *essential* before the chest x-ray is done?
○ 1. Make sure the client does not eat food.
○ 2. Remove the metal necklace he is wearing.
○ 3. Have the client swallow x-ray dye.
○ 4. Administer a parenteral analgesic.

The client with pneumonia has difficulty raising his respiratory secretions.

34 If all of the following nursing measures are possible, which one helps *most* when planning to obtain the sputum specimen?
○ 1. Providing the client with a generous fluid intake.
○ 2. Encouraging the client to change positions regularly.
○ 3. Asking the dietitian to send the client food high in fiber.
○ 4. Seeing to it that the client has sufficient rest.

35 At what time of the day is it *best* for the nurse to attempt obtaining a sputum specimen?
○ 1. Before bedtime
○ 2. After a meal
○ 3. Between meals
○ 4. Upon awakening

36 The *best evidence* that the client understands the nurse's instruction on how to handle the sputum specimen container is when the client says
○ 1. he should don gloves before opening the container.
○ 2. he should wipe the container with an alcohol swab.
○ 3. he cannot touch the outside of the container.
○ 4. he must not touch the inside of the container.

37 After collecting the sputum specimen, which nursing action is *most appropriate*?
○ 1. Administer oxygen
○ 2. Provide mouth care
○ 3. Offer nourishment
○ 4. Encourage ambulation

38 While the nurse conducts a physical assessment, which one of the following findings *most indicates*

that the client with pneumonia also has developed pleurisy?

- ○ 1. The client has a productive cough.
- ● 2. The client has pain when breathing.
- ○ 3. The client's nailbeds are cyanotic.
- ○ 4. The client's heart rate is rapid.

A client with pneumococcal pneumonia is receiving penicillin by intramuscular injection and asks the nurse why the physician chose penicillin to treat the pneumonia.

39 The *best response* from the nurse is that

- ● 1. the sensitivity report showed the organism was easily killed by penicillin.
- ○ 2. most viral infections respond well when treated with penicillin drugs.
- ○ 3. penicillin is one of the safest yet most effective antibiotics.
- ○ 4. all antibiotics are similar; the choice of drug is not that important.

The nurse chooses to inject the prescribed dose of penicillin into the dorsogluteal site.

40 If the nurse selects the site *correctly*, the injection is administered into the

- ○ 1. hip.
- ○ 2. arm.
- ○ 3. thigh.
- ● 4. buttock.

41 The *recommended technique* to help reduce discomfort when giving an intramuscular injection into the dorsogluteal site is to have the client

- ● 1. point his toes inward.
- ○ 2. tighten his muscles.
- ○ 3. cross his legs.
- ○ 4. flex his knees.

42 If a client is allergic to penicillin, to which other group of antibiotics can the nurse anticipate that the client may also be hypersensitive?

- ○ 1. Aminoglycosides, like kanamycin sulfate (Kantex)
- ● 2. Tetracyclines, like doxycyline (Vibramycin)
- ○ 3. Cephalosporins, like ceftriaxone sodium (Rocephin)
- ○ 4. Floroquinolones, like ciprofloxacin (Cipro)

A nurse volunteer administers influenza vaccine to older adults during a community-wide immunization campaign.

43 Which question is *essential* to ask before administering the influenza vaccine?

- ○ 1. Have you had influenza in the past year?
- ○ 2. Did you receive pneumonia vaccine last year?
- ● 3. Are you allergic to eggs or egg products?
- ○ 4. Do you have a history of respiratory disease?

The nurse notes that an elderly resident with influenza has a fever of 104.6°F, headache, dry cough, and sore muscles.

44 In the absence of any pre-existing cardiovascular or renal disease, if the nurse instructs the nursing assistant to encourage the client to consume extra fluids, what is an *appropriate goal* for oral intake in the next 24-hour period?

- ○ 1. 500 mL
- ○ 2. 1000 mL
- ● 3. 1500 mL
- ○ 4. 3000 mL

The physician orders the nurse to give two aspirin tablets orally every 4 hours p.r.n. if the client with influenza has a fever over 102°F and to administer a tepid sponge bath at this time.

45 The nurse is *most accurate* in explaining to the client that the sponge bath is being given to

- ○ 1. maintain skin integrity.
- ○ 2. remove microorganisms.
- ● 3. promote heat loss.
- ○ 4. provide comfort.

The nursing assistant helping with the sponge bath asks the nurse to explain what the word tepid means.

46 The *best explanation* of the word "tepid" is that it means

- ○ 1. hot.
- ● 2. warm.
- ○ 3. cool.
- ○ 4. cold.

47 If the client with influenza develops all of the following, which one is an indication that the sponge bath should be discontinued?

- ○ 1. Nausea
- ● 2. Chills
- ○ 3. Flushing
- ○ 4. Confusion

48 Which of the following is the *best indication* that the tepid sponge bath is having a therapeutic effect?

- ● 1. The client is feeling more comfortable.
- ○ 2. The client feels like eating lunch.
- ○ 3. The client's rectal temperature is 102.4°F.
- ○ 4. The client's headache is somewhat relieved.

49 Other than obtaining a vaccination against influenza, what is the *best advice* the nurse can give to high-risk persons for avoiding influenza?

- ○ 1. Consume adequate vitamin C.
- ● 2. Avoid going to crowded places.
- ○ 3. Dress warmly in cold weather.
- ○ 4. Reduce daily stress and anxiety.

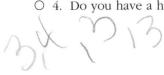

The nurse in a nursing home is required by the state's law to test all newly admitted clients for tuberculosis. The agency's policy is to administer a Mantoux intradermal skin test.

50 The nurse's injection technique is *correct* if the needle is inserted at a
- ● 1. 10-degree angle.
- ○ 2. 45-degree angle.
- ○ 3. 90-degree angle.
- ○ 4. 180-degree angle.

51 The nurse is *correct* in assessing the site of the tuberculin skin test
- ○ 1. in one week.
- ○ 2. the next day.
- ● 3. in 48 hours.
- ○ 4. in 5 days.

52 When it is determined that a tuberculin skin test is positive, the *most accurate* explanation is that
- ○ 1. there is an active infection present.
- ● 2. antibodies are present in the blood.
- ○ 3. the client is immune to this type of disease.
- ○ 4. the client needs to be in strict isolation.

53 When a previously negative client has a positive reaction to a tuberculin skin test, the nurse is *most correct* in explaining to the client that
- ○ 1. skin tests will be performed every 6 months.
- ○ 2. he or she will need to quit his or her job.
- ○ 3. he or she will need to live alone temporarily.
- ● 4. antituberculosis drug(s) will be prescribed.

A client with tuberculosis continues to have evidence of the tubercle bacilli in his sputum after 6 weeks of drug therapy.

54 Which one of the following questions is *most important* to ask at this time?
- ○ 1. When did you last take your prescribed medications?
- ● 2. Have you taken all your medications as prescribed?
- ○ 3. How many drug refills have you obtained?
- ○ 4. Have you experienced any drug side effects?

Efforts at obtaining a sputum specimen from a client who is suspected of having tuberculosis have been unsuccessful. The physician orders a gastric lavage.

55 The *best explanation* from the nurse as to the reason for performing a gastric lavage is that the organism
- ● 1. may be found in swallowed sputum.
- ○ 2. also infects gastric tissue.
- ○ 3. migrates from the lungs to the stomach.
- ○ 4. can be destroyed by instilling fluid.

56 Which health teaching measure is *most important* to emphasize when instructing the client with tuberculosis on ways to prevent transmission of the disease?
- ○ 1. Eating a nutritious diet.
- ○ 2. Getting adequate sleep.
- ● 3. Covering the nose and mouth when coughing.
- ○ 4. Handwashing before and after elimination.

The nurse follows up on the dietitian's instructions with a client with tuberculosis who must manage his needs on a very low income.

57 If the client identified that his lunches often included the following menus, which meal is the *most nutritious?*
- ○ 1. Tossed salad, vinaigrette dressing, iced tea
- ● 2. Jelly sandwich on whole wheat bread, coffee
- ○ 3. Meatless chili with beans, cornbread, milk
- ○ 4. Chicken bouillon, gelatin, sweetened lemonade

The physician prescribes a combination of aminosalicylate (Teebacin) and isoniazid (Laniazid) to treat a client with tuberculosis.

58 When the client asks the nurse why he is taking two drugs, the *best explanation* is that when these drugs are combined
- ○ 1. one diminishes the side effects of the other.
- ● 2. one kills the live organism, the other its spores.
- ○ 3. their dosages can be reduced.
- ○ 4. bacterial resistance is slowed.

59 To avoid the gastrointestinal side effects associated with aminosalicylate (Teebacin), the *best action* the nurse can plan is to
- ○ 1. administer the drug on an empty stomach.
- ● 2. give the drug with food or at mealtimes.
- ○ 3. encourage the client to drink lots of water.
- ○ 4. provide the client with a carbonated beverage.

NURSING CARE OF CLIENTS WITH CHRONIC OBSTRUCTIVE PULMONARY DISEASE

An adult male client who has had asthma since early childhood comes to the emergency department in respiratory distress.

60 The *best position* for the client when the nurse prepares to assess lung sounds is to have him
- ● 1. sit up.
- ○ 2. stand.
- ○ 3. lie on his back.
- ○ 4. lie on his side.

61 When the nurse listens to the asthma client breathe, the *most characteristic* lung sound during the onset of an asthma attack is
○ 1. wet bubbling.
○ 2. dry crackling.
○ 3. soft blowing.
◉ 4. noisy wheezing.

Pulse oximetry is used to monitor the oxygenation status of the asthmatic client.

62 The nurse is *most correct* in applying the sensor of the pulse oximeter to the client's
○ 1. arm.
○ 2. lip.
◉ 3. ear.
○ 4. leg.

63 If the client with asthma is diffusing sufficient oxygen from the lungs to the blood, the pulse oximeter displays a range between
○ 1. 80 to 100 mm Hg.
○ 2. 95 to 100 mm Hg.
○ 3. 80% to 100%.
◉ 4. 95% to 100%.

A blood sample is taken from the asthmatic client's radial artery to measure blood gases.

64 Immediately after the specimen is drawn, the *most essential* nursing action is to
◉ 1. apply direct pressure to the site for 5 minutes.
○ 2. warm the blood in the specimen tube for 5 minutes.
○ 3. assess the client's blood pressure in 5 minutes.
○ 4. elevate the client's arm for at least 5 minutes.

The physician orders 60% oxygen administration with a partial rebreathing mask and bag reservoir for the client having an asthma attack.

65 When administering oxygen with a partial rebreather mask, which of the following observations is *most important* to report to the respiratory therapy department?
○ 1. Moisture accumulates inside the mask.
◉ 2. The bag collapses during inspiration.
○ 3. The mask covers the mouth and nose.
○ 4. The strap about the head is snug.

The physician orders 0.1 mg of epinephrine subcutaneously for the asthmatic client. The label indicates that the epinephrine is a 1:1000 dilution, which means that 1 g of epinephrine has been mixed with 1000 mL of liquid.

66 The *correct volume* needed to administer the prescribed dose of 0.1 mg of epinephrine is
◉ 1. 0.1 mL.
○ 2. 1.0 mL.
○ 3. 10 mL.
○ 4. 0.001 mL.

67 Which one of the following nursing measures helps *most* to reduce the anxiety the client is experiencing during an asthma attack?
○ 1. Close the door to the examination room.
◉ 2. Remain within the client's view.
○ 3. Pull the bedside privacy curtain.
○ 4. Cover the client with a light sheet.

The physician orders pulmonary function tests for a client who has smoked cigarettes for many years.

68 The *best evidence* that the client understands the procedure involved in a pulmonary function test is that the client states this test involves
○ 1. having an x-ray.
○ 2. drawing blood.
◉ 3. breathing into a mouthpiece.
○ 4. examining expectorated sputum.

The condition of a client with emphysema worsens when he develops a respiratory infection.

69 While assisting the client with emphysema into a hospital gown, the nurse is *most likely* to find that his chest appears
○ 1. funnel-shaped.
◉ 2. barrel-shaped.
○ 3. slender.
○ 4. muscular.

The nurse prepares to administer oxygen to the client with emphysema with a nasal cannula.

70 Which one of the following oxygen flow rates is *most appropriate* for a client with emphysema?
◉ 1. 2 L/min
○ 2. 5 L/min
○ 3. 8 L/min
○ 4. 10 L/min

The client with emphysema is receiving intravenous fluid that contains aminophylline.

71 The nurse is *accurate* in explaining to the client that the *primary purpose* for using this drug is to
○ 1. relieve persistent coughing.
○ 2. lessen sputum production.
◉ 3. reduce respiratory distress.
○ 4. dilute thick secretions.

72 Which one of the following side effects can the nurse expect when a person receives aminophylline?
○ 1. Bronchospasm
○ 2. Hypotension
○ 3. Drowsiness
◉ 4. Tachycardia

73 When assisting the client with emphysema perform postural drainage, which one of the following nursing actions helps *most* to loosen secretions?
○ 1. Tell the client to take deep breaths.
◉ 2. Strike the back with a cupped hand.
○ 3. Apply pressure below the diaphragm.
○ 4. Place the client in a sitting position.

74 Which of the following nursing observations is the *best evidence* that postural drainage is effective?
○ 1. The client's respiratory rate is increased.
○ 2. The client's appetite is much improved.
○ 3. The client's sputum culture is negative.
◉ 4. The client expels a large volume of sputum

The physician orders 2 puffs of albuterol sulfate (Ventolin) four times a day using a metered dose inhaler.

75 After administering the first puff of aerosol, the *best evidence* that the client is using the inhaler correctly is that the client
○ 1. depresses the canister a second time before exhaling.
◉ 2. holds his or her breath for up to 10 seconds before exhaling.
○ 3. cleans the mouthpiece with a clean paper tissue or cloth.
○ 4. bends from the waist to increase the exhaled volume.

Before being discharged, the client with emphysema says to the nurse, "This disease made me a prisoner in my own home."

76 The *best response* from the nurse is
◉ 1. "Tell me more about how you're feeling."
○ 2. "There are lots of things you can still do."
○ 3. "You're just having a bad day today."
○ 4. "You'll probably feel better tomorrow."

77 Which discharge instruction is *best* for reducing fatigue and shortness of breath the client with chronic obstructive pulmonary disease experiences when eating?

○ 1. "Eat simple carbohydrates to obtain quick energy."
○ 2. "Eat fatty foods to get maximum caloric intake."
◉ 3. "Eat frequent small meals to reduce energy use."
○ 4. "Eat the largest meal late at night before sleep."

NURSING CARE OF CLIENTS WITH LUNG CANCER

An older adult male is undergoing diagnostic tests to determine if he has cancer of the lung.

78 If the client is typical of most others with cancer of the lung, which one of the following *early warning signs* did he most likely ignore?
○ 1. Difficulty swallowing
○ 2. Gradual weight loss
◉ 3. Persistent cough
○ 4. Unusual bleeding

The physician requests a sputum specimen from the client with possible lung cancer to see if it contains tumor cells.

79 Which one of the following nursing actions ensures that an appropriate specimen is collected?
○ 1. Have the client gargle and expectorate the liquid.
○ 2. Tell the client to provide a large volume of saliva.
◉ 3. Explain that he should attempt a deep, forceful cough.
○ 4. Swab the back of his throat to stimulate gagging.

A bronchoscopy is scheduled for the client with suspected lung cancer.

80 Which one of the following is *most important* for the nurse to plan prior to the bronchoscopy?
◉ 1. Keep the client from eating and drinking.
○ 2. Have the client empty his bowel and bladder.
○ 3. Ensure that the client gets adequate sleep.
○ 4. Scrub the upper chest with an antiseptic.

81 Which one of the following assessments is *most important* for the nurse to make following a bronchoscopy?
○ 1. Level of consciousness
○ 2. Condition of mouth
◉ 3. Respiratory effort
○ 4. Ability to speak

The nurse observes blood when suctioning the secretions that accumulate in the client's mouth after the bronchoscopy.

82 Which other additional assessment is *most important* for the nurse to make at this time to evaluate the significance of the bleeding?
- ◑ 1. Count the pulse rate.
- ○ 2. Listen to heart sounds.
- ○ 3. Check the pupil response.
- ○ 4. Measure chest expansion.

83 When the nurse empties the secretions from the suction container, which one of the following infection control measures is *most important* to perform?
- ○ 1. Wear a mask.
- ○ 2. Wear a gown.
- ○ 3. Wear goggles.
- ◑ 4. Wear gloves.

84 Which one of the following assessment techniques is *most important* for the nurse to perform before allowing a client food or fluids following a bronchoscopy?
- ○ 1. Touch the arch of the palate with a tongue blade.
- ○ 2. Listen to the abdomen for active bowel sounds.
- ○ 3. Inspect the oral mucous membranes for moisture.
- ◉ 4. Palpate the throat while the client swallows.

A client with lung cancer is scheduled for a pneumonectomy.

85 If the client has an *accurate understanding* of the explanation the surgeon provided, he tells the nurse that during surgery
- ○ 1. one of his lungs will be removed.
- ◉ 2. one lobe of his lung will be removed.
- ○ 3. a sample of tissue from his lung will be biopsied.
- ○ 4. a lung will be opened and examined during surgery.

86 While helping to develop the postoperative plan of care for the client who is undergoing a pneumonectomy, it is *essential* to stress that this client lie with his
- ◉ 1. healthy lung uppermost.
- ○ 2. head lower than his heart.
- ○ 3. legs gatched at the knees.
- ○ 4. arms elevated on pillows.

87 If the client who has a pneumonectomy manifests all of the following, which one is a *temporary, expected outcome* of thoracic surgery?

- ◑ 1. Persistent cough
- ○ 2. Chest numbness
- ○ 3. Impaired swallowing
- ○ 4. Prolonged anorexia

88 Following the administration of morphine sulfate to the client with a pneumonectomy, which assessment is *most important* to make?
- ○ 1. Color of wound drainage
- ○ 2. Temperature of the skin
- ○ 3. Range of motion
- ◉ 4. Respiratory rate

The nurse prepares a client with advanced lung cancer and pleural effusion for a thoracentesis.

89 Which position is *most correct* for the nurse to place a client undergoing a thoracentesis?
- ○ 1. Lithotomy
- ○ 2. Sitting
- ○ 3. Prone
- ◉ 4. Supine

NURSING CARE OF CLIENTS WITH CHEST INJURIES

90 Before treating and releasing a client with fractured ribs from the emergency department, which one of the following instructions is *most important* for the nurse to provide?
- ◉ 1. Breathe deeply several times every hour.
- ○ 2. Breathe shallowly to avoid discomfort.
- ○ 3. Breathe rapidly to promote ventilation.
- ○ 4. Breathe into a paper bag every hour.

A nurse stops to assist after witnessing a motorcycle accident.

91 When assessing the accident victim, which finding is *most indicative* that the individual has a flail chest?
- ○ 1. Sucking air is heard near the chest.
- ◉ 2. The trachea deviates from midline.
- ○ 3. A portion of chest moves inward during inspiration.
- ○ 4. The victim has severe chest pain during expiration.

During a mugging, a victim is stabbed in the chest, causing his lung to collapse. Two chest tubes are inserted in the emergency department.

92 Where is it *most likely* that the nurse will see bloody drainage?
- ○ 1. From the victim's nose
- ○ 2. From the victim's mouth
- ○ 3. From the tube in the upper chest
- ◉ 4. From the tube in the lower chest

Once the two chest tubes are inserted, they are connected to a commercial waterseal drainage system.

93   When the nurse monitors the chamber with the water-seal, which finding suggests that the system is functioning *appropriately*?
   ○ 1. The fluid rises and falls with respirations.
   ○ 2. The fluid level is lower than when first filled.
   ● 3. The fluid bubbles continuously.
   ○ 4. The fluid looks frothy white.

94   When caring for the client with a hemothorax, it is *essential* that the chest drainage tube
   ● 1. hangs below the opening in the drainage collector.
   ○ 2. hangs straight from the bed into the container.
   ○ 3. is wrapped so as to encircle the client's chest.
   ○ 4. is tucked securely under the bed's mattress.

95   Which one of the following is *most indicative* that air is leaking into the tissue around a chest tube insertion site?
   ○ 1. The tissue appears pale or almost colorless.
   ○ 2. There is a hissing sound like a leaking tire.
   ● 3. The skin crackles when touched.
   ○ 4. Air is felt as it escapes.

A client with waterseal drainage is transported for a chest x-ray.

96   Which of the following nursing actions is *most appropriate* at this time?
   ○ 1. Clamp the chest tubes before leaving the room.
   ● 2. Keep the drainage system below the insertion site.
   ○ 3. Attach a portable suction machine to the chest tubes.
   ○ 4. Provide mechanical ventilation during transport.

97   What is the *best method* for determining the amount of drainage from a chest tube when a closed waterseal system is used?
   ○ 1. Empty the collection chamber and measure the volume.
   ○ 2. Subtract the client's fluid intake from his output.
   ○ 3. Instill sterile irrigation solution and measure the drainage.
   ● 4. Subtract the previously marked volume from the current amount.

NURSING CARE OF CLIENTS WITH PULMONARY EMBOLISM

Following an abdominal hysterectomy, a client suddenly experiences severe chest pain and dyspnea. A pulmonary embolism is suspected.

98   When the client whose condition has changed suddenly says, "Nurse, I'm dying," what is the *best* nursing response?
   ○ 1. "You'll be just fine in a few minutes."
   ● 2. "I'll stay with you while we wait for the doctor."
   ○ 3. "Why would you even think something like that?"
   ○ 4. "Let's talk about something more pleasant."

99   During the time the client with a suspected pulmonary embolism is experiencing chest pain and dyspnea, which nursing action is *most important*?
   ● 1. Administer oxygen by face mask.
   ○ 2. Turn on the television for distraction.
   ○ 3. Offer the client a sip of water.
   ○ 4. Wipe the client's face with a cool cloth.

The client with a pulmonary embolism becomes unresponsive, stops breathing, and is pulseless. The nurse initiates cardiopulmonary resuscitation (CPR).

100   How many breaths per minute are administered to an adult when performing cardiopulmonary resuscitation?
   ○ 1. 8 per minute
   ● 2. 12 per minute
   ○ 3. 15 per minute
   ○ 4. 20 per minute

NURSING CARE OF CLIENTS WITH A TRACHEOSTOMY

101   Which of the following assessments provides the *best indication* that the nurse needs to suction the client with a tracheostomy?
   ○ 1. Respirations are deep.
   ○ 2. Pulse rate is slow.
   ● 3. Wet lung sounds are heard.
   ○ 4. Blood pressure is low.

102   Which nursing action is *essential* before suctioning the client with a tracheostomy tube?
   ○ 1. Provide mouth care.
   ○ 2. Moisten the catheter.
   ○ 3. Clean around the stoma.
   ● 4. Remove the inner cannula.

103 When is the *best time* to occlude the vent on the suction catheter when suctioning a client with a tracheostomy?
- ○ 1. Before inserting the catheter
- ○ 2. When inside the inner cannula
- ● 3. While withdrawing the catheter
- ○ 4. When the client begins coughing

104 When suctioning the airway of a client with a tracheostomy, the nurse applies suction for *no longer than*
- ○ 1. 5 to 7 seconds.
- ● 2. 10 to 15 seconds.
- ○ 3. 15 to 20 seconds.
- ○ 4. 20 to 30 seconds.

105 While withdrawing the suction catheter from a client's tracheostomy tube, which one of the following nursing techniques is *most correct*?
- ○ 1. Remove the catheter slowly.
- ○ 2. Pinch and pull the catheter.
- ○ 3. Plunge the catheter up and down.
- ● 4. Twist and rotate the catheter.

106 Which assessment is best for determining if the client with a tracheostomy is becoming hypoxemic while being suctioned?
- ○ 1. Monitoring level of consciousness
- ○ 2. Assessing skin color and temperature
- ● 3. Watching pulse oximetry levels
- ○ 4. Counting the respiratory rate

A nurse has been asked to be a peer evaluator when other nurses practice the procedure for tracheostomy care during an inservice program.

107 When performing the tracheostomy care demonstration, it is *correct* for each nurse to
- ○ 1. cut a gauze square to fit around the stoma.
- ○ 2. secure the ties at the back of the neck.
- ● 3. attach new ties before removing the old.
- ○ 4. replace the cannula after changing the ties.

108 Which one of the following explanations is the *most accurate* reason for using a cuffed tracheostomy tube?
- ● 1. The cuff prevents skin breakdown.
- ○ 2. The cuff prevents aspiration.
- ○ 3. The cuff provides more comfort.
- ○ 4. The cuff reduces infection.

NURSING CARE OF CLIENTS WITH A SUDDEN AIRWAY OCCLUSION

A frantic person calls the physician's office because a family member is choking on a piece of hard candy.

109 What information in the following list does the physician's office nurse need to know *first* before recommending further action?
- ○ 1. Is the person able to walk?
- ● 2. Is the person able to cough?
- ○ 3. In what position is the person?
- ○ 4. Can the person still swallow?

During a school banquet a piece of meat becomes lodged in a person's airway.

110 The *most accurate* placement of the hands when performing the Heimlich maneuver is to place the thumb side of the fist
- ○ 1. on the manubrium.
- ○ 2. on the xiphoid process.
- ● 3. below the navel.
- ○ 4. below the sternum.

Directions: Two numbers appear in parentheses following each rationale. The first number identifies the textbook listed in the references, page 512, and the second number identifies the page(s) in that textbook on which the correct answer can be verified. Occasionally two or more textbooks are given to verify the correct answer.

NURSING CARE OF CLIENTS WITH UPPER RESPIRATORY INFECTIONS

1 1. The common cold is a viral infection of the nasal passages and throat. Antibiotics are only useful in treating bacterial infections. No drug cures the common cold. A head cold without additional secondary complications is self-limiting. (18:1191; 21:279)
Nursing Process—Implementation
Client Need—Health promotion/maintenance

2 3. A high fever suggests that the client with a common cold has acquired a secondary bacterial infection, such as bronchitis or pneumonia. Viral infections like the common cold generally are associated with a low-grade fever. Symptoms of the common cold are generally confined to the head and throat. They include nasal congestion and discharge, discomfort in the nose and throat, sneezing, and watery eyes. The person also may have a headache, feel chilled, and experience fatigue and loss of appetite. A dry cough is due to nasal drainage passing into the pharynx causing irritation. A productive cough is more indicative that the infection involves the lower respiratory tract. (18:1191)
Nursing Process—Data collection
Client Need—Physiological integrity

3 3. Nonprescription decongestants are contraindicated for individuals with hypertension and heart disease. Most contain adrenergic drugs like ephedrine sulfate, which stimulate the sympathetic nervous system. They cause tachycardia and increase blood pressure, even in normal individuals. Adrenergic drugs are not contraindicated in individuals with arthritis, asthma, or diabetes unless they had accompanying cardiovascular disease. (17:378; 20:242)
Nursing Process—Data collection
Client Need—Physiological integrity

4 1. Using nasal decongestants, which have a vasoconstricting action, more frequently than recommended tends to result in nasal congestion from rebound vasodilation. Decongestants do not cause physical dependence nor microbial drug resistance. Ulcer-
ation of the nasal mucosa is more likely a consequence of irritation and trauma from blowing and wiping the nose. (17:378; 20:242)
Nursing Process—Implementation
Client Need—Health promotion/maintenance

5 2. Excessive or forceful nose blowing can propel infectious secretions into the eustachian tube, causing a secondary ear infection. Keeping the head elevated when asleep, the ears covered, or placing cotton in the ear canal does not reduce the potential for developing an ear infection. (17:378)
Nursing Process—Implementation
Client Need—Health promotion/maintenance

6 3. The maxillary sinuses are located in the cheek. Pain from maxillary sinusitis is described as being in the cheek or the upper teeth. If the frontal sinuses are infected, the pain is felt near the eyes. (18:1205; 21:276)
Nursing Process—Data collection
Client Need—Physiological integrity

7 2. Overuse of nasal decongestants leads to "rebound phenomenon." This means that the congestion becomes worse and recurs in less time after using the drug. Discontinuing the use of the drug causes the client to experience the original nasal congestion, but systemic withdrawal symptoms typical of addiction do not occur. Most decongestants are adrenergic drugs, which cause vasoconstriction, not bleeding. The mucous membrane may sting, burn, or feel dry. The immune system is unaffected by nasal decongestants. (17:378; 20:242)
Nursing Process—Implementation
Client Need—Health promotion/maintenance

8 3. Tilting the head backward allows gravity and head positioning to locate and maintain the liquid nasal medication within the nasopharynx. Bending forward causes loss of medication before it can provide a therapeutic effect. None of the other described positions help distribute nasal medications where they are intended for use. (17:384; 20:244)

Nursing Process—Implementation
Client Need—Health promotion/maintenance

9 3. The greatest danger in using a steam vaporizer is the potential for accidental scalding. Steam vaporizers do saturate the air with moisture and may cause a fire if the heating element comes in contact with flammable materials. It is more appropriate to suggest using a cool mist humidifier rather than a steam vaporizer. (16:579)

Nursing Process—Implementation
Client Need—Safe, effective care environment

NURSING CARE OF CLIENTS WITH INFLAMMATORY AND ALLERGIC DISORDERS OF THE UPPER AIRWAYS

10 3. The throat is swabbed with a sterile applicator to obtain a sample of infectious organisms in the inflamed tissue of the pharynx. A sputum specimen is obtained by expectoration. A throat culture is obtained from the posterior pharynx rather than the mouth and tongue. Organisms in saliva would not necessarily indicate the pathogen causing pharyngitis. (18:1178; 25:214)

Nursing Process—Implementation
Client Need—Safe, effective care environment

11 1. Glomerulonephritis, rheumatic fever, and rheumatic heart disease are but a few of the consequences following untreated or undertreated infections caused by the beta hemolytic Streptococcus organism. To ensure that the organism is destroyed, the American Heart Association recommends that streptococcal infections be treated with penicillin or erythromycin for a full 10 days. The other three diseases are infectious but are not caused by this particular organism. (18:1191; 21:278)

Nursing Process—Implementation
Client Need—Health promotion/maintenance

12 2. Speaking in a normal voice or whispering prolongs laryngitis. Resting swollen vocal cords allows the local edema to subside. Laryngitis is not associated with a vitamin deficiency. Simple laryngitis does not usually require bed rest. Massaging the throat provides comfort for some people, but it does not relieve hoarseness. (18:1192; 21:279)

Nursing Process—Implementation
Client Need—Health promotion/maintenance

13 3. Persistent hoarseness is the earliest symptom of cancer of the larynx. Nagging cough or hoarseness is one of the seven early warning signs of cancer identified by the American Cancer Society. The

other diseases cause respiratory symptoms, none of which is hoarseness. (18:1192; 21:297)

Nursing Process—Evaluation
Client Need—Health promotion/maintenance

14 3. Antihistamines commonly cause people to feel drowsy and fall asleep easily. Anyone taking an antihistamine is warned to use caution if driving or operating machinery while taking a drug in this category. If there is any effect on weight, it is more likely to be weight gain due to a reduction in activity. Gastrointestinal side effects include increased appetite, nausea, and diarrhea, but not constipation. (17:377; 20:238)

Nursing Process—Implementation
Client Need—Health promotion/maintenance

15 1. Many hypersensitive people are allergic to more than one substance. Testing does not promote the production of blocking antibodies. Even though skin testing is considered a standard of practice among allergy specialists and insurance companies partially or completely pay for this service, most clients generally want to know how the proposed medical care benefits them personally. (18:1160; 21:487)

Nursing Process—Implementation
Client Need—Health promotion/maintenance

16 4. An area of local erythema, or redness, indicates a positive reaction to the antigen applied to the scratched skin. Swelling, known as induration, also may accompany a reaction. A positive reaction does not appear pale or feel especially painful or numb. (18:1160; 21:487)

Nursing Process—Data collection
Client Need—Physiological integrity

17 2. The client undergoing desensitization stays in the physician's office for observation for at least 20 minutes following the injection. Occasionally, a person has a severe allergic reaction to even the small amount of antigen used in the desensitization injection. The client's safety is endangered if a severe reaction occurs and medical assistance is not immediately available. Antihistamines may reduce allergic symptoms, but aspirin has no direct effect. If a client waits 20 minutes, driving is not contraindicated. The client need not call the office when arriving home. (18:1161)

Nursing Process—Implementation
Client Need—Physiological integrity

18 1. Signs of anaphylaxis include labored breathing, hives, and loss of consciousness as blood pressure falls. Headache, sore throat, and urinary incontinence are not associated with an anaphylactic reaction. (4:1153; 18:357; 21:490)

    Nursing Process—Data collection
    Client Need—Physiological integrity

19 4. Epinephrine is the drug of choice when a client experiences a severe allergic reaction. This drug helps raise the blood pressure by constricting blood vessels and dilates the bronchi, thereby facilitating breathing. Without emergency treatment, persons experiencing severe allergic reactions can die in 5 to 10 minutes. Codeine and morphine are central nervous system depressants. They potentiate hypotension. Dopamine is an adrenergic drug in the same family as epinephrine, but it is not the drug of choice during anaphylaxis. It is more often given later to maintain the blood pressure of individuals in shock. (18:357; 21:491)

    Nursing Process—Planning
    Client Need—Physiological integrity

20 3. Because shock is one of the major problems during a severe allergic reaction, monitoring blood pressure is the most important assessment for evaluating the effectiveness of treatment. The nurse expects the blood pressure to rise, breathing becomes less labored, and the person becomes alert. Maintaining adequate urine output indicates that a person's circulatory volume is sufficient, but this assessment is difficult unless a urinary catheter is in place. Skin color is not as valid an assessment, but it should go from pale to appropriate ethnic color once blood flow is restored to the periphery. As long as the brain is receiving adequate oxygen, the pupils continue to respond by constricting when stimulated with direct light. (4:1153; 21:491)

    Nursing Process—Data collection
    Client Need—Physiological integrity

21 3. Establishing or maintaining an open airway is the first step in resuscitation. Administering a precordial thump is appropriate in a witnessed cardiac arrest, but this is not generally the case in a severe allergic reaction. Raising the head is inappropriate because it interferes with resuscitation efforts and reduces blood flow to the brain. Covering normothermic individuals with blankets diverts blood to the skin rather than internal organs. (18:1154; 21:402)

    Nursing Process—Implementation
    Client Need—Physiological integrity

NURSING CARE OF CLIENTS HAVING A TONSILLECTOMY

22 1. Frequent swallowing often accompanies hemorrhage following nasal or oral surgery. Belching, coughing, and grinding the teeth are not associated with blood loss. (4:897; 18:904)

    Nursing Process—Data collection
    Client Need—Physiological integrity

23 2. Until a client is awake and alert after a tonsillectomy the client is maintained in a side-lying or prone position. This position enables blood to drain from the mouth rather than swallowed or aspirated. Once the client is alert and can control his or her own secretions, a semi-Fowler's position is appropriate. (18:904; 21:277)

    Nursing Process—Implementation
    Client Need—Physiological integrity

NURSING CARE OF CLIENTS WITH CANCER OF THE LARYNX

24 2. Of the choices provided, restlessness is the most indicative sign of early hypoxia. Blood loss is expected; if it is profuse or prolonged, it eventually affects the red blood cells' oxygen-carrying capacity. Clients with compromised oxygenation are more likely to manifest tachycardia than an irregular heart rhythm. Thirst is a sign of hypovolemia. (25:402; 26:875)

    Nursing Process—Data collection
    Client Need—Physiological integrity

25 4. Until the laryngectomy client learns esophageal speech or the use of a mechanical vibrator, providing paper and pencil or a magic slate is the best alternative for communication. Lip reading is often frustrating for nursing personnel who are unaccustomed to this technique. The client has a permanent loss of natural voice as a result of a total laryngectomy. (4:891; 21:287)

    Nursing Process—Planning
    Client Need—Physiological integrity

26 3. Looking at the tracheostomy tube is interpreted as dealing with the reality of the loss. This is a positive step toward acceptance and adaptation. Grieving follows a cycle of denial or disbelief, anger, depression, bargaining, and acceptance. Believing that there has been a misdiagnosis is an example of denial. Social isolation indicates a state of depression characterized by withdrawal from human interaction. Asking the nurse to help him bathe and

shave suggests that the client perceives himself as helpless. (4:1571)
> Nursing Process—Evaluation
> Client Need—Psychosocial integrity

NURSING CARE OF CLIENTS WITH INFLAMMATORY AND INFECTIOUS DISORDERS OF THE LOWER AIRWAYS

27 3. When assessing a cough, the nurse determines if the cough is nonproductive or productive. If the cough is productive, it is important to document the color, odor, amount, and viscosity of sputum that is raised. Other data that may aid the physician in making a diagnosis include the onset, duration, precipitating factors, and relief measures. (4:880; 17:390)
> Nursing Process—Data collection
> Client Need—Physiological integrity

28 1. A patient taking a narcotic (codeine) is warned not to exceed the recommended dose. Extra self-administration leads to sedation and habituation. Because narcotic antitussives do not interfere with sleep, their administration is not contraindicated before retiring. Expectorants, not sedative antitussives, are taken with extra fluids to thin mucoid secretions facilitating their expectoration. Chilling substances, rather than warming them, is more likely to disguise an unpleasant taste. (20:248)
> Nursing Process—Planning
> Client Need—Health promotion/maintenance

29 3. The approximate equivalent of 5 mL is one teaspoon in household measurements. Some manufacturers of nonprescription cough medications include a dosing cup marked with various household equivalents. To ensure safety, however, the nurse includes an explanation of the equivalent during discharge instructions. Four or five mL is the approximate equivalent of one dram in the apothecary system of measurements, but the apothecary system of measurements is not usually used when instructing lay persons on self-administration of medications. (17:35; 20:33)
> Nursing Process—Implementation
> Client Need—Health promotion/maintenance

30 4. Syrups are given last and are not followed by water or other liquids for a period of time because they are intended to have a soothing effect on the mucosa of the pharynx. Waiting 15 minutes after giving the syrup shortens the time of local effectiveness. The remaining alternatives involve swallowing water immediately after administering the cough syrup. (17:391–392)
> Nursing Process—Implementation
> Client Need—Physiological integrity

31 1. Aerosol therapy involves depositing small droplets of moisture onto respiratory tissue. The warmed moist air soothes the respiratory passages and liquefies secretions produced as a result of the inflammation. Other benefits are obtained by adding medications to the vaporized water. Individuals with acute bronchitis are generally bothered initially by a nonproductive cough that is aggravated by dry air. Oral or parenteral antibiotic therapy is used to kill infectious organisms. Respiratory mucosa is moist. The respiratory rate is lowered as ventilation is improved. However, this is a secondary benefit of aerosol therapy and not its primary purpose. (18:1218; 25:776)
> Nursing Process—Evaluation
> Client Need—Health promotion/maintenance

32 3. Codeine depresses the cough center in the brain. Antitussives that contain codeine or a similar synthetic chemical, dextromethorphan, are called sedative antitussives. They are indicated when a person's lungs are clear, but persistent coughing continues that serves no good purpose or adversely affects recovery from other conditions. Bronchodilators open respiratory passages. Salicylates and steroids are types of drugs that reduce inflammation. (17:388–390; 20:246–247)
> Nursing Process—Implementation
> Client Need—Health promotion/maintenance

33 2. Any article containing metal is removed before a chest x-ray is performed. The image of a metal object that remains in place during an x-ray may be misinterpreted as diseased tissue. Fasting is not required before a chest x-ray. No radiopaque dye is given for a chest x-ray. Analgesia is not necessary because there is no accompanying discomfort. (7:191))
> Nursing Process—Planning
> Client Need—Safe, effective care environment

34 1. Respiratory secretions that are difficult to raise are thinned when fluid intake is increased. Increasing moisture in inspired air through humidification also helps. Changing positions improves circulation and prevents pooling of respiratory secretions. High-fiber foods help to reduce or prevent constipation. Frequent rest relieves fatigue and activity intolerance. (25:775–776)
> Nursing Process—Planning
> Client Need—Safe, effective care environment

35 4. It is easiest to obtain a sputum specimen when the client first awakens in the morning or following an aerosol treatment. Secretions tend to accumulate in the respiratory tract during the night. Pooled secretions are more easily raised, especially if the individual is not fatigued from activity. Forced coughing after a meal can lead to vomiting. (7:753; 25:776)

    Nursing Process—Planning
    Client Need—Safe, effective care environment

36 4. The client must not touch the inside of the sputum specimen container or the inside of its lid. The inside of the container is kept sterile so that no other sources of microorganisms, other than what is present in the sputum, are collected. The hands contain abundant pathogens and nonpathogens. It is not necessary to don gloves because the outside of the container can be touched. Wiping the outside of the container is not necessary because it is considered unclean anyway. (18:559; 21:271)

    Nursing Process—Evaluation
    Client Need—Health promotion/maintenance

37 2. Mouth care is an appropriate hygiene measure after obtaining a sputum specimen. Expectorating sputum often causes a residual foul taste in the mouth or an unpleasant odor to the breath. Oxygen is appropriate if the client is short of breath. Eating is delayed until the client is rested and unlikely to become nauseous. Walking may cause further fatigue after the effort of coughing. (25:776)

    Nursing Process—Implementation
    Client Need—Physiological integrity

38 2. The most classic symptom associated with pleurisy is feeling a sharp, stabbing pain when taking a deep breath. Pleurisy is an inflammation of the pleural membranes surrounding the lungs. If a cough is present, it is due to some other pulmonary problem. Cyanotic nailbeds and tachycardia are caused by any number of cardiopulmonary diseases that interfere with tissue oxygenation. (4:909; 18:1194)

    Nursing Process—Data collection
    Client Need—Physiological integrity

39 1. Antibiotics are selected on the basis of their effect on the infectious organism. This information is obtained by performing a culture and sensitivity. The organism is first encouraged to grow in the laboratory medium. Then small disks of various drugs are placed in the growing colonies. If growth is inhibited around a certain disk, it is a good drug to use. Antibiotics are ineffective in treating viral infections. Though widely used, penicillin, like any other drug, has dangerous side effects. Such things as drug effectiveness, cost, route of administration, the client's history of drug allergy, and other factors affect the physician's choice. (17:104–105; 20:52)

    Nursing Process—Implementation
    Client Need—Health promotion/maintenance

40 4. The dorsogluteal site is located in the buttock. The hip is the location of the ventrogluteal site. The deltoid site is located in the arm. The vastus lateralis and rectus femoris are injection sites located in the thigh. (18:740; 25:739)

    Nursing Process—Implementation
    Client Need—Physiological integrity

41 1. Pointing the toes inward reduces the discomfort when giving an injection into the dorsogluteal site. Tightening muscles increases discomfort. Crossing the legs and flexing the knees places the client in an awkward position and does not relieve discomfort. (18:734; 25:745)

    Nursing Process—Implementation
    Client Need—Physiological integrity

42 3. Cephalosporins are chemically similar to penicillins. Therefore, it is appropriate for nurses to anticipate that a person who is allergic to penicillin may also react adversely when given a cephalosporin type of antibiotic. Before administering a cephalosporin to a client with a pencillin allergy, it is best to consult the physician and observe the client closely if the medical order is not changed. Although allergic reactions occur with the administration of any antibiotic, the other antibiotic groups do not demonstrate the same cross-sensitivity with penicillin. (17:110; 20:60)

    Nursing Process—Data collection
    Client Need—Physiological integrity

43 3. Influenza vaccine contains albumin from the eggs in which the virus is cultured. Individuals who are allergic to egg or egg products may react adversely. Influenza vaccinations are repeated yearly to provide immunity against viral strains identified during the previous year. Having had a pneumococcal pneumonia vaccine, which also is recommended for older adults, has no correlation with administering the influenza vaccine. Although influenza and pneumococcal vaccines are recommended for anyone with a chronic disease, it is not an essential criterion. (3:247)

    Nursing Process—Data collection
    Client Need—Physiological integrity

44 4. An intake of 3000 mL is safe in the absence of any pre-existing cardiovascular or renal problems. The additional fluid helps to keep the client hydrated and aids in temperature regulation. Less than 3000 mL is insufficient due to the increased metabolic rate secondary to the extremely elevated body temperature. (18:160; 25:253)

Nursing Process—Planning
Client Need—Physiological integrity

45 3. A sponge bath enhances loss of body heat by promoting evaporation from the skin's surface. Soap is not used when giving a sponge bath to a feverish client. Therefore, its purpose is not to remove microorganisms nor to maintain skin integrity. For some clients, a sponge bath feels soothing. However, comfort is not the primary purpose for administering the sponge bath to a feverish patient. (4:279; 18:573; 25:585, 590)

Nursing Process—Implementation
Client Need—Health promotion/maintenance

46 3. Tepid means a temperature that is cool or lukewarm. Most authorities recommend that a tepid temperature is in the range of 80°F to 93°F. It is not appropriate to use bath water that is hot or warm when trying to reduce a fever. Cold or icy water is only used if the client has severe hyperthermia, for example, from heat stroke. (18:573; 25:583)

Nursing Process—Implementation
Client Need—Health promotion/maintenance

47 2. Chilling is an indication that the body temperature is falling too rapidly. The muscle contraction that accompanies chilling produces heat and interferes with reducing body temperature. It is best to temporarily discontinue the sponge bath, dry the skin, and protect the client from any drafts. Nausea is not an adverse effect associated with sponge bathing. A feverish individual is likely to appear flushed and may become disoriented. These signs indicate that nursing measures, such as the sponge bath, need to proceed to relieve the fever. (18:573; 25:145)

Nursing Process—Data collection
Client Need—Physiological integrity

48 3. A decrease in the client's temperature is the best evidence that the tepid sponge bath is having a therapeutic effect. Feeling more comfortable and hungry, along with relief of the headache, are subjective responses that correlate with fever reduction. However, objective data are more reliable indicators. (4:279; 18:573)

Nursing Process—Evaluation
Client Need—Physiological integrity

49 2. All of the options provided help reduce the potential for infection. However, because respiratory infections are primarily spread by direct contact with another sick individual, avoiding crowds is the best advice. The U.S. Public Health Service Advisory Committee on Immunization recommends annual vaccination against influenza for people over the age of 65 and those with other chronic health problems. (18:1192)

Nursing Process—Implementation
Client Need—Health promotion/maintenance

50 1. When administering an intradermal injection, the needle is inserted between the layers of skin at approximately a 10- to 15-degree angle. Subcutaneous injections are given at either a 45- or 90-degree angle depending on the size of the client. Intramuscular injections are given at a 90-degree angle. It is incorrect to give any injection by inserting the needle at a 180-degree angle. (18:730; 25:733)

Nursing Process—Implementation
Client Need—Physiologic integrity

51 3. The standard length of time for reading a tuberculin skin test is 48 to 72 hours after the test is administered. The nurse observes for signs of redness and measures any evidence of an indurated (hard) area of tissue. Some individuals who are immunosuppressed do not always respond positively to the initial skin test, yet they are symptomatic. A second skin test that is more strongly concentrated is administered to immunosuppressed clients and additional diagnostic tests, like a sputum examination and chest x-ray, are performed to definitively diagnose the disease. (4:902; 21:303)

Nursing Process—Implementation
Client Need—Health promotion/maintenance

52 2. A positive tuberculin skin test indicates that at some time, the person became infected with the microorganism that causes tuberculosis and developed antibodies. It does not necessarily mean that there is a currently active infectious process taking place, nor does it mean that there is not an active infection. Anyone with a positive tuberculin skin test without any known history of having had the disease, must have a subsequent chest x-ray and sputum examinations. Drugs are administered prophylactically to individuals who suddenly test positive after having a history of being negative. A positive skin test does not indicate protective immunity. This infectious disease is transmitted by inhaling moist droplets or dried spores containing the infectious organism. The Centers for Disease Control and Prevention recommends following Airborne Precautions,

which requires wearing a particulate air filter respirator when caring for hospitalized clients who are actively contagious. (16:251; 14:815, 842)
   Nursing Process—Implementation
   Client Need—Health promotion/maintenance

53 4. Prophylactic drug therapy with isoniazid (INH) is initiated whenever a person with a previously negative skin test demonstrates a positive reaction. Isoniazid is combined with other drugs if the disease is confirmed with additional diagnostic tests like sputum examinations and chest x-ray. Once a skin test is positive, it remains positive life-long. Most individuals with active tuberculosis become noninfectious within two weeks with appropriate drug therapy; therefore unemployment is not a realistic consequence. Immediate family members also are tested and treated prophylactically so that living separately is unnecessary. (20:93)
   Nursing Process—Implementation
   Client Need—Health promotion/maintenance

54 2. Noncompliance is one of the leading causes of treatment failures. All clients who must take one or more drugs need to be informed that their medications should be taken consistently throughout the treatment period. (4:903; 20:95; 21:303)
   Nursing Process—Data collection
   Client Need—Health promotion/maintenance

55 1. Gastric lavage is used to obtain a specimen from a person who swallows respiratory secretions rather than expectorating them. Tuberculosis is spread to other tissues besides the lungs. However, the spread is generally by means of the bloodstream. The gastric secretions tend to destroy organisms. The instilled fluid provides sufficient liquid volume in the stomach to aid in removing the desired specimen. (21:303; 26:299)
   Nursing Process—Implementation
   Client Need—Health promotion/maintenance

56 3. To prevent the transmission of infectious microorganisms that cause tuberculosis, it is appropriate to instruct clients to cover the nose and mouth when coughing or sneezing, dispose of paper tissues appropriately, and perform frequent handwashing. Although handwashing is important for everyone following elimination, there is no logical correlation between preventing tuberculosis which is spread through respiratory secretions and washing the hands before and after elimination. Eating nutritiously and obtaining adequate sleep promote healing and early resolution of the active disease process. (4:903; 26:299)
   Nursing Process—Implementation
   Client Need—Health promotion/maintenance

57 3. Combining beans and a grain is an economic means of consuming all essential amino acids found in an animal source. Drinking milk also improves the nutrition of this meal choice. The alternative meals are economic. However, because they do not provide adequate sources of protein, they are not considered nutritious choices. (6:177–178; 25:228–229)
   Nursing Process—Evaluation
   Client Need—Physiological integrity

58 4. Bacterial resistance occurs more slowly when antitubercular drugs are used in combination rather than singly. Side effects are not reduced; they do not act at different periods during the organism's life cycle; and their dosage is not altered when given in combination. (17:130; 20:93; 21:303)
   Nursing Process—Implementation
   Client Need—Health promotion/maintenance

59 2. Giving medication with food protects the stomach from becoming upset. The potential for gastric upset is increased if irritating medications are administered on an empty stomach. Drinking water does not necessarily reduce gastrointestinal side effects. Though a carbonated beverage may relieve stomach distention, it is not the best approach for reducing the irritation caused by many drugs, including aminosalicylate. (17:131; 20:97)
   Nursing Process—Planning
   Client Need—Physiological integrity

NURSING CARE OF CLIENTS WITH CHRONIC OBSTRUCTIVE PULMONARY DISEASE

60 1. A sitting position is preferred when auscultating the chest. This allows the nurse access to the anterior, lateral, and posterior areas of the chest. Changing positions during auscultation further taxes an already dyspneic client. A client in respiratory distress generally does not tolerate lying flat or on his side. Standing is unsafe for a client who is having extreme difficulty breathing. (25:188)
   Nursing Process—Planning
   Client Need—Physiological integrity

61 4. As air passages become narrowed, as in the onset of an asthmatic attack, the nurse is most likely to hear wheezing. This generally is noted during expiration. Wet bubbling sounds indicate accumulated secretions. This is more likely heard during recovery from the asthmatic attack when thick secretions are able to move. Dry crackling sounds indicate that air is moving into and opening small airways, such as the terminal bronchioles and alveoli. Soft blowing sounds are normal in open, distal small airways of the lungs. (18:1201; 21:308)

Nursing Process—Data collection
Client Need—**Physiological integrity**

62 3. The sensor of a pulse oximeter is applied to the earlobe, finger, thumb, toe, or bridge of the nose. The arm or leg is too dense to allow light to transilluminate from tissue to the sensor. Applying the sensor to the lip causes discomfort or is dislodged easily. (4:884; 25:402)

Nursing Process—Implementation
Client Need—**Safe, effective care environment**

63 4. A normal oxygen saturation is 95% to 100%. Supplemental oxygen administration is appropriate if the oxygen saturation is sustained below 90%. The normal level of the partial pressure of oxygen (PaO_2), which is measured by arterial blood gas analysis, is 80 to 100 mm Hg. (4:884; 25:402)

Nursing Process—Data collection
Client Need—**Physiological integrity**

64 1. To avoid excessive blood loss and a painful hematoma from a punctured arterial site, it is essential to apply direct pressure for a minimum of 3 to 5 minutes. The specimen is cooled in ice once it is collected. The blood pressure is not likely to be affected by the loss of 5 to 10 mL of blood. Elevating the arm is one way to control bleeding from a vein, but it is not likely to be effective in the case of bleeding from an artery. (7:124)

Nursing Process—Implementation
Client Need—**Physiological integrity**

65 2. The reservoir bag of a nonrebreathing mask remains partially filled during inspiration. If the bag collapses completely, the equipment may be faulty. This information is reported to the respiratory therapy department. The mask is applied properly if it covers the mouth and nose and the strap fits the head snugly. Moisture is likely to accumulate because the oxygen is being humidified. This is not significant information to report. The nurse can temporarily wipe the moisture away and reapply the mask. (4:926; 18:1217)

Nursing Process—Implementation
Client Need—**Physiological integrity**

66 1. The volume of epinephrine 1:1000 needed to administer 0.1 mg is 0.1 mL. To solve the problem using a ratio and proportion method, use the following steps (20:28; 25:699):

$$\frac{1000 \text{ mg (1 g)}}{1000 \text{ mL}} = \frac{0.1 \text{ mg}}{\text{X mL}}$$

$$1000X = 100$$

$$X = 0.1 \text{ mL}$$

Nursing Process—Implementation
Client Need—**Physiological integrity**

67 2. Remaining with the client in respiratory distress provides reassurance that someone is available. Anxiety is best reduced by being with another supportive individual. Closing the door, pulling the privacy curtain, and covering the client are confining actions. They are apt to increase the feeling of being suffocated. (21:317; 23:290)

Nursing Process—Implementation
Client Need—**Psychosocial integrity**

68 3. A pulmonary function test is performed by having the client breathe in and out through a mouthpiece. A tube connects the mouthpiece to an air-filled drum. The drum rises and falls with ventilation. A graphic recording of the volume of air exchanged during breathing is obtained. (4:882; 7:675; 21:273)

Nursing Process—Evaluation
Client Need—**Health promotion/maintenance**

69 2. Individuals with longstanding emphysema develop a barrel-shaped appearance to their chest. The physical change is probably due to chronic overdistention of the lungs due to impaired ability to exhale air. A person with emphysema does not usually have a funnel-shaped, slender, or muscular chest. (4:928; 18:1203)

Nursing Process—Data collection
Client Need—**Physiological integrity**

70 1. Giving oxygen at greater than 3 L to a client with chronic respiratory disease interferes with the brain's response to the hypoxic drive. The stimulus to breathe in a person with chronic obstructive lung disease comes from low levels of oxygen rather than higher than normal levels of carbon dioxide. Administering high concentrations of oxygen depresses the respiratory center. (4:929)

Nursing Process—Implementation
Client Need—**Physiological integrity**

71 3. The therapeutic action of aminophylline is the reduction of respiratory distress. Aminophylline is classified as a bronchodilator. Aminophylline does not relieve coughing, decrease sputum production, or thin secretions. (17:397; 20:239–240)

Nursing Process—Implementation
Client Need—**Health promotion/maintenance**

72 4. Aminophylline is likely to cause tachycardia because it affects the sympathetic nervous system. Other side effects include hypertension, insomnia, and restlessness. The therapeutic action of aminophylline is bronchodilation, not bronchospasm. (17:397; 20:240)

Nursing Process—Data collection
Client Need—**Physiological integrity**

73 2. Administering rhythmic gentle blows with a cupped hand, known as percussion, causes thick secretions to break loose from within the airways. This technique also is combined with vibration. Vibration involves producing wave-like tremors to the chest by making firm, circular movements with open hands. For draining all but the upper lobes of the lung, the client is positioned so that the lower chest is elevated higher than the head. Deep breathing improves ventilation, but it does not necessarily move secretions. Applying pressure below the diaphragm is an emergency measure for relieving an obstructed airway. (4:929; 25:776–777)

   Nursing Process—Implementation
   Client Need—Physiological integrity

74 4. Expectorating a large volume of sputum is the best evidence that postural drainage is effective. The respiratory rate is lowered if hypoxia is relieved. Although the return of an appetite is a good sign, it is not the best evidence that postural drainage is effective. A negative sputum culture indicates only that an infectious process is not present. (4:929; 18:1181–1182)

   Nursing Process—Evaluation
   Client Need—Physiological integrity

75 2. To promote maximum distribution of inhaled medication, it is best to hold the breath for up to 10 seconds and then slowly exhale through pursed lips. If a second puff is ordered, it is best to wait several minutes before self-administering another dose. The mouthpiece is cleaned in warm water, rinsed, and allowed to air dry at least once each day. Using pursed-lip breathing rather than bending from the waist is the preferred method for increasing exhaled volume. (3:251))

   Nursing Process—Evaluation
   Client Need—Health promotion/maintenance

76 1. It is therapeutic to encourage a person to express his or her feelings. It shows that the nurse has empathy with the person's emotional condition and is willing to listen. Disagreeing with the client, belittling feelings, and using a reassuring cliché block the therapeutic effectiveness of communication. (9:151; 25:79–80)

   Nursing Process—Implementation
   Client Need—Psychosocial integrity

77 3. Eating several small meals each day promotes adequate intake of calories without becoming overly tired. Simple carbohydrates provide quick energy, but this recommendation is not better than eating a variety of foods at frequent intervals. Dietary fats are higher in calories than carbohydrates and pro-

tein, but fat consumption contributes to hyperlipidemia and increases the risks of cardiovascular disease. Most people have more energy early in the day; consequently, eating the largest meal at night is counterproductive. (3:245)

   Nursing Process—Implementation
   Client Need—Health promotion/maintenance

NURSING CARE OF CLIENTS WITH LUNG CANCER

78 3. A cough and dyspnea are generally the earliest signs of lung cancer. Most tend to ignore these signs, rationalizing that they are a consequence of chronic smoking. Therefore, early diagnosis and treatment of lung cancer often are delayed. Later signs of lung cancer include unexplained weight loss, blood-tinged sputum, fatigue, and respiratory distress. (4:917; 21:318)

   Nursing Process—Data collection
   Client Need—Physiological integrity

79 3. Coughing is the best method for raising sputum. Saliva is not sputum. Gargled solution is not likely to contain adequate secretions or cells from the bronchial or deeper pulmonary structures. Stimulating a gag reflex is more likely to cause the client to vomit. (4:326–327; 7:755; 25:776)

   Nursing Process—Implementation
   Client Need—Safe, effective care environment

80 1. Preparation for a bronchoscopy includes keeping the client from eating or drinking for at least 4 to 8 hours prior to the procedure. This reduces the risk of aspiration. Though emptying the bowel and bladder promotes comfort, the accidental loss of urine or stool is not as life-threatening as aspiration. Adequate rest is desirable but not essential. The instrument used for bronchoscopy is introduced through the mouth. Therefore, scrubbing the upper chest is unnecessary. (7:146; 21:273)

   Nursing Process—Planning
   Client Need—Safe, effective care environment

81 3. Respiratory effort is the most critical assessment to make following a bronchoscopy. It is one of the first responses to change if the client experienced edema and trauma in the airway. All the other assessment alternatives are appropriate but not as likely to indicate life-threatening consequences. (7:148; 21:272)

   Nursing Process—Data collection
   Client Need—Physiological integrity

82 1. The pulse rate is the best indication at this time as to whether the nurse should be concerned about the presence of blood in the secretions. Slight bleeding is expected following bronchoscopy due to trauma. If hemorrhage or impaired ventilation is occurring, the pulse rate is rapid. Pupillary changes are an indication of brain function. Heart sounds indicate how effectively blood is circulating through the chambers of the heart. Chest expansion is more likely to change if one lung is not filling adequately with air. (4:881; 18:1185)

> Nursing Process—Data collection
> Client Need—Physiological integrity

83 4. Gloves are the most important barrier garment in this situation. Gloves are worn whenever there is a possibility for contact with body fluids containing blood. Because the nurse is involved in holding the container, the hands need protection. In addition to the gloves, it is acceptable to don any or all of the other items. The choice of additional items is based on the nurse's judgment as to the potential for contact with blood by some other means such as splashing into the eyes, nose, or mouth or onto the uniform. (18:335; 25:451–452)

> Nursing Process—Implementation
> Client Need—Safe, effective care environment

84 1. The nurse establishes that the gag reflex is present before the client is given food or oral fluids following a bronchoscopy. Stimulating the palatal arch causes the client to gag if the effects of the local anesthetic have worn off. The other choices are techniques of physical assessment but are unlikely to be affected by a bronchoscopy. (7:792)

> Nursing Process—Data collection
> Client Need—Physiological integrity

85 1. The prefix "pneumo" refers to lung; the suffix "ectomy" means removal. The name of the procedure in which only a lobe of the lung is removed is "lobectomy." The other two choices are not as accurate an explanation. They do not include the main purpose for performing the surgical procedure. (25:325)

> Nursing Process—Evaluation
> Client Need—Safe, effective care environment

86 1. The client with a pneumonectomy lies with the unoperative lung uppermost. Maintaining the collection of postoperative drainage within the empty cavity from which the lung is removed promotes consolidation. Also ventilation is facilitated by avoiding compression of the remaining healthy lung between the mattress and body weight. Lying with the head lowered interferes with breathing because abdominal contents press against the diaphragm. Gatching the knees is a comfort measure

but is not necessarily essential to this client's care. Elevating the arms on pillows is an optional position to use if and when the client's breathing becomes labored. However, it is not specified in the routine postoperative plan for care. (26:315)

> Nursing Process—Implementation
> Client Need—Physiological integrity

87 2. Removal of the lung is often accompanied by interruption of the intercostal nerves. As a consequence, clients who undergo a pneumonectomy may experience numbness in the operative area, which tends to be temporary. It is unusual for the postoperative client to manifest impaired swallowing or prolonged anorexia. If the client has a persistent cough, it is more likely due to pre-existing disease rather than an expected outcome of the surgical procedure. (26:315)

> Nursing Process—Data collection
> Client Need—Physiological integrity

88 4. Morphine sulfate depresses respiratory rate and depth. If the respiratory rate is severely compromised, the client may not have adequate gas exchange. Assessing the characteristics of wound drainage, skin temperature, and range of motion are all important, but they are not generally affected by the administration of a narcotic analgesic. (17:183; 20:133)

> Nursing Process—Data collection
> Client Need—Physiological integrity

89 2. It is best to place a client undergoing a thoracentesis in a sitting position so that the physician has access to the eighth or ninth rib space. Once sitting, it is helpful for the client to rest his head and elevate his arms on the over-bed table. If this position is impossible, the nurse may alternatively place the client on his unaffected side. Lithotomy position is used for procedures in which the caregiver needs access to structures in the area of the vaginal or urinary meatus and for some rectal procedures. It is incorrect to place the client in a prone or supine position for a thoracentesis. (18:1182; 26:271)

> Nursing Process—Implementation
> Client Need—Safe, effective care environment

NURSING CARE OF CLIENTS WITH CHEST INJURIES

90 1. To prevent the widespread collapse of alveoli, known as atelectasis, clients with fractured ribs are instructed to breathe deeply several times every hour. People with fractured ribs have a natural tendency to breathe shallowly to avoid discomfort. Shallow breathing promotes atelectasis. Breathing

rapidly leads to respiratory alkalosis. Breathing into a paper bag promotes an increased level of carbon dioxide in the blood. This is appropriate for individuals who are hyperventilating and becoming lightheaded. (25:319)
  Nursing Process—Implementation
  Client Need—Health promotion/maintenance

91 3. Flail chest is a condition in which three or more ribs are broken in two or more places, making the chest wall unstable. This condition is characterized by a paradoxic movement of the unstable section during inspiration and expiration. In other words, when the client takes a breath, an area of the chest wall moves inward; when the client exhales, the area moves outward. A sucking chest wound and tracheal deviation are associated with a pneumothorax. Chest pain only during expiration is not a common finding. (26:308)
  Nursing Process—Data collection
  Client Need—Physiological integrity

92 4. When a person experiences a hemothorax, blood collects and drains by gravity through the tube in the lower chest. Air in the chest rises and exits through the tube in the upper chest. It is unlikely that blood comes from the victim's nose or mouth. If the client has a productive cough, the sputum may be blood-tinged. (4:910–911)
  Nursing Process—Data collection
  Client Need—Physiological integrity

93 1. The fluid in the waterseal chamber tidals, i.e., rises and falls in synchrony with respirations, or bubbles intermittently when it has just been inserted. If the lung has expanded, if the drainage system is connected to suction, or if the tubing is kinked or plugged, tidaling and intermittent bubbling are not seen. If the fluid level falls below the filling line of 2 cm, more fluid is added. Continuous bubbling indicates that there is a leak in the system. The fluid in the waterseal chamber looks clear and transparent. (25:418–419)
  Nursing Process—Data collection
  Client Need—Safe, effective care environment

94 2. To facilitate gravity drainage the chest tubes hang straight from the bed into the drainage collector. If the tubes hang below the collector, drainage is slowed or stopped. Wrapping the chest tube around the client's chest or tucking it under the bed's mattress compresses the lumen of the tubes and impairs drainage. (18:733; 14:828)
  Nursing Process—Implementation
  Client Need—Safe, effective care environment

95 3. Air that is leaking and becoming trapped within the local tissue at the insertion site crackles when touched. The crackling sound, called crepitus or subcutaneous emphysema, resembles that of crisp rice cereal when mixed with milk. Puffs of air are not felt. There is no hissing sound because the air does not escape into the atmosphere. The air tends to diffuse into the tissue and rise to the upper part of the body. Eventually the face and neck may appear swollen. The tissue around the chest may appear pale, but this is not a phenomenon that can be directly linked to an air leak. (21:328; 25:417)
  Nursing Process—Data collection
  Client Need—Physiological integrity

96 2. The drainage collector is always kept below the tubes' insertion sites to facilitate drainage. As long as the waterseal is maintained, the current status of lung function is unaffected. Clamping the chest tubes for an appreciable amount of time leads to a tension pneumothorax. Suction is not applied directly to the chest tubes. Suction may be added to the waterseal system, but the tube connecting to the suction source is disconnected when the client ambulates or is transported from the room. Mechanical ventilation is necessary only if a client cannot maintain adequate oxygenation even with supplemental oxygen. (4:912; 26:316)
  Nursing Process—Implementation
  Client Need—Physiological integrity

97 4. Each nurse marks the level of drainage on the calibrated collection chamber with the date and time. The volume of drainage is calculated by subtracting the previously marked volume from the current total volume. The drainage compartment is never emptied while the chest tube is in place. Chest tubes are not irrigated. Subtracting fluid intake from output only helps in evaluating the status of the client's total fluid balance. (25:421)
  Nursing Process—Implementation
  Client Need—Physiological integrity

NURSING CARE OF CLIENTS WITH PULMONARY EMBOLISM

98 2. Staying with a frightened client is one of the best methods for relieving or reducing anxiety. Telling her she will be fine is a nontherapeutic communication technique called offering false reassurance. Asking a "why" question is a nontherapeutic technique because rather than accept the client's feeling, it demands that the client provide an explana-

tion. Changing the subject also is an example of nontherapeutic communication. (23:244; 25:83)
Nursing Process—Implementation
Client Need—Psychosocial integrity

99 1. Administering oxygen is the most significant immediate action for reducing the client's dyspnea and chest pain. In this anxious state the client is not easily distracted. Oral fluids are avoided in case cardiopulmonary resuscitation is needed. Recently ingested fluids or food could be aspirated. Wiping the client's face shows concern, but it is not likely to alter symptoms or the client's perception of the seriousness of the situation. (4:921; 21:310)
Nursing Process—Implementation
Client Need—Physiological integrity

100 2. Anyone over the age of 8 is given rescue breaths at a rate of 10 to 12 per minute or once every 5 seconds. Infants and children up to the age of 8 years old are given 20 breaths per minute. (25:806)
Nursing Process—Implementation
Client Need—Physiological integrity

NURSING CARE OF CLIENTS WITH A TRACHEOSTOMY

101 3. Wet lung sounds indicate that secretions are accumulating within the airway. Because a client with a tracheostomy lacks the ability to cough effectively, the nurse protects and maintains an open airway for him. Deep respirations are not undesirable. A rapid pulse rate is more likely to indicate impaired ventilation. A low blood pressure is unrelated to the need for oxygenation. (4:892; 25:779)
Nursing Process—Data collection
Client Need—Physiological integrity

102 2. Moistening the catheter by immersing it in sterile normal saline and suctioning solution through the lumen tests the function of the suction machine and reduces the surface tension inside the plastic catheter. Clients with artificial airways need frequent mouth care, but it is not essential before performing tracheal suctioning. The stoma is cleaned from time to time, but this does not have to be done before suctioning the airway. The airway is suctioned before removing the inner cannula for cleaning. (4:892; 25:780)
Nursing Process—Implementation
Client Need—Physiological integrity

103 3. The vent on a suction catheter is not occluded until after the catheter is fully inserted and is being withdrawn. This reduces the potential for causing hypoxemia. Closing the vent before insertion or when just inside the inner cannula prolongs the time during which oxygen is removed from the airway. Coughing may or may not coincide with the proper time to occlude the vent. Therefore, it is not used as a criterion for this action. (4:893; 18:1222)
Nursing Process—Implementation
Client Need—Physiological integrity

104 2. Suctioning does not extend beyond 10 to 15 seconds. Some suggest holding one's own breath during suctioning promotes awareness of the air hunger the client is experiencing. Suctioning for too little time does not effectively clear the airway. Suctioning beyond 10 to 15 seconds causes hypoxemia. (18:1222; 25:782)
Nursing Process—Implementation
Client Need—Physiological integrity

105 4. Twisting and rotating the catheter during its withdrawal helps remove secretions that are located in all directions within the airway. Withdrawing the catheter slowly causes the nurse to exceed the recommended time for suctioning. Neither pinching and pulling nor plunging the catheter up and down are acceptable techniques during suctioning. (25:782; 26:273)
Nursing Process—Implementation
Client Need—Physiological integrity

106 3. Pulse oximetry monitoring is useful for detecting the saturation of hemoglobin with oxygen. It takes a prolonged state of hypoxemia to alter the level of consciousness, skin color, and respiratory rate. (25:402; 26:323)
Nursing Process—Data collection
Client Need—Physiological integrity

107 3. To prevent the possibility that the client may cough the tracheostomy tube out of his airway, the old ties are not removed until the replacement ties are secured. Gauze squares are not cut to fashion a stomal dressing. The cut threads may enter the airway and irritate the tissue. Special drain gauze or tracheostomy dressing material are used, or gauze is folded rather than cut to fit around the stoma. The inner cannula is replaced as soon as it is cleaned, rinsed, and dried, or within at least 5 minutes. If there is a delay in replacing the inner cannula, mucous secretions may accumulate and dry in the outer cannula. This alters the size of the opening and interferes with replacement. (18:1222–1223; 25:789)
Nursing Process—Implementation
Client Need—Physiological integrity

108 2. A cuff on a tracheostomy tube forms a tight seal, preventing liquid nasopharyngeal secretions, stomach contents, or tube feeding formula from entering the lower respiratory passages. If the person is receiving mechanical ventilation, the cuff ensures that the oxygenated air does not escape before it is delivered to the lower areas of the lungs. An inflated cuff may lead to tissue breakdown because the pressure occludes capillary blood flow. Using a cuffed tracheostomy tube does not provide more comfort or reduce infection any better than an uncuffed tracheostomy tube. (25:785)

> **Nursing Process—Implementation**
> **Client Need—Health promotion/maintenance**

NURSING CARE OF CLIENTS WITH A SUDDEN AIRWAY OCCLUSION

109 2. The ability to cough indicates that the foreign object in the airway is not totally obstructing the passage of air. As long as the person has only a partial obstruction, he is allowed to cough to clear his own airway. The ability to walk is not important except to verify that the person's brain is still receiving oxygen and he has not lost consciousness. The position of the victim is not the most important data to obtain at this time. The ability to swallow will not relieve the lodged object if it is in the airway. (18:371; 25:794)

> **Nursing Process—Data collection**
> **Client Need—Physiological integrity**

110 4. The thumb side of the fist is placed against the abdomen above the navel and below the xiphoid process. The xiphoid process is the tip of the sternum. The manubrium is the upper portion of the sternum. (18:371; 25:795)

> **Nursing Process—Implementation**
> **Client Need—Physiological integrity**

Classification of Test Items

Unit I   Review Test 4

Directions: After each question the correct answer is given, as well as a classification of each test question. Compare the correct answer with your answer. If a question has been answered incorrectly, draw a line to the end of all the columns. When finished, add up the number of your correct answers in each column and place that number in the respective box at the end in the area identified as *Number Correct*.

To determine the percentage of questions you answered correctly and your performance in each of the test plan categories, divide the *Number Correct* in each column by the *Number Possible* in each column. Then multiply the decimal by 100. For example:

$$\frac{\text{Number Correct: 86}}{\text{Number Possible: 110}} = 0.781 \times 100 = 78\%$$

Any score that is less than 75% indicates an area where further review would be beneficial.

KEY TO ITEM CLASSIFICATION:

NURSING PROCESS

D = Data collection
P = Planning
I = Implementation
E = Evaluation

CLIENT NEEDS

S = Safe, effective care environment
P = Physiological integrity
M = Psychosocial integrity
H = Health promotion/maintenance

Question #	Answer #	D	P	I	E	S	P	M	H
1	1			I					H
2	3	D					P		
3	3	D					P		
4	1			I					H
5	2			I					H
6	3	D					P		
7	2			I					H
8	3			I					H
9	3			I		S			
10	3			I		S			
11	1			I					H
12	2			I					H
13	3				E				H
14	3			I					H
15	1			I					H

Question #	Answer #	Nursing Process				Client Needs			
		D	P	I	E	S	P	M	H
16	4	D					P		
17	2			I			P		
18	1	D					P		
19	4		P				P		
20	3	D					P		
21	3			I			P		
22	1	D					P		
23	2			I			P		
24	2	D					P		
25	4		P				P		
26	3				E			M	
27	3	D					P		
28	1		P						H
29	3			I					H
30	4			I			P		
31	1				E				H
32	3			I					H
33	2		P			S			
34	1		P			S			
35	4		P			S			
36	4				E				H
37	2			I			P		
38	2	D					P		
39	1			I					H
40	4			I			P		
41	1			I			P		
42	3	D					P		
43	3	D					P		
44	4		P				P		
45	3			I					H
46	3			I					H

Question #	Answer #	Nursing Process				Client Needs			
		D	P	I	E	S	P	M	H
47	2	D					P		
48	3				E		P		
49	2			I					H
50	1			I			P		
51	3			I					H
52	2			I					H
53	4			I					H
54	2	D							H
55	1			I					H
56	3			I					H
57	3				E		P		
58	4			I					H
59	2		P				P		
60	1		P				P		
61	4	D					P		
62	3			I		S			
63	4	D					P		
64	1			I			P		
65	2			I			P		
66	1			I			P		
67	2			I				M	
68	3				E				H
69	2	D					P		
70	1			I			P		
71	3			I					H
72	4	D					P		
73	2			I			P		
74	4				E		P		
75	2				E				H
76	1			I				M	
77	3			I					H

Question #	Answer #	Nursing Process				Client Needs			
		D	P	I	E	S	P	M	H
78	3	D					P		
79	3			I		S			
80	1		P			S			
81	3	D					P		
82	1	D					P		
83	4			I		S			
84	1	D					P		
85	1				E	S			
86	1			I			P		
87	2	D					P		
88	4	D					P		
89	2			I		S			
90	1			I					H
91	3	D					P		
92	4	D					P		
93	1	D				S			
94	2			I		S			
95	3	D					P		
96	2			I			P		
97	4			I			P		
98	2			I				M	
99	1			I			P		
100	2			I			P		
101	3	D					P		
102	2			I			P		
103	3			I			P		
104	2			I			P		
105	4			I			P		
106	3	D					P		
107	3			I			P		
108	2			I					H

Question #	Answer #	Nursing Process				Client Needs			
		D	P	I	E	S	P	M	H
109	2	D					P		
110	4			I			P		
Number Correct	89	25	9	50	5	8	51	3	27
Number Possible	110	31	10	59	10	13	61	4	32
Percentage Correct	81	81	90	85	50	62	84	75	84

The Nursing Care of Clients with Disorders of the Reproductive System

Directions: With a pencil, blacken the circle in front of the option you have chosen for your correct answer.

NURSING CARE OF CLIENTS WITH BREAST DISORDERS

A 30-year-old female has a routine pelvic examination and asks the nurse who prepares her when she should begin to have routine mammography done.

1 If the client is asymptomatic and does not have any high-risk factors for developing breast cancer, the nurse would be *accurate* in telling her that a baseline mammogram is recommended at the age of
   - 1. 35.
   - 2. 40.
   - ● 3. 45.
   - 4. 50.

The office nurse uses the opportunity to teach breast self-examination.

2 The nurse is *most accurate* in identifying that the breasts should be examined during a shower, lying down, and
   - ● 1. bending from the waist.
   - 2. standing before a mirror.
   - 3. while arching the back.
   - 4. leaning side-to-side.

3 The client demonstrates *correct* breast palpation technique when she uses
   - 1. the heel of her hand.
   - 2. the index finger only.
   - 3. the index finger and thumb.
   - ● 4. the pads of her fingertips.

4 The nurse is correct in explaining that the *best* technique for palpating breast tissue during BSE is in small circles or as spokes of a wheel from
   - ● 1. the nipple to the outer margins of the breast.
   - 2. the outer margins of the breast toward the nipple.
   - 3. the sternum toward each axilla.
   - 4. each axilla toward the sternum.

5 The premenopausal client has a correct understanding of how frequently to perform BSE if she says it is appropriate to examine her breasts
   - 1. on a weekly basis.
   - 2. every 6 months.
   - 3. 1 week before each menses.
   - ● 4. 1 week after each menses.

A 35-year-old female makes an appointment with her physician because she has felt several lumps in her right breast. She is scheduled for a mammogram.

6 When the office nurse gives the client instructions on how to prepare for the mammogram, which is *most accurate*?
   - 1. Shave the hair from your axillae.
   - 2. Avoid using any underarm deodorant.
   - 3. Wipe each breast with an antiseptic pad.
   - ● 4. Refrain from wearing a brassiere.

7 If the nurse obtains all of the following data before the mammogram, which one is a *high-risk factor* for developing breast cancer?
○ 1. The client started menstruating at age 16.
○ 2. The client has been pregnant three times.
● 3. The client's sister has had breast cancer.
○ 4. The client's children were all breast-fed.

The radiologist interprets the findings on the mammogram as benign fibrocystic disease.

8 It is *correct* for the nurse to explain that fibrocystic lesions may become larger and more tender
○ 1. after the menstrual cycle.
○ 2. following sexual intercourse.
○ 3. nearer to menopause.
● 4. just before menstruation.

9 Although its efficacy has not been conclusively proven, the nurse is *correct* in explaining that some women with fibrocystic disease get relief from their symptoms by eliminating their intake of
○ 1. alcohol.
● 2. caffeine.
○ 3. saturated fat.
○ 4. refined sugar.

A home-health nurse visits a postpartum client with a breast abscess. The client has purulent drainage from one breast and is on antibiotic therapy.

10 What information is *most appropriate* for preventing the spread of the infectious microorganisms elsewhere?
○ 1. Include more sources of protein in your diet.
○ 2. Keep your breasts supported in a tight brassiere.
● 3. Shower daily and wash your hands frequently.
○ 4. Apply warm compresses at least four times a day.

During a presurgical assessment, a 67-year-old female tells the nurse that she has felt a lump in her left breast for the past 6 months.

11 If the lump has all of the following characteristics when the nurse palpates the breast tissue, which one is *most suggestive* that the lump may be cancerous?
○ 1. The lump can be moved about.
○ 2. The lump is about 0.5 cm (1 inch).
● 3. The lump is irregularly shaped.
○ 4. The lump is near the areola.

The physician recommends an excisional biopsy followed by an immediate modified radical mastectomy if the biopsy shows malignant cells.

12 If the client tells the nurse that she would prefer to postpone the mastectomy until the biopsy has been more thoroughly examined, which action is most appropriate for the nurse to take *first?*
○ 1. Explain that most biopsies are accurate.
● 2. Help advocate for her choice of treatment.
○ 3. Discourage her from opposing the physician.
○ 4. Recommend that she seek a second opinion.

The client's breast tumor is malignant and she undergoes a left modified radical mastectomy.

13 Which one of the following nursing orders is *most appropriate* to add to the client's *immediate* postoperative plan for care?
○ 1. Maintain the client in a dorsal recumbent position.
○ 2. Limit oral fluid intake to no more than 2000 mL/day.
● 3. Use the right arm when assessing blood pressures.
○ 4. Inspect the incision at least once each shift.

14 Based upon the location and extent of this client's surgery, it is *most appropriate* to closely assess the client for
● 1. shallow breathing.
○ 2. inadequate nutrition.
○ 3. impaired bowel motility.
○ 4. signs of pressure sores.

15 Which activity of daily living (ADL) is *most therapeutic* for the nurse to recommend for preserving muscle strength and joint flexibility in the arm on the operative side?
○ 1. Feeding herself
● 2. Brushing her hair
○ 3. Writing letters
○ 4. Washing her chest

16 When adding to the postoperative plan for care, which nursing measure is *most appropriate* for preventing the arm on the operative side from swelling?
○ 1. Applying an ice pack
○ 2. Applying warm compresses
● 3. Keeping the arm elevated
○ 4. Ambulating frequently

17 If the client asks for information on brassieres and other aspects of life following her mastectomy, the *best resource* to recommend is the local chapter of the
○ 1. American Garment Industry.
○ 2. American Cancer Society.
◉ 3. Breast Prosthetics Association.
○ 4. Organization for Mammary Cosmetics.

18 Before discharging the mastectomy client, which instruction concerning breast self-examination is *most correct*?
○ 1. Examine your breast upon awakening from sleep.
◉ 2. Examine your breast on the first day of the month.
○ 3. Examine your breast after you finish your shower.
○ 4. Examine your breast before your yearly mammogram.

NURSING CARE OF CLIENTS WITH DISTURBANCES IN MENSTRUATION

A nurse obtains a history from a 20-year-old client who says she does not menstruate.

19 Which question is most important for the nurse to ask *next*?
◉ 1. Have you ever had any menstrual periods?
○ 2. Do you have any pubic hair growth?
○ 3. Have you ever been sexually attracted to males?
○ 4. Are there any siblings with a similar problem?

An 18-year-old female confides to the nurse that she has cramps that accompany the onset of menstruation.

20 Besides a mild analgesic, like ibuprofen (Motrin), it is appropriate for the nurse to recommend
○ 1. obtaining a prescription for an oral contraceptive.
○ 2. switching from menstrual pads to tampons.
◉ 3. using local applications of heat.
○ 4. reducing her physical activity.

A 34-year-old female makes an appointment with a physician concerning her pattern of heavy menstrual bleeding. A pelvic examination is scheduled.

21 Which of the following instructions is *most appropriate* if a Papanicolaou (Pap) smear will be obtained at the time of the pelvic examination?
◉ 1. Do not douche for several days before your appointment.

○ 2. Stop using any and all forms of contraception temporarily.
○ 3. Drink at least one quart of liquid an hour before your appointment.
○ 4. Take a mild laxative the night before your scheduled appointment.

22 Before taking the client to the room where the pelvic examination will be performed, which nursing action is *most appropriate*?
○ 1. Ask the client to sign a consent form.
◉ 2. Give the client an opportunity to void.
○ 3. Offer the client a mild analgesic.
○ 4. Help the client instill a vaginal lubricant.

23 Which question is *most important* to ask to ensure valid analysis of the vaginal specimen?
○ 1. When did you last have sexual intercourse?
○ 2. How old were you when you had your first pregnancy?
◉ 3. What was the date of your last menstrual period?
○ 4. Have you ever used oral contraceptives in your life?

24 The nurse is correct in placing the client in which position when the physician is ready to perform the pelvic examination?
○ 1. Sims position
○ 2. Trendelenberg position
○ 3. Fowler's position
◉ 4. Lithotomy position

25 Before sending the vaginal specimen for examination, it is *most important* for the nurse to
○ 1. rinse the slide in plain water.
○ 2. wipe the slide with antiseptic.
◉ 3. apply a chemical fixative to the slide.
○ 4. enclose the slide in a sterile tube.

A 22-year-old female calls a physician's office and reports to the nurse that she is bleeding vaginally at a time other than her expected menses.

26 If the nurse collects all of the following data, which one is *most likely* contributing to her bleeding.
◉ 1. The client has been taking an oral contraceptive for two months.
○ 2. The client has just changed employment and is under unusual stress.
○ 3. The client's sexual partner is uncircumcised.
○ 4. The client has been constipated for 2 days.

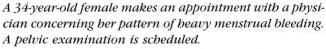

NURSING CARE OF CLIENTS WITH INFECTIOUS AND INFLAMMATORY DISORDERS OF THE FEMALE REPRODUCTIVE SYSTEM

A 25-year-old female has repeated vaginal infections. The symptoms suggest that the client has moniliasis caused by the yeast-like microorganism, **Candida albicans.**

27 After the infectious organism is confirmed as being *Candida albicans*, which nonprescription product is *best* for the nurse to recommend?
- ○ 1. Miconazole (Monistat 7)
- ○ 2. Nitrofurazone (Furacin)
- ○ 3. Hydrocortisone (HydroCort)
- ○ 4. Neomycin (Myciquent)

28 Which instruction is *best* to offer when teaching the client about inserting vaginal medication?
- ○ 1. Place the applicator just inside the vaginal opening.
- ○ 2. Insert the applicator while sitting on the toilet.
- ○ 3. Instill the medication just before retiring for sleep.
- ○ 4. Don disposable latex gloves before applying the drug.

29 Which one of the following health practices is it *most appropriate* for the nurse to teach this client?
- ○ 1. Take showers rather than tub baths if possible.
- ○ 2. Wipe away from the vagina following a bowel movement.
- ○ 3. Use a lanolin-based soap for genital cleansing.
- ○ 4. Avoid sexual intercourse more than once a week.

30 What information is *best* for the client who says she plans on administering a vaginal irrigation (douche) twice a week?
- ○ 1. Use a concentrated solution of vinegar and water.
- ○ 2. Frequent douching removes helpful microorganisms.
- ○ 3. Use no more than 8 to 16 ounces of irrigant.
- ○ 4. Discontinue the instillation if cramping occurs.

31 To reduce the potential for toxic shock syndrome, the *most appropriate* health teaching a nurse can offer menstruating women is to
- ○ 1. avoid using superabsorbent brands of tampons.
- ○ 2. use a nondeodorized type of sanitary product.
- ○ 3. refrain from taking tub baths while menstruating.
- ○ 4. report menses that last longer than seven days.

A 21-year-old client is recovering from acute pelvic inflammatory disease (PID).

32 When assigning a nursing assistant to this client's care, which instruction for disposing of soiled drainage pads is *most correct?*
- ○ 1. Flush all perineal pads down the toilet.
- ○ 2. Double-wrap the pads in infectious waste bags.
- ○ 3. Place the pads in the client's waste basket.
- ○ 4. Enclose the soiled pads in a clean paper bag.

33 If the client with PID asks what, if any, long-term consequences are associated with this disorder, the nurse is *most accurate* in identifying which one of the following reproductive sequela?
- ○ 1. Cancer of the cervix
- ○ 2. Premature labors
- ○ 3. Spontaneous abortions
- ○ 4. Infertility

A 24-year-old female is being treated for endometriosis. A laporoscope will be used to remove ectopic tissue.

34 When the client asks where the laporoscope is inserted, the nurse is *most correct* in identifying which structure?
- ○ 1. Abdomen
- ○ 2. Vagina
- ○ 3. Uterine cervix
- ○ 4. Uterine fundus

35 Following the laporoscopy, if the client experiences all of the following, which one can the nurse attribute *directly* to the endoscopic procedure?
- ○ 1. The client says she feels nauseous.
- ○ 2. The client has shoulder discomfort.
- ○ 3. The client has urinary frequency.
- ○ 4. The client develops leg cramps.

A 68-year-old female who is asymptomatic except for experiencing painful intercourse asks the nurse if this is an indication of reproductive disease.

36 Based on this client's age, which one of the following is the *best* explanation for the client's discomfort?
- ○ 1. The pelvic muscles are more sensitive to pressure after menopause.
- ○ 2. The clitoris is less responsive to sexual foreplay as women age.
- ○ 3. The vagina atrophies if intercourse is infrequent.
- ○ 4. The mucous-producing glands decrease with aging.

NURSING CARE OF FEMALE CLIENTS WITH BENIGN AND MALIGNANT DISORDERS OF THE UTERUS AND OVARIES

The cause of a 42-year-old female's symptoms is fibroid tumors (myomas).

37 In addition to pressure in the pelvic region, which sign or symptom is the client with the diagnosis of myoma *most likely* to reveal during a nursing history?
○ 1. Heavy menstrual bleeding
◉ 2. Irregular menstrual bleeding
○ 3. Abdominal pain at the time of ovulation
○ 4. Breast tenderness during menstruation

A pelvic ultrasound (sonogram) using a transabdominal approach is scheduled for the client with fibroid tumors.

38 When preparing the client for the sonogram, which one of the following instructions is *most important* for the nurse to stress?
◉ 1. Avoid voiding for several hours before the test.
○ 2. Remain fasting from midnight before the test.
○ 3. Take a mild analgesic, like aspirin, before the test.
○ 4. Use an antiseptic soap when showering before the test.

After the diagnosis of the client with fibroid tumors is confirmed, she is scheduled for a dilation and curretage (D&C) in the ambulatory surgery department.

39 Before the client is allowed to return home, which one of the following is *most important* for the nurse to document?
○ 1. The client's ability to eat without nausea
◉ 2. The client's ability to empty her bladder
○ 3. The client's pelvic pain has been relieved
○ 4. The client's perineal pad has been changed

A client with an abnormal Papanicolaou (Pap) smear has a colposcopy performed in her physician's office.

40 Before the client leaves, the nurse is *most correct* in instructing her to report which one of the following *common* problems associated with this procedure?
◉ 1. Excessive bleeding
○ 2. Inability to void
○ 3. Pressure during bowel elimination
○ 4. Pain in the right lower quadrant

A premenopausal female makes an appointment with her physician because she has been having vaginal bleeding following sexual intercourse.

41 To determine the extent of the client's symptomatic bleeding, which question is *most important* to ask?
○ 1. Has your energy level changed remarkably?
○ 2. Do you have intercourse more than once a week?
◉ 3. How many sanitary pads do you use?
○ 4. Is the bleeding light or dark red?

42 If the physician wants to perform a Schiller's test on the client with abnormal vaginal bleeding, what substance should the nurse have available?
○ 1. Silver nitrate
○ 2. Hydrogen peroxide
○ 3. Acetone
◉ 4. Iodine

The client is scheduled for electrocauterization when a battery of diagnostic tests indicate that she has cancer of the cervix in an early stage.

43 After the electrocauterization procedure, which of the following discharge instructions is *most appropriate?*
○ 1. Douche in 24 hours to remove debris and blood clots.
◉ 2. Avoid heavy lifting until after a surgical follow-up.
○ 3. Stay in bed for most of the next 5 days.
○ 4. Sexual activity can be resumed in 1 week.

Internal radiation therapy is used to treat a 54-year-old client with cancer of the cervix. An applicator containing radioactive material is inserted into the client's vagina.

44 Based on the fact that the client is receiving this type of radiation therapy, the nurse is *most correct* in adding which of the following nursing orders on the client's plan for care.
○ 1. Elevate head of bed to 90 degrees.
◉ 2. Maintain strict bed rest.
○ 3. Offer nourishment q 2h.
○ 4. Weigh daily before breakfast.

45 If the nurse finds the radioactive insert in the bed, the *best action* to take is to
○ 1. return it to the nuclear medicine department.
○ 2. discard it in the infectious waste receptacle.
○ 3. reinsert it immediately.
◉ 4. place it in a lead container.

46 If the nurse must handle the radioactive implant, which action is *best* to take?
- ○ 1. Use sterile vinyl gloves.
- ○ 2. Perform handwashing first.
- ◉ 3. Employ long-handled forceps
- ○ 4. Enclose it in a glass jar.

47 Considering the fact that the implant emits radioactivity, which staff nurse is *best* to care for the client with the radioactive implant?
- ○ 1. A male nurse with oncology nursing experience
- ◉ 2. A female nurse who has had a hysterectomy
- ○ 3. A female nurse who has survived cancer herself
- ○ 4. A male nurse whose mother died of cancer

A 64-year-old client with cancer of the uterus will undergo an abdominal hysterectomy under general anesthesia. The nurse will insert a retention catheter prior to surgery.

48 The correct length to which the nurse inserts the catheter into the urinary meatus is approximately
- ○ 1. ½ inch.
- ○ 2. 1 inch.
- ◉ 3. 2 to 3 inches.
- ○ 4. 5 to 6 inches.

Before the client returns from the post-anesthesia reacting room, the registered nurse asks the practical nurse to help revise the hysterectomy client's care plan.

49 Which one of the following diagnoses is most appropriate for the nurse to add to the client's problem list *at this time*?
- ○ 1. Risk for Ineffective Airway Clearance
- ○ 2. Risk for Altered Nutrition
- ◉ 3. Ineffective Individual Coping
- ○ 4. Impaired Verbal Communication

There are postoperative orders for applying antiembolic stockings on the legs of the client with the hysterectomy.

50 When managing the care of the client with antiembolic stockings, which one of the following routines is *best* to follow?
- ◉ 1. They are worn continuously, but removed and reapplied at least twice a day.
- ○ 2. They are worn continuously during the day hours and removed at night.
- ○ 3. They are applied just before the client gets up to ambulate.
- ○ 4. The are applied only when the client is in bed.

51 When the practical nurse observes a nursing assistant giving postoperative care to the client with a hysterectomy, which action indicates that the nursing assistant needs further instruction?
- ○ 1. The nursing assistant offers a variety of oral fluids frequently.
- ○ 2. The nursing assistant helps the client ambulate in the hall.
- ◉ 3. The nursing assistant raises the knee-gatch on the bed.
- ○ 4. The nursing assistant helps the client with her menu selections.

52 When the physician indicates that the retention catheter can be removed, which action is *most important* for the nurse to perform *first*?
- ○ 1. Cleanse the labia with soap and water.
- ○ 2. Measure the urine in the drainage bag.
- ◉ 3. Remove the fluid from the balloon.
- ○ 4. Disconnect the catheter and drainage bag.

The client's bladder is distended after the catheter is removed despite the fact that she is urinating approximately 100 mL with each voiding. The physician instructs the nurse to catheterize the client and measure the residual urine.

53 Which one of the following is *most correct* when the nurse carries out the medical order?
- ○ 1. The nurse catheterizes the client as soon as possible.
- ◉ 2. The nurse catheterizes the client after her next voiding.
- ○ 3. The nurse connects the catheter to gravity drainage.
- ○ 4. The nurse uses a small gauge catheter to drain the bladder.

A 59-year-old client with ovarian cancer is receiving antineoplastic chemotherapy following a total hysterectomy.

54 Which of the following assessments are *most important* for the nurse to obtain to determine the client's dose of most antineoplastic drugs?
- ○ 1. The client's blood pressure and pulse
- ◉ 2. The client's body weight and height
- ○ 3. The client's age and date of surgery
- ○ 4. The client's history of allergies to foods and drugs

55 Since many antineoplastic drugs affect bone marrow function, which one of the following tests is *most important* for the nurse to monitor for the safety of the client?
- ○ 1. Mean cell volume
- ○ 2. Total leukocyte count
- ○ 3. Differential cell count
- ◉ 4. Complete blood count

56 When the nurse administers the parenteral form of the prescribed antineoplastic drug, which nursing action is *best* for preventing accidental self-absorption of the drug?
- ○ 1. Use only prefilled syringes.
- ◉ 2. Wear disposable latex gloves.
- ○ 3. Dilute the drug with saline.
- ○ 4. Mix the drug in a closed vial.

The client experiences almost total hair loss as antineoplastic drug therapy progresses.

57 Which of the following statements is *most accurate* when discussing this side effect with the client?
- ○ 1. The hair loss is permanent, but attractive wigs are available.
- ○ 2. The hair loss is permanent, but hair transplantation is a possible solution.
- ○ 3. The hair loss is temporary; it may grow back in several years.
- ◉ 4. The hair loss is temporary; it will regrow after chemotherapy is finished.

NURSING CARE OF FEMALE CLIENTS WITH MISCELLANEOUS DISORDERS OF THE REPRODUCTIVE SYSTEM

When a 72-year-old client is admitted to a nursing home, the transfer form indicates that the client has a prolapsed uterus.

58 When the nurse does a physical assessment, which technique is *best* for determining the extent of the prolapse?
- ○ 1. Examine the perineum when the client rolls from side to side.
- ○ 2. Examine the perineum as the client stands and bears down.
- ◉ 3. Examine the perineum with the client in a dorsal recumbent position.
- ○ 4. Examine the perineum with a lubricated speculum and flashlight.

A cystocele begins to cause symptoms for a 53-year-old female.

59 If this client is typical of others with this condition, she will most likely report to the nurse that she experiences urinary incontinence when she

- ○ 1. awakens.
- ○ 2. walks.
- ○ 3. sleeps.
- ◉ 4. sneezes.

60 If the cystocele is not severe, the *best* nursing suggestion for relieving the client's incontinence is to
- ○ 1. recommend the purchase of absorbent underwear.
- ○ 2. show her how to apply an external catheter.
- ◉ 3. teach her to exercise her perineal muscles.
- ○ 4. instruct her to limit her intake of fluids.

The client with the cystocele chooses to have an anterior colporrhaphy when her symptoms persist. She will catheterize herself for approximately a week after being discharged.

61 Which one of the following is the *best* indication that the client is performing self-catheterization appropriately?
- ○ 1. She empties 50 mL of urine from her bladder each time.
- ◉ 2. She is free of signs of a urinary tract infection.
- ○ 3. She inserts the catheter for 30 minutes each time.
- ○ 4. She catheterizes herself every four hours.

NURSING CARE OF CLIENTS WITH INFLAMMATORY DISORDERS OF THE MALE REPRODUCTIVE SYSTEM

A physician prescribes an oral antibiotic for a client with prostatitis.

62 When the nurse gives the client his prescription, which of the following is *most important* to teach him?
- ○ 1. Drink a glass of milk when taking the medication.
- ○ 2. Report if your urine becomes a lighter color.
- ◉ 3. Take all the medication until it is completely gone.
- ○ 4. Monitor your body temperature on a daily basis.

In addition to a mild analgesic, the physician recommends that the client with prostatitis use a sitz bath as a comfort measure.

63 Which of the following nursing instructions concerning this client's sitz bath regimen is *accurate*?
- ○ 1. Use cool tepid water.
- ◉ 2. Soak for 20 minutes.
- ○ 3. Add mild liquid soap to the water.
- ○ 4. Massage your scrotum while bathing.

A 22-year-old client presents with a swollen scrotum that is painful. The physician suspects epididymitis and orders a clean catch urine specimen for a culture and sensitivity test.

64 When the nurse asks the client to repeat the instructions for collecting a clean-catch urine specimen, which statement indicates the client needs further clarification?
- ○ 1. The client says he must clean his penis.
- ◉ 2. The client says he must collect all his urine.
- ○ 3. The client says he must retract his foreskin.
- ○ 4. The client says he must use a sterile container.

65 Which of the following is *best* for the nurse to recommend for promoting this client's comfort?
- ◉ 1. Using a scrotal support
- ○ 2. Wearing cotton briefs
- ○ 3. Buying larger underwear
- ○ 4. Applying a hot water bag

A client develops orchitis.

66 When the nurse gathers all of the following information, which is *most suggestive* as the etiology for the client's condition?
- ○ 1. The client has multiple sexual partners.
- ◉ 2. The client is an active homosexual.
- ○ 3. The client was never immunized for mumps.
- ○ 4. The client is a Gulf War veteran.

When the client with orchitis recovers, the nurse uses the opportunity to teach him how to perform testicular self-examination.

67 Which statement is *accurate* when explaining the technique for testicular self-examination?
- ○ 1. Palpate each testicle simultaneously.
- ◉ 2. Roll each testicle between the thumb and fingers.
- ○ 3. Examine your testicles at least yearly.
- ○ 4. Perform the self-examination in a cool room.

NURSING CARE OF CLIENTS WITH STRUCTURAL DISORDERS OF THE MALE REPRODUCTIVE SYSTEM

During a physical assessment, the nurse notes that a 25-year-old male client has an undescended testicle.

68 When the client asks how this condition affects his masculinity, the nurse is *most accurate* in stating
- ◉ 1. It has little effect whatsoever.
- ○ 2. You are most likely impotent.
- ○ 3. Your breasts may enlarge later.
- ○ 4. Your libido is probably reduced.

A 56-year-old client for whom the foreskin does not retract easily over the glans penis has a circumcision performed.

69 Besides assessing the dressing for bleeding, which other postoperative nursing assessment is a *priority* following this surgical procedure?
- ○ 1. The client's efforts at deep breathing
- ○ 2. The client's ability to achieve an erection
- ◉ 3. The client's volume of urinary output
- ○ 4. The client's pattern of bowel elimination

A client with a hydrocele has the fluid aspirated from his scrotum. The physician orders a cold application to the area.

70 When carrying out this intervention, which action is *most appropriate?*
- ○ 1. The nurse applies ice in a sealed plastic bag.
- ◉ 2. The nurse places a covered ice pack to the scrotum.
- ○ 3. The nurse positions him on a hypothermia blanket.
- ○ 4. The nurse seats him on an ice-filled ring.

NURSING CARE OF CLIENTS WITH BENIGN AND MALIGNANT DISORDERS OF THE MALE REPRODUCTIVE SYSTEM

A 65-year-old client makes an appointment for a routine physical examination.

71 If the physician asks the nurse to prepare the client for an assessment of the client's prostate gland, which position is *preferred?*
- ○ 1. Lithotomy position
- ◉ 2. Modified standing position
- ○ 3. Dorsal recumbent position
- ○ 4. Fowler's position

A 72-year-old client with a history of benign prostatic hypertrophy (BPH) phones the nurse at his physician's office.

72 If the reason for this client's call is the fact that he has not been able to urinate in 16 hours, which one of the following suggestions is *most appropriate?*
- ○ 1. If you are unable to urinate within 8 hours, go to an emergency department.
- ○ 2. Use a sterile, lubricated cotton applicator to dilate your urethra.
- ○ 3. Stop drinking any more beverages until you are able to urinate.
- ◉ 4. Try to release urine while relaxing in a tub of warm water.

The client with BPH is unsuccessful in voiding naturally, and he is catheterized in the emergency department.

73 Unless the physician specifies otherwise, what is the *maximum* volume the nurse should withdraw *at this time*?
   ○ 1. 500 mL
   ● 2. 1000 mL
   ○ 3. 1500 mL
   ○ 4. 2000 mL

The client with BPH is scheduled for a sonogram of his prostate.

74 When the nurse provides pretest information, which statement is *most correct*?
   ○ 1. You will need to fast from midnight the night before the test.
   ● 2. You will need to empty your bladder just before the test begins.
   ○ 3. You will need to consume at least a quart of water an hour before the test.
   ○ 4. You will need to self-administer an enema an hour before the test.

A transurethral prostatectomy (TURP) is performed and the client is returned to the nursing unit with a 3-way catheter for administering intermittent bladder irrigations.

75 When the client's spouse asks the nurse about the catheter drainage, it is correct to explain that *immediately* after a TURP, it is expected that the urine will be
   ○ 1. light pink.
   ● 2. dark amber.
   ○ 3. dark red.
   ○ 4. light yellow.

76 To calculate the client's urinary output, which one of the following techniques is *correct*?
   ○ 1. Measure the total volume in the urinary drainage bag.
   ○ 2. Add the volume of irrigant and the urinary drainage.
   ○ 3. Divide the urinary drainage by the volume of irrigant.
   ● 4. Subtract the volume of irrigant from the urine drainage.

77 To promote patency of the urinary catheter, which nursing order is *most appropriate* to add to the plan of care?
   ● 1. Milk the urinary catheter every hour and *p.r.n.*

   ○ 2. Deflate the catheter balloon once each shift.
   ○ 3. Empty the drainage container every 4 hours.
   ○ 4. Maintain an oral intake of at least 2 L/day.

78 When the client with a TURP complains of bladder discomfort and a feeling of urgency to void, which nursing action is best to take *first*?
   ● 1. Check that the urinary drainage catheter is patent.
   ○ 2. Administer a prescribed analgesic as soon as possible.
   ○ 3. Change the client to a semi-Fowler's position.
   ○ 4. Get the client out of bed to ambulate for a while.

79 The discharge plan for the client with a TURP should include which measure for reducing episodes of urinary incontinence?
   ● 1. Void at least every 2 hours when awake.
   ○ 2. Start and stop the urinary stream when voiding.
   ○ 3. Avoid drinking beverages that contain caffeine.
   ○ 4. Sit rather than stand when attempting to void.

A 68-year-old client with cancer of the prostate undergoes a suprapubic prostatectomy. He returns to the nursing unit with a Foley catheter in his urethra and a cystostomy tube in his abdomen.

80 Which one of the following nursing orders is *most appropriate* to add to the client's *initial* postoperative plan for care?
   ○ 1. Connect the cystostomy tube to a leg bag for drainage.
   ○ 2. Secure the cystostomy tube to the client's thigh.
   ● 3. Ensure that the cystostomy tube is unclamped at all times.
   ○ 4. Clamp the Foley catheter when the cystostomy tube is irrigated.

81 What special instruction concerning the technique for taking vital signs is *most important* when assigning this task to a nursing assistant?
   ○ 1. Take the client's respirations while he is resting.
   ○ 2. Take the client's pulse at the radial artery.
   ○ 3. Take the client's blood pressure with an aneroid manometer.
   ● 4. Take the client's temperature other than rectally.

A radical inguinal orchiectomy is performed on a 22-year-old client with testicular cancer.

82 If the client makes all of the following comments, which one indicates that he has *misinterpreted* the consequences of his surgery.
- ○ 1. The client says his beard will continue to grow.
- ● 2. The client says his voice will sound higher.
- ○ 3. The client says his sperm count will be lower.
- ○ 4. The client says his sex drive will be unaffected.

NURSING CARE OF CLIENTS WITH SEXUALLY TRANSMITTED DISEASES

83 When a nurse discusses healthy behaviors with an 18-year-old, which one of the following is most important to stress as a *major* risk factor for acquiring sexually transmitted diseases?
- ○ 1. Experiencing early puberty
- ○ 2. Attending R-rated movies
- ● 3. Having multiple sex partners
- ○ 4. Getting limited sex education

A male client reports symptoms that are suggestive of a gonorrhea infection.

84 If a culture is ordered to detect the causative organism, which body substance will the nurse collect?
- ○ 1. Venous blood
- ○ 2. Sterile urine
- ○ 3. Ejaculated semen
- ● 4. Urethral drainage

85 When collecting a specimen from the client who may have a gonorrhea infection, which nursing action is *correct*?
- ● 1. The nurse wears latex gloves.
- ○ 2. The nurse uses a disinfectant.
- ○ 3. The nurse asks the client to provide the specimen.
- ○ 4. The nurse refrigerates the specimen immediately.

86 When a nurse counsels a female client with herpes genitalis, which instruction is *accurate*?
- ○ 1. Have a Pap test done at least every 6 months.
- ● 2. Avoid vaginal intercourse for at least 6 months.
- ○ 3. If you take your medicine, you won't infect anyone else.
- ○ 4. Your infection confers immunity for any future children.

87 While assessing a male client with tertiary syphilis, which finding is *most associated* with this stage of the disease?
- ○ 1. The client has sharp leg pains.
- ○ 2. The client has a red skin rash.
- ● 3. The client has a penile ulcer.
- ○ 4. The client has patchy hair loss.

88 If the client with primary stage syphilis makes all of the following comments, which one indicates that he *lacks* a clear understanding of this disease?
- ○ 1. The client says he can be cured using antibiotic therapy.
- ○ 2. The client says his sexual partner(s) should be tested.
- ○ 3. The client says syphilitic lesions may be present in the vagina.
- ● 4. The client says one infection confers lifelong immunity.

89 When the nurse teaches a client who has been diagnosed with a chlamydia infection, which statement is *accurate*?
- ● 1. Your sexual partner(s) need simultaneous treatment.
- ○ 2. There is no known cure for this kind of infection.
- ○ 3. This is a rare type of sexually transmitted disease.
- ○ 4. Males manifest symptoms, but infected women do not.

90 When a female client describes her gynecological symptoms, which one is *most suggestive* that her problem is trichomoniasis?
- ○ 1. The client describes having a series of fluid-filled vesicles on her vagina.
- ○ 2. The client describes having vaginal drainage that causes intense itching.
- ○ 3. The client describes her vaginal drainage as appearing like it contains milk curds.
- ● 4. The client says she has tenderness and pressure in her lower abdomen.

A client with trichomoniasis is treated with oral metronidazole (Flagyl).

91 Which nursing instruction is *essential* for preventing a drug-food interaction while the client is taking metronidazole?
- ○ 1. Use plain salt rather than the iodized type.
- ○ 2. Stop eating anything with aspartame (NutraSweet)
- ○ 3. Eliminate sources of monosodium glutamate (MSG).
- ● 4. Avoid consuming alcohol in any form.

A nurse refers a client with genital warts to a gynecologist who confirms that they are caused by the human papillomavirus.

92   When the client asks if there is any danger associated with this condition, the *most correct* response is that they
   ○ 1. can be treated with an antibiotic, such as penicillin or tetracycline.
   ◉ 2. appear to increase the risk of cancer of the vulva, vagina, and cervix.
   ○ 3. can be prevented if the individual takes birth control pills.
   ○ 4. are of no danger and need not be treated.

To prevent infection with the human immunodeficiency virus (HIV), a client says he uses a condom when having intercourse.

93   To provide additional protection it is *accurate* for the nurse to recommend that the client also
   ○ 1. remove the condom immediately after intercourse.
   ○ 2. wash his penis with a dilute vinegar solution.
   ◉ 3. use a spermicide containing nonoxynol-9.
   ○ 4. apply copious amounts of vaginal lubricant.

94   The best method for the nurse to evaluate the effectiveness of the drug zidovudine (AZT) used to treat a client with acquired immunodeficiency syndrome (AIDS), is to monitor
   ○ 1. vital signs.
   ◉ 2. blood counts.
   ○ 3. culture reports.
   ○ 4. urine output.

NURSING CARE OF CLIENTS PRACTICING FAMILY PLANNING

A female client receives a 6-month supply of oral contraceptives.

95   The nurse is correct to include which one of the following when providing drug teaching?
   ◉ 1. It is best to take oral contraceptives at the same time each day.
   ○ 2. For optimum effect, oral contraceptives must be taken on an empty stomach.
   ○ 3. Begin taking oral contraceptives on the first day of menstruation.
   ○ 4. Oral contraceptives are best taken in the morning with food.

96   While a client is taking oral contraceptives, what information is *most appropriate* for reducing the risk of developing blood clots?
   ○ 1. Stop smoking while taking oral contraceptives.
   ○ 2. Drink a high volume of fluid to dilute the blood.
   ○ 3. Keep your legs elevated while sitting in a chair.
   ○ 4. Eat more garlic and onions on a weekly basis.

A pregnant client is considering a tubal ligation after the birth of her child.

97   If the client makes all of the following statements, which one indicates that the client is *misinformed*?
   ○ 1. "I will have a small abdominal incision."
   ○ 2. "This procedure is not easily reversed."
   ◉ 3. "I will no longer menstruate afterward."
   ○ 4. "Recovery should occur in a brief time."

98   If a female client with an intrauterine device describes all of the following, which one is *most likely* related to her choice for family planning?
   ○ 1. The client says she experiences breast tenderness.
   ◉ 2. The client says her menstrual flow is quite heavy.
   ○ 3. The client says she has been steadily gaining weight.
   ○ 4. The client says her acne seems to be getting worse.

99   Immediately after a vasectomy, the nurse is correct in telling the client to use an alternative birth control method for *at least*
   ○ 1. 1 week.
   ◉ 2. 1 month.
   ○ 3. 6 weeks.
   ○ 4. 6 months.

100   When teaching a male client about how to use a condom, which one of the following instructions is *correct*?
   ○ 1. Wait until the penis becomes limp to remove it from the vagina.
   ○ 2. You can reuse a condom as long as you wash it between uses.
   ◉ 3. Leave a small space between the end of the condom and the penis.
   ○ 4. Apply a condom before the penis is in an erect state.

Directions: Two numbers appear in parentheses following each rationale. The first number identifies the textbook listed in the references, page 512, and the second number identifies the page(s) in that textbook on which the correct answer can be verified. Occasionally two or more textbooks are given for verifying the correct answer.

NURSING CARE OF CLIENTS WITH BREAST DISORDERS

1 1. The American Cancer Society recommends that all women have an initial baseline mammogram between the ages of 35 and 39. Between the ages of 40 and 49, women should have mammograms every 1 to 2 years and yearly after the age of 50. (4:996)
Nursing Process—Implementation
Client Need—Health promotion/maintenance

2 2. While standing before a mirror, the contour of the breasts are inspected. Ominous signs include a change in the size of one breast, dimpling of the skin, or an altered nipple appearance. (4:1022; 21:860; 25:186)
Nursing Process—Implementation
Client Need—Health promotion/maintenance

3 4. The pads of the four fingertips are used to feel for breast abnormalities during a BSE. (21:860; 25:186)
Nursing Process—Evaluation
Client Need—Health promotion/maintenance

4 2. There is more than one correct description for the manner in which breast self-examination is performed, but they all include that the breasts are palpated from the outer margins toward the nipple. (18:1319; 21:860; 25:186)
Nursing Process—Implementation
Client Need—Health promotion/maintenance

5 4. Premenopausal females should perform BSE every month, 1 week after the end of menstruation. When a client is past menopause, BSE should be performed on a selected date each month, for example the first day of the month. (4:1022; 18:1318)
Nursing Process—Evaluation
Client Need—Health promotion/maintenance

6 2. Underarm deodorant, body powder, or ointments on the breast can produce artifacts on the mammogram film. The artifacts may be misinterpreted as pathologic findings. A brassiere may be worn before and after, but not during, a mammogram. Shaving underarm hair is a cultural choice; it is not a test requirement. Normal hygiene measures are appropriate, but it is not necessary to wipe the breasts with an antiseptic before the test. (4:996; 7:726).
Nursing Process—Implementation
Client Need—Health Promotion/maintenance

7 3. Having a close blood relative with breast cancer places a female at high risk for also developing this disease. Menstruating before the age of 12 and being nulliparous are additional predisposing factors. Breast feeding has many advantages, but protection against breast cancer is not one. (4:1021; 18:1324)
Nursing Process—Data collection
Client Need—Health promotion/maintenance

8 4. Fibrocystic lesions cause more discomfort before menstruation since they are affected by increasing levels of estrogen. There is relief of symptoms when menstruation occurs. Symptoms do not commonly increase with aging. Fibrocystic lesions are not influenced by sexual activity. (4:1020; 21:860)
Nursing Process—Implementation
Client Need—Health promotion/maintenance

9 2. Some women report that their breast discomfort has been reduced by eliminating coffee, tea, cola, and chocolate. Objectively there is no evidence that the fibrocystic lesions become smaller or disappear with any particular diet modification. Consuming a high-fat diet seems to have a relationship in developing breast cancer. Refined sugar and alcohol are not linked to breast disease. (4:1020; 18:1324)
Nursing Process—Implementation
Client Need—Health promotion/maintenance

10 3. Cleaning with soap and water is one of the best methods for reducing the transmission of microorganisms. Eating more sources of protein is a healthful measure, but it is not as specific as maintaining intact skin. Supporting the breasts and applying warm compresses provide comfort, but have no effect on preventing the transmission of microorganisms elsewhere. (25:430)

Nursing Process—Implementation
Client Need—Health promotion/maintenance

11 3. Cancerous tumors tend to be irregularly shaped and attached firmly to surrounding tissue. Benign breast tumors tend to have a well-defined border and be freely movable. Neither the size nor the location of the lump can necessarily predict if the lump is benign or malignant. Cancerous tumors in nulliparous females or those who have not breast-fed infants, however, are more commonly located in the upper outer quadrant of the breast. (4:1021; 18:1323)

Nursing Process—Data collection
Client Need—Physiological integrity

12 2. Competent adult clients have the right to self-determination once they have all the pertinent information on which to make a decision. Once that occurs, nurses have a duty to facilitate whatever choices clients make. Discouraging her from opposing the physician's recommendation promotes passivity. Even if most biopsies are accurate, some are not. A second opinion may eventually be appropriate, but many times the treatment plan can be modified to suit the client's wishes by facilitating open communication between the client and the physician. (4:28)

Nursing Process—Implementation
Client Need—Safe, effective care environment

13 3. Since this surgery compromises the client's vascular and lymphatic circulation, blood pressures and any other invasive procedures involving an arm are performed on the opposite upper extremity. Postmastectomy patients are generally not restricted to any one particular position; however, a sitting position tends to promote incisional drainage. Fluids are not commonly restricted. It is appropriate to assess the dressing and drainage, but the incisional wound is inspected only at the time of a dressing change, which may take place several days later. (4:1026; 21:866)

Nursing Process—Planning
Client Need—Physiological integrity

14 1. Breathing may be compromised due to the thoracic incision and restrictive (pressure) dressing that is applied. This type of dressing prevents movement of the chest muscles and thus reduces lung capacity until the dressing is removed. Having the client take deep breaths and encouraging coughing every 2 hours is of major importance in the prevention of respiratory problems, such as atelectasis and hypostatic pneumonia. (4:1026; 21:866)

Nursing Process—Data collection
Client Need—Physiological integrity

15 2. Most mastectomy clients tend to avoid raising the arm on the operative side following surgery. If this practice is prolonged, they tend to lose their full range of motion. Using the affected arm for hair brushing requires using muscles that elevate the arm and extend the chest muscles. Although self-feeding, writing, and washing the chest are good activities, they are not as likely to exercise the muscle groups to the same extent as brushing the hair. (18:1327; 21:867)

Nursing Process—Planning
Client Need—Physiological integrity

16 3. In postmastectomy clients, the standard of practice is to elevate the affected arm on pillows while in bed, to raise the arm and exercise the hand muscles, and to support the arm in a sling while ambulating. Applying ice reduces swelling and warm compresses dilate blood vessels, but because this surgery tends to compromise the client's circulation and sensory perception, they are not the most appropriate measures to use. (18:1326; 21:866)

Nursing Process—Planning
Client Need—Physiological integrity

17 2. The American Cancer Society provides volunteers who offer personal support and printed materials for postmastectomy clients in its program called Reach to Recovery. None of the other associations or organizations in the incorrect options exist to this author's knowledge. (4:1026; 21:867)

Nursing Process—Implementation
Client Need—Health promotion/maintenance

18 2. Clients who have had breast cancer are at risk for cancer in the opposite breast. Therefore, they must be conscientious about performing monthly breast self-examinations. Postmenopausal females pick an arbitrary date and perform breast self-examination on that date each month. The time of day is not pertinent. Breasts are examined during a shower, not afterward, when it is easier for the fingers to glide over the breast tissue. Breasts are examined monthly rather than once a year. (4:1022)

Nursing Process—Implementation
Client Need—Health promotion/maintenance

NURSING CARE OF CLIENTS WITH DISTURBANCES IN MENSTRUATION

19 1. It is important to differentiate between primary amenorrhea, a condition in which a female has never menstruated, and secondary amenorrhea, in

which menstruation has occurred but has been absent for more than 3 months. Although the other questions are pertinent, none is the most important question to ask next. (4:998–999)
>   Nursing Process—Data collection
>   Client Need—Health promotion/maintenance

20 3. Local applications of heat and mild analgesics are the first line of treatment for minor symptoms of dysmenorrhea. It is premature to seek a prescription for an oral contraceptive at this time, although they are effective in certain cases for relieving dysmenorrhea. There is no correlation between the choice of hygiene products and their relationship to dysmenorrhea. (4:999)
>   Nursing Process—Implementation
>   Client Need—Health promotion/maintenance

21 1. Douching in the days preceding a Pap smear interferes with accurate test results because it removes exfoliated cells. None of the other instructions are necessary when preparing a client for a pelvic examination. (7:764; 25:202)
>   Nursing Process—Implementation
>   Client Need—Safe, effective care environment

22 2. Pelvic organs are more easily palpated if the bladder is empty. The client experiences less discomfort if her bladder is empty. It is inappropriate to instill a vaginal lubricant before the examination. Analgesia is generally unnecessary. No special consent form is required. (25:202)
>   Nursing Process—Implementation
>   Client Need—Safe, effective care environment

23 3. It is best to document the date of a client's last menstrual period to assist the pathologist in determining if the microscopic cells are appropriate for the current stage in the luteal cycle. Answers to the other questions are immaterial to the results of the Pap smear. (25:202)
>   Nursing Process—Data collection
>   Client Need—Safe, effective care environment

24 4. A lithotomy position is preferred when performing a pelvic examination. In unusual circumstances, a Sims position is used. Neither a Trendelenberg nor a Fowler's position facilitates access to the vagina. (25:203)
>   Nursing Process—Implementation
>   Client Need—Safe, effective care environment

25 3. To preserve the integrity of the specimen, the slide on which the secretions have been deposited must be sprayed or immersed in a chemical fixative. (25:205)
>   Nursing Process—Implementation
>   Client Need—Safe, effective care environment

26 1. Breakthrough bleeding or spotting may occur among clients who take oral contraceptives with low dosages of estrogen or progesterone. Stress has been implicated in delaying menses or causing irregularity in a previously regular cycle, but it is uncommon for stress to cause mid-cyle bleeding. Having sexual intercourse with an uncircumcised partner is not a common cause of vaginal bleeding. Straining to have a stool is not a common cause of vaginal bleeding other than in one who recently had vaginal surgery or a vaginal delivery. (18:1327; 20:371)
>   Nursing Process—Data collection
>   Client Need—Health promotion/maintenance

NURSING CARE OF CLIENTS WITH INFECTIOUS AND INFLAMMATORY DISORDERS OF THE FEMALE REPRODUCTIVE SYSTEM

27 1. Several former antifungal prescription drugs are now available without a prescription. Drugs like miconazole come in forms such as vaginal tablets, creams, and suppositories. The other drugs, although manufactured for topical use, are not effective for treating vaginal infections caused by *C. albicans*. (21:835)
>   Nursing Process—Implementation
>   Client Need—Health promotion/maintenance

28 3. Instilling the drug before bedtime aids in retaining the medication within the vagina for a substantial period of time. If that is not possible, the client is instructed to recline for 10 to 30 minutes afterward. The applicator is inserted 2 to 4 inches within the vagina. The best position for instilling the drug is reclining in a dorsal recumbent position. Latex gloves are a matter of personal choice when self-administering vaginal medication. They are required when instilling the drug into someone else. Good handwashing is important in either case. (25:722)
>   Nursing Process—Implementation
>   Client Need—Health promotion/maintenance

29 2. Yeasts are present in the intestinal tract and are introduced into the vagina if stool is wiped across rather than away from the vaginal opening. This is often a common etiological factor in urinary tract infections as well. Showers versus tub baths are a matter of personal preference as long as the tub is cleaned on a routine basis. Some types of vaginal infections are spread from infected sexual partners, but limiting intercourse to once a week is not likely to prevent them. Lanolin soap is not more effective than antiseptic body soaps for reducing the growth of microorganisms. (4:1007)

> Nursing Process—Implementation
> Client Need—Health promotion/maintenance

30 2. Douching for the purpose of hygiene is unnecessary and can be harmful since it depletes helpful microorganisms that tend to prevent vaginal infections. A vinegar solution alters the pH of the vagina and makes it an inhospitable environment for microbial growth, but it is better to use a dilute solution rather than one that is concentrated. The volume of douche solutions can be more than 8 to 16 ounces. The solution drains out by gravity when the capacity of the vagina is reached. Cramping is not common. (25:582)

> Nursing Process—Implementation
> Client Need—Health promotion/maintenance

31 1. Toxic shock syndrome is caused by *Staphlococcus aureus*. The use of superabsorbent tampons tends to result in less frequent changing of tampons. Retention of the organism in a confined area where there is access to a rich blood supply promotes the growth and proliferation of the organism. It is appropriate to report prolonged menses since they can lead to anemia from blood loss, but that has no connection with toxic shock syndrome. Hygiene is never neglected regardless of whether a woman is menstruating or not. Some individuals are sensitive to scents used in sanitary products, but they have no relationship to toxic shock syndrome. (4:1009; 18:1328)

> Nursing Process—Implementation
> Client Need—Health promotion/maintenance

32 2. It is essential to contain any and all infectious drainage from a client with PID within specially marked infectious waste bags. Double wrapping soiled items prior to disposal or terminal cleaning protects other health care workers from accidental contamination with infectious microorganisms. Flushing absorbent pads down the toilet could cause plumbing problems. Neither an open wastebasket nor paper bags are sufficient barriers for containing the infectious microorganisms. (4:210,212; 18:605–606; 25:452–453)

> Nursing Process—Implementation
> Client Need—Safe, effective care environment

33 4. Infertility is a common consequence of PID. It results from scarring of fallopian tubes, which subsequently block the passages for both sperm and ova. With early and aggressive treatment, the sequela may be prevented or minimized. Cancer of the cervix, premature labors, and spontaneous abortions are not directly related to a prior incidence of PID. (4:1009)

> Nursing Process—Implementation
> Client Need—Health promotion/maintenance

34 1. A laparoscope is inserted through the abdominal wall. Once inserted, the endoscope is used to visualize the intra-abdominal and pelvic organs, obtain biopsies of tissue, and perform therapeutic treatment procedures. (4:994; 7:811; 18:1315)

> Nursing Process—Implementation
> Client Need—Health promotion/maintenance

35 2. Shoulder or abdominal discomfort may be experienced for 1 to 2 days after a laparoscopy. The discomfort is caused by the bolus of carbon dioxide that is instilled to distend the abdominal cavity. Nausea and leg cramps are unrelated to the laparoscopic procedure. Urinary urgency may occur following removal of the retention catheter that is used to keep the bladder empty during the laparoscopy, but it is not a direct effect of the endoscopy. (7:814)

> Nursing Process—Implementation
> Client Need—Health promotion/maintenance

36 4. Decreased estrogen production after menopause reduces the potential for vaginal lubrication. A dry vaginal mucous membrane is a common etiological factor in painful intercourse after menopause. Pelvic muscles do not become more sensitive to pressure with age. The amount of foreplay, no matter how long it continues, cannot stimulate mucus secretion if mucus cannot be produced. The vagina atrophies from age-related changes and has no relationship to the frequency of intercourse. (1:240; 18:1332; 27:94)

> Nursing Process—Implementation
> Client Need—Health promotion/maintenance

NURSING CARE OF FEMALE CLIENTS WITH BENIGN AND MALIGNANT DISORDERS OF THE UTERUS AND OVARIES

37 1. Fibroid tumors respond to estrogen stimulation. Heavy menstrual bleeding is a common complaint of clients with myomas. If pain occurs, it usually accompanies menstruation. Irregular menses and breast tenderness, if they are present, are not associated with fibroid tumors. (21:846)

> Nursing Process—Data collection
> Client Need—Physiological integrity

38 1. A full bladder is essential when performing a pelvic sonogram. Clients must consume at least a quart of water one hour before the examination and refrain from urinating until the examination is completed. Fasting is not necessary. The examination is not

painful so an analgesic is unnecessary. No special skin preparation is required prior to the examination. (7:843; 25:208)
  Nursing Process—Implementation
  Client Need—Safe, effective care environment

39 2. All of the data described are valid facts to document. But documenting that this client has voided in a sufficient amount to empty her bladder is most pertinent to the safety of the client after discharge. (18:1316)
  Nursing Process—Implementation
  Client Need—Safe, effective care environment

40 1. It is common to have slight bleeding after a colposcopy. If excessive bleeding occurs, it is reported. None of the other options describes a common problem following colposcopy. (7:805)
  Nursing Process—Implementation
  Client Need—Health promotion/maintenance

41 3. Identifying the number of sanitary pads that are used helps to quantify the extent of bleeding that is occurring. It provides more information than asking how often the client has sexual intercourse or if her energy level has changed. The color of the blood provides a characteristic of the blood loss, but it does not indicate the extent of bleeding. (4:1017; 21:850)
  Nursing Process—Data collection
  Client Need—Physiological integrity

42 4. Schiller's test is used to make a differential diagnosis of cervical cancer while the malignancy is in its superficial stage. When the cervix is painted with iodine, cells that do not stain suggest a malignancy. Further diagnostic tests like a cervical biopsy are performed in addition to the Schiller's test before treatment is initiated. (4:1017; 21:850)
  Nursing Process—Implementation
  Client Need—Safe, effective care environment

43 2. Following electrocauterization, the client is told to avoid straining and heavy lifting because these activities may cause bleeding from the cauterized site. The physician usually re-examines the client in 2 to 4 weeks. Absolute bed rest is not necessary, but the client should rest more than usual. Neither douching nor sexual intercourse are permitted until the physician indicates it is safe to do so. (21:836)
  Nursing Process—Implementation
  Client Need—Health promotion/maintenance

44 2. Bed rest must be maintained to retain the applicator within the vagina. In fact, the head of the bed is not raised more than 45 degrees while the radioactive applicator is in place. Nourishment is important, but it is related more to the client's nutritional status

than to radiation therapy. Weighing the client is postponed while the radioactive applicator is in place. (4:1197)
  Nursing Process—Planning
  Client Need—Safe, effective care environment

45 4. Displaced radioactive materials are placed in a lead container as soon as they are discovered. Lead blocks the transmission of radioactivity. The nuclear medicine department then manages the substance appropriately. Radioactive substances are never discarded. The physician, not the nurse, is responsible for reinserting the implant. (4:1197; 21:152)
  Nursing Process—Implementation
  Client Need—Safe, effective care environment

46 3. Distance is one of the measures used to reduce exposure to radiation. Therefore, radioactive substances are never handled with the hands. A long-handled forceps and lead container should be in the room of a client with a radioactive implant in a body orifice. Neither handwashing, vinyl gloves, nor using a glass jar controls exposure to radiation. (4:1197; 21:152)
  Nursing Process—Implementation
  Client Need—Safe, effective care environment

47 2. All of the described nurses have strengths that may be helpful to this client. However, since exposure to radiation can affect male and female gametes, it is best that the client be cared for by a nurse for whom pregnancy is unlikely or a male nurse who has had a vasectomy. (21:152)
  Nursing Process—Planning
  Client Need—Safe, effective care environment

48 3. The female urethra is approximately 1½ to 2 inches long. Inserting the catheter 2 to 3 inches places the tip of the catheter into the bladder and urine should flow. Once urine flows, the catheter is advanced another ½ to 1 inch to ensure that the balloon of the indwelling catheter is well past the bladder neck. (18:651; 25:652)
  Nursing Process—Implementation
  Client Need—Physiological integrity

49 1. All clients who receive general anesthesia are prone to respiratory complications. Since a clear airway and breathing are higher priorities than nutrition to maintain immediately postoperatively, Risk for Altered Airway Clearance is the most appropriate addition at this time. It is too premature to make the diagnosis of Ineffective Individual Coping. The client should have no difficulty communicating verbally once she is returned from the post-anesthesia room (PAR). (21:852)

Nursing Process—Implementation
Client Need—Safe, effective care environment

50 1. To accomplish their purpose, antiembolism stockings are worn continuously except when they are removed for assessment and hygiene. (18:565; 25:553)
Nursing Process—Implementation
Client Need—Physiological integrity

51 3. Abdominal surgery clients are prone to developing blood clots in their lower extremities. Therefore, the knees are not elevated since that promotes stasis of blood flow. All of the other activities are appropriate for a client recovering from a hysterectomy. (21:240)
Nursing Process—Evaluation
Client Need—Safe, effective care environment

52 3. It is important to deflate the balloon first. Cleansing the perineum and measuring the urinary output are essential actions, but they can be postponed until after the catheter has been removed. It is not necessary to separate the catheter from the drainage bag. After the bag is emptied, both can be disposed of in an appropriate waste receptacle. (25:662)
Nursing Process—Implementation
Client Need—Physiological integrity

53 2. To measure the volume of urine that is being retained in the bladder, it is important to catheterize the client within 10 minutes after voiding. The size of the catheter is relative to the size of the client. The size is not pertinent to the purpose of the procedure. The catheter is connected to gravity drainage only if the physician orders a retention catheter based upon a certain retained volume. (4:317)
Nursing Process—Implementation
Client Need—Physiological integrity

54 2. The dosages of many toxic drugs that are administered to adults as well as drugs administered to children are calculated on the basis of the client's body surface area. Body surface area is calculated by using both body weight and height. The other data is important to obtain, but they have no relationship to the dosage of the drug that will be administered. (17:27, 618)
Nursing Process—Data collection
Client Need—Safe, effective care environment

55 4. A complete blood count provides information about all the cells that the bone marrow produces. The mean cell volume, total leukocyte count, and differential cell count are all important, but none is as comprehensively informative as a complete blood cell count. (17:628; 20:445)

Nursing Process—Data collection
Client Need—Physiological integrity

56 2. Latex gloves act as a barrier against contact between the drug and the nurse's skin. Regardless of the drug manufacturer's directions for preparing the drug, wearing gloves reduces the risk for accidentally absorbing the medication. (17:637; 20:444)
Nursing Process—Implementation
Client Need—Physiological integrity

57 4. The hair that is lost with some antineoplastic drugs returns after chemotherapy is terminated. The return of hair growth varies from client to client, but in all cases it is restored in less than 2 years. (17:634; 20:445)
Nursing Process—Implementation
Client Need—Health promotion/maintenance

NURSING CARE OF FEMALE CLIENTS WITH MISCELLANEOUS DISORDERS OF THE REPRODUCTIVE SYSTEM

58 2. Standing and bearing down is the best technique for determining the extent of uterine prolapse. Using this technique, the nurse can evaluate the effect of gravity in relation to the relaxed pelvic muscles. The other assessment techniques are used if the client is unable to stand. (18:1330)
Nursing Process—Data collection
Client Need—Physiological integrity

59 4. The majority of clients with a cystocele experience stress incontinence. Stress incontinence is manifested by a slight loss of urine when abdominal pressure increases as with sneezing, coughing, laughing, and lifting heavy objects. (18:1329; 21:841)
Nursing Process—Data collection
Client Need—Physiological integrity

60 3. Perineal exercises, known also as Kegel exercises, strengthen the muscles that help suspend the bladder. Purchasing absorbent underwear is an option if the cystocele is more serious or if the client chooses not to proceed with a surgical repair. Applying an external catheter is an option, but not a very effective or popular one. It is inappropriate to limit oral fluid intake as a means of controlling adult incontinence. (18:1329–1330; 21:842, 941)
Nursing Process—Implementation
Client Need—Health promotion/maintenance

61 2. Absence of a urinary tract infection is the best indication that the client is following appropriate aseptic principles when performing self-catheterization. The volume of urine is more than 50 mL if the bladder is being emptied completely. The catheter is removed immediately after the bladder is emptied. The frequency of catheterization depends on the client's rate of urine formation and sensation of a need to void. Frequency of catheterization is not an indication of appropriate technique. (4:838; 18:1283)

Nursing Process—Evaluation
Client Need—Health promotion/maintenance

NURSING CARE OF CLIENTS WITH INFLAMMATORY DISORDERS OF THE MALE REPRODUCTIVE SYSTEM

62 3. Inadequate treatment leads to developing a chronic condition. Whenever an antibiotic is prescribed, it is important to stress that all of the medication should be taken. Taking only a portion of the medication may not be of sufficient quantity to destroy the infectious microorganism. It also contributes to the development of resistant strains. Drinking milk, reporting significant information, and monitoring body temperature may be important in some cases. The latter recommendations are based more on factors such as the side effects of the drug, the condition for which the drug is prescribed, and the client's physical condition. (17:50–51, 18:1307; 20:57)

Nursing Process—Implementation
Client Need—Health promotion/maintenance

63 2. A sitz bath is more effective if it lasts approximately 20 minutes. The water is approximately 110°F, which is considered warm, not tepid. Soap is omitted since a sitz bath is a technique for applying heat. The prostate surrounds the urethra. Massaging the scrotum has no direct benefit in relieving the client's symptoms. (21:872; 25:586–587)

Nursing Process—Implementation
Client Need—Health promotion/maintenance

64 2. Only a small portion of urine that is voided in midstream, that is, after the first release of urine is wasted, is collected. The procedure does require cleansing of the penis, retracting the foreskin if the client is uncircumcised, and depositing the urine directly into a sterile container. (4:316; 25:635)

Nursing Process—Evaluation
Client Need—Safe, effective care environment

65 1. Elevating and supporting the scrotum helps to relieve the discomfort of epididymitis. Analgesics are also prescribed. The choice of larger underwear or wearing cotton briefs is a personal choice and does not inherently relieve the client's symptoms. Heat

is contraindicated since it can damage sperm. (4:1030; 21:880)

Nursing Process—Implementation
Client Need—Health promotion/maintenance

66 3. The mumps virus can infect the testes of males who have not been adequately immunized before puberty. A sexually transmitted disease is likely if the testes and the epididymis are co-infected, but that is not the case in this situation. Although Gulf War veterans have developed many and varied symptoms, orchitis has not been a commonly occurring disorder among them. (18:1310; 21:879)

Nursing Process—Data collection
Client Need—Physiological integrity

67 2. The testicle is rolled between the thumb and fingers when performing a self-examination. Each testicle is examined separately. It is easier to palpate the testes when the scrotum is warm, like during or after a shower. Testicular self-examination should be performed monthly. (4:1031; 25:192)

Nursing Process—Implementation
Client Need—Health promotion/maintenance

NURSING CARE OF MALE CLIENTS WITH STRUCTURAL DISORDERS OF THE MALE REPRODUCTIVE SYSTEM

68 1. As long as there is one descended testicle, it most likely produces sufficient testosterone to produce normal secondary sexual characteristics, adequate sperm for conception, and a healthy sexual drive. Impotence, the inability to achieve an erection, is not generally compromised. (18:1307)

Nursing Process—Implementation
Client Need—Health promotion/maintenance

69 3. The priority nursing assessments following a circumcision include checking on the amount of local bleeding and the client's ability to void. Swelling can obstruct the urethra and interfere with the release of urine. Deep breathing and bowel patterns are routine assessments for surgical clients who have received general anesthesia. It would be inappropriate to assess the client's erectile function at this time. (4:1030)

Nursing Process—Data collection
Client Need—Physiological integrity

70 2. Whenever a device that is cold or warm is placed on a client's body, it is placed within some type of fabric cover. A plastic bag is not an appropriate cover. A hypothermia blanket is too large for the local effect that is desired. An ice-filled ring is not located in the best area for producing a local effect. (25:584)

> Nursing Process—Implementation
> Client Need—Physiological integrity

NURSING CARE OF CLIENTS WITH BENIGN AND MALIGNANT DISORDERS OF THE MALE REPRODUCTIVE SYSTEM

71 2. The best position for assessing the characteristics of the prostate gland is one in which the client leans forward from the waist while standing. The body is braced against the examination table for support. The rectum is examined with clients in lithotomy and dorsal recumbent positions, but these are not the preferred positions. A Fowler's position does not facilitate a rectal examination. (25:199–200)

> Nursing Process—Implementation
> Client Need—Safe, effective care environment

72 4. Relaxing in a tub of warm water may help the client with BPH urinate. However, if the technique is unsuccessful, catheterization becomes necessary. Waiting 24 hours is unsafe. It also is unsafe and inappropriate to suggest dilating the urethra and to restrict oral intake until urination takes place. (18:1309)

> Nursing Process—Implementation
> Client Need—Health promotion/maintenance

73 2. After draining 1000 mL of urine, the client should feel relief. Withdrawing any more than 1000 mL in a short amount of time can contribute to rupture of mucosal blood vessels. More urine is drained after waiting a period of time. The physician may override this rule of thumb in special circumstances. (4:851)

> Nursing Process—Implementation
> Client Need—Physiological integrity

74 4. When a prostate sonogram is performed, a rectal probe is inserted. The presence of stool can interfere with imaging the prostate as well as contribute to discomfort. Therefore, it is important that the rectum be empty. The client may wish to empty his bladder, but that is not a necessity when this test is performed. The test does not require fasting. Water may be instilled within the sheath surrounding the rectal probe, but the client is not required to consume a large volume of water. (7:862)

> Nursing Process—Implementation
> Client Need—Safe, effective care environment

75 3. Dark red urine is expected after a TURP. The color gets lighter and clearer during or after bladder irri-

gations and as the postoperative time passes. (4:851)

> Nursing Process—Implementation
> Client Need—Health promotion/maintenance

76 4. The irrigation solution is a part of the volume that collects in the drainage bag. Therefore, to find the true urine output, the amount of instilled irrigant is subtracted from the volume in the drainage bag. (4:851)

> Nursing Process—Implementation
> Client Need—Physiological integrity

77 4. In the absence of fluid precautions, increasing the oral intake helps to dilute the urine and reduce the potential for obstruction. Milking the tubing helps to dislodge clots, but it is not as effective as keeping the urine dilute. It is inappropriate to deflate the balloon. Emptying the drainage container does not maintain catheter patency. (21:878; 26:678)

> Nursing Process—Planning
> Client Need—Physiological integrity

78 1. Obstructions in the drainage catheter are the chief cause of bladder discomfort following TURP. A belladonna and opium suppository may be helpful, but this option is not the first course of action. Sitting can increase intraabdominal pressure and contribute to more bleeding. Ambulating may or may not improve drainage through the catheter, but it is not the first choice of actions. (4:851; 26:679)

> Nursing Process—Implementation
> Client Need—Physiological integrity

79 2. The tendency to dribble urine is reduced or prevented by alternately stopping the flow of urine and resuming urination during voiding. Caffeine is a bladder irritant, but eliminating it is not the best measure for promoting urinary control. Standing is the most natural position for males when voiding. Sitting does not affect urinary control. (21:878)

> Nursing Process—Planning
> Client Need—Health promotion/maintenance

80 3. In the immediate postoperative period, all urinary drainage catheters, including the cystostomy tube, are unclamped to facilitate drainage. The suprapubic cystostomy tube is clamped later when bladder retraining is begun. A cystostomy catheter is too short to attach to the thigh or a leg bag. (21:876; 26:678)

> Nursing Process—Planning
> Client Need—Physiological integrity

81 4. The temperature is taken by any route other than rectal for the first postoperative week when a client has had prostatic surgery. Inserting a rectal thermometer can result in perforation of the rectal mucosa and damage to the prostatic capsule, which has been left behind when the prostate is removed. All the other instructions are correct, but they are not the most important instruction to give the nursing assistant. (21:878)
Nursing Process—Implementation
Client Need—Safe, effective care environment

82 2. One functioning testis ought to produce enough testosterone to sustain all of a male's secondary sex characteristics and his libido. However, after this surgery, the sperm count is reduced and their mobility is impaired. (4:1031)
Nursing Process—Evaluation
Client Need—Health promotion/maintenance

NURSING CARE OF CLIENTS WITH SEXUALLY TRANSMITTED DISEASES

83 3. Intimate sexual contact with one or more sexual partners is the highest risk factor on the list for acquiring a sexually transmitted disease. Developing sexually at an early age does not necessarily affect a person's sexual choices. Movies that are objectionable for children and adolescents does not necessarily mean that the movies are rated exclusively on the basis of sexual scenes. Sex education is important and too little of it does predispose individuals to making poor sexual choices. However, it is not as great a risk factor as having multiple sexual partners. (4:1032)
Nursing Process—Implementation
Client Need—Health promotion/maintenance

84 4. The most likely substance that will be cultured if a client has gonorrhea is urethral drainage. However, the organism might also be cultured from swabs taken from the rectum, vagina, pharynx and so on. The organism causing gonorrhea is not generally found in blood or urine. It is found in semen, but the collection is more involved since it requires masturbation and ejaculation to produce the specimen. (7:470; 21:890)
Nursing Process—Implementation
Client Need—Safe, effective care environment

85 1. Gloves are worn as a standard precaution when collecting body substances from any client regardless of the tentative diagnosis. Using a disinfectant is not appropriate for any specimen collection. As long as gloves are worn, the nurse can touch the client. Cultures for the gonorrhea organism are inoculated onto a culture medium as soon as possible;

therefore, refrigeration is undesirable. (21:893)
Nursing Process—Implementation
Client Need—Safe, effective care environment

86 1. Females infected with the herpes simplex type 2 virus are at greater risk for developing cervical cancer. Males infected with the virus are at greater risk for developing prostatic cancer. Clients may have vaginal intercourse but a condom should be used and all sexual partners should be informed of their potential for infection. Drugs may decrease the frequency of outbreaks and reduce the length of time when symptoms are manifested. Therefore, taking medication does not confer protection for others. Spontaneous abortions increase among infected pregnant women. Infants can acquire the herpes virus at the time of vaginal delivery. (18:853; 21:891)
Nursing Process—Implementation
Client Need—Health promotion/maintenance

87 1. One of the manifestations of tertiary syphilis is sharp stabbing leg pains. There may also be other organ system damage to the heart, brain, liver, bones, and eyes. A painless ulcer is a characteristic of primary-stage syphilis. The secondary stage of syphilis is accompanied by a red skin rash and patchy loss of hair. (4:1033; 18:853)
Nursing Process—Data collection
Client Need—Physiological integrity

88 4. There is no lifelong immunity to syphilis. Each new incident is treated with antibiotic therapy. Antibiotic therapy destroys the microorganism and prevents further consequences from the disease. Sexual partners are tested and treated if they are infected. Syphilitic lesions can appear on the penis, outside and inside the vagina, around the mouth, and even the nipple. (4:1033; 18:852–853)
Nursing Process—Evaluation
Client Need—Health promotion/maintenance

89 1. To avoid a continuous cycle of reinfection, the sexual partner(s) are simultaneously treated with the same drug therapy. Appropriate treatment can cure this sexually transmitted disease, but it does not prevent reinfection. Chlamydial infections are extremely common. A large proportion of both genders are asymptomatic and go undiagnosed until a complication of the infection is manifested. (4:1035–1036; 18:855)
Nursing Process—Implementation
Client Need—Health promotion/maintenance

90 2. Vaginal pruritus is a common problem experienced by females infected with *Trichomonas vaginalis*. Fluid-filled vesicles are associated with herpetic lesions. Vaginal drainage that seems to contain flecks of milk is characteristic of candidiasis (moniliasis). Among several possible etiologies, abdominal discomfort is experienced by females with gonorrhea or chlamydia infections. (4:1035)

    Nursing Process—Data collection
    Client Need—Physiological integrity

91 4. Consuming alcohol while taking metronidazole can cause disorientation, headache, cramps, vomiting, and convulsions. There are no known food-drug interactions with this drug and iodized salt, monosodium glutamate, or aspartame. (4:1035)

    Nursing Process—Implementation
    Client Need—Health promotion/maintenance

92 2. There is a relationship between genital warts and an increased risk of cancer of the vulva, vagina, and cervix. Genital warts are treated with topical applications of chemicals or surgical removal. If sexual partners are not treated, the virus can be retransmitted. The use of a condom is recommended until the warts disappear. (18:855; 21:892)

    Nursing Process—Implementation
    Client Need—Health promotion/maintenance

93 3. Nonoxynol-9 has been shown to inhibit the HIV virus and reduce the potential for infection. Removing the condom immediately, washing with a dilute solution of vinegar, and using vaginal lubricant are not techniques for preventing an HIV infection. (4:1172; 21:497)

    Nursing Process—Implementation
    Client Need—Health Promotion/maintenance

94 2. Blood counts reveal if the CD4 and CD8 cells are increasing, decreasing, or staying the same. Changes in vital signs signal complications such as infections, but this is not the best method for monitoring drug effectiveness. Viruses can only be cultured in living tissue. Consequently this approach is not used except in research. The effectiveness of zidovudine is not related to urine output. (20:103)

    Nursing Process—Data collection
    Client Need—Physiological integrity

NURSING CARE OF CLIENTS PRACTICING FAMILY PLANNING

95 1. Oral contraceptives are taken at approximately the same time each day, preferably in the evening. They do not need to be taken on an empty stomach. An oral contraceptive is started on the fifth day of

menstruation and, depending on the type used, is taken for 20 or 21 days. (20:375)

    Nursing Process—Implementation
    Client Need—Health promotion/maintenance

96 1. Smoking increases the risk for developing blood clots in women who take oral contraceptives. Maintaining a high fluid volume and elevating the legs are ways of preventing venous stasis, but they are not directly related to the cause and effect nature of the question. There are claims that garlic and onions have an anticoagulant effect, but the claims have not been thoroughly documented in scientific research. (18:848; 20:375)

    Nursing Process—Implementation
    Client Need—Health promotion/maintenance

97 3. Menstruation continues because the ovarian hormones are circulated in the blood, not through the fallopian tubes. A tubal ligation performed through the abdomen leaves only a small incisional scar. Hospitalization is brief. Although tubal ligations have been reversed, they are still considered a permanent form of contraception. (4:1037)

    Nursing Process—Evaluation
    Client Need—Health promotion/maintenance

98 2. After an IUD is inserted, many women experience menstrual cramps, an increase in blood loss, and longer duration of menstrual periods. Breast tenderness, weight gain, and acne are more common with hormonal methods of birth control. (18:849)

    Nursing Process—Data collection
    Client Need—Physiological integrity

99 3. Having a vasectomy does not ensure sterility immediately. A sperm count is done at 6 weeks, 6 months, and yearly thereafter. When the sperm count is zero for 6 weeks, the chances for conception are almost impossible. (18:850)

    Nursing Process—Implementation
    Client Need—Health promotion/maintenance

100 3. Leaving a space between the tip of the condom and penis allows an area where the ejaculate can be contained. Condoms are designed for one use only. A new condom is applied with each new erection. To prevent leakage of semen, the condom is grasped as the erect penis is withdrawn from the vagina. Condoms are applied as the penis becomes erect. (25:193)

    Nursing Process—Implementation
    Client Need—Health promotion/maintenance

Classification of Test Items

Unit I   Review Test **5**

The Nursing Care of Clients with Disorders of the Reproductive System

Directions: After each question, the correct answer is given as well as a classification of each test question. Compare the correct answer with your answer. If a question has been answered *incorrectly*, draw a line to the end of all the columns. When finished, add up the number of your correct answers in each column and place that number in the respective box at the end in the area identified as *Number Correct*.

To determine the percentage of questions you answered correctly and your performance in each of the test plan categories, divide the *Number Correct* in each column by the *Number Possible* in each column. Then multiply the decimal by 100. For example:

$$\frac{\text{Number Correct: 75}}{\text{Number Possible: 100}} = 0.750 \times 100 = 75\%$$

Any score that is less than 75% indicates an area where further review would be beneficial.

KEY TO ITEM CLASSIFICATION:

NURSING PROCESS

D = Data collection
P = Planning
I = Implementation
E = Evaluation

CLIENT NEEDS

S = Safe, effective care environment
P = Physiological integrity
M = Psychosocial integrity
H = Health promotion/maintenance

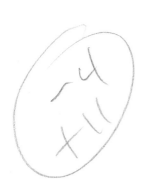

Question #	Answer #	Nursing Process				Client Needs			
		D	P	I	E	S	P	M	H
1	1			I					H
2	2			I					H
3	4				E				H
4	2			I					H
5	4				E				H
6	2			I					H
7	3	D							H
8	4			I					H
9	2			I					H
10	3			I					H
11	3	D					P		
12	2			I		S			
13	3		P				P		
14	1	D					P		
15	2		P				P		

153

Question #	Answer #	Nursing Process				Client Needs			
		D	P	I	E	S	P	M	H
16	3		P				P		
17	2			I					H
18	2			I					H
19	1	D							H
20	3			I					H
21	1			I		S			
22	2			I		S			
23	3	D				S			
24	4			I		S			
25	3			I		S			
26	1	D							H
27	1			I					H
28	3			I					H
29	2			I					H
30	2			I					H
31	1			I					H
32	2			I		S			
33	4			I					H
34	1			I					H
35	2			I					H
36	4			I					H
37	1	D					P		
38	1			I		S			
39	2			I		S			
40	1			I					H
41	3	D					P		
42	4			I		S			
43	2			I					H
44	2		P			S			
45	4			I		S			
46	3			I		S			
47	2		P			S			

Question #	Answer #	D	P	I	E	S	P	M	H
		Nursing Process				**Client Needs**			
48	3			I			P		
49	1			I		S			
50	1			I			P		
51	3				E	S			
52	3			I			P		
53	2			I			P		
54	2	D				S			
55	4	D					P		
56	2			I			P		
57	4			I					H
58	2	D					P		
59	4	D					P		
60	3			I					H
61	2				E				H
62	3			I					H
63	2			I					H
64	2				E	S			
65	1			I					H
66	3	D					P		
67	2			I					H
68	1			I					H
69	3	D					P		
70	2			I			P		
71	2			I		S			
72	4			I					H
73	2			I			P		
74	4			I		S			
75	3			I					H
76	4			I			P		
77	4		P				P		
78	1			I			P		
79	2		P						H

Question #	Answer #	Nursing Process				Client Needs			
		D	P	I	E	S	P	M	H
80	3		P				P		
81	4			I		S			
82	2				E				H
83	3			I					H
84	4			I		S			
85	1			I		S			
86	1			I					H
87	1	D					P		
88	4				E				H
89	1			I					H
90	2	D					P		
91	4			I					H
92	2			I					H
93	3			I					H
94	2	D					P		
95	1			I					H
96	1			I					H
97	3				E				H
98	2	D					P		
99	3			I					H
100	3			I					H
Number Correct	83	13	6	56		21	21		41
Number Possible	100	18	8	66	8	23	27	0	50
Percentage Correct	83	72	75	85	100	91	78		82

The Nursing Care of Clients with Disorders of the Neurologic System

Directions: With a pencil, blacken the circle in front of the option you have chosen for your correct answer.

NURSING CARE OF CLIENTS WITH INFECTIOUS AND INFLAMMATORY CONDITIONS

A 23-year-old male is brought to the hospital after efforts to relieve his fever are unsuccessful. The tentative diagnosis is meningitis.

1 If the tentative diagnosis is accurate, which assessment finding is the nurse likely to document?
- ○ 1. The client says he has double vision.
- ● 2. The client says he has a stiff neck.
- ○ 3. The client says his joints ache.
- ○ 4. The client says he is very thirsty.

The physician plans to do a lumbar puncture (spinal tap) on the client who may have meningitis.

2 To facilitate performing the lumbar puncture, it is *best* for the nurse to place the client
- ● 1. in a knee-chest (genupectoral) position.
- ○ 2. sitting up in an orthopneic position.
- ○ 3. in a side-lying position with his neck flexed.
- ○ 4. in a left lateral position with right knee flexed.

3 After the lumbar puncture has been performed, it is *best* for the nurse to
- ○ 1. keep the client positioned on his side.
- ○ 2. ambulate the client about the room.
- ○ 3. withhold food and fluids for an hour.
- ● 4. keep the client flat for several hours.

4 While awaiting the results of diagnostic tests, it is *best* to care for the client with possible meningitis following which *transmission-based* precautions?
- ○ 1. Droplet precautions
- ● 2. Airborne precautions
- ○ 3. Contact precautions
- ○ 4. Standard precautions

The physician orders an aquathermia pad (K-pad) to reduce the fever of the client with meningitis.

5 When implementing the medical order, the nurse is *most correct* to
- ○ 1. place the blanket on top of the client.
- ● 2. enclose the blanket in a light cloth cover.
- ○ 3. add normal saline to the fluid chamber.
- ○ 4. replace crushed ice periodically as it melts.

6 To reduce the potential for seizures and promote comfort for the client with meningitis, it is *best* for the nurse to keep the room
- ● 1. dark and quiet.
- ○ 2. warm and sunny.
- ○ 3. cool and well-ventilated.
- ○ 4. warm and well-humidified.

The care plan of a client with viral encephalitis indicates that the nurse should perform neurological checks every 2 hours.

7 If the client had been unresponsive except to painful stimuli, which one of the following new assessments indicate that the client is *improving*?
- ○ 1. The client's pupils remain fixed when stimulated with light.
- ○ 2. The client's pupils dilate when stimulated with light.
- ● 3. The client opens his eyes when his name is called.
- ○ 4. The client swallows when his cheek is stroked with a swab.

The nursing team discusses the case of a new client who has Guillain-Barré syndrome.

8 When the medical history is reviewed, which one of the following facts is most likely related to the client's diagnosis?
  - ○ 1. The client had an immunization in the last week.
  - ○ 2. The client was bitten by a spider two days ago.
  - ◑ 3. The client drinks fresh unpasteurized milk from his cows.
  - ○ 4. The client sprayed his garden with insecticide this week.

9 When the nursing team plans the care of a client with Guillain-Barré syndrome, which nursing assessment is *most accurate* for determining if the client is developing ineffective breathing?
  - ○ 1. Pulse rate
  - ○ 2. Skin color
  - ○ 3. Red cell count
  - ◉ 4. Pulse oximetry

The client with Guillain-Barré syndrome begins to have difficulty swallowing food.

10 When the nurse is asked to recommend a technique for nourishing the client, which method is most appropriate *at this time*?
  - ○ 1. Administering crystalloid intravenous fluid
  - ◉ 2. Administering nasogastric tube feedings
  - ○ 3. Administering total parenteral nutrition
  - ○ 4. Administering gastrostomy tube feedings

The nurse assigned to a client with post-polio syndrome reads the client's health history.

11 If the nurse finds all of the following information documented in the client's medical record, which one best explains how the client first contracted poliomyelitis?
  - ○ 1. The client was immunized with killed injectable polio vaccine (IPV) as an infant.
  - ◉ 2. The client was immunized with live oral polio vaccine (OPV) as an infant.
  - ○ 3. The client received his polio immunization before he was 9 months old.
  - ○ 4. The client received his polio and rubella immunization at the same time.

A hospice nurse makes a visit to the home of a client with acquired immunodeficiency syndrome (AIDS) dementia complex.

12 The *best* advice the nurse can give the family when the client becomes confused is to
  - ○ 1. turn the television on so the client can hear human voices.

  - ○ 2. play some of the client's favorite music when he is disturbed.
  - ◉ 3. tell the client where he is at, who you are, and what is happening.
  - ○ 4. bathe the client so he can experience the touch of another person.

NURSING CARE OF CLIENTS WITH CONVULSIVE DISORDERS

A 23-year-old female who experienced a seizure while at work is undergoing diagnostic tests.

13 When preparing a client for an electroencephalogram (EEG), which nursing action is appropriate to perform?
  - ○ 1. Administer a pretest sedative an hour before.
  - ○ 2. Withhold food and water after midnight.
  - ◉ 3. Assist the client with shampooing her hair.
  - ○ 4. Take her blood pressure lying and sitting.

Seizure precautions are ordered on the plan of care for the client undergoing an EEG.

14 When implementing this order, which of the following nursing actions is *most appropriate*?
  - ○ 1. The client is moved to a room close to the nursing station.
  - ○ 2. The client's food is served in paper and plastic containers.
  - ○ 3. The overhead light is left on at all times.
  - ◉ 4. The side rails on the bed are softly padded.

15 When the client who has had an EEG begins to have a seizure, which action should the nurse take *first*?
  - ○ 1. Administer oxygen by nasal cannula.
  - ○ 2. Take her blood pressure and pulse.
  - ○ 3. Restrain her arms and upper body.
  - ◉ 4. Place her in a side-lying position.

16 When documenting a seizure, which of the following is *most important* to identify?
  - ○ 1. The time the seizure started
  - ◉ 2. The duration of the seizure
  - ○ 3. The client's mood just prior to the seizure
  - ○ 4. The client's comments after the seizure

17 When a client is injured during a seizure, assuming all of the following are true, which one is *most important* to document on the accident report to reduce the risk for liability?
  - ○ 1. The client was assigned to a licensed nurse.
  - ◉ 2. The signal cord was within the client's reach.
  - ○ 3. The client's vital signs had been stable.
  - ○ 4. The client was last observed to be reading.

The medical record of a client with epilepsy indicates that he has had two previous episodes of status epilepticus.

18 Which emergency drug should the nurse plan to have available in case the client has a similar episode?
- ○ 1. Diazepam (Valium)
- ◉ 2. Phenytoin (Dilantin)
- ○ 3. Magnesium sulfate
- ○ 4. Phenobarbital sodium

19 When a client takes phenytoin sodium (Dilantin), which hygiene measure is *especially important* to perform?
- ○ 1. Shampooing the hair
- ○ 2. Trimming fingernails
- ◉ 3. Brushing the teeth
- ○ 4. Bathing the skin

NURSING CARE OF CLIENTS WITH NEUROLOGIC TRAUMA

A nurse who witnesses a motor vehicle accident stops to provide emergency assistance to the injured people.

20 When the nurse assesses a male victim who has been thrown from the vehicle, which one of the following is *most suggestive* that he has a serious head injury?
- ○ 1. The accident victim says he has a bad headache.
- ○ 2. The accident victim asks the nurse, "What happened?"
- ○ 3. The accident victim holds his head with his hands.
- ◉ 4. The accident victim has serous drainage from his ears.

21 Which one of the following actions is *most important* for the nurse to do *next*?
- ◉ 1. Maintain the accident victim's present position.
- ○ 2. Assist the accident victim to the shade of a tree.
- ○ 3. Cover the client with a light blanket.
- ○ 4. Give the client some water to drink.

22 To reduce the risk for liability, it is *most appropriate* for the nurse to
- ○ 1. avoid giving the accident victim any personal identification.
- ○ 2. remain with the accident victim until paramedics arrive.
- ◉ 3. conceal the fact that he or she is a nurse.
- ○ 4. let others at the scene provide direct care.

The accident victim is evaluated in the emergency department.

23 While waiting for the physician to examine the client, it is *best* for the emergency department nurse to keep the client in
- ○ 1. dorsal recumbent position with his legs elevated.
- ◉ 2. supine position with his head slightly elevated.
- ○ 3. left lateral position with his knees flexed.
- ○ 4. right lateral position with his neck flexed.

The client with a head injury is admitted after x-rays are taken of his head, neck, and spine.

24 If the nurse assigned to this client's care performs all of the following assessments, which one is *most important*?
- ○ 1. The nurse assesses the client's lung sounds.
- ○ 2. The nurse assesses the client's skin integrity.
- ○ 3. The nurse assesses the client's urine characteristics.
- ◉ 4. The nurse assesses the client's pupillary responses.

25 If the nurse obtains all of the following data, which one is reported to the physician *immediately*?
- ○ 1. The client rates his headache as "3" on a scale of 0 to 10.
- ○ 2. The client leaves most of the food on his dietary tray.
- ◉ 3. The client is difficult to arouse.
- ○ 4. The client says he feels exhausted.

26 If the nurse notes all of the following when assessing the client with the head injury, which one is most likely contributing to the change in his condition?
- ○ 1. The client has been disturbed every hour.
- ○ 2. The client has had very little fluid intake.
- ◉ 3. The client's neck is flexed toward his chest.
- ○ 4. The client's bladder is becoming quite full.

The client with the head injury is treated with mannitol (Osmitrol).

27 Which of the following is *most appropriate* for the nurse to assess while the client is receiving mannitol?
- ○ 1. Urinary output
- ◉ 2. Respiratory rate
- ○ 3. Level of pain
- ○ 4. Skin condition

A 22-year-old male acquires a complete transection of his spinal cord at the level of the 5th thoracic (T5) vertebrae at the time of a diving accident.

28 Which one of the following statements indicates that the client with the spinal injury has an *accurate understanding* of his prognosis?
- ○ 1. The client says, "After surgery, I can expect full function."
- ○ 2. The client says, "My recovery depends on my rehabilitation efforts."
- ○ 3. The client says, "I will retain functions above my chest."
- ● 4. The client says, "No one can predict my potential outcome at this time."

The client with the spinal cord injury is stable and he is transferred to a rehabilitation unit.

29 When the nursing team discusses the management of the client with the spinal injury, which plan has the *highest priority*?
- ○ 1. Relieving the client's physical discomfort.
- ○ 2. Strengthening the client's upper body muscles.
- ○ 3. Confronting the client's denial of his condition.
- ● 4. Letting the client verbalize his feelings.

The client with the spinal cord injury develops a severe headache and hypertension. Autonomic dysreflexia is suspected.

30 Besides helping the client to sit up, which other nursing action is *most appropriate* at this time?
- ○ 1. Talking quietly to the client to relieve his anxiety.
- ○ 2. Inserting an oral airway in case he has a seizure.
- ○ 3. Compressing the client's abdomen with firm pressure.
- ● 4. Checking to see if his urinary catheter is patent.

31 When planning a bowel retraining program for the client with the spinal cord injury, which one of the following is *most appropriate* to include?
- ○ 1. Administer a tap-water enema just before bedtime.
- ● 2. Encourage a high-fiber diet to increase stool bulk.
- ○ 3. Change disposable absorbent undergarments when soiled.
- ○ 4. Pad the rim of the bedpan to prevent skin breakdown.

32 Prior to discharge, which one of the following home care suggestions is best for promoting the mobility of the client with a spinal cord injury?
- ○ 1. Rent or buy a conventional hospital bed.
- ● 2. Build a wheelchair ramp to the door.
- ○ 3. Apply for a handicapped parking sticker.
- ○ 4. Purchase a pair of supportive shoes.

NURSING CARE OF CLIENTS WITH DEGENERATIVE DISORDERS

An older adult female with Parkinson's disease is placed in a nursing home for basic nursing care.

33 Which one of the following is *most important* to assess before developing the client's plan for care?
- ● 1. The client's ability to perform activities of daily living
- ○ 2. The client's preferences and dislikes of various foods
- ○ 3. The client's family members and her network of social support
- ○ 4. The client's feelings about giving up her independent living

The client with Parkinson's disease takes levodopa (Dopar) b.i.d.

34 When the nurse observes that the client has difficulty swallowing the capsule of medication, which action is best to take?
- ● 1. Soak the capsule in water until soft.
- ○ 2. Tell her to chew the capsule a while.
- ○ 3. Empty the capsule in the client's mouth.
- ○ 4. Offer water before giving her the capsule.

The physician prescribes a stool softener, a multivitamin, and a drug to counteract osteoporosis for the client who takes levodopa (Dopar).

35 Which of the following nursing actions is *best* when preparing to administer the prescribed medications?
- ● 1. Administer them all at the prescribed time.
- ○ 2. Question the order for the multivitamin.
- ○ 3. Withhold the stool softener until it is needed.
- ○ 4. Give the anti-osteoporitic drug with milk.

*The registered nurse adds the nursing diagnosis "**Risk for injury related to propulsive gait**" to the care plan of the client with Parkinson's disease.*

36 If all of the following interventions are possible, which one is *best*?
- ○ 1. Ambulate with assistance only.
- ○ 2. Restrain in geriatric chair.
- ● 3. Have client use a quad cane.
- ○ 4. Dress with supportive shoes.

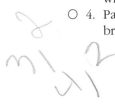

37 Since the client with Parkinson's disease is prone to constipation, it is best for the nurse to encourage her to eat
- ◉ 1. raw fruits.
- ○ 2. wheat pasta.
- ○ 3. cured meat.
- ○ 4. canned peas.

An older female client with dementia is admitted to the dedicated Alzheimer's unit in an extended-care facility.

38 When the client is observed to wander about the facility, which nursing intervention is *most appropriate* for the client's safety?
- ○ 1. Keep the client confined to her room.
- ○ 2. Attach an identity tag with a phone number.
- ◉ 3. Lock all the outside doors in the facility.
- ○ 4. Make sure she is dressed appropriately.

39 What approach is *best* when managing the care of a client with dementia who insists on carrying a purse with her at all times?
- ○ 1. Ask the client where her purse can be stored.
- ○ 2. Ensure that she has her purse with her.
- ○ 3. Inform the client that her purse may be lost.
- ◉ 4. Find out why the client feels the need for a purse.

40 To prevent frustrating and agitating the older client with dementia when she asks for her mother, it is *best* for the nurse to
- ○ 1. explain that her mother has been dead several years.
- ○ 2. tell her that her mother will visit a little later.
- ◉ 3. say, "You miss your mother. What was she like?"
- ○ 4. ask the client when she last saw her mother.

A 48-year-old female client experiences an exacerbation of multiple sclerosis from which she has been asymptomatic for the past 6 months.

41 Which one of the following is *best* for helping the client deal with her fears at this time?
- ◉ 1. Encourage the client to verbalize her feelings.
- ○ 2. Provide an accurate explanation of the disease.
- ○ 3. Tell her about her physical assessment findings.
- ○ 4. Explain the disease may become periodically acute.

42 When assisting the client with multiple sclerosis with her activities of daily living (ADL) which approach is *best*?
- ○ 1. Complete all ADL as quickly as possible.
- ○ 2. Eliminate whatever the client cannot perform.

- ◉ 3. Let the client rest between the activities.
- ○ 4. Perform all the client's ADL for her.

43 Which one of the following should the client with multiple sclerosis be warned to avoid?
- ○ 1. Hot weather
- ○ 2. Wet climates
- ○ 3. Dry environments
- ◉ 4. Cold temperatures

The physician prescribes interferon beta-1b (Betaseron) by the subcutaneous route for the client with multiple sclerosis.

44 When the nurse alternates the injections in the client's upper arms, it is *best* to choose a site that is no closer to a previous one than
- ○ 1. ¼ inch.
- ○ 2. ½ inch.
- ○ 3. 1 inch.
- ◉ 4. 2 inches.

45 When the client is taught to self-administer her own subcutaneous injections before discharge, the nurse is *most correct* in instructing her to rotate the injections in the
- ○ 1. thighs and hips.
- ○ 2. forearms and hips.
- ◉ 3. thighs and abdomen.
- ○ 4. abdomen and buttocks.

46 The *best* nursing action when the client who is receiving interferon develops anorexia and nausea is to
- ○ 1. withhold the medication.
- ○ 2. offer frequent mouth care.
- ○ 3. administer the drug after meals.
- ◉ 4. provide small, frequent meals.

During a physical assessment, the nurse notes that in addition to the client's weakness, the client with multiple sclerosis also has numbness in parts of her body.

47 Which measure for preventing impaired skin integrity is appropriate to add to the plan of care *at this time*?
- ○ 1. Use an air-fluidized (Clinitron™) bed.
- ◉ 2. Change positions every 2 hours.
- ○ 3. Rub reddened areas every 2 hours.
- ○ 4. Add alcohol to the bath water.

An older male develops myasthenia gravis.

48 When the nurse reviews the client's medical history, which sign or symptom is the client most likely to have experienced when his disease became manifested?
- ○ 1. Sudden hearing loss
- ○ 2. Sensitivity to light
- ◉ 3. Drooping eyelids
- ○ 4. Protruding tongue

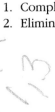

49 When the nurse cares for the client with myasthenia gravis, which one of the following assessments is *most appropriate* to make?
○ 1. The client's ability to breathe
◉ 2. The client's range of motion
○ 3. The client's level of appetite
○ 4. The client's quality of hygiene

50 When planning the care of a client with myasthenia gravis, which equipment item is *most important* to place at the bedside?
○ 1. A pole for administering intravenous fluid
○ 2. A cardiac defibrillator in case of cardiac arrest
◉ 3. A suction machine in case of compromised swallowing
○ 4. An electronic pump for administering tube feedings

The client with myasthenia gravis is treated with pyridostigmine bromide (Mestinon). The dosage will be adjusted according to the client's response.

51 If the nurse observes all of the following, which one is an indication that the dose of pyridostigmine is excessive for this client?
○ 1. The client cannot open his mouth.
○ 2. The client cannot make a fist.
○ 3. The client has urinary incontinence.
◉ 4. The client talks incoherently.

52 Which nursing action is *best* for controlling the symptoms of the client with myasthenia gravis?
○ 1. Ensure that the client has regular bowel and bladder elimination.
◉ 2. Administer each dose of medication at the precise scheduled time.
○ 3. Encourage a half-hour of active exercise twice each day.
○ 4. Provide nutritional supplements between each meal and at bedtime.

The care plan for the client with myasthenia gravis indicates that the client uses the Credé method to promote urination.

53 If the client performs the Credé method correctly, the nurse will observe him
○ 1. run tap water in the sink by the toilet.
○ 2. hold his hand in a bowl of cool water.
○ 3. pour warm water over his lower abdomen.
◉ 4. apply hand pressure over his bladder.

A 60-year-old client in the late stage of amyotrophic lateral sclerosis (Lou Gehrig's disease) is admitted to the hospital.

54 Based on the course of this disease, which one of the following nursing diagnoses is *most likely* included on the client's plan of care?

○ 1. Altered Growth and Development
◉ 2. Body Image Disturbance
○ 3. Impaired Adjustment
○ 4. Total Self-Care Deficit

55 When teaching the children of a client diagnosed with Huntington's chorea, which one of the following instructions is *most appropriate*?
◉ 1. Genetic testing is advisable before having children.
○ 2. It is wise to store sperm in a bank for the future.
○ 3. Have children before you reach the age of 30.
○ 4. You should consider adopting all your children.

NURSING CARE OF CLIENTS WITH CEREBROVASCULAR DISORDERS

56 When a nurse makes a home visit to evaluate a 79-year-old client, which symptom suggests that the client is having transient ischemic attacks (TIAs)?
◉ 1. The client reports having brief periods of unilateral weakness.
○ 2. The client reports having brief periods of mental depression.
○ 3. The client reports having brief periods of photosensitivity.
○ 4. The client reports having brief periods of stabbing head pain.

57 After the nurse gathers more data concerning the TIAs, which action is *most appropriate*?
○ 1. Explain the phenomenon in understandable language.
◉ 2. Refer the client for immediate medical evaluation.
○ 3. Recommend taking a baby aspirin once each day.
○ 4. Teach the client to avoid dietary sources of fat.

An older adult male is admitted after emergency medical personnel are called to examine a client who was found unconscious at home.

58 When the nurse checks the client's pupils, which technique is *correct*?
○ 1. The nurse asks the client to look at the light source.
○ 2. The nurse rotates occluding each of the client's eyes.
◉ 3. The nurse dims the lights in the examination area.
○ 4. The nurse observes for extraocular eye movement.

A computed tomography (CT) of the brain with contrast dye is ordered on the unconscious client.

59 If the client's wife reports that the client is allergic to all of the following, which one must be reported to the physician before the CT?
- ○ 1. Tomatoes
- ● 2. Shellfish
- ○ 3. Chocolate
- ○ 4. Strawberries

It is determined that the unconscious client has had a cerebral vascular accident (CVA).

60 As the nursing team develops a plan of care for the client with a CVA, which area of nursing management is *most important* to the client's rehabilitation?
- ○ 1. Regulating bowel and bladder elimination
- ● 2. Preventing contractures and joint deformities
- ○ 3. Dealing with problems of altered body image
- ○ 4. Facilitating positive outcomes from grieving

61 When the nurse monitors the neurological status of the client with the CVA, which finding is most suggestive that the client's intracranial pressure is increasing?
- ● 1. Systolic pressure increases and diastolic decreases.
- ○ 2. Systolic pressure decreases and diastolic increases.
- ○ 3. Apical heart rate is greater than the radial rate.
- ○ 4. Radial pulse rate is greater than the apical rate.

*The charge nurse enters the nursing diagnosis of "**Risk for Ineffective Airway Clearance related to decreased level of consciousness and inability to swallow**" on the nursing care plan of the client with a CVA.*

62 Which nursing intervention is most appropriate for managing the identified problem?
- ○ 1. Keeping the client supine
- ○ 2. Removing all head pillows
- ● 3. Performing oral suctioning
- ○ 4. Providing oral hygiene

The nurse instructs the wife of the client with a CVA on how to perform passive range-of-motion exercises.

63 When teaching the client's wife, which instruction is *most accurate*?
- ○ 1. Move the paralyzed limbs in as many directions as possible.
- ● 2. Move all extremities in as many directions as possible.
- ○ 3. Move the upper extremities in as many directions as possible.
- ○ 4. Move the lower extremities in as many directions as possible.

The nurse applies a footboard to the bed of the client with a CVA.

64 Which statement *best describes* how the nurse positions the feet when a footboard is used?
- ○ 1. The soles of the feet are perpendicular to the board.
- ● 2. The soles of the feet are parallel to the board.
- ○ 3. The ankles of each foot are flexed less than 90 degrees toward the head.
- ○ 4. The ankles of each foot are extended more than 90 degrees away from the head.

The nurse determines that the client with the CVA has expressive aphasia.

65 Which nursing intervention is *best* for communicating with this client?
- ○ 1. Stimulate the client aurally by turning on the television.
- ● 2. Have the client point to key phrases printed on a clipboard.
- ○ 3. Avoid talking to the client since conversation is impossible.
- ○ 4. Encourage the client to speak rather than using gestures.

The client with a CVA has hemianopia.

66 Which nursing order is most appropriate to add to the client's plan of care in relation to this post-CVA problem?
- ● 1. Apply dark glasses to the client in bright light.
- ○ 2. Cover the client's affected eye with a dark patch.
- ○ 3. Approach the client from his unaffected side.
- ○ 4. Have the client look from near to far to see clearly.

67 When the client with the CVA is stable enough to transfer from his bed to a wheelchair, which of the nurse's actions is *correct*?
- ○ 1. Instruct the client on how to balance with a walker.
- ○ 2. Position the wheelchair perpendicular to the bed.
- ○ 3. Stand behind the locked wheelchair.
- ● 4. Brace the paralyzed foot and knee.

A client with a leaking cerebral aneurysm is being treated conservatively with complete rest, anticonvulsants, and sedatives.

68 If the nurse observed all of the following when caring for the client with a cerebral aneurysm, for which one is it *most important* to intervene?
○ 1. The client has a chronic cough.
○ 2. The client is becoming bored.
○ 3. The client has a diminished appetite.
○ 4. The client wants to talk with his wife.

The client with the cerebral aneurysm tells the nurse that the nonnarcotic analgesic he received 2 hours ago has not adequately relieved his headache.

69 Which nursing action is *most appropriate* in response to the client's statement?
○ 1. Administer another dose of the nonnarcotic analgesic immediately.
○ 2. Explain that frequent analgesia administration will mask symptoms.
○ 3. Consult the physician about ordering a narcotic analgesic.
○ 4. Utilize a non-drug intervention such as listening to a guided imagery tape.

NURSING CARE OF CLIENTS WITH TUMORS OF THE NEUROLOGIC SYSTEM

A client with symptoms that suggest a brain tumor is scheduled for positron emission tomography (PET).

70 When the nurse provides test preparation instructions, which substance is it important for the client to avoid the day before the test?
○ 1. Caffeine
○ 2. Food dyes
○ 3. Diuretics
○ 4. Antibiotics

71 Before the client is discharged after the PET is completed, which instruction is *most appropriate*?
○ 1. Take a mild laxative tonight.
○ 2. Increase your fluid intake.
○ 3. Get at least 8 hours of sleep.
○ 4. Report any abdominal discomfort.

The PET confirms a brain tumor and the client is scheduled for a craniotomy.

72 Which preoperative assessment is *most important* to document as a basis for postoperative comparison?
○ 1. The client's motor strength in all extremities
○ 2. The client's anterior and posterior skin integrity

○ 3. The client's knowledge of potential surgical risks
○ 4. The client's appetite and choice of food preferences

73 When the nurse inserts a retention catheter in the male client undergoing a craniotomy, the nurse is correct in inserting the catheter to a depth of
○ 1. 2 to 4 inches.
○ 2. 4 to 6 inches.
○ 3. 6 to 8 inches.
○ 4. 8 to 10 inches.

74 The skin preparation which will include shaving the hair from the client's head is *best* implemented
○ 1. the night before surgery.
○ 2. after the morning shower.
○ 3. before preoperative sedation.
○ 4. in the operating room area.

75 After the hair has been shaved from the head of the client undergoing a craniotomy, it is best for the nurse to
○ 1. dispose of it in a biologic waste container.
○ 2. place it in a plastic-lined waste basket.
○ 3. put it in a paper bag and give it to the family.
○ 4. flush the hair away in a large waste hopper.

The client who underwent a craniotomy returns to the nursing unit after 6 hours of surgery.

76 During the immediate postoperative assessment, when the nurse notes that the client's dressing is moist, which action is *most appropriate* to take *first*?
○ 1. The nurse changes the dressing.
○ 2. The nurse reinforces the dressing.
○ 3. The nurse removes the dressing.
○ 4. The nurse documents the findings.

Following the craniotomy, the client has periods of confusion.

77 Which nursing intervention is best during the client's periods of confusion?
○ 1. Read a newspaper or magazine to the client.
○ 2. Inform the client that confusion is temporary.
○ 3. Withhold verbal communication temporarily.
○ 4. Reorient the client to place and situation.

78 Before requesting the clear liquid diet prescribed by the physician, which assessment is essential?
○ 1. The condition of the oral mucous membranes
○ 2. The ability of the client to feed himself
○ 3. The status of the client's dental hygiene
○ 4. The client's ability to swallow effectively

The physician restricts the client's oral fluid intake to no more than 1000 mL.

79 When the client asks why he cannot drink fluids freely, the *best explanation* is that
○ 1. oral fluid may contribute to vomiting.
○ 2. the kidneys need to conserve fluid output.
◉ 3. it reduces the fluid volume in the cranium.
○ 4. the prescribed volume is sufficient for relieving thirst.

NURSING CARE OF CLIENTS WITH NERVE DISORDERS

A client is diagnosed with trigeminal neuralgia (tic douloureux).

80 Based on factors that cause the client to experience paroxysmal pain, which nursing order is *most appropriate* on this client's plan for care?
○ 1. Direct a fan toward the client's face.
◉ 2. Avoid care that involves touching the face.
○ 3. Keep ice chips available at the bedside.
○ 4. Apply warm facial compresses for pain.

The physician treats the client with trigeminal neuralgia with carbamzepine (Tegretol).

81 Since this drug can cause liver dysfunction, it is appropriate in the discharge teaching to tell this client to report
○ 1. unusual bleeding.
○ 2. black stools.
○ 3. pale urine.
◉ 4. mottled skin.

Drug therapy is unsuccessful for the client with trigeminal neuralgia. The physician severs one of the branches of the trigeminal nerve and orders eye irrigations postoperatively.

82 If the eye irrigation is performed correctly, the nurse directs the flow of solution from the
○ 1. lower conjunctiva toward the corneal surface.
◉ 2. outer canthus of the eye to the inner canthus.
○ 3. nasal corner of the eye toward the temple.
○ 4. margin of the eyelashes to the folds of the lids.

A female client develops Bell's palsy due to inflammation around the seventh cranial nerve.

83 When the nurse performs a physical assessment, which finding is *most closely associated* with this client's disorder?

○ 1. Quivering movement of the eyes
○ 2. Muscle spasms about the lips
○ 3. Sudden loss of olfactory function
◉ 4. Unilateral facial paralysis

84 Which one of the following is the *most appropriate* addition to the care plan for the client with Bell's palsy?
○ 1. Reduce the amount of light within the room.
○ 2. Advise the client to drink liquids from a cup.
◉ 3. Inspect the buccal pouch for food after eating.
○ 4. Discourage the client from looking in a mirror.

A home health nurse evaluates a client's response to treatment for postherpetic neuralgia following an outbreak of shingles (herpes zoster).

85 When the client asks the nurse about the source of her condition, the *most accurate* explanation is that the symptoms result from a reactivation of the infectious agent that causes
○ 1. rubella.
○ 2. rubeola.
◉ 3. chickenpox.
○ 4. influenza.

A client experiences recurrent pain along the sciatic nerve. The client is scheduled for a myelogram.

86 When the nurse describes the myelogram procedure to the client, which statement is *most accurate*?
◉ 1. Part of the test involves a lumbar puncture.
○ 2. You will be asked to change positions frequently.
○ 3. Dye will be instilled into a vein in your arm.
○ 4. Light anesthesia is administered during the test.

The myelogram shows that the client with sciatic pain has a herniated intervertebral lumbar disk.

87 Which one of the following instructions is *best* when the client obtains relief from his symptoms?
○ 1. Carry heavy objects away from your center of gravity.
◉ 2. Lift with your knees bent and your back straight.
○ 3. Create a base of support by keeping the feet together.
○ 4. Select a soft, spongy mattress for your bed.

The client with the herniated lumbar disk eventually has spinal surgery.

88 When changing the client's position postoperatively it is *best* to
○ 1. raise the client with a mechanical lift.
◉ 2. log-roll the client from side to side.
○ 3. have the client flex his legs and lift.
○ 4. pull the client's arms and then his legs.

The client who has had spinal surgery is fitted with a thoracolumbar sacro-orthotic (TCSO) brace.

89 The *best evidence* that the client understands how to prevent skin breakdown while wearing the TLSO brace is the statement,
○ 1. "I need to dust my skin with talc every morning."
○ 2. "I should apply a lubricant to the brace hinges."
◉ 3. "I need to wear a cotton shirt under my brace."
○ 4. "I should rub my skin with alcohol every night."

Correct Answers and Rationale

Directions: Two numbers appear in parentheses following each rationale. The first number identifies the textbook listed in the references, page 512, and the second number identifies the page(s) in that textbook on which the correct answer can be verified. Occasionally two or more textbooks are given for verifying the correct answer.

NURSING CARE OF CLIENTS WITH INFECTIOUS AND INFLAMMATORY CONDITIONS

1 2. Neck stiffness, also called nuchal rigidity, is a common symptom among those who contract meningitis. Another symptom is photosensitivity, but not double vision. Meningeal irritation may be accompanied by a severe headache, but not joint aches. Thirst may be a consequence of a high fever and dehydration, but it is not a common complaint. (21:524)
  Nursing Process—Data collection
  Client Need—Physiological integrity

2 3. A lumbar puncture is usually performed with the client in a side-lying position with the neck and knees acutely flexed. It is anatomically difficult for the physician to perform this test with the client in a knee-chest, othopneic, or left lateral position. (4:1105; 25:213)
  Nursing Process—Implementation
  Client Need—Safe, effective care environment

3 4. To prevent complications and allow time for more cerebrospinal fluid to form, clients are kept flat in bed for several hours. Increasing fluids helps reform cerebrospinal fluid at a faster rate. A supine position is preferred so as to apply pressure on the puncture site. Ambulating the client is unsafe; it can lead to a severe headache or neurological complications. (4:1105; 25:214)
  Nursing Process—Implementation
  Client Need—Physiological integrity

4 1. There are only three categories of transmission-based precautions. They include airborne, droplet, and contact precautions. Since most forms of meningitis are spread from the droplets of infected persons, airborne and contact precautions are inappropriate. Standard precautions are followed when caring for *all* clients regardless of their infectious status. (4:1133; 25:451–453)
  Nursing Process—Planning
  Client Need—Safe, effective care environment

5 2. To protect the client's skin, there should be a layer of light cloth between the client and the aquathermia pad. The pad is placed beneath the client. Distilled water is used to fill the fluid chamber. Ice is not used; the distilled water is chilled electronically. (4:531; 25:483–484)
  Nursing Process—Implementation
  Client Need—Safe, effective care environment

6 1. Photophobia is relieved and the potential for seizures reduced by keeping the room dark and quiet. It also is appropriate to keep the room cool and well-ventilated, but these conditions help to restore and maintain normal body temperature. A warm environment is least appropriate for clients with meningitis. (4:1133; 26:617)
  Nursing Process—Implementation
  Client Need—Physiological integrity

7 3. The best sign of improvement is when a previously unresponsive client now responds when hearing his or her name called. When checking the pupils, a normal finding is that they constrict when stimulated with light. A swallowing reflex is just that—a reflex. It is not a measure of cognitive improvement. (18:589–590; 21:513)
  Nursing Process—Evaluation
  Client Need—Physiological integrity

8 1. The exact cause of Guillain-Barré is unknown, but there seems to be a relationship to prior exposure to infectious agents via an actual infection or their attenuated form in an immunization. This condition is not associated with spider bites, unpasteurized milk, or insecticides. (4:1132; 21:525)
  Nursing Process—Data collection
  Client Need—Health promotion/maintenance

9 4. Pulse oximetry readings which can be monitored continuously is the most accurate technique for monitoring if a client is breathing effectively. The pulse rate increases with hypoxemia, but tachycardia can be due to other causes such as anxiety. Cyanosis is not an early sign of hypoxemia. The red cell count may increase in response to hypoxemia, but this occurs more in chronic conditions than in acute situations. (4:884; 25:402–404)
> Nursing Process—Planning
> Client Need—Physiological integrity

10 2. Tube feedings utilize the normal route for digestion, absorption, and elimination of nutrients. Nasogastric tube feedings are less invasive than creating a gastrostomy. Crystalloid intravenous fluid does not supply all the nutrients that a person needs to maintain a healthy state. Total parenteral nutrition requires a more invasive technique for administration than nasogastric tube feedings. (6:600, 603)
> Nursing Process—Planning
> Client Need—Physiological integrity

11 2. Although oral polio vaccination is the preferred method for immunizing infants against poliomyelitis, there have been rare cases when children immunized in this way have actually developed vaccine-related paralysis. The theory is that the live virus in the oral vaccine is capable of causing the disease. Killed virus is unable to cause the disease. If immunizations are followed, OPV is given at 2, 4, 6 months of age. A booster is given before entry to school. Although OPV is usually given at the same time as diphtheria, pertussis, and tetanus immunizations, there is nothing in the literature to suggest that if it is given with rubella vaccine that the disease can develop. (22:451)
> Nursing Process—Data collection
> Client Need—Health promotion/maintenance

12 3. The best technique to clear up the client's confusion is to reorient him to person, place, and circumstances. Reorientation may have to be repeated frequently. Encouraging the family to turn the television on, play the client's favorite music, and touch the client are techniques for providing sensory stimulation. (4:1133)
> Nursing Process—Implementation
> Client Need—Health promotion/maintenance

NURSING CARE OF CLIENTS WITH CONVULSIVE DISORDERS

13 3. To ensure that the electrodes remain attached to the skull, the hair should be clean and dry. Fasting is not required, although beverages containing caffeine are restricted 8 hours before an EEG. The blood pressure is assessed before the test but it is not necessary to have the client lie down and then sit during the assessment. Drugs that affect brain activity, like sedatives, are not usually administered because they can affect the outcome of the test. (7:932–933)
> Nursing Process—Implementation
> Client Need—Safe effective care environment

14 4. With a client with known or suspected seizure disorder, the side rails are padded with bath blankets to prevent injury. Keeping the room brightly lit can be disturbing to the client and is not necessary. In some, seizures are precipitated by bright lights and noise. Although a client may be injured by glass or metal utensils on a tray, they are not usually restricted. The client is observed more closely by the nurse if near the nursing station, but room arrangements like this are not always available. (21:542; 26:572)
> Nursing Process—Implementation
> Client Need—Safe, effective care environment

15 4. When a client begins to convulse, the highest priority is establishing a patent airway. This can most easily be done by turning this client on her side, allowing saliva and vomitus (if present) to drain from the mouth. Turning also prevents the tongue from blocking the airway. Oxygen is administered after the airway is open and clear. Vital signs are taken after the seizure is completed. A client is *never* restrained while having a seizure since this could cause musculoskeletal injuries. (21:542; 26:572)
> Nursing Process—Implementation
> Client Need—Physiological integrity

16 2. Although the time the seizure started is important information to document, it is not as valuable to the diagnostic process as identifying the duration of the seizure. The client's mood prior to the seizure and comments afterward may be diagnostic, but they are not higher priorities than documenting the duration of the seizure. (26:571–572)
> Nursing Process—Implementation
> Client Need—Physiological integrity

17 2. If sued, it is important to prove that safety standards were being followed. The best evidence is noting that the signal cord was within the client's reach. This information may relieve the nurse from liability. It is important to document the vital signs when the client was found. The time the client was last

observed is more pertinent legally than what the client was doing when observed. (25:31–33)
> Nursing Process—Implementation
> Client Need—**Safe, effective care environment**

18 1. All of the drugs listed are used as anticonvulsants to treat a variety of seizure disorders. However, the drug of choice for treating *status epilepticus* is diazepam (Valium) by the intravenous route. (17:361)
> Nursing Process—Planning
> Client Need—**Physiological integrity**

19 3. Phenytoin causes gingival hyperplasia. Therefore brushing the teeth becomes especially important for preventing oral infections. (4:1118; 17:369)
> Nursing Process—Implementation
> Client Need—**Health promotion/maintenance**

NURSING CARE OF CLIENTS WITH NEUROLOGIC TRAUMA

20 4. All of the assessment findings identified in the options are possible with a head injury, but the most serious of them all is seeing serous drainage from the ears. Serous drainage from the ears or nose suggests that the meninges have been lacerated and the drainage is cerebrospinal fluid. (4:1136; 21:569)
> Nursing Process—Data collection
> Client Need—**Physiological integrity**

21 1. As long as the accident victim is breathing and alert, it is best to keep the head and neck from moving. Movement may further damage the neck and spinal cord. Ambulating or moving the accident victim before he or she is immobilized in a neck brace is potentially unsafe. Covering the accident victim with a light blanket is appropriate if the environmental temperature is cold or the client is manifesting signs of shock. Water is generally withheld until the need for surgery is overruled. (21:576)
> Nursing Process—Planning
> Client Need—**Physiological integrity**

22 2. According to most Good Samaritan laws, after stopping to provide aid, nurses have an obligation to remain with the victim until someone else with comparable knowledge and skills arrives. The other options describe actions that are legal, but not ethical. (4:1550)
> Nursing Process—Implementation
> Client Need—**Safe, effective care environment**

23 2. Keeping the head elevated 30 to 45 degrees aids in promoting venous return, which helps to reduce intracranial pressure. None of the other described positions results in elevation of the accident victim's head. (4:1112)
> Nursing Process—Implementation
> Client Need—**Physiological integrity**

24 4. Changes in pupil response indicate increasing intracranial pressure. The other assessments are appropriate when caring for any client, but they do not provide information as to the client's neurologic status. (21:569)
> Nursing Process—Data collection
> Client Need—**Physiological integrity**

25 3. A change in the client's level of consciousness is an indication that intracranial pressure is increasing. The information in the other options is important to document, but they are not significant enough to notify the physician. (18:1043)
> Nursing Process—Data collection
> Client Need—**Physiological integrity**

26 3. Flexing the neck interferes with venous outflow from the brain. Venous congestion raises intracranial pressure. Fluids are generally restricted for a client with a head injury to reduce the potential for raising intracranial pressure. Being frequently disturbed interferes with the client's sleep pattern, but that is not as significant a consequence as identifying the relationship between neck flexion and increased intracranial pressure. A full bladder causes autonomic dysreflexia in a client with a spinal cord injury. (4:1112, 1136)
> Nursing Process—Data collection
> Client Need—**Physiological integrity**

27 1. Mannitol is a potent osmotic diuretic. Monitoring urinary output is one of the data that indicates the client's response to drug therapy. Side effects associated with mannitol therapy include dehydration, electrolyte loss, vomiting, and diarrhea. (4:1112; 17:489)
> Nursing Process—Data collection
> Client Need—**Physiological integrity**

28 3. The client with a complete transection of the spinal cord at the T5 level will be a permanent paraplegic. At the present time, there has been little success in restoring neuromuscular functions that have been lost in spinal injuries. (4:1137)
> Nursing Process—Evaluation
> Client Need—**Health promotion/maintenance**

29 2. All of the goals are appropriate, but the one that has the highest priority is maintaining as much upper body function as possible. Upper body strength is the key to the client's ability to maintain mobility and self-care. (21:578)

> Nursing Process—Planning
> Client Need—Physiological integrity

30 4. Autonomic dysreflexia is often triggered by a full bladder or fecal impaction. Therefore, of the four options, checking the client's catheter for patency is the most appropriate action to take. Autonomic dysreflexia can have life-threatening consequences if unrelieved. An alert client is not likely to tolerate an oral airway. Relieving the client's anxiety is appropriate, but it is not the most appropriate action to take first. Compressing the client's abdomen will not relieve the symptoms of autonomic dysreflexia. (4:1137; 21:578)

> Nursing Process—Implementation
> Client Need—Physiological integrity

31 2. Adding bulk to the stool promotes regular stool elimination. Fiber makes a moister stool, which reduces or prevents fecal impaction. The presence of a fecal impaction also may cause autonomic dysreflexia. Some paraplegics perform manual disimpaction on a regular basis to promote bowel elimination. Daily enemas are excessive; but if an enema is necessary, it is more effective if administered after a meal when the gastrocolic reflex is more active. Changing disposable undergarments and padding the bed pan promote skin integrity, but these measures will not help manage bowel elimination. (18:1032; 21:591)

> Nursing Process—Planning
> Client Need—Physiological integrity

32 2. A wheelchair ramp allows the client to get in and out of the house. A hospital bed assists with positioning the client. A handicapped parking sticker ensures that the client would not have to travel long distances to get in and out of public facilities, but it does not ultimately promote mobility. Supportive shoes help to prevent contractures, but the client will most likely never use his or her legs for ambulating again. (26:595)

> Nursing Process—Implementation
> Client Need—Health promotion/maintenance

NURSING CARE OF CLIENTS WITH DEGENERATIVE DISORDERS

33 1. Assessing the client's ability to carry out various ADL facilitates planning those interventions for which the client requires assistance. All of the other data are important to the care of the client, but physiological needs have a higher priority. (17:355; 21:537)

> Nursing Process—Data collection
> Client Need—Physiological integrity

34 4. Offering a few sips of water before placing the capsule in her mouth moistens the oral cavity and helps in swallowing an oral medication. Capsules are never softened by placing them in water before administration or by having the client hold the capsule in the mouth. An opened capsule at the least is unpleasant to taste. At the worst, an opened capsule may be absorbed at an undesirable rate. (20:14)

> Nursing Process—Implementation
> Client Need—Physiological integrity

35 2. Pyridoxine (vitamin B$_6$), which is present in most multivitamins, reduces the effectiveness of levodopa. Therefore it is best to hold the multivitamin while checking the drug order with the physician. Stool softeners are generally given on a routine basis to facilitate the ease of passing feces. The antiosteoporitic drug can be given with milk, or not. (17:350; 26:603)

> Nursing Process—Implementation
> Client Need—Physiological integrity

36 3. The best approach is to promote the client's independence and opportunity for active exercise for as long as possible. An ambulation aid, such as a quad cane, meets both objectives. If the client is only allowed to ambulate with assistance, mobility may be limited by the number of staff. It is even better to provide gait training concurrently. Applying restraints to this client violates the tenets of the Omnibus Budget Reconciliation Act (OBRA). Using supportive shoes is a good nursing measure, but by itself it is not the best intervention. (26:603; 21:536)

> Nursing Process—Planning
> Client Need—Physiological integrity

37 1. Raw fruits and vegetables are good sources of fiber, which increases the bulk and water content of the stool. Almost all pasta is made from some type of refined wheat flour. Whole grains are a better source of fiber. Cured meat, like frankfurters and ham, contain fiber and a great deal of sodium. The serving size of meat is likely to be smaller in volume and less healthy than a piece of raw fruit. The fiber in vegetables and fruit is softened by cooking. Consequently, the cooking process reduces the undigestible bulk. (6:574)

> Nursing Process—Implementation
> Client Need—Physiological integrity

38 2. It is best to make sure the client can be identified and returned to the care-providing agency. The Alzheimer's Association distributes identification tags and keeps a registry of client names as well. Confining the client to her room is inappropriate. Locking the outside doors is a safety hazard. It is better to install doors that sound an alarm when opened. Keeping the client dressed appropriately preserves the client's dignity, but does not ensure safety. (27:760; 18:1356)
   Nursing Process—Implementation
   Client Need—Safe, effective care environment

39 2. The purse may be a symbol of security for the client. Therefore, it is best to accommodate the client's idiosyncrasy. Trying to alter the client's behavior may increase her confusion and lead to aggressive behavior. The client may not have the cognitive ability to offer a reason, choose a storage place, or understand the concept of loss. (1:329–330)
   Nursing Process—Implementation
   Client Need—Psychosocial integrity

40 3. Clients with dementia can sometimes be distracted from their original thoughts. Reminding the client that her mother is dead may distress the client. Lying to the client is not ethical. The client whose memory is impaired may become frustrated when asked to identify when she last saw her mother. (1:329)
   Nursing Process—Implementation
   Client Need—Psychosocial integrity

41 1. Fears can be less irrational if and when they are shared with someone else. Giving accurate information, identifying assessment findings, and validating that her health experience is common are appropriate nursing measures once the client verbalizes her fears. (23:234–235; 26:605)
   Nursing Process—Implementation
   Client Need—Psychosocial integrity

42 3. Providing periods of rest between activities can accommodate for the client's symptoms of fatigue and weakness. Using this type of schedule may facilitate more self-care and elevate her self-esteem. All clients are entitled to have their basic needs met; if not by themselves, then staff must carry out that responsibility. The client may tire and become more fatigued by being hurried. Doing tasks that the client is capable of performing is demeaning. (4:1120, 1530; 26:604)
   Nursing Process—Planning
   Client Need—Physiological integrity

43 1. Hot weather, even hot baths, increase the weakness that is common among clients with multiple sclerosis. They are not as adversely affected by rainy, dry, or cold environments. (4:1120; 26:606)
   Nursing Process—Implementation
   Client Need—Health promotion/maintenance

44 3. Subcutaneous injections are placed no closer than 1 inch in all directions from another recent injection. (18:734)
   Nursing Process—Implementation
   Client Need—Physiological integrity

45 3. The thighs and abdomen are sites that are used for administering subcutaneous injections. These sites are more accessible for self-administration than the arms. (18:734; 25:736)
   Nursing Process—Implementation
   Client Need—Health promotion/maintenance

46 4. Interferon beta-1b is essential for reducing the frequency of exacerbations of multiple sclerosis. Therefore, withholding the drug because of anorexia and nausea is not an option. Mouth care improves the client's appetite, but it is not a technique that will relieve nausea. Administering the drug after meals will not improve the client's appetite, nor will it relieve nausea. Therefore, the best approach is to meet the client's nutritional needs by providing small, frequent meals. (28:595)
   Nursing Process—Planning
   Client Need—Physiological integrity

47 2. Changing the client's position every two hours is sufficient in most circumstances to maintain the skin that is currently intact. An air-fluidized bed is appropriate when a client is totally immobile or already has stage 3 or 4 pressure sores. It is inappropriate to rub reddened skin areas since this further damages the skin. (25:568, 473–474)
   Nursing Process—Planning
   Client Need—Physiological integrity

48 3. Ptosis, which is drooping of the eyelids, is one of the more common signs of myasthenia gravis. Generalized weakness is also evidenced by difficulty swallowing and inarticulate speech. Hearing is unaffected, as is the pupillary reflex. The client may have some problems moving his tongue during speech, but it does not generally protrude. (4:1156; 21:529)
   Nursing Process—Data collection
   Client Need—Physiological integrity

49 1. Clients with myasthenia gravis are prone to upper body muscular weakness which can compromise the ability to breathe. Since ventilation is critical to life, this assessment is most appropriate and important for the nurse to make. The others are components of any client's assessment. (4:1156; 21:529; 26:607)

> Nursing Process—Data collection
> Client Need—Physiological integrity

50 3. An oral suction machine is best kept at the bedside of a client with myasthenia gravis. Suctioning may be needed quickly if the client cannot clear his or her own airway. A tube feeding pump may be needed eventually, but its acquisition could be delayed temporarily. An intravenous pole is easily acquired when and if it is needed. A cardiac defibrillator should remain centrally located near the nursing station when not in use. (18:1038)

> Nursing Process—Planning
> Client Need—Physiological integrity

51 1. Signs of pyridostigmine overdose include clenched jaws, abdominal cramps, and muscle rigidity. An inability to make a fist is a sign that the dose is insufficient. Neither urinary incontinence nor talking incoherently are drug-related. (21:529)

> Nursing Process—Data collection
> Client Need—Physiological integrity

52 2. Administering medications for myasthenia gravis at precise times prevents the worsening of symptoms as the medication wears off. Getting adequate nourishment is a healthy behavior, but dietary measures do not affect the symptoms of myasthenia gravis. Exercise may actually precipitate muscular weakness. Ensuring elimination is an appropriate nursing measure for managing the consequences of myasthenia gravis, but not for controlling the muscular weakness that causes elimination problems. (18:1038)

> Nursing Process—Implementation
> Client Need—Physiological integrity

53 4. The Credé method is performed by leaning forward from the waist and pressing over the bladder area. The other options describe methods for promoting urination, but none describe the Credé method. (25:640, 642)

> Nursing Process—Evaluation
> Client Need—Health promotion/maintenance

54 4. As amyotrophic lateral sclerosis progresses, clients generally become totally dependent on family or health-care workers for all of their basic needs. Death usually is a consequence of respiratory failure or pneumonia. (21:530)

> Nursing Process—Planning
> Client Need—Physiological integrity

55 1. Huntington's chorea is a fatal hereditary disease that manifests around the age of 30. Genetic testing can identify which of the client's children eventually will develop the disease and pass it on to their children. Those who have inherited the gene can take measures to prevent conception of infants who also may be affected. (18:1038)

> Nursing Process—Implementation
> Client Need—Health promotion/maintenance

NURSING CARE OF CLIENTS WITH CEREBROVASCULAR DISORDERS

56 1. Besides weakness, clients who are experiencing TIAs may describe feeling dizzy, having speech disturbances, visual loss or double vision, Depression is common among older adults, but it is not unique to a TIA. There are visual changes during a TIA, but photosensitivity is not one of them. Stabbing head pain is more characteristic of a cerebral hemorrhage. (18:1122; 21:552)

> Nursing Process—Data collection
> Client Need—Physiological integrity

57 2. One or more TIAs warn that a stroke may occur in the very near future; it therefore is unwise to ignore the symptoms. Although providing an explanation is appropriate, it does not have greater priority than an immediate referral. A baby aspirin taken daily is a measure that may prevent vascular thrombosis, but evaluating and treating the etiology of the symptoms supersedes techniques for prevention at this time. A low-fat diet is a healthy lifestyle, but the atherosclerosis that has been progressing for a long time is not likely to be eliminated with this measure alone. (18:1122)

> Nursing Process—Implementation
> Client Need—Physiological integrity

58 3. To obtain valid assessment data, the light in the client's environment is dimmed. The client is instructed to stare into the distance, not directly at the light. Both eyes are open and the response of each eye is observed separately before the opposite eye is directly stimulated. The nurse is primarily observing whether the stimulated pupil constricts. (25:179)

> Nursing Process—Implementation
> Client Need—Physiological integrity

59 2. An allergy to shellfish indicates a sensitivity to iodine, which is a component in many contrast dyes. To avoid a reaction, an allergy to shellfish must be reported. None of the other allergic substances affects the CT procedure. (25:206)

> Nursing Process—Implementation
> Client Need—Safe, effective care environment

60 2. The long-term outcomes following a stroke are often determined by aggressive nursing efforts to maintain musculoskeletal function. Rehabilitation begins on admission with functional positioning, active and passive exercise, and early physical and occupational therapy. Managing bowel and bladder elimination does not have the same impact as preventing the development of musculoskeletal deformities. Helping the client cope with altered body image and grieving are appropriate nursing responsibilities. But even if they are positively resolved, the client's rehabilitation is delayed if he or she develops contractures and immobile joints. (21:554)
   Nursing Process—Planning
   Client Need—Physiological integrity

61 1. A widened pulse pressure is an ominous sign that accompanies increased intracranial pressure. Pulse pressure is the difference between systolic and diastolic blood pressure. A pulse pressure between 30 to 50 mm Hg is considered normal. A widened pulse pressure is one that exceeds 50 mm Hg. If a trend is developing, however, it is reported early rather than waiting until the pulse pressure equals or exceeds 50 mm Hg. (25:155)
   Nursing Process—Data collection
   Client Need—Physiological integrity

62 3. Clients who are unable to clear their own airways are suctioned. An unconscious client also is positioned on his or her side rather than supine. Removing pillows is inconsequential to maintaining a clear airway. Oral hygiene is an appropriate nursing measure for meeting the client's basic needs, but it does not clear the client's airway. (21:555)
   Nursing Process—Planning
   Client Need—Physiological integrity

63 2. Passive range-of-motion exercises are performed on all joints the client does not move actively. For an unconscious client, this principle applies to all extremities. (25:495)
   Nursing Process—Implementation
   Client Need—Health promotion/maintenance

64 2. To ensure the maximum potential use of the feet, they are maintained in a functional position. A functional position correlates with a person's position when standing. When standing, the soles of the feet are flat against the supporting surface. Therefore, the soles of the feet are parallel to the footboard when the client is in bed. The ankles are neither flexed less than 90 degrees, nor extended more than 90 degrees. (25:471; 26:579–580)
   Nursing Process—Implementation
   Client Need—Physiological integrity

65 2. Expressive aphasia means the client can understand what is said, but cannot respond using spoken language. An appropriate alternative is to utilize some nonverbal method by which the client can communicate. Using a written or printed list of key words can be substituted. The television is used for diversion, but its use is not therapeutic in restoring speech. Encouraging speech is likely to cause frustration since the loss of language is not from a lack of effort or practice. Despite the client's inability to respond verbally, it is still appropriate for the nurse to speak to the client. (18:1107; 21:556)
   Nursing Process—Implementation
   Client Need—Psychosocial integrity

66 3. Hemianopia is a visual problem in which the client loses the nasal half of the visual field in the eye on the unaffected side, and the temporal half of the field of vision on the paralyzed side of the body. Therefore, to accommodate the client's residual peripheral vision, it is best to approach the client from his or her unaffected side. The actions in the other options have no therapeutic value when caring for a client with hemianopia. (18:1129; 21:554)
   Nursing Process—Planning
   Client Need—Safe, effective care environment

67 4. A client with hemiplegia is best assisted from bed to a wheelchair by bracing the disabled foot and knee. The client with hemiplegia is unable to use a walker unless there is some residual strength in the paralyzed arm. The wheelchair is placed parallel to the bed. The nurse stands in front of the client to facilitate bracing and balancing the client. (18:484; 25:484)
   Nursing Process—Implementation
   Client Need—Physiological integrity

68 1. Coughing increases intracranial pressure and increases the potential for cerebral bleeding. The other identified problems require nursing management, but reducing or eliminating coughing has the highest priority for intervention. (21:559)
   Nursing Process—Planning
   Client Need—Physiological integrity

69 4. Non-drug interventions, when used in combination with analgesics, increase the therapeutic effect. Most oral analgesics are scheduled for administration at 3- or 4-hour intervals. In most neurological conditions, narcotics are avoided because they may alter pupil response, level of consciousness, or breathing. Mild analgesics can be safely used when treating pain experienced by neurological clients. (21:169)
   Nursing Process—Implementation
   Client Need—Physiological integrity

NURSING CARE OF CLIENTS WITH TUMORS OF THE NEUROLOGIC SYSTEM

70 1. Before a PET, clients are informed to eliminate caffeine, alcohol, tobacco, tranquilizers, and sedatives for 24 hours prior to the test. The results of the PET are not affected by sugar, diuretics, or antibiotics. (4:314; 7:636)

Nursing Process—Implementation
Client Need—Safe, effective care environment

71 2. Consuming extra fluids helps excrete the radioisotope used during the examination. There is no specific reason to recommend taking a laxative, getting sleep, or reporting abdominal discomfort. (4:314; 7:736)

Nursing Process—Implementation
Client Need—Physiological integrity

72 1. The client's postoperative neurological status is monitored frequently. One of the pertinent assessments is the client's ability to move each extremity and his or her motor strength in each. Changes in either are indications that the intracranial pressure is increasing. The other assessment data are appropriate to document, but they are not as significant to the client's safety as assessing the client's motor strength. (18:1019; 21:572)

Nursing Process—Data collection
Client Need—Physiological integrity

73 3. When catheterizing an adult male, the catheter is usually inserted a distance of 6 to 8 inches or until urine begins to flow. A catheter that is inserted less than 6 inches or inflated before urine flows might not be located in the bladder. Urethral damage may occur if the tip of the catheter and the bulb are not totally within the bladder. (25:656)

Nursing Process—Implementation
Client Need—Physiological integrity

74 4. To preserve the client's dignity and to reduce the potential for infection, the hair usually is shaved after the client has been transferred from the nursing unit to the surgical department. Shaving the night before facilitates colonization of microorganisms within the skin abrasions. If the skin preparation is done on the nursing unit, it is better to do so before administering sedation and to shave the head after a shower so loose hair can be rinsed away. (4:1134; 18:1020)

Nursing Process—Implementation
Client Need—Safe, effective care environment

75 3. The client's hair is bagged in a paper bag and offered to the client's family. They may wish to retain it for sentimental reasons or have it used for constructing a wig. If the family is not interested in keeping the hair, the information is documented. The hair is then disposed according to the agency's policies. (4:1020; 18:1134)

Nursing Process—Implementation
Client Need—Safe, effective care environment

76 2. To reduce the potential for a wound infection, it is best to reinforce a moist dressing. Usually the surgeon performs the first dressing change unless otherwise specified in the medical orders. The condition of the dressing and the action taken are important information to document. It is inappropriate to remove or change the dressing. (21:574)

Nursing Process—Implementation
Client Need—Physiological integrity

77 4. Reorientation is appropriate during periods of confusion. It may be necessary to repeat information several times. Providing an explanation and withholding communication are not nursing actions that are useful in the management of a confused client. Reading to a client may help to raise the client's consciousness. (4:1135; 18:1020)

Nursing Process—Implementation
Client Need—Psychosocial integrity

78 4. Before the client receives oral fluids, it is essential for the nurse to assess the client's ability to swallow. Clients undergoing neurological surgery may have residual muscular weakness, which creates the potential for aspiration. The other assessments are appropriate, but they are not as important to consuming liquids as the ability to swallow. (21:574)

Nursing Process—Data collection
Client Need—Physiological integrity

79 3. Limiting fluids controls the potential for developing cerebral edema. Limiting fluids also reduces the potential for vomiting, but controlling intracranial pressure is more important. The kidneys automatically adjust the volume of urine excreted according to the fluid status of the client. Thirst is a subjective phenomenon. Restricting oral fluids to 1000 mL does not ensure that the client's thirst will be relieved. (21:574)

Nursing Process—Implementation
Client Need—Health promotion/maintenance

NURSING CARE OF CLIENTS WITH NERVE DISORDERS

80 2. Measures are taken to avoid stimulating trigger points that provoke pain along the ophthalmic, mandibular, and maxillary branches of the trigeminal nerve. Therefore, anything that involves touching the face is avoided. Even air drafts can initiate an attack of pain. (4:1131; 21:532)

> Nursing Process—Planning
> Client Need—Physiological integrity

81 1. Since the liver produces prothrombin, a substance that is important to clot formation, signs of unusual bleeding indicate adverse effects to the liver. This drug also causes hematologic changes that also may be evidenced as abnormal bleeding. Clay-colored stools and dark brown urine are associated with liver disturbances, but not pale urine and black stools. Mottled skin is not a sign of liver impairment. (28:212)

> Nursing Process—Implementation
> Client Need—Health promotion/maintenance

82 3. Directing the flow across the conjunctiva from the nasal to temporal corners of the eye helps keep the solution from dripping down the client's nose. It also keeps debris from entering the nasolacrimal duct. None of the other anatomical descriptions are accurate. (4:1070)

> Nursing Process—Implementation
> Client Need—Physiological integrity

83 4. The seventh cranial nerve is the facial nerve. Inflammation around the facial nerve results in sudden paralysis of skeletal muscles about the face. The paralysis is usually unilateral. None of the other assessment findings are commonly associated with Bell's palsy. (21:533)

> Nursing Process—Data collection
> Client Need—Physiological integrity

84 3. Food may become trapped in the buccal pouch of a client with Bell's palsy. Therefore, the nurse inspects this area after each meal, assesses for mechanical trauma, and removes debris. Controlling light has no therapeutic value. Drinking from a cup does not promote better facial muscle function. Although looking in a mirror may be distressing, dealing with the reality of the situation is a component of the grieving process. The nurse may wish to stress that some clients recover muscular function, although the period of recovery may be quite slow. (21:533)

> Nursing Process—Planning
> Client Need—Physiological integrity

85 3. The same virus that causes chickenpox is implicated in the condition called shingles. Latent virus cells apparently are harbored within peripheral nerves. The virus becomes activated by a variety of means, such as a concurrent infection, injury, or injection. (18:1026)

> Nursing Process—Implementation
> Client Need—Health promotion/maintenance

86 1. To allow room for instilling dye or air within the vertebral column, approximately 15 mL of spinal fluid is withdrawn via a lumbar puncture. The client is instructed to lie prone on the examination table. The table, however, is tilted to promote movement of the dye. Local anesthesia is used at the site of the lumbar puncture, but no other forms of anesthesia are commonly given. (7:564)

> Nursing Process—Implementation
> Client Need—Health promotion/maintenance

87 2. Bending the knees while keeping the back straight is an excellent technique for using good body mechanics. The back is often strained by lifting objects with the waist bent. Heavy objects are carried close to the center of gravity. (25:467)

> Nursing Process—Implementation
> Client Need—Health promotion/maintenance

88 2. Until healing takes place, clients are log rolled following spinal surgery. Log-rolling involves moving the client's shoulders and hips as a unit so as to avoid twisting the spine. None of the other turning options describes a log-rolling technique. (18:1001)

> Nursing Process—Implementation
> Client Need—Physiological integrity

89 3. The most effective technique for maintaining the integrity of the skin is to wear a knit cotton shirt under the brace. Talc helps to absorb moisture from the skin. Alcohol dries the skin and reduces the presence of microorganisms. The brace does not have hinges that require lubrication. (18:1001–1002)

> Nursing Process—Evaluation
> Client Need—Health promotion/maintenance

Classification of Test Items

Unit I   Review Test **6**

The Nursing Care of Clients with Disorders of the Neurologic System

Directions: After each question, the correct answer is given as well as a classification of each test question. Compare the correct answer with your answer. If a question has been answered *incorrectly*, draw a line to the end of all the columns. When finished, add up the number of your correct answers in each column and place that number in the respective box at the end in the area identified as *Number Correct*.

To determine the percentage of questions you answered correctly and your performance in each of the test plan categories, divide the *Number Correct* in each column by the *Number Possible* in each column. Then multiply the decimal by 100. For example:

$$\frac{\text{Number Correct: } 70}{\text{Number Possible: } 89} = 0.786 \times 100 = 79\%$$

Any score that is less than 75% indicates an area where further review would be beneficial.

KEY TO ITEM CLASSIFICATION:

NURSING PROCESS

D = Data collection
P = Planning
I = Implementation
E = Evaluation

CLIENT NEEDS

S = Safe, effective care environment
P = Physiological integrity
M = Psychosocial integrity
H = Health promotion/maintenance

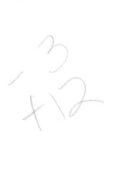

Question #	Answer #	Nursing Process				Client Needs			
		D	P	I	E	S	P	M	H
1	2	D					P		
2	3			I		S			
3	4			I			P		
4	1		P			S			
5	2			I		S			
6	1			I			P		
7	3				E		P		
8	1	D							H
9	4		P				P		
10	2		P				P		
11	2	D							H
12	3			I					H
13	3			I		S			
14	4			I		S			
15	4			I			P		

Question #	Answer #	Nursing Process				Client Needs			
		D	P	I	E	S	P	M	H
16	2			I			P		
17	2			I		S			
18	1		P				P		
19	3			I					H
20	4	D					P		
21	1		P				P		
22	2			I		S			
23	2			I			P		
24	4	D					P		
25	3	D					P		
26	3	D					P		
27	1	D					P		
28	3				E				H
29	2		P				P		
30	4			I			P		
31	2		P				P		
32	2			I					H
33	1	D					P		
34	4			I			P		
35	2			I			P		
36	3		P				P		
37	1			I			P		
38	2			I		S			
39	2			I				M	
40	3			I				M	
41	1			I				M	
42	3		P				P		
43	1			I					H
44	3			I			P		
45	3			I					H
46	4		P				P		
47	2		P				P		

−11

−14
+33

2 3 8 1 4 6 1 3

Question #	Answer #	Nursing Process				Client Needs			
		D	P	I	E	S	P	M	H
48	3	D					P		
49	1	D					P		
50	3		P				P		
51	1	D					P		
52	2			I			P		
53	4				E				H
54	4		P				P		
55	1			I					H
56	1	D					P		
57	2			I			P		
58	3			I			P		
59	2			I		S			
60	2		P				P		
61	1	D					P		
62	3		P				P		
63	2			I					H
64	2			I			P		
65	2			I				M	
66	3		P			S			
67	4			I			P		
68	1		P				P		
69	4			I			P		
70	1			I		S			
71	2			I			P		
72	1	D					P		
73	3			I			P		
74	4			I		S			
75	3			I		S			
76	2			I			P		
77	4			I				M	
78	4	D					P		
79	3			I					H

Question #	Answer #	Nursing Process				Client Needs			
		D	P	I	E	S	P	M	H
80	2		P				P		
81	1			I					H
82	3			I			P		
83	4	D					P		
84	3		P				P		
85	3			I					H
86	1			I					H
87	2			I					H
88	2			I			P		
89	3				E				H
Number Correct	68	13	14	35	3	7	42	4	14
Number Possible	100	17	19	49	4	13	54	5	17
Percentage Correct	76%	76	74	71	75	54	78	80	82

The Nursing Care of Clients with Cardiac Disorders

Nursing Care of Clients with Hypertensive Heart Disease

Nursing Care of Clients with Coronary Artery Disease

Nursing Care of Clients with Myocardial Infarction

Nursing Care of Clients with Congestive Heart Failure

Nursing Care of Clients with Conduction Disorders

Nursing Care of Clients with Valvular Disorders

Nursing Care of Clients with Infectious and Inflammatory Disorders of the Heart

Correct Answers and Rationale

Classification of Test Items

Directions: With a pencil, blacken the circle in front of the option you have chosen for your correct answer.

NURSING CARE OF CLIENTS WITH HYPERTENSIVE HEART DISEASE

A nurse volunteers to do blood pressure screenings during a local community hospital's annual health fair.

1 What *modification* is *most appropriate* when taking the blood pressure of a person who weighs 225 lb?
○ 1. The nurse takes the blood pressure on the client's thigh.
○ 2. The nurse has the client lie down during the assessment.
○ 3. The nurse pumps the manometer up to 225 mm Hg.
● 4. The nurse uses an extra-large blood pressure cuff.

2 If the nurse obtains the following adult blood pressure recordings on four separate clients, which one is it *most appropriate* to recommend rechecking within two months?
○ 1. Client A whose blood pressure is 138/88 mm Hg
● 2. Client B whose blood pressure is 132/98 mm Hg
○ 3. Client C whose blood pressure is 120/80 mm Hg
○ 4. Client D whose blood pressure is 90/60 mm Hg

A nurse teaches a spouse how to assess her hypertensive husband's blood pressure.

3 To be consistent with the American Heart Association's recommendations for measuring the *diastolic blood pressure*, the nurse is accurate in instructing the spouse to record the pressure at which
○ 1. the loud knocking sounds become muffled.
● 2. the last loud knocking sound is heard.
○ 3. the swishing sound becomes loud.
○ 4. the swishing sound becomes faint.

4 The *best response* when a client asks why it is important to control hypertension is that sustained hypertension
○ 1. decreases the life span of many blood cells.
○ 2. leads to the formation of venous blood clots.
● 3. compromises blood flow to many vital organs.
○ 4. predisposes to narrowing of the cardiac valves.

5 If a client reports all of the following, which one is *most suggestive* that the client is hypertensive.
● 1. The client says he has had unexplained nosebleeds.
○ 2. The client says he has difficulty sleeping all night.
○ 3. The client says he has observed blood in his urine.
○ 4. The client says he experiences abdominal fullness.

6 If a hypertensive client is willing to implement lifestyle changes to reduce his blood pressure, which is *best* for the nurse to encourage?
○ 1. Eating more complex carbohydrates
○ 2. Balancing rest with exercise
○ 3. Utilizing more leisure activities
● 4. Giving up smoking cigarettes

7 When the nurse reviews a 55-year-old hypertensive client's medical record, which finding is *most indicative* that the client's heart has become affected by sustained high blood pressure?
○ 1. The client has a strong S_1 heart sound.
○ 2. The client's heart rate is 100 when active.
● 3. The client's heart is moderately enlarged.
○ 4. The client has an irregular heart rhythm.

A hypertensive client's physician recommends that he follow a low-sodium diet.

8 The *best evidence* that the client understands his dietary restrictions is if the client says he must avoid
  ○ 1. soy sauce.
  ○ 2. lemon juice.
  ○ 3. maple syrup.
  ○ 4. onion powder.

A client with hypertension will begin taking furosemide (Lasix) 40 mg orally every day.

9 When the nurse instructs him about his medications, at what time of the day is it *best* to tell him to take the furosemide?
  ○ 1. Before bedtime
  ○ 2. When arising
  ○ 3. With his main meal
  ○ 4. In the late afternoon

10 If the client who takes furosemide (Lasix) likes all of the following fruit in his packed lunch, which one is *best* for him to eat to maintain an adequate potassium level?
  ○ 1. Apples
  ○ 2. Grapes
  ○ 3. Bananas
  ○ 4. Pineapple

NURSING CARE OF CLIENTS WITH CORONARY ARTERY DISEASE

11 If the nurse finds all of the following data in a client's health history, which one is the *most significant* risk factor for developing coronary artery disease?
  ○ 1. The client is employed as an architect.
  ○ 2. The client's ethnic origin is British.
  ○ 3. The client had rheumatic fever as a child.
  ○ 4. The client is seriously overweight.

The physician tells a client at risk for coronary artery disease that his high cholesterol level needs to be lowered.

12 When the client asks the nurse to explain how cholesterol acts as a cardiac risk factor, the *best explanation* is that excess fat in the blood
  ○ 1. expands the circulating blood volume.
  ○ 2. thickens the lining of the arteries.
  ○ 3. interferes with the excretion of urine.
  ○ 4. stimulates the heart to beat faster.

The physician advises the client who is at risk for coronary artery disease to follow a low cholesterol diet.

13 If the client tells the nurse that his usual breakfast is eggs, sausage, and white bread and butter, the *healthiest change* the nurse could suggest is to substitute

  ○ 1. wheat toast for bread.
  ○ 2. margarine for butter.
  ○ 3. cereal for eggs.
  ○ 4. ham for sausage.

The client who is attempting to control his cardiac risk factors is given a prescription for nicotinic acid tablets to help lower his triglyceride level.

14 The nurse is *accurate* in telling the client that an unpleasant side effect he may experience while taking nicotinic acid is
  ○ 1. discolored urine.
  ○ 2. frequent belching.
  ○ 3. flushing of the skin.
  ○ 4. foul-smelling feces.

Lifestyle changes prove insufficient for reducing a client's cholesterol level, and the physician prescribes an antihyperlipidemic drug, colestipol (Colestid).

15 After providing medication instructions, the *best evidence* that the client knows this drug's potential side effects is when he says this drug may cause
  ○ 1. constipation.
  ○ 2. palpitations.
  ○ 3. visual changes.
  ○ 4. weight loss.

A middle-aged adult is scheduled for a stress electrocardiogram (EKG).

16 When the client asks of what use the EKG will be, it is *most correct* for the nurse to explain that a stress EKG
  ○ 1. shows how the heart performs during exercise.
  ○ 2. determines his potential target heart rate.
  ○ 3. verifies how much he needs to improve his fitness.
  ○ 4. can predict if he will have a heart attack soon.

A client with coronary artery disease experiences periodic chest pain.

17 If the client is typical of others who have angina pectoris, he will tell the nurse that his chest pain is relieved by
  ○ 1. aspirin.
  ○ 2. rest.
  ○ 3. heat.
  ○ 4. ice.

The client takes nitroglycerin sublingual tablets when he experiences angina.

18 The client administers the nitroglycerin correctly if he places the tablet
○ 1. between his gum and cheek.
○ 2. at the back of his throat.
● 3. under his tongue.
○ 4. between his teeth.

19 If the client experiences all of the following after taking his nitroglycerin, which one is a side effect of his medication?
● 1. Headache
○ 2. Backache
○ 3. Diarrhea
○ 4. Vomiting

The nurse explains that nitroglycerin tablets lose their potency if exposed to light and air.

20 The client has a *correct understanding* of how to assess when the tablets need replacing if he says that they
○ 1. smell like vinegar.
○ 2. become discolored.
● 3. no longer tingle when used.
○ 4. disintegrate when touched.

21 It is *correct* for the nurse to tell the client that if his chest pain is not relieved after taking one nitroglycerin tablet he should
● 1. take another tablet in 5 minutes.
○ 2. drive to the emergency department.
○ 3. call his physician without delay.
○ 4. swallow two more additional tablets.

An obese client who has angina has been advised to reduce his consumption of saturated fat and calories to control the progression of his coronary artery disease.

22 The *best evidence* that the client is compliant with his diet therapy is that he reports using which one of the following fats for cooking?
● 1. Margarine
○ 2. Shortening
○ 3. Coconut oil
○ 4. Corn oil

The obese client with angina asks the nurse how many calories are in one hot apple pie like those sold at a fast-food restaurant.

23 If the literature supplied by the fast-food chain indicates that one hot apple pie contains 2 g of protein, 14 g of fat, and 31 g of carbohydrates, the nurse is *correct* in telling the client that one hot apple pie is *equal* to

○ 1. 47 calories.
○ 2. 199 calories.
● 3. 255 calories.
○ 4. 343 calories.

The physician prescribes an oral long-acting nitrate, isosorbide dinitrate (Isordil), for the obese client to reduce the incidence of angina that he has been experiencing.

24 Which one of the following symptoms, if identified by the client, is an indication that his dosage of isosorbide dinitrate needs to be adjusted?
○ 1. The client says he experiences nausea.
○ 2. The client says he experiences anorexia.
○ 3. The client says he experiences drowsiness.
● 4. The client says he experiences dizziness.

A client who has been experiencing chest pain will undergo a heart catheterization and coronary arteriogram.

25 To reduce the client's anxiety, it is *best* for the nurse to
○ 1. teach the client how coronary artery disease is best treated.
● 2. listen to the client express his feelings about his condition.
○ 3. explain to the client how well others have done having this test.
○ 4. avoid discussing the heart catheterization until he has relaxed.

The nurse carries out the teaching plan for cardiac catheterization and coronary arteriogram.

26 Which of the following indicates that the client understands what will happen during the testing procedure?
○ 1. The client says that he will be able to hear his heart beating in his chest.
○ 2. The client says that he will experience a heavy sensation all over his body.
○ 3. The client says that he will be anesthetized and won't feel any discomfort.
● 4. The client says that he will feel a warm sensation as the dye is instilled.

27 Prior to the heart catheterization and coronary arteriogram, it is essential that the nurse ask the client if he is allergic to iodine or
○ 1. penicillin.
○ 2. morphine.
● 3. shellfish.
○ 4. eggs.

The femoral artery is the site used to thread the heart catheter.

28 When the coronary arteriogram is completed, the nurse is *most correct* in keeping the client flat in bed with the leg used for the catheterization

1. extended.
2. flexed.
3. abducted.
4. adducted.

29 The *most important* physical assessment the nurse should plan to perform after the femoral artery has been cannulated is to
1. palpate the client's distal peripheral pulses.
2. auscultate the client's heart and lung sounds.
3. percuss all four quadrants of the client's abdomen.
4. inspect the skin integrity on the client's back.

Based on the results of the coronary arteriogram, the physician recommends that the client undergo percutaneous transluminal coronary angioplasty (PTCA).

30 If the client understands his physician's explanation of the PTCA procedure, he will describe that a
1. balloon-tipped catheter will be inserted into a coronary artery.
2. Teflon graft will be used to replace an area of weakened heart muscle.
3. section of vein from his leg will be grafted around a narrowed coronary artery.
4. battery-operated pacemaker will be implanted to maintain his heart rate.

While waiting to undergo percutaneous transluminal coronary angioplasty (PTCA), the client takes propranolol hydrochloride (Inderal).

31 When the client asks the nurse how this drug helps prevent angina, the *best explanation* is that it
1. promotes excretion of body fluid.
2. reduces the rate of heart contraction.
3. alters pain receptors in the brain.
4. dilates the major coronary arteries.

32 While the client takes propranolol hydrochloride, the nurse can expect that his pulse rate will be
1. faster than usual.
2. weaker than before.
3. temporarily irregular.
4. slower than in the past.

On advice of his physician, the client who will undergo percutaneous transluminal coronary angioplasty has been taking one baby aspirin daily.

33 The *best explanation* for the drug therapy in this situation is that aspirin tends to

1. relieve chest pain.
2. prevent blood clots.
3. reduce muscle spasms.
4. promote well-being.

34 When the client returns to his room following the PTCA procedure, which one of the following is reported immediately to the physician?
1. Urine output of 100 mL/h
2. Blood pressure of 108/68
3. Dry mouth
4. Chest pain

A client who has had a previous percutaneous transluminal angioplasty (PTCA) undergoes coronary artery bypass graft (CABG) surgery.

35 When assessing the client postoperatively, the nurse is *most correct* in attaching the sensor from a pulse oximeter to the client's
1. chest.
2. thigh.
3. arm.
4. finger.

The nurse delegates taking vital signs on the client who has undergone a coronary artery bypass graft to a nursing assistant.

36 Which one of the following actions indicates that the nursing assistant who assesses the client's pulse rate needs more instruction?
1. The nursing assistant places her thumb over the radial artery.
2. The nursing assistant counts the pulse rate for 1 full minute.
3. The nursing assistant rests the client's arm on his abdomen.
4. The nursing assistant presses the artery against the bone.

After the coronary artery bypass graft (CABG) surgery, the client experiences acute pain in his incisional area.

37 The nurse could expect that *acute pain* may have which one of the following effects on the client's vital signs?
1. The temperature may be elevated.
2. The pulse rate may become rapid.
3. The respiratory rate may slow.
4. The blood pressure may fall.

The physician orders a patient-controlled analgesia (PCA) infuser pump for the client following coronary artery bypass graft (CABG) surgery.

38 What information is *best* for the nurse to provide the client regarding the use of a PCA infuser pump?
○ 1. Press the control button when pain medication is needed.
○ 2. Call the nurse each time the PCA infuser needs to be used.
○ 3. Use the PCA infuser only when the pain is severe.
○ 4. Frequent use of the PCA infuser can cause addiction.

39 Which of the following information about the client's use of a PCA pump infuser is *most important* for the nurse to communicate to the staff on the next shift?
○ 1. The name of the client's physician
○ 2. The purpose for using the infuser
○ 3. The number of doses administered
○ 4. The client's sense of independence

40 After the coronary artery bypass graft surgery, which nursing assessment finding is evidence that collateral circulation at the *donor* graft site is adequate?
○ 1. The client is free of chest pain.
○ 2. The toes are warm and normal size.
○ 3. The client moves his leg easily.
○ 4. The heart rate remains regular.

NURSING CARE OF CLIENTS WITH MYOCARDIAL INFARCTION

A 65-year-old client with severe chest pain is evaluated in the emergency department. The tentative diagnosis is acute myocardial infarction.

41 If the client is found to have all of the following signs and symptoms, which assessment finding correlates most with an evolving myocardial infarction?
○ 1. The client is sweating profusely.
○ 2. The client's face is flushed.
○ 3. The client says he is thirsty.
○ 4. The client has a moist cough.

42 Which of the following questions is *least* helpful when assessing the client with the possible myocardial infarction about his pain?
○ 1. "How long have you been in pain?"
○ 2. "Where is your pain located?"
○ 3. "What were you doing when your pain started?"
○ 4. "Do you think an injection for pain would help?"

43 If the client with severe chest pain is typical of other people who experience a myocardial infarction, he is likely to tell the nurse that his discomfort radiates to his
○ 1. flank.
○ 2. groin.
○ 3. abdomen.
○ 4. shoulder.

44 Which of the following statements can the nurse expect the client who may be having a myocardial infarction to use when describing his pain?
○ 1. "The pain comes and goes."
○ 2. "The pain came on slowly."
○ 3. "The pain is tingling in nature."
○ 4. "The pain has remained continuous."

45 If the client's pain is due to a myocardial infarction, which prescribed medication is *best* for the nurse to administer?
○ 1. A nonsteroid, such as ibuprofen (Advil)
○ 2. A nonsalicylate, such as acetaminophen (Tylenol)
○ 3. A salicylate, such as acetylsalicylic acid (aspirin)
○ 4. A narcotic, such as meperidine hydrochloride (Demerol)

The wife of the client with the possible myocardial infarction says her husband delayed seeking medical attention because he thought his discomfort was due to having strained muscles from doing yard work.

46 The nurse is *most correct* in explaining to the client's wife that her husband's hesitation in going to the hospital is an example of a coping technique called
○ 1. regression.
○ 2. projection.
○ 3. denial.
○ 4. undoing.

47 If the wife of the client with the severe chest pain reports all of the following, which one is *least* likely to have predisposed her husband to having a myocardial infarction?
○ 1. Smoking cigarettes
○ 2. Eating fatty foods
○ 3. Working under emotional stress
○ 4. Drinking an occasional cocktail

A 57-year-old client comes to the emergency department for what he says is acute indigestion or food poisoning, which he states began several hours ago.

48 If the client who complains of acute indigestion has had an acute myocardial infarction, which one of the following laboratory test results can the nurse expect to be abnormally high?

○ 1. Alkaline phosphatase
○ 2. Alphafetoprotein (AFP)
◉ 3. Creatinine phosphokinase (CPK)
○ 4. Gamma-glutamyl transferase

Based on the laboratory test results and because the client has been experiencing symptoms for only a few hours, the physician plans to administer the drug streptokinase (Streptase).

49 The nurse is *most correct* in explaining to the client that streptokinase is given to
◉ 1. dissolve blood clots.
○ 2. slow his heart rate.
○ 3. improve heart contraction.
○ 4. lower his blood pressure.

50 For which adverse effect is it *essential* for the nurse to monitor when a client receives streptokinase or another similar drug?
○ 1. Hypertension
○ 2. Constipation
◉ 3. Bleeding
○ 4. Vomiting

51 Which one of the following drugs should the nurse plan to have on hand in case the client who receives streptokinase (Streptase) develops an allergic reaction?
○ 1. vitamin K (Synkavite)
○ 2. heparin sodium (Liquaemin sodium)
◉ 3. diphenhydramine (Benadryl)
○ 4. warfarin sodium (Coumadin)

52 Which one of the following findings is *most indicative* to the nurse that the client who is receiving streptokinase (Streptase) is having an allergic reaction?
◉ 1. The client develops urticaria.
○ 2. The client develops dysuria.
○ 3. The client develops hemoptysis.
○ 4. The client develops dyspepsia.

A 55-year-old female collapses in a chair when visiting a hospitalized client.

53 The *first action* the nurse who discovers her should take, is to
◉ 1. open her airway.
○ 2. give two breaths.
○ 3. shake her gently.
○ 4. lay her on the floor.

54 The *best method* the nurse can use to open the airway of the person who is not breathing is to
○ 1. elevate the neck.
◉ 2. lift the chin.
○ 3. press on the jaws.
○ 4. clear the mouth.

55 The *best method* for determining if rescue breathing should be performed is to
○ 1. observe the victim's skin color.
○ 2. feel for pulsations at the neck.
◉ 3. listen for spontaneous breathing.
○ 4. blow air into the victim's mouth.

56 To deliver an *effective volume* of air into the lungs of the person who is not breathing, the nurse
○ 1. presses on the victim's trachea.
○ 2. removes the victim's dentures.
◉ 3. pinches the victim's nose shut.
○ 4. squeezes the victim's cheeks.

A post-myocardial infarction client is unresponsive and pulseless.

57 The correct placement for the nurse's hands before administering cardiac compressions is
◉ 1. on the lower half of the sternum.
○ 2. below the tip of the xiphoid process.
○ 3. over the costal cartilage.
○ 4. directly above the manubrium.

58 During cardiopulmonary resuscitation (CPR), the nurse compresses the chest of an adult victim at a rate of *no less than*
○ 1. 15 compressions per minute.
○ 2. 40 compressions per minute.
○ 3. 60 compressions per minute.
◉ 4. 80 compressions per minute.

A second person arrives to assist the nurse with cardiopulmonary resuscitation (CPR).

59 When two rescuers perform CPR, the rate of compressions to ventilations is
○ 1. 15 compressions to 2 breaths.
◉ 2. 5 compressions to 1 breath.
○ 3. 1 compression for each breath.
○ 4. 1 compression to 5 breaths.

60 The *best* evidence for determining that the cardiac compressions can be discontinued is that
○ 1. the victim's color improves.
○ 2. the pupils become dilated.
◉ 3. a pulse can be palpated.
○ 4. the victim begins to vomit.

61 After a client has been successfully resuscitated, the best position during the recovery period is
○ 1. supine with head elevated.
◉ 2. on the victim's side.
○ 3. prone with the head lowered.
○ 4. flat with knees raised.

The nurse attaches electrocardiogram leads to the chest of a client who has experienced a myocardial infarction in the last 12 hours.

62 When the client is startled by an alarm caused by a loose lead, the *best approach* for relieving his anxiety is to
○ 1. describe his current heart rhythm.
◉ 2. explain the reason the alarm sounded.
○ 3. give him a prescribed tranquilizer.
○ 4. provide him with a magazine to read.

The physician orders nitroglycerin in a transdermal patch form (Nitrodisc).

63 Which of the following nursing actions is *essential* when applying the transdermal patch?
◉ 1. Rotate the site of application.
○ 2. Squeeze the drug reservoir.
○ 3. Tape the patch to the chest.
○ 4. Apply ice to the skin area.

64 The nurse is acting *correctly* by withholding the application of the nitroglycerin patch and notifying the physician when the client's
○ 1. temperature is 99.8°F (37.7°C).
○ 2. respiratory rate is 24 at rest.
○ 3. apical heart rate is 90.
◉ 4. blood pressure is 94/62.

The physician of the client who had a myocardial infarction subsequently prescribes diltiazem hydrochloride (Cardizem) once a day a.c.

65 The nurse carries out the drug order *accurately* by administering the medication
○ 1. at his bedtime.
◉ 2. before a meal.
○ 3. with some food.
○ 4. as necessary.

The client who had the myocardial infarction says to the nurse, "This scares me. I'm concerned about what could happen to me."

66 Of the following comments, which one is *best* for the nurse to make *at this time*?
◉ 1. "What are your concerns?"
○ 2. "Why are you so scared?"
○ 3. "Your doctor says you're doing just fine."
○ 4. "You need to concentrate on getting well."

The physician requests that the client receive diet teaching for a calorie-restricted, low-fat, low-sodium diet.

67 The *best evidence* that the client understands his diet instructions is that he says he should avoid using

○ 1. catsup.
○ 2. vinegar.
○ 3. onions.
○ 4. lemon.

68 If the nurse observes the client who had a myocardial infarction do all of the following, which one should the nurse caution him to avoid because of its potentially dangerous consequences?
○ 1. Reading a murder mystery
◉ 2. Straining to have a stool
○ 3. Washing his hands and face
○ 4. Playing a game of solitaire

To evaluate the damage done to the heart of the client who had a myocardial infarction, the physician orders an echocardiogram.

69 The client has a *correct understanding* of an echocardiogram if he tells the nurse that this examination involves imaging the heart using
○ 1. heat waves.
◉ 2. sound waves.
○ 3. radiation waves.
○ 4. electric waves.

NURSING CARE OF CLIENTS WITH CONGESTIVE HEART FAILURE

A 78-year-old female is admitted to the hospital with left-sided congestive heart failure.

70 When obtaining a health history from the client, the nurse is *most likely* to find that the *earliest* symptom was
○ 1. anorexia.
◉ 2. dyspnea.
○ 3. nausea.
○ 4. headaches.

71 When the lungs of the client in left-sided congestive heart failure are auscultated, the nurse is *most likely* to hear
○ 1. clear breath sounds.
○ 2. reduced breath sounds.
◉ 3. crackling sounds.
○ 4. rumbling sounds.

72 The position the nurse should plan to use to help the client in left-sided congestive heart failure feel most comfortable is a
○ 1. back-lying position.
○ 2. face-lying position.
○ 3. side-lying position.
◉ 4. semisitting position.

73 The *most likely* emotional response in clients like the one experiencing left-sided congestive heart failure is

○ 1. depression.
◉ 2. anxiety.
○ 3. apathy.
○ 4. stoicism.

The client in left-sided congestive heart failure is to receive oxygen by mask.

74 After attaching the tubing to the oxygen supply, the nurse starts the flow of oxygen to the mask
○ 1. before applying the mask to the client's face.
◉ 2. after the mask is secured to the client's face.
○ 3. just as the mask is placed on the client's face.
○ 4. whenever the client says she is short of breath.

The physician prescribes 80 mg of intramuscular furosemide (Lasix) stat for a resident in a nursing home who has congestive heart failure and pulmonary edema.

75 If the furosemide comes prepared in an ampule labeled 40 mg/2 mL, the nurse is *accurate* in administering
○ 1. 0.25 mL.
○ 2. 0.4 mL.
○ 3. 1 mL.
◉ 4. 4 mL.

76 As the nurse prepares to withdraw the furosemide, the *best technique* for removing the medication from the stem of the glass ampule is to
○ 1. allow the ampule to stand undisturbed for a few minutes.
◉ 2. tap the stem of the ampule with the fingernail a few times.
○ 3. hold the ampule upside down, then flip it right side up.
○ 4. roll the ampule gently between the palms of the hands.

77 The *best evidence* that furosemide (Lasix) has had a therapeutic effect is that the client's
○ 1. pulse becomes slower.
○ 2. blood pressure stabilizes.
◉ 3. urinary output increases.
○ 4. anxiety is diminished.

The client in congestive heart failure and pulmonary edema is prepared to be transferred by ambulance to the emergency department.

78 If the nurse believes that the client is extremely frightened, what is the *best action* for the nurse to take at this time?
◉ 1. Stay with the client.
○ 2. Notify the physician.
○ 3. Tell him he'll be okay.
○ 4. Record the collected data.

79 While the client continues to receive furosemide daily, it is *essential* for the nurse to monitor the serum level of
○ 1. calcium.
○ 2. magnesium.
◉ 3. potassium.
○ 4. bicarbonate.

80 Which one of the following physical assessments is *most important* for a nurse to monitor daily on a client with congestive heart failure?
○ 1. Pupil response
○ 2. Bowel sounds
○ 3. Appetite
◉ 4. Weight

A 63-year-old female sees her physician, who has been treating her for chronic obstructive pulmonary disease (COPD).

81 Which one of the following findings is *most suggestive* that the client with COPD is developing right-sided congestive heart failure?
○ 1. Her urine contains glucose.
◉ 2. Her ankles are swollen.
○ 3. She has an irregular pulse.
○ 4. She has a chronic cough.

82 An additional finding during the nurse's assessment of the client with COPD that supports the possibility of right-sided congestive heart failure is
◉ 1. neck vein distension.
○ 2. burning during urination.
○ 3. periodic constipation.
○ 4. chronic indigestion.

The physician admits the client in right-sided congestive heart failure to the hospital to digitalize her.

83 If the client develops digitalis toxicity, the nurse is *most likely* to detect
◉ 1. anorexia and nausea.
○ 2. dizziness and insomnia.
○ 3. pinpoint pupils and double vision.
○ 4. ringing in the ears and itchy skin.

After the digitalizing loading doses have achieved their therapeutic effect, the physician prescribes a daily maintenance dose of 0.125 mg of digoxin (Lanoxin) by mouth.

84 If each tablet of digoxin contains 0.25 mg, how much should the nurse administer to the client each day?
◉ 1. ½ tablet
○ 2. 1 tablet
○ 3. 2 tablets
○ 4. 4 tablets

85 Before administering the digoxin (Lanoxin) to the client in right-sided congestive heart failure, it is *essential* that the nurse assess her
 ● 1. pulse rate.
 ○ 2. blood pressure.
 ○ 3. heart sounds.
 ○ 4. lung sounds.

The client in right-sided congestive heart failure is on a low-sodium diet.

86 If the client understands the restrictions of a low-sodium diet, she will tell the nurse that of the following list of foods, the one that she *may* consume is
 ○ 1. canned chicken soup.
 ○ 2. frozen sausage pizza.
 ● 3. fresh garden salad.
 ○ 4. smoked ocean fish.

NURSING CARE OF CLIENTS WITH CONDUCTION DISORDERS

The physician attaches a Holter monitor to a client who has been experiencing brief fainting spells.

87 Which one of the following instructions is *most important* for helping the physician interpret the information being collected by the Holter monitor?
 ● 1. Record the time and type of physical activities performed.
 ○ 2. Take the radial pulse rate every hour during the next day.
 ○ 3. Try to relax and limit exercise as much as possible.
 ○ 4. Eat lightly and avoid hot or spicy foods.

88 To prevent electrical interference, it is *most appropriate* to recommend that the client whose heart rhythm is being assessed with a Holter monitor avoid
 ○ 1. standing close to a microwave oven.
 ○ 2. driving under overhead power lines.
 ○ 3. shaving with an electric razor.
 ● 4. using a cellular telephone.

The physician admits a client with an abnormal heart rhythm for the insertion of an artificial pacemaker.

89 If the client understands the nurse's explanation of the heart's conduction system, which structure will he identify as the site of the *natural* pacemaker?
 ○ 1. Purkinje fibers
 ○ 2. Bundle of His
 ○ 3. Atrioventricular (AV) node
 ● 4. Sinoatrial (SA) node

90 To assesses the area where the permanent pacemaker battery has been implanted, the nurse is *most correct* in examining the skin
 ○ 1. beneath the left nipple.
 ○ 2. near the brachial artery.
 ○ 3. in the midsternum.
 ● 4. below the clavicle.

91 As part of the discharge instructions, the nurse is *most correct* in telling the client with an artificial pacemaker that a sign of pacemaker malfunction is
 ○ 1. tingling in the chest area.
 ● 2. dizziness during activity.
 ○ 3. pain radiating to the arm.
 ○ 4. tenderness beneath the skin.

Cardioversion will be performed on a female client who has developed a rapid atrial heart rate.

92 The client has a *correct understanding* of the cardioversion procedure if she tells the nurse that it involves
 ● 1. administering an electric current to the heart.
 ○ 2. threading a thin, plastic catheter into her heart.
 ○ 3. evaluating blood flow to areas of heart muscle.
 ○ 4. scanning the heart after injecting a radioisotope.

93 Before cardioversion is attempted, the nurse is *most correct* in *withholding* which one of the following prescribed medications?
 ○ 1. Diazepam (Valium)
 ● 2. Digoxin (Lanoxin)
 ○ 3. Cimetidine (Tagamet)
 ○ 4. Glyburide (Diabeta)

94 The *best evidence* that the cardioversion procedure has been successful is
 ○ 1. the client regains consciousness immediately.
 ● 2. normal sinus cardiac rhythm is restored.
 ○ 3. the apical heart rate equals the radial rate.
 ○ 4. the pulse pressure is approximately 40 mm Hg.

NURSING CARE OF CLIENTS WITH VALVULAR DISORDERS

During a routine pre-employment physical examination a physician discovers that a 28-year-old female has a heart murmur.

95 If the heart murmur is related to valve damage caused by a childhood infection, which of the following diseases can the nurse *most likely* expect this client to report having?
 ○ 1. Varicella (chickenpox)
 ○ 2. Rubella (German measles)
 ● 3. Rheumatic fever
 ○ 4. Whooping cough

After a diagnostic workup, the physician informs the client with the heart murmur that she has mitral stenosis.

96 The nurse is *most correct* in explaining to the client that the mitral valve is located between the
   ○ 1. right ventricle and the pulmonary artery.
   ◉ 2. left atrium and left ventricle.
   ○ 3. right atrium and right ventricle.
   ○ 4. left ventricle and the aorta.

97 The *best location* for the nurse to auscultate the sounds from the mitral valve is
   ○ 1. at the fifth intercostal space in the left midclavicular line.
   ◉ 2. at the fourth intercostal space to the left of the sternum.
   ○ 3. at the second intercostal space to the right of the sternum.
   ○ 4. at the second intercostal space to the left of the sternum.

The physician prescribes 250 mg of nafcillin sodium (Unipen) P.O. q.i.d. for the client with mitral stenosis.

98 What is the *best explanation* the nurse can give the client for taking this prescribed medication?
   ○ 1. It may destroy the virus causing her disease.
   ○ 2. It may reduce the scar tissue on the valve.
   ◉ 3. It may stop blood clots from forming.
   ○ 4. It may prevent future bacterial infections.

A 49-year-old male client who has been taking diuretics and digitalis for the long-term treatment of mitral stenosis becomes progressively worse. He plans to have surgery to replace his mitral valve.

99 Which one of the following statements indicates that the client understands the surgical procedure involving mitral valve replacement?
   ◉ 1. The client says his blood will be circulated through a heart-lung machine.
   ○ 2. The client says the surgeon will enlarge his valve by inserting his finger.
   ○ 3. The client says his chest will be opened during surgery but not his heart.
   ○ 4. The client says a piece of his leg vein will be used to replace his valve.

100 Which one of the following signs is *most often manifested* by adults who have had chronic cardiac or pulmonary disease most of their lives?
   ○ 1. Deviated nasal septum
   ○ 2. Flushed facial skin
   ◉ 3. Clubbed fingertips
   ○ 4. Hoarse vocal sounds

Postoperatively, the client with the mitral valve replacement is short of breath with moderate activity.

101 Which nursing intervention is *best* to add to the care plan to reduce the client's energy expenditure?
   ◉ 1. Administer oxygen when the client is dyspneic.
   ○ 2. Distribute routine care over several hours.
   ○ 3. Provide analgesic medications when necessary.
   ○ 4. Restrict visitors to brief periods of time.

The physician writes an order stating the client with a mitral valve replacement can be up in the chair if he can tolerate the increased activity.

102 Which of the following criteria is the *best evidence* that the client is able to tolerate the activity involved in getting out of bed?
   ○ 1. His appetite has improved.
   ○ 2. He has more restful sleep.
   ◉ 3. His heart rate is stable.
   ○ 4. He says he is very bored.

The client who had cardiac surgery to replace his mitral valve, is disappointed that his progress is so slow. One day he pushes away his lunch tray, and it falls to the floor.

103 At this time, it is *best* for the nurse to
   ○ 1. clean up the floor and say nothing.
   ○ 2. find out what food he would prefer.
   ◉ 3. let the client talk about his fears.
   ○ 4. leave him alone until he feels better.

NURSING CARE OF CLIENTS WITH INFECTIOUS AND INFLAMMATORY DISORDERS OF THE HEART

A pulmonary artery catheter is used to monitor pressure within the heart of a client following cardiac surgery. The client is now suspected of having bacterial endocarditis.

104 Which one of the following nursing assessment findings is the *best evidence* that the client is experiencing an infectious process?
   ○ 1. The client has chest pain.
   ○ 2. The client has a dry cough.
   ◉ 3. The client has a fever.
   ○ 4. The client has dyspnea.

A 63-year-old female with cancer of the liver is admitted with pericarditis.

105 When the nurse auscultates the client's chest, which action best facilitates hearing the client's heart and lung sounds?
   ◉ 1. Ask the client to hold her breath.
   ○ 2. Turn the oxygen off momentarily.
   ○ 3. Lay the client flat in bed.
   ○ 4. Locate the point of the xiphoid.

106 While auscultating the chest of a client with pericarditis, which one of the following is the nurse *most likely* to hear?
○ 1. Expiratory wheezes
○ 2. Inspiratory gurgles
● 3. A cardiac friction rub
○ 4. A clicking heart murmur

107 Which nursing assessment finding supports the assumption that the client's cardiac stroke volume is *reduced*?
○ 1. The client faints with activity.
○ 2. The client develops hypertension.
● 3. The client manifests bradycardia.
○ 4. The client has a bounding pulse.

The client undergoes a pericardiocentesis and is placed on fluid restrictions.

108 Which nursing intervention is *best* to add to the plan of care for alleviating the client's thirst?
○ 1. Chill all oral fluids.
○ 2. Offer hard, sour candy.
○ 3. Puree all solid food.
● 4. Give ice chips often.

Directions: Two numbers appear in parentheses following each rationale. The first number identifies the textbook listed in the references, page 512, and the second number identifies the page(s) in that textbook on which the correct answer can be verified. Occasionally, two or more textbooks are given to verify the correct answer.

NURSING CARE OF CLIENTS WITH HYPERTENSIVE HEART DISEASE

1 4. One can assume that a person who is obese will need a larger than usual adult cuff. A common guide is to select a cuff the bladder of which encircles at least two-thirds of the limb at its midpoint and is as wide as 40% of the mid-limb circumference. If the cuff is too narrow, the blood pressure will be higher than its true measurement; if too wide, the measurement will be lower than the true pressure. (25:156)
  Nursing Process—Planning
  Client Need—Physiological integrity

2 2. The Joint National Committee on Detection, Evaluation, and Treatment of High Blood Pressure (1993) recommends that an initial diastolic pressure between 90 and 99 mm Hg be rechecked in two months even if the systolic pressure is normal, i.e., less than 140 mm Hg. (25:164–165)
  Nursing Process—Data collection
  Client Need—Health promotion/maintenance

3 2. *Phase V* of Korotkoff sounds, the point at which the last sound is heard before a period of continuous silence, is considered the best reflection of adult diastolic pressure. In some cases, two diastolic pressures are recorded: the pressure at which the loud knocking sound becomes muffled and the last sound that is heard. (4:160; 19:503)
  Nursing Process—Implementation
  Client Need—Health promotion/maintenance

4 3. Untreated hypertension tends to cause fibrous tissue to form in systemic arterioles. The fibrous quality leads to decreased tissue perfusion, which is especially dangerous when it affects target organs like the heart, kidneys, and brain. Hypertension is not linked to a shortened life cycle of blood cells, venous clots, nor stenosis of cardiac valves. (4:765; 21:406)
  Nursing Process—Implementation
  Client Need—Health promotion/maintenance

5 1. Some of the earliest manifestations of hypertension include spontaneous nosebleeds, awakening with a headache, and blurred vision. Complications of hypertension, such as congestive heart failure, are manifested by dyspnea when lying down, but not early awakening from sleep. Hematuria is not a sign that generally is associated with hypertension. Abdominal fullness may have multiple etiologies. (4:766; 21:406)
  Nursing Process—Data collection
  Client Need—Physiological integrity

6 4. Smoking cessation is the single most therapeutic health change for anyone who has or is at risk for cardiopulmonary disease. Although increasing the intake of complex carbohydrates such as oatmeal and other whole grains has healthy benefits in lowering blood cholesterol, smoking cessation provides more dramatic results in less time. Striking a healthy balance between rest and exercise and taking advantage of more leisure activities are also beneficial, but any one of these still cannot compare with the beneficial effects on arterioles from smoking cessation. (18:1108)
  Nursing Process—Implementation
  Client Need—Health promotion/maintenance

7 3. Myocardial hypertrophy is the direct consequence of having to pump against increased peripheral resistance due to hypertension. A strong S_1 heart sound is a healthy finding. A heart rate of 100 during aerobic activity is within normal limits for a client who is 55. An irregular heart rhythm may have multiple etiologies, but etiologies other than hypertension are usually more common. (4:1108; 21:406)
  Nursing Process—Data collection
  Client Need—Physiological integrity

8 1. Soy sauce is high in sodium and therefore is restricted on a low-sodium diet. Lemon juice and onion powder (not salt) can be used liberally. Maple syrup is not restricted for its sodium content, but may be limited if the client needs to lose weight. (6:544)

> Nursing Process — Evaluation
> Client Need — Health promotion/maintenance

9 2. To avoid disturbing sleep with a need for urination, a daily dose of a diuretic like furosemide is administered in the early morning. (20:315)

> Nursing Process — Implementation
> Client Need — Health promotion/maintenance

10 3. People who take potassium-depleting diuretics like furosemide should eat foods that replace this electrolyte. One banana contains approximately 10 mEq of potassium. Other fruits that are rich sources include oranges and orange juice, cantaloupe, and nectarines. (4:511; 6:205)

> Nursing Process — Implementation
> Client Need — Health promotion/maintenance

NURSING CARE OF CLIENTS WITH CORONARY ARTERY DISEASE

11 4. Obesity, which often is linked with hyperlipidemia, is a risk factor for developing coronary artery disease. As an ethnic group, people from Great Britain do not experience an unusually high predisposition to coronary artery disease. Occupations in which workers experience anxiety, such as air traffic controllers, but not architects, are more likely to develop stress-related disorders such as hypertension and cardiac disorders. Rheumatic fever is more likely to cause valvular disease than coronary artery disease. (21:374)

> Nursing Process — Data collection
> Client Need — Health promotion/maintenance

12 2. A buildup of cholesterol causes atherosclerosis. Fat becomes deposited within the lining of arteries. The deposits enlarge to form plaque. The fatty plaque thickens the arterial walls, causing the passageway for blood to become narrowed. Eventually the plaque is infiltrated with calcium, which causes the vessel to become hard and inelastic. When the normal volume of blood is forced to pass through narrow and inelastic vessels, the pressure within the vessels increases. The heart is prone to failure because it must work very hard to pump against the vascular resistance. (4:740; 21:373)

> Nursing Process — Implementation
> Client Need — Health promotion/maintenance

13 3. In keeping with a low-cholesterol diet, the healthiest change is to eat cereal rather than eggs for breakfast. Egg yolk is a rich source of cholesterol. There is not much, if any, appreciable change in levels of cholesterol by substituting the foods listed in the other options. (6:517, 521)

> Nursing Process — Implementation
> Client Need — Health promotion/maintenance

14 3. In doses large enough to lower blood fat components, nicotinic acid causes relaxation of peripheral vascular smooth muscle. This causes some people to experience flushing of the skin. The flushing, primarily in the head, neck, and ears, is accompanied by a sensation of warmth, tingling, itching, and headache. This effect tends to subside as therapy continues. (6:513; 20:294)

> Nursing Process — Implementation
> Client Need — Health promotion/maintenance

15 1. Bile acid sequestrants, of which colestipol is one, can cause constipation, bleeding tendencies, abdominal pain and distention, hypersensitivity reactions, headache, and backache. (20:292)

> Nursing Process — Evaluation
> Client Need — Health promotion/maintenance

16 1. A stress EKG demonstrates the extent to which the heart tolerates and responds to the additional demands placed on it during exercise. The heart's ability to continue adapting is related to the adequacy of blood supplied to the myocardium through the coronary arteries. If the client develops chest pain, dangerous cardiac rhythm changes, or significantly elevated blood pressure, the diagnostic testing is stopped. (20:343)

> Nursing Process — Implementation
> Client Need — Health promotion/maintenance

17 2. Angina is generally relieved by rest. The chest pain is caused by an inadequate supply of oxygenated blood to the myocardium due to partially occluded coronary arteries. Once the myocardium's demand for additional oxygen is reduced through inactivity, the chest pain is relieved. Aspirin, heat, or ice are not appropriate measures for relieving the pain of angina pectoris. (4:741; 21:379)

> Nursing Process — Data collection
> Client Need — Physiological integrity

18 3. Sublingual means under the tongue. Clients are instructed not to chew or swallow the tablets. They dissolve in the mouth. The drug is absorbed through the rich blood supply beneath the tongue. Tablets for buccal administration are placed between the gum and cheek. A tablet intended for swallowing is placed on the tongue at the back of the throat. A chewable tablet is placed between the teeth. (25:718)

> Nursing Process — Evaluation
> Client Need — Health promotion/maintenance

19 1. Side effects of nitroglycerin include headache, flushing, and dizziness. These effects are the direct result of vasodilation. Relief is obtained by decreasing the dosage of the drug or by taking a mild pain reliever. (20:284–285)
Nursing Process—Evaluation
Client Need—Physiological integrity

20 3. The client experiences a fizzing or tingling in the mouth if nitroglycerin tablets are still fresh. Tablets need to be replaced approximately every 3 months. Old aspirin tends to smell like vinegar. Nitroglycerin tablets do not become discolored or disintegrate when touched when they have lost their potency. (17:464)
Nursing Process—Evaluation
Client Need—Health promotion/maintenance

21 1. The dose of nitroglycerin may be repeated in 5 minutes. However, the client is told to call the physician if the pain is not relieved after three successive doses, because other treatment may be necessary. A person having chest pain should never drive himself to the hospital. Sublingual tablets are not swallowed. (17:464)
Nursing Process—Implementation
Client Need—Health promotion/maintenance

22 4. Corn oil is an example of a polyunsaturated oil. Using unsaturated fats helps lower blood cholesterol. In limited amounts it is healthier to consume polyunsaturated fats than saturated fats, such as grease or lard, or hydrogenated fats, such as solid vegetable shortenings and hard margarines. Coconut and palm oil are more highly saturated than lard. (6:164–165)
Nursing Process—Evaluation
Client Need—Health promotion/maintenance

23 3. Protein and carbohydrate both have 4 calories per gram; fat contains 9 calories per gram. Thus, the total calorie count for a piece of pie containing 2 g of protein, 14 g of fat, and 31 g of carbohydrate is 255 calories. (4:592)
Nursing Process—Implementation
Client Need—Health promotion/maintenance

24 4. Dizziness is a common side effect of nitrate drugs. Nitrates have a direct relaxing effect on the smooth muscle of blood vessels producing vasodilation. When blood vessels dilate, blood pressure falls, and the client experiences vertigo. Isosorbide dinitrate is administered in a range of 5 to 40 mg. Once the data are reported, the physician may wish to lower the dosage the client is receiving or have him take the drug at night before going to sleep. In some instances, the side effects diminish or disappear after taking the drug over a period of time. (17:459; 20:287)
Nursing Process—Data collection
Client Need—Physiological integrity

25 2. When a person is worried and fearful, the nurse encourages and listens as the client expresses his feelings. Verbalization often lifts the mental burden that a client is experiencing. Most clients feel alone, overwhelmed, and helpless during a crisis. Listening is an active process even if the nurse does not make many verbal contributions. Learning is impaired during times of mild to severe anxiety. How others have done disregards the uniqueness of the situation for this person. Avoiding the subject communicates that the nurse does not care. (23:291)
Nursing Process—Implementation
Client Need—Psychosocial integrity

26 4. The contrast dye used during the coronary arteriogram causes vasodilation and is experienced as a brief flush or warmth that spreads over the skin surface. It is possible to feel fluttering or what some describe as "butterflies" as the catheter is passed into the heart, disturbing its rhythm. Chest pain, if it is experienced, is generally treated with nitroglycerin. The client receives sedation prior to the diagnostic testing but is not anesthetized. (21:343)
Nursing Process—Evaluation
Client Need—Health promotion/maintenance

27 3. People who are allergic to shellfish also may be sensitive to iodine. The radiopaque dye used during the arteriogram is iodine based. The physician is notified if the client indicates a history of allergies to either of these substances. The physician may cancel the procedure or be prepared to administer an antihistamine or other emergency drugs. (7:959, 18:580)
Nursing Process—Data collection
Client Need—Safe, effective care environment

28 1. When the femoral artery is the site used for inserting the heart catheter, the nurse makes sure that the client does not bend his leg or flex his hip for 6 to 8 hours. Flexing the hip may lead to bleeding and clot formation. Sandbags may be placed over the pressure dressing to decrease discomfort and control bleeding. (4:309; 18:1106)
Nursing Process—Implementation
Client Need—Physiological integrity

29 1. Peripheral pulses distal to the catheter insertion site are assessed frequently. The injury to the artery and subsequent bleeding can lead to clot formation.

The thrombus could totally occlude the flow of oxygenated blood through the vessel. Absence of a distal pulse is reported immediately because this is an emergency situation. (7:960; 18:1106)

    Nursing Process—Planning
    Client Need—Physiological integrity

30 1. A PTCA procedure involves dilating narrowed or occluded coronary arteries with a double lumen balloon catheter. The pressure from the inflated balloon compresses the fatty plaque that has narrowed the artery. A CABG procedure uses a piece of leg vein to bypass a narrowed area of coronary artery. A pacemaker is used when it is difficult to maintain the heart rate in the normal range with drug therapy. Grafting skeletal muscle, not Teflon, over scarred areas of myocardium is just now in experimental stages. (4:742; 21:375)

    Nursing Process—Evaluation
    Client Need—Health promotion/maintenance

31 2. Propranolol hydrochloride is a beta-blocker. It blocks the sympathetic receptors for epinephrine. Epinephrine speeds the heart rate, which requires a great deal of oxygen. By blocking the effect of epinephrine, the heart rate is slowed, and not as much oxygen is needed by the myocardium. In addition, at a slower rate the heart fills with a greater volume of blood. Thus, each time the heart contracts, it delivers a substantial amount of blood to the coronary arteries. As long as the coronary arteries deliver an adequate amount of oxygenated blood to the myocardium, chest pain is prevented. (17:443)

    Nursing Process—Implementation
    Client Need—Health promotion/maintenance

32 4. Beta-blockers interfere with the action of epinephrine. They reduce heart rate. Therefore, the pulse rate tends to be slower than in the unmedicated period. Some clients become bradycardic while taking propranolol. (20:266)

    Nursing Process—Data collection
    Client Need—Physiological integrity

33 2. Aspirin is recommended in low daily doses to reduce the potential for forming a blood clot, which could occlude the narrowed opening in a diseased coronary artery. Aspirin interferes with platelet aggregation or clumping; therefore, it acts as a prophylactic antithrombotic agent. Aspirin is more useful in relieving headaches and musculoskeletal pain than chest pain, and it is not a muscle relaxant.

There is no scientific evidence that aspirin improves mood or causes euphoria. (17:475; 20:124)

    Nursing Process—Implementation
    Client Need—Health promotion/maintenance

34 4. Signs of complications following PTCA include chest pain, bleeding from the catheter insertion site, and abnormal heart rhythms. Chest pain indicates that the dilated coronary artery has suddenly closed again. If untreated, a myocardial infarction could occur. An hourly urine output of 30 to 50 mL or more is adequate. A blood pressure of 108/68 is in the low ranges of normal. A dry mouth is a consequence of fluid restriction and medication administered prior to the procedure. As long as the blood pressure continues to remain in normal ranges, the nurse relieves the discomfort of a dry mouth by giving oral care and administering oral fluids. (21:376)

    Nursing Process—Implementation
    Client Need—Physiological integrity

35 4. The sensor for pulse oximetry is applied to the fingertip, toe, ear, or tip of the nose. A pulse oximeter measures the oxygen saturation of hemoglobin. It is a convenient, noninvasive monitoring technique of a client's oxygenation. The sensor does not fit on the chest, thigh, or arm. (4:631; 25:402–403)

    Nursing Process—Implementation
    Client Need—Safe, effective care environment

36 1. Using the thumb to obtain a pulse rate can result in inaccurate data. It is possible that the health care worker could feel his or her own pulse rather than the client's. It is best to rest or support the client's arm and compress the artery against the bone using the fingertips. It is not incorrect to count the pulse for 1 full minute, in fact, it is preferred if the pulse is abnormal in any way. (18:464; 25:150)

    Nursing Process—Evaluation
    Client Need—Safe, effective care environment

37 2. A client in acute pain is most likely to have a rapid pulse rate, rapid respiratory rate, and rising blood pressure. Pain is least likely to influence body temperature. (4:154)

    Nursing Process—Data collection
    Client Need—Physiological integrity

38 1. Each time a client feels the need for medication he presses a control button releasing a very low dose of narcotic. The low dosage is administered at frequent intervals. Usually, less total narcotic is actually used because, with frequent use, the discomfort rarely falls below a tolerable range. It is best to use the PCA infuser before pain becomes severe. PCA infusers are used only for a few days postoperatively, making it unlikely that narcotic addiction would occur. Because the client can use the machine independently, it frees the nurse to perform other responsibilities. (25:373)

    Nursing Process—Implementation
    Client Need—Health promotion/maintenance

39 3. The number of doses the client administered during the current shift is important information to communicate. It indicates how much pain the client is experiencing and his understanding of how best to use the machine. The name of the client's physician is readily available on multiple records. There is only one use for a PCA infuser pump, and that is to relieve pain. Because the client controls the use of the machine, it promotes a sense of independence. However, that is not the most important information for the nurse to report. (25:374)

    Nursing Process—Implementation
    Client Need—Safe, effective care environment

40 2. The saphenous vein is the most common blood vessel used for coronary artery bypass grafting. Removing a portion of this leg vein can temporarily impair the return of venous blood to the heart. Impaired venous return is manifested by edema and cool skin temperature in the toes, foot, or ankle of the operative leg. Therefore, the fact that the toes are warm and of normal size is the best evidence that venous blood is adequately returning to the heart through other blood vessels in the leg. The ability to move the leg is evidence that neurologic function is intact. A regular heart rate and absence of chest pain is evidence that the newly attached graft is supplying the heart muscle with adequate oxygenated blood. (18:226; 25:436)

    Nursing Process—Evaluation
    Client Need—Physiological integrity

NURSING CARE OF CLIENTS WITH MYOCARDIAL INFARCTION

41 1. The chest pain accompanying a myocardial infarction is often of such severity that the client becomes extremely diaphoretic. Hypotension is apt to make the client's skin appear pale or ashen. Thirst is associated with hypovolemia or diabetes mellitus. A moist cough is more likely found in clients with respiratory disease and congestive heart failure. (4:746; 25:377)

    Nursing Process—Data collection
    Client Need—Physiological integrity

42 4. The most pertinent data to assess concerning pain are its onset, quality, intensity, location, and dura-

tion and what makes the pain better or worse. Although it is important to collaborate with the client on treatment approaches, the ultimate decision as to the route and prescribed drug to administer is a decision that is best made on the basis of the nurse's education and experience. (25:367)

    Nursing Process—Data collection
    Client Need—Physiological integrity

43 4. A client experiencing a myocardial infarction is likely to describe the pain as being substernal or radiating to the shoulder, arm, teeth, jaw, or throat. (4:746; 21:376)

    Nursing Process—Data collection
    Client Need—Physiological integrity

44 4. Unlike angina pectoris, the pain caused by an acute myocardial infarction is not relieved by rest, sublingual nitroglycerin, or other oral nitrate drugs. Many describe the pain associated with a myocardial infarction using such terms as squeezing, suffocating, or crushing. The pain comes on suddenly. (4:746; 21:377)

    Nursing Process—Data collection
    Client Need—Physiological integrity

45 4. A narcotic analgesic, such as meperidine hydrochloride or morphine sulfate, usually is required to relieve the severe pain associated with a myocardial infarction. Nonsteroidal, nonsalicylate, and salicylate analgesics generally are prescribed for minor pain that is other than cardiac in origin. (4:748; 18:1115)

    Nursing Process—Planning
    Client Need—Physiological integrity

46 3. Denial shuts out the painful awareness of reality. The person refuses to believe that an event is really happening. Regression occurs when a person resorts to a pattern of behavior characteristic of an earlier age. Projection involves blaming a negative situation on someone or something else. Undoing often takes on the form of offering a verbal apology or gift to make up for unacceptable behavior. (23:15; 25:60)

    Nursing Process—Implementation
    Client Need—Psychosocial integrity

47 4. Of the factors listed in this item, having an occasional alcoholic beverage is least likely to predispose to a myocardial infarction. Small amounts of alcohol may increase the good kind of cholesterol called high-density lipoprotein. However, alcohol does elevate triglyceride levels. Because the relationship of elevated triglycerides to heart disease has not been conclusively established, consuming small amounts of alcohol generally is not recommended for preventing atherosclerosis and the potential for a heart attack. Smoking, working under stress, and eating a diet high in fat and cholesterol are definite risk factors in developing a myocardial infarction. (4:283; 18:685)

    Nursing Process—Data collection
    Client Need—Health promotion/maintenance

48 3. CPK is an enzyme found in high concentrations in the heart and skeletal muscles and in much smaller amounts in brain tissue. The CPK blood level, especially its isoenzyme CPK-MB, becomes elevated within 2 hours after a myocardial infarction. An elevated alkaline phosphatase is associated primarily with liver and bone diseases. AFP is a substance produced and secreted by tumor cells. The presence of AFP indicates that a person has cancer. Gamma-glutamyl transferase is a test used to determine liver cell dysfunction and to detect alcohol-induced liver disease. (4:747; 25:377)

    Nursing Process—Data collection
    Client Need—Physiological integrity

49 1. Streptokinase is a thrombolytic enzyme. It is used to dissolve deep vein and arterial thromboemboli. This and other thrombolytic agents, such as urokinase (Abbokinase), anistreplase (Eminase), alteplase (Activase), and tissue plasminogen activator, activate plasminogen and convert it to plasmin. Plasmin breaks down the fibrin of a blood clot. Thrombolytic agents do not slow the heart rate, improve heart contraction, or lower blood pressure. (4:748; 21:377)

    Nursing Process—Implementation
    Client Need—Health promotion/maintenance

50 3. Bleeding is the most common adverse reaction associated with thrombolytic drug therapy. Blood loss may be internal, involving the gastrointestinal or genitourinary tract, or may result in bleeding within the brain. Bleeding also may be external or superficial, manifested as oozing from venipuncture or injection sites, nosebleeds, and skin bruising. Recent trauma, childbirth, or surgery are contraindications for using a thrombolytic agent. (25:378)

    Nursing Process—Planning
    Client Need—Physiological integrity

51 3. The antihistamine drug diphenhydramine (Benadryl) is prescribed in the event that a client develops an allergic reaction. Vitamin K is given as an antidote when prothrombin levels are beyond therapeutic range, as in the case when oral anticoagulants like warfarin sodium (Coumadin) are prescribed. Both heparin sodium (Liquaemin so-

dium) and warfarin sodium are administered to prevent future blood clots from developing. (26:190)

    Nursing Process—Planning
    Client Need—Physiological integrity

52 1. Urticaria is a term for hives. Hives, welts, and skin rashes are common manifestations of an allergic reaction. In addition, the nurse may observe difficulty breathing, wheezing, and hypotension. Dysuria is a term for painful urination. Hemoptysis indicates that the client is coughing bloody sputum. Dyspepsia is another word for indigestion. Neither dysuria, hemoptysis, nor dyspepsia are commonly associated with allergic reactions. (17:475, 481; 20:272)

    Nursing Process—Data collection
    Client Need—Physiological integrity

53 3. To properly assess the need for resuscitation, the first action is to gently shake the victim and shout, "Are you OK?" If the victim remains unresponsive, it is important for the rescuer to call loudly for additional help. If the victim cannot be aroused and is not breathing, the rescuer gives two breaths. The victim is on a firm, flat surface before cardiac compressions are given. (25:800)

    Nursing Process—Implementation
    Client Need—Physiological integrity

54 2. The nurse uses the chin lift/head tilt method for opening the airway when neck trauma is not suspected. This is performed by using one hand to lift the chin upward. The position is maintained by placing the other hand across the forehead. The jaw thrust method is used if the chin lift/head tilt method does not open the airway adequately or if there is a possible neck injury. Placing a hand under the neck is no longer a recommended practice. The mouth is cleared with a finger sweep after opening the airway. (25:803)

    Nursing Process—Implementation
    Client Need—Physiological integrity

55 3. Once the airway is open, some victims begin breathing spontaneously. The nurse assesses for spontaneous breathing by leaning over the victim's head and listening or feeling for the movement of air from the nose or mouth. The chest or abdomen also is observed for rising and falling. Skin color is not a dependable assessment finding because hypotension, for whatever reason, is likely to cause the victim to appear pale or ashen. A carotid pulse is checked to determine the need for performing heart compressions. Administering rescue breath-

ing is unnecessary if the victim is spontaneously breathing. (25:800)
> Nursing Process—Data collection
> Client Need—Physiological integrity

56 3. Pinching the nose shut allows maximum ventilation with no loss of air through the nostrils. If there is a mouth injury or it is impossible to prevent air from leaking in an adult victim, the rescuer may use the mouth-to-nose technique for giving ventilations. When resuscitating an infant or small child, a seal is made by covering both the victim's nose and mouth with the rescuer's mouth. Once the breath is given, the rescuer allows the air to be exhaled passively. Pressing on the trachea may interfere with the passage of air. Removing dentures and squeezing the victim's cheeks may interfere with maintaining a tight seal during rescue breathing. (18:364; 25:800)
> Nursing Process—Implementation
> Client Need—Physiological integrity

57 1. Both of the rescuer's hands are on top of one another on the lower half of the sternum two finger breadths above the xiphoid process. Placing the hands below the tip of the xiphoid process could cause the liver to be lacerated. The costal cartilage connects the ribs to the sternum. Compressing over the costal cartilage could fracture the victim's ribs. The manubrium is the upper portion of the sternum. The hands are placed too high on the chest if positioned above the manubrium. (25:805)
> Nursing Process—Implementation
> Client Need—Physiological integrity

58 4. The adult chest is compressed during CPR at a rate between 80 to 100 times per minute. The sternum is depressed approximately 1½ to 2 inches with each compression. Rates below 80/min are not likely to circulate blood adequately. (25:806)
> Nursing Process—Implementation
> Client Need—Physiological integrity

59 2. The American Heart Association recommends that when two rescuers perform CPR, they administer five compressions and then a breath. The ratio for a single rescuer is 15 compressions to two breaths. CPR is never interrupted for longer than 7 seconds. (25:804)
> Nursing Process—Implementation
> Client Need—Physiological integrity

60 3. If the pulse returns, cardiac compressions are stopped. The carotid pulse is assessed for a full 5 seconds after the first minute of resuscitation and

thereafter every 4 to 5 minutes unless consciousness is restored. The victim's color may improve as a consequence of effective resuscitation efforts. Dilated and fixed pupils are an indication that the brain is not adequately oxygenated. Vomiting can occur in a nonbreathing and pulseless victim. It can occur from distending the stomach with air. (4:1543; 25:802)
> Nursing Process—Evaluation
> Client Need—Physiological integrity

61 2. The recovery position following successful cardiopulmonary resuscitation is a side-lying position. This position helps to protect and maintain the airway. (4:1543; 25:801)
> Nursing Process—Implementation
> Client Need—Physiological integrity

62 2. Hospitalization, for most people, is a unique experience. Anxiety is relieved by providing people in an unfamiliar environment with information about hospital equipment, clinical procedures, and agency routines. All explanations are given in simple, understandable terms. Once informed, the client has a basis for interpreting the reality of his experiences. The client is not likely to understand a description of heart rhythm. Administering a tranquilizer at this time or distracting him with a magazine does not help prevent a similar reaction in the future. (21:106)
> Nursing Process—Implementation
> Client Need—Psychosocial integrity

63 1. Application sites are rotated when topical nitroglycerin ointment or transdermal patches are used. The drug reservoir is not touched or manipulated in any way. The patch is self-adhering once the adhesive backing is removed. Ointment application papers are covered with kitchen plastic wrap and taped in place to prevent soiling clothing and to promote drug absorption. The patch is placed on the chest, back, upper abdomen, or arms. It is not necessary to apply ice to the skin. (20:284, 286)
> Nursing Process—Implementation
> Client Need—Physiological integrity

64 4. Nitroglycerin dilates arterial vessels. This action lowers the blood pressure. Therefore, if the client's blood pressure is already low, as in 94/62, the nurse checks with the physician before applying the patch. It is not uncommon for the temperature of a client with a myocardial infarction to be slightly elevated. This is probably due to the inflammatory response from the injury to the myocardium. A

respiratory rate of 24 and an apical heart rate of 90 are within normal limits. (20:287)
> Nursing Process—Implementation
> Client Need—Physiological integrity

65 2. The abbreviation *a.c.* means that a medication should be administered before meals. The abbreviation for a bedtime administration is *h.s.* If the physician wanted the drug administered with food, the abbreviation *p.c.*, which means *after meals*, is used. Administering a drug as necessary or as needed is indicated with the abbreviation *p.r.n.* (4:407)
> Nursing Process—Implementation
> Client Need—Physiological integrity

66 1. Asking open-ended questions encourages the client to elaborate, which eventually may relieve emotional tension. The best approach is to listen actively, remain nonjudgmental, and avoid offering any personal opinions. Asking a client a "why" question is often nontherapeutic, because the client may not be consciously aware of what is motivating his feelings or behavior. Telling the client that his physician believes he is doing fine implies that his fears are unfounded. A nonempathetic response may cause the client to terminate further discussion. Giving advice, as in "You need to concentrate on getting well," also is nontherapeutic because it blocks continued communication on the subject. (23:87; 25:79)
> Nursing Process—Implementation
> Client Need—Psychosocial integrity

67 1. One tablespoon of catsup contains 156 mg of sodium. Its use is generally omitted on a sodium-controlled diet. Vinegar, onions, and lemons are used freely by a person on a low-calorie, low-fat, low-sodium diet. (6:544)
> Nursing Process—Evaluation
> Client Need—Health promotion/maintenance

68 2. Straining involves holding one's breath and bearing down against a closed glottis. This action, sometimes called Valsalva's maneuver, increases abdominal and arterial pressure. The increase in arterial pressure acts as resistance to the pumping action of the heart. The flow of blood through the coronary arteries is temporarily reduced, causing ischemia and chest pain. If the wall of the heart is necrotic, the increase in pressure could cause the weakened muscle to rupture, and the client could hemorrhage to death. Stool softeners generally are ordered prophylactically to eliminate straining when having a stool. Reading a murder mystery and playing solitaire are passive activities that ought not to affect the cardiovascular system. People who experience heart attacks participate in their own self-care provided that they do not develop signs of activity intolerance. Signs that indicate that the client should rest include becoming short of breath, developing a rapid or irregular heart rate, and experiencing increased blood pressure. (18:1116; 21:380)
> Nursing Process—Implementation
> Client Need—Health promotion/maintenance

69 2. An echocardiogram uses ultrasonic (sound) waves to image the heart's structure. The sound waves are reflected back in various ways, depending on the density of the tissues, to produce a replication of the heart that is later evaluated. An x-ray uses radiation. An EKG picks up electric activity from the heart muscle. Thermography tests sense heat and variations in temperature to formulate images from body structures. (21:342)
> Nursing Process—Evaluation
> Client Need—Safe, effective care environment

NURSING CARE OF CLIENTS WITH CONGESTIVE HEART FAILURE

70 2. Early left-sided congestive heart failure is manifested by dyspnea and fatigue. Other classic signs and symptoms include a moist cough, orthopnea, tachycardia, restlessness, and confusion. (18:1111; 21:414)
> Nursing Process—Data collection
> Client Need—Safe, effective care environment

71 3. A complication of congestive heart failure is pulmonary edema. In this condition, fluid occupies space within the small airways. As air is moved through the fluid-filled airways, the examiner is likely to hear crackles, also called rales. Crackles are high-pitched sounds heard in distant lung areas during inspiration. Some compare this abnormal sound to that made by a popular rice cereal as it comes in contact with milk. (21:414)
> Nursing Process—Data collection
> Client Need—Physiological integrity

72 4. A client with dyspnea usually is most comfortable and has the least amount of difficulty with breathing when placed in either a semisitting (semi- or mid-Fowler's), sitting (high-Fowler's), or a standing position. Sitting and standing positions cause organs to fall away from the diaphragm, giving more room for the lungs to expand. (21:418)
> Nursing Process—Planning
> Client Need—Physiological integrity

73 2. People who are having difficulty breathing, a common symptom in left-sided congestive heart failure, typically feel anxious, apprehensive, and fearful. They are much less likely to feel depressed, apathetic, or stoic. (21:419–420)
Nursing Process—Data collection
Client Need—Psychosocial integrity

74 1. Oxygen is started before applying a mask to the client's face. Flooding the mask with oxygen provides a readily available supply for the client to begin breathing immediately. If the flow of oxygen is begun after the mask is in place, it can intensify the client's breathless feeling. Placing an oxygen mask on a client's face without simultaneously giving oxygen is likely to cause hypoxemia. (25:413)
Nursing Process—Implementation
Client Need—Physiological integrity

75 4. The correct volume needed to administer 80 mg of furosemide when the dosage strength is 40 mg/2 mL is 4 mL. A common formula to compute proper dosage is as follows: (20:36; 25:699)

$$\frac{\text{dosage desired}}{\text{dosage on hand}} \times \text{quantity}$$

$$= \text{amount to administer}$$

$$\frac{80 \text{ mg}}{40 \text{ mg}} \times 2 \text{ mL} = \frac{160}{40} = 4 \text{ mL}$$

Nursing Process—Implementation
Client Need—Physiological integrity

76 2. The best technique for bringing medication to the base of an ampule is to tap the stem several times with a fingernail. Allowing the ampule to stand, flipping it back and forth, or rolling the ampule does not bring medication trapped in the stem of an ampule into the base of the container. (25:728)
Nursing Process—Implementation
Client Need—Physiological integrity

77 3. An increase in urinary output indicates that the drug furosemide is achieving its desired effect. By eliminating excessive water from the blood volume, the work of the heart is reduced. Less fluid will accumulate in the lungs. Furosemide may lower the blood pressure due to the change in fluid volume. The pulse rate is not changed appreciably when furosemide is given. Once breathing is improved, anxiety is reduced. However, this is not the best evidence for assessing the effectiveness of furosemide. (20:308)
Nursing Process—Evaluation
Client Need—Physiological integrity

78 1. The presence of another person does much to relieve anxiety. This is especially true when a person perceives himself or herself in a helpless and powerless situation. It is essential that a fearful person is not left alone. The physician cannot do anything more than the nurse in this situation. Telling him he'll be OK is perhaps false reassurance because the outcome of his condition is not predictable. Recording the data can be postponed temporarily or reported verbally if it is needed. (23:290)
Nursing Process—Implementation
Client Need—Psychosocial integrity

79 3. It is essential that the nurse monitor the serum potassium level of clients for whom a loop diuretic, like furosemide, is prescribed. A loop diuretic increases the excretion of sodium, chloride, and potassium. Low levels of potassium can cause a disturbance in the conduction system of the heart. Many clients who take a loop diuretic replace the lost potassium by eating foods that contain appreciable amounts of this electrolyte, or potassium supplements are prescribed. (20:311)
Nursing Process—Data collection
Client Need—Physiological integrity

80 4. Significant weight gain or loss, such as a difference of 2 lb or more in 24 hours, indicates major changes in body fluid distribution. Weight gain indicates fluid retention and impaired renal excretion. Weight loss indicates a therapeutic response to medical and drug therapy. Pupil response, bowel sounds, and appetite are appropriate to monitor in the daily assessments, but congestive heart failure is not likely to cause major changes in these findings. (4:751; 26:147–148)
Nursing Process—Data collection
Client Need—Physiological integrity

81 2. Swelling of the feet and ankles accompanies right-sided congestive heart failure. Dependent edema occurs because the pumping action of the heart is impaired, decreasing blood flow to the kidneys. The combination of heart and kidney impairments causes fluid retention. Excess fluid builds up in the lower extremities and abdomen. Glucose in the urine is associated with diabetes mellitus. An irregular pulse is not unusual in an older adult, but its significance should be evaluated. A client with congestive heart failure may coincidentally be depressed. However, this is not a common finding among all people with congestive heart failure. (4:751; 26:147)
Nursing Process—Data collection
Client Need—Physiological integrity

82 1. If neck veins distend with the head elevated 45 degrees or more, it is an indication that an increased volume of blood is not being circulated well through the right side of the heart. Burning on urination is a symptom of a bladder infection or trauma to the urethra. Periodic constipation and chronic indigestion are due to any number of factors. They are not common findings associated with congestive heart failure. (4:751; 26:147)

    Nursing Process—Data collection
    Client Need—Physiological integrity

83 1. Gastrointestinal symptoms associated with digitalis toxicity include anorexia, nausea, vomiting, and diarrhea. The client may become drowsy and confused. There are visual changes, such as blurred vision, disturbance in seeing yellow and green colors, and a halo effect around dark objects. Toxic doses of digitalis drugs also can increase cardiac automaticity, causing a rapid heart rate, or depress the conduction of cardiac impulses, causing a slow heart rate. Serum drug levels are used to monitor the client's metabolism of digitalis. Pinpoint pupils are associated with opiate toxicity. Ringing in the ears is a symptom of salicylate toxicity. (20:255)

    Nursing Process—Data collection
    Client Need—Physiological integrity

84 1. Half of a 0.25-mg tablet is the correct amount of drug to administer to give 0.125 mg. The formula for determining the correct number of tablets is as follows: (20:36; 25:699)

$$\frac{\text{dosage desired}}{\text{dosage on hand}} \times \text{quantity}$$
$$= \text{amount to administer}$$

$$\frac{0.125 \text{ mg}}{0.25 \text{ mg}} \times 1 \text{ tablet} = \frac{0.125}{0.25} = 0.5 \text{ or } \tfrac{1}{2} \text{ tablet}$$

    Nursing Process—Implementation
    Client Need—Physiological integrity

85 1. Because digitalis preparations affect cardiac automaticity and the conduction system, it is essential that the nurse monitor the client's apical or radial pulse before each administration of the drug. Assessment of blood pressure, heart sounds, and lung sounds is part of a comprehensive cardiopulmonary assessment, but they are not directly affected by the administration of digitalis. (20:258)

    Nursing Process—Data collection
    Client Need—Physiological integrity

86 3. People on sodium-restricted diets may consume fresh vegetables or vegetables that are canned or frozen without salt. Canned and dehydrated soups contain between 630 and 1300 mg of sodium per cup. Pizza and other convenience foods have sodium added to the crust and sauce. Sodium also is present in the cheese topping. In addition, salt is used when preparing sausage. Smoked fish are salted prior to smoking to promote their preservation. (6:541–542)

    Nursing Process—Evaluation
    Client Need—Health promotion/maintenance

NURSING CARE OF CLIENTS WITH CONDUCTION DISORDERS

87 1. A Holter monitor is used to collect data on a person's heart rhythm patterns during normal daily activity. For an accurate interpretation, it is important to correlate the recorded data with the performance of physical activity. The client need not assess his radial pulse; the heart rate is determined from the rhythm strip. The client should not alter his usual activities of daily living to obtain pertinent data. There are no dietary restrictions when using a Holter monitor. (7:453; 21:342–343)

    Nursing Process—Implementation
    Client Need—Safe, effective care environment

88 3. Using electrical devices like electric razors and toothbrushes may alter the data being recorded with a Holter monitor. The other activities are not known to cause electrical interference with a Holter monitor. (7:454)

    Nursing Process—Implementation
    Client Need—Safe, effective care environment

89 4. The SA node is the site of the heart's natural pacemaker. The SA node is called the pacemaker of the heart because it creates the electric impulses that cause the heart to contract. This specialized tissue is located in the wall of the right atrium between the openings for the inferior and superior vena cavae. A properly functioning SA node initiates regular impulses at a rate of 60 to 100 beats per minute. Once an impulse is sent from the SA node, it then travels down several internodal pathways to the AV node, the Bundle of His, the right and left bundle branches, and the Purkinje fibers. (12:176–177; 21:337)

    Nursing Process—Evaluation
    Client Need—Health promotion/maintenance

90 4. A permanent pacemaker battery is usually implanted beneath the skin below the right clavicle. However, the area below the left clavicle sometimes is used. The wire for a temporary pacemaker is inserted through a peripheral vein. It is then threaded into the right atrium and the right ventricle. Pacemaker wires are placed during cardiac surgery in case a client needs pacing postoperatively.

The wires are seen externally from the skin on the chest. (21:398)
>Nursing Process—Data collection
>Client Need—Physiological integrity

91 2. If the artificial pacemaker does not support a heart rate sufficiently high enough to maintain an adequate cardiac output, the client feels dizzy and possibly faints. Tingling in the chest is unrelated to the artificial pacemaker. Pain that radiates to the arm is a symptom of angina pectoris or myocardial infarction. Tenderness may be caused by an infectious process. (21:401)
>Nursing Process—Implementation
>Client Need—Health promotion/maintenance

92 1. Cardioversion is similar to defibrillation. It involves administering a mild electric shock to the heart. Cardiac catheterization and angiography involve threading a catheter into the heart. Several types of cardiac imaging, such as multigated acquisition and thallium-201 scans, can be used to assess blood flow to the heart muscle. (4:736; 21:398–399)
>Nursing Process—Evaluation
>Client Need—Health promotion/maintenance

93 2. Digitalis and diuretics are withheld for 24 to 72 hours before elective cardioversion to avoid altering the ability to restore normal conduction. Diazepam is generally prescribed as a preprocedural sedative. There are no contraindications for administering cimetidine, a histamine antagonist, or glyburide, an oral hypoglycemic agent. (21:399)
>Nursing Process—Implementation
>Client Need—Physiological integrity

94 2. The purpose of cardioversion is to stop the rapid cardiac rhythm and reestablish the SA node as the pacemaker. If this occurs, the heart beats regularly between 60 to 100 beats per minute. Drugs such as diazepam (Valium) or midazolam (Versed) are used to produce conscious sedation. The client remains awake but usually has no memory of the experience. Equal apical and radial pulse rates are desirable, but this is not an indication of successful cardioversion. The normal difference between the systolic and diastolic blood pressures, also known as the pulse pressure, is approximately 40 mm Hg. Adequate cardiac output generally is reflected in a normal blood pressure measurement. However, the primary expected outcome of cardioversion is the restoration of normal cardiac rhythm. (21:399)
>Nursing Process—Evaluation
>Client Need—Physiological integrity

NURSING CARE OF CLIENTS WITH VALVULAR DISORDERS

95 3. Rheumatic fever often causes permanent damage to the heart and valves. About half who had rheumatic fever have narrowed mitral valves. Varicella, rubella, and whooping cough are acute infections, but they are not known to cause damage to heart valves. Intrauterine rubella infection causes congenital heart defects, deafness, blindness, and mental retardation. (18:884; 21:363)
>Nursing Process—Data collection
>Client Need—Health promotion/maintenance

96 2. The mitral valve is an atrioventricular valve. It is located between the left atrium and left ventricle. The pulmonic valve is between the right ventricle and the pulmonary artery. The tricuspid valve is between the right atrium and right ventricle. The aortic valve is located between the left ventricle and the aorta. (12:174; 21:365)
>Nursing Process—Implementation
>Client Need—Health promotion/maintenance

97 1. The sound from the mitral valve is best heard by auscultating the apical area, which is at the fifth intercostal space in the left midclavicular line. When assessing heart sounds, the auscultatory areas are not directly over the anatomic locations of the heart valves. The aortic valve is best heard at the second intercostal space to the right of the sternum. The pulmonic valve is best heard at the second intercostal space to the left of the sternum. The tricuspid valve is best heard at the fourth intercostal space to the left of the sternum. (25:186–187)
>Nursing Process—Data collection
>Client Need—Physiological integrity

98 4. A daily maintenance dose of penicillin, like nafcillin sodium, is prescribed for some people with a history of rheumatic heart disease, to prevent future streptococcal infections. Subsequent streptococcal infections continue to damage the heart. If daily doses of antibiotic are not taken, they are prescribed before oral surgery, tooth extractions, or other invasive procedures are performed. Nafcillin sodium will not destroy a virus, reduce scar tissue, or stop blood clots from forming. (18:1113; 21:366)
>Nursing Process—Implementation
>Client Need—Health promotion/maintenance

99 1. To maintain adequate perfusion of all the cells in the body during any open heart surgery, blood is oxygenated and circulated by cardiopulmonary bypass using a heart-lung machine. A mitral commissurotomy is a procedure in which the surgeon blindly inserts a finger into the narrowed valve and dilates the opening. When a mitral commissurotomy is performed, the damaged valve is not replaced. Porcine (pork) valves and mechanical valves are used for replacing diseased valvular tissue. (21:427)

> Nursing Process—Evaluation
> Client Need—Safe, effective care environment

100 3. Clubbing of the fingertips is a physical change that occurs after years of poor oxygenation. It is found in people with long-term cardiopulmonary diseases. As the name suggests, the fingertips appear like clubs; they are wider than normal at the distal end. The angle at the base of the nail is greater than the normal 160 degrees. A deviated nasal septum is most often congenital or caused by trauma. Flushed facial skin is seen in people who are feverish, have hypertension, or excess blood volume. A hoarse voice is symptomatic of diseased or inflamed vocal cords. (4:525; 25:189–190)

> Nursing Process—Data collection
> Client Need—Physiological integrity

101 2. Providing rest between periods of routine nursing care measures such as bathing, oral hygiene, and ambulation, helps clients adapt to activity intolerance. Administering oxygen is appropriate to prevent hypoxemia, but it does not reduce energy expenditure. Analgesic medications do relieve pain, but they do not relieve shortness of breath. Visitors are likely to tire a client, but since most clients benefit from the emotional support of significant others, it is not the first intervention to use to reduce the expenditure of energy. (21:269)

> Nursing Process—Planning
> Client Need—Physiological integrity

102 3. Evidence of activity intolerance includes rapid or irregular heart rate, hypotension, chest pain, dyspnea, and severe fatigue. If any of these are noted, the nurse is correct in limiting any further activity. An improved appetite, restful sleep, and an interest in further activity are all positive signs, but they are not appropriate physiologic criteria of a person's ability to tolerate activity. (25:492)

> Nursing Process—Data collection
> Client Need—Physiological integrity

103 3. When a person is emotionally upset, it is most therapeutic to allow an opportunity to express feelings. Saying nothing or leaving the room are of little help because these actions do not provide any support. The client, in this case, is not unhappy with the food. Rather, he is displacing his anger and frustration onto an inanimate object. Finding out a food

preference avoids dealing with the emotional issues. (26:154)

> Nursing Process—Implementation
> Client Need—Psychosocial integrity

NURSING CARE OF CLIENTS WITH INFECTIOUS AND INFLAMMATORY DISORDERS OF THE HEART

104 3. A fever is one of the classic ways that the body fights an infection. An elevated body temperature tends to destroy or inhibit the growth and reproduction of microorganisms. Chemicals present in white blood cells, which fight infection, trigger a heat-producing response in the hypothalamus. Chest pain usually is caused by inadequate blood supply to the myocardium. Pneumonia is more likely to cause a moist cough. Dyspnea is a common finding in many cardiopulmonary diseases. (18:77–78; 25:132, 144)

> Nursing Process—Data collection
> Client Need—Physiological integrity

105 2. To enhance the ability to hear auscultated sounds, it is best to reduce or eliminate sources of noise in the room. The humidifier attached to the flow meter of the oxygen is likely to cause extra noise, which may interfere with identifying normal and abnormal sounds. Holding the breath may aggravate a client's already compromised ventilation. Giving sips of water and locating the xiphoid will not promote the auscultation of heart or lung sounds. (18:172)

> Nursing Process—Data collection
> Client Need—Physiological integrity

106 3. A pericardial friction rub is a grating or leathery sound most often heard in people with pericarditis. It is caused by two layers of tissue moving roughly over one another. Wheezes and gurgles are evidence of pulmonary problems, such as asthma or pneumonia. A clicking sound is associated with pathology of the cardiac valves. A murmur is an abnormal sound made by the turbulent flow of blood through narrow or incompetent valves. (4:760; 21:353)

> Nursing Process—Data collection
> Client Need—Physiological integrity

107 1. Fainting indicates that the volume of blood ejected from the left ventricle is inadequate to keep the brain oxygenated. Reduced stroke volume also is manifested by hypotension, tachycardia, and a weak pulse. (21:354–355)

> Nursing Process—Data collection
> Client Need—Physiological integrity

108   2. Sucking on hard, sour candy facilitates the production of saliva that keeps the mouth moist and promotes the perception that thirst is quenched. Chilling fluids increases pleasure when consuming oral fluids, but it does not alleviate thirst. Clients may consider pureed food unpalatable; the same moisture is present in the food whether pureed or not. Ice chips are not given liberally to clients on fluid restrictions. The ice is calculated within the restricted volume of fluid. (21:355)

Nursing Process—Planning
Client Need—Physiological integrity

The Nursing Care of Clients with Cardiac Disorders

Directions: After each question, the correct answer is given as well as a classification of each test question. Compare the correct answer with your answer. If a question has been answered *incorrectly*, draw a line to the end of all the columns. When finished, add up the number of your correct answers in each column and place that number in the respective box at the end in the area identified as *Number Correct.*

To determine the percentage of questions you answered correctly and your performance in each of the test plan categories, divide the *Number Correct* in each column by the *Number Possible* in each column. Then multiply the decimal by 100. For example:

$$\frac{\text{Number Correct: } 88}{\text{Number Possible: } 108} = 0.814 \times 100 = 81\%$$

Any score that is less than 75% indicates an area where further review would be beneficial.

KEY TO ITEM CLASSIFICATION:

NURSING PROCESS

D = Data collection
P = Planning
I = Implementation
E = Evaluation

CLIENT NEEDS

S = Safe, effective care environment
P = Physiological integrity
M = Psychosocial integrity
H = Health promotion/maintenance

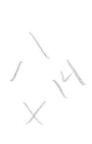

Question #	Answer #	Nursing Process				Client Needs			
		D	P	I	E	S	P	M	H
1	4		P				P		
2	2	D							H
3	2			I					H
4	3			I					H
5	1	D					P		
6	4			I					H
7	3	D					P		
8	1				E				H
9	2			I					H
10	3			I					H
11	4	D							H
12	2			I					H
13	3			I					H
14	3			I					H
15	1				E				H

Question #	Answer #	Nursing Process				Client Needs			
		D	P	I	E	S	P	M	H
16	1			I					H
17	2	D					P		
18	2	D					P		
19	1				E				H
20	3				E		P		
21	3				E				H
22	4				E				H
23	3			I					H
24	4	D					P		
25	2			I				M	
26	4				E				H
27	3	D				S			
28	1			I			P		
29	1		P				P		
30	1				E				H
31	2			I					H
32	4	D					P		
33	2			I					H
34	4			I			P		
35	4			I		S			
36	1				E	S			
37	2	D					P		
38	1			I					H
39	3			I		S			
40	2				E		P		
41	1	D					P		
42	4	D					P		
43	4	D					P		
44	4	D					P		
45	4		P				P		
46	3			I				M	
47	4	D							H

Question #	Answer #	Nursing Process				Client Needs			
		D	P	I	E	S	P	M	H
48	3	D					P		
49	1			I					H
50	3		P				P		
51	3		P				P		
52	1	D					P		
53	3			I			P		
54	2			I			P		
55	3	D					P		
56	3			I			P		
57	1			I			P		
58	4			I			P		
59	2			I			P		
60	3				E		P		
61	2			I			P		
62	2			I				M	
63	1			I			P		
64	4			I			P		
65	2			I			P		
66	1			I				M	
67	1				E				H
68	2			I					H
69	2				E	S			
70	2	D				S			
71	3	D					P		
72	4		P				P		
73	2	D						M	
74	1			I			P		
75	4			I			P		
76	2			I			P		
77	3				E		P		
78	1			I				M	
79	3	D					P		

Question #	Answer #	Nursing Process				Client Needs			
		D	P	I	E	S	P	M	H
80	4	D					P		
81	2	D					P		
82	1	D					P		
83	1	D					P		
84	1			I			P		
85	1	D					P		
86	3				E				H
87	1			I		S			
88	3			I		S			
89	4				E				H
90	4	D					P		
91	2			I					H
92	1				E				H
93	2			I			P		
94	2				E		P		
95	3	D							H
96	2			I					H
97	1	D					P		
98	4			I					H
99	1				E	S			
100	3	D					P		
101	2		P				P		
102	3	D					P		
103	3			I				M	
104	3	D					P		
105	2	D					P		
106	3	D					P		
107	1	D					P		
108	2		P				P		
Number Correct	96	33	6	40	17	8	52	7	29
Number Possible	108	36	8	45	19	9	59	7	33

8   3 2 5 2 1 7 88 100 4

89 %   92 75 89 89 89 88 88

Question #	Answer #	Nursing Process				Client Needs			
		D	P	I	E	S	P	M	H
Percentage Correct									

The Nursing Care of Clients with Endocrine Disorders

Nursing Care of Clients with Disorders of the Pituitary Gland

Nursing Care of Clients with Disorders of the Thyroid Gland

Nursing Care of Clients with Disorders of the Parathyroid Glands

Nursing Care of Clients with Disorders of the Adrenal Glands

Nursing Care of Clients with Pancreatic Endocrine Disorders

Correct Answers and Rationale

Classification of Test Items

Directions: With a pencil, blacken the circle in front of the option you have chosen for your correct answer.

NURSING CARE OF CLIENTS WITH DISORDERS OF THE PITUITARY GLAND

Following head trauma, a female client develops signs and symptoms of diabetes insipidus.

1 When the nurse assesses the client, which finding is *most characteristic* of this client's disorder?
- ○ 1. Polyphagia
- ◉ 2. Polyuria
- ○ 3. Glycosuria
- ○ 4. Hyperglycemia

2 The urine that the nurse collects for a routine urinalysis is *most likely* to appear
- ○ 1. dark amber.
- ○ 2. pale yellow.
- ◉ 3. colorless.
- ○ 4. light green.

3 When the nurse adds to the plan of care for the client with diabetes insipidus, which one of the following is *essential* for monitoring the client's condition?
- ◉ 1. Measuring intake and output
- ○ 2. Measuring blood glucose levels
- ○ 3. Counting caloric intake
- ○ 4. Assessing vital signs

The care plan of the client with diabetes insipidus indicates that the client must be weighed each day.

4 When directing the nursing assistant to weigh the client, which instruction is *most important* for obtaining accurate data?
- ○ 1. Have the patient stand on a scale at the bedside.
- ◉ 2. Weigh the client at the same time as on previous days.
- ○ 3. Ask the client to remove her slippers when weighed.
- ○ 4. Ask the client to identify her predisease weight.

The client with diabetes insipidus is treated with intranasal lypressin (Diapid), 2 sprays q.i.d. and p.r.n.

5 When the nurse observes the client self-administer her medication, which action indicates that the client is performing the procedure correctly?
- ○ 1. The client assumes a supine position.
- ○ 2. The client tilts her head to the side.
- ○ 3. The client inverts the drug container.
- ◉ 4. The client inhales with each spray.

6 If the client experiences any of the following, which one is the *best* indication that the client should self-administer a *p.r.n.* dose of lypressin?
- ◉ 1. Increased thirst
- ○ 2. Onset of headache
- ○ 3. Abdominal cramping
- ○ 4. Frequent stools

The cause of a male client's visual problems is determined to be just one of many signs and symptoms he is manifesting as a result of acromegaly.

7 Which finding is the nurse most likely to acquire when performing a physical assessment of the client with acromegaly?
- ○ 1. Exceptional height
- ◉ 2. Enlarged hands
- ○ 3. Gonadal atrophy
- ○ 4. Loss of teeth

8 When the nursing team develops the plan for this client's care, which problem is this client *most likely* to manifest?
○ 1. Activity intolerance
○ 2. Diminished intelligence
○ 3. Ineffective breathing
○ 4. Impaired swallowing

The client with acromegaly will undergo a transsphenoidal hypophysectomy after a short course of therapy with bromocriptine (Parlodel).

9 Since bromocriptine may cause postural hypotension, which one of the following nursing instructions is *most appropriate?*
○ 1. Lay down for ½ hour after taking bromocriptine.
○ 2. Avoid taking elevators in tall buildings.
○ 3. Rise slowly from a sitting or lying position.
○ 4. Have your blood pressure taken once a week.

10 Which one of the following statements indicates that the client has *misunderstood* the expected outcome of his surgery?
○ 1. The client says that his appearance will gradually become normal.
○ 2. The client says that he will need to take replacement hormones.
○ 3. The client says that he will need to see his physician regularly.
○ 4. The client says that the surgical incision will be inconspicuous.

11 Immediately after surgery, where is the *best* location for assessing for bleeding?
○ 1. The skull
○ 2. The pharynx
○ 3. Behind the ear
○ 4. Above the eyelid

NURSING CARE OF CLIENTS WITH DISORDERS OF THE THYROID GLAND

A 35-year-old female is undergoing tests to determine why she has stopped menstruating. One of the tests that the client undergoes is a radioactive iodine uptake test.

12 When the test is completed, which of the nurse's statements is *accurate?*
○ 1. You must remain isolated until your radiation is decreased.
○ 2. You are free to go since the amount of radiation is harmless.
○ 3. You must follow special urine precautions for a short time.
○ 4. You will be given an antidote for reducing the radioactivity.

The results of the diagnostic tests confirms that the client has myxedema.

13 In addition to amenorrhea, which other sign of myxedema is the nurse likely to observe when assessing the client with myxedema?
○ 1. The client's voice is hoarse.
○ 2. The client's skin is oily.
○ 3. The client is quite thin.
○ 4. The client is very restless.

14 When conducting a nursing history, which one of the following subjective symptoms is the client likely to describe?
○ 1. Difficulty in urinating
○ 2. Intolerance to cold
○ 3. Profuse perspiration
○ 4. Excessive appetite

The client with myxedema is treated with levothyroxine (Synthroid), one tablet, q.d.

15 Which one of the following statements is the *best evidence* that the client with myxedema understands her drug therapy?
○ 1. The client says she must take this drug after each meal.
○ 2. The client says she should avoid driving if sleepy.
○ 3. The client says she must take this drug for life.
○ 4. The client says she can skip a dose if she is nauseous.

A client makes an appointment with a physician because she has noticed an area of fullness in her neck. The physician diagnoses the problem as an endemic (colloid or simple) goiter.

16 To prevent this condition from developing in other family members, the nurse is *accurate* in recommending that their diet include
○ 1. green leafy vegetables.
○ 2. iodized table salt.
○ 3. whole grains.
○ 4. citrus fruits.

17 When the nurse reads the medical history of the client with an endemic (colloid or simple) goiter, which one of the following is this client *most likely* to have experienced?
○ 1. Gradual weight loss
○ 2. Slight hand tremors
○ 3. Trouble swallowing
○ 4. Sparse hair loss

A female client is undergoing treatment for Graves disease (thyrotoxicosis or toxic diffuse goiter).

18 When the nurse assesses the client with Graves disease, which is the nurse *most likely* to find?

○ 1. Bulging eyes
○ 2. Bulbous nose
○ 3. Thick lips
○ 4. Large tongue

The physician considers treating the client with Graves disease with propylthiouracil (Propyl-Thyracil).

19 Before the client obtains the drug prescription, it is *essential* for the nurse to ask if the client
○ 1. has trouble swallowing.
○ 2. prefers a liquid form.
○ 3. has digestive disorders.
○ 4. might be pregnant now.

20 Since propylthiouracil can cause agranulocytosis, it is *essential* that the nurse inform the client to report having
○ 1. persistent sore throat.
○ 2. occasional heart palpitations.
○ 3. intolerance to fatty foods.
○ 4. prolonged bleeding with trauma.

A subtotal thyroidectomy is planned for a client with Graves' disease that has induced a euthyroid state. One of the prescribed preoperative drugs is strong iodine solution (Lugol's solution), 4 gtt, p.o., for 10 days.

21 When the nurse instructs the client on how to self-administer the strong iodine solution, which of the following directions is *best*?
○ 1. Swallow the drug quickly.
○ 2. Take the drug before meals.
○ 3. Dilute the drug in fruit juice.
○ 4. Chill the drug before taking it.

22 The *best answer* when the client asks the nurse to explain the purpose for the preoperative drug therapy is that it
○ 1. firms the gland so it is easily removed.
○ 2. decreases the postoperative recovery time.
○ 3. decreases the risk of postoperative bleeding.
○ 4. eliminates the need for hormone replacement.

23 Preoperatively, which of the following is *most important* for the nurse to teach the client who will be undergoing a subtotal thyroidectomy?
○ 1. The techniques for changing positions
○ 2. The reasons for performing leg exercises
○ 3. The purpose for measuring intake and output
○ 4. The schedule at which food will be offered

24 To prepare for potential postoperative complications, it is *most appropriate* for the nurse to place which item in the room of the client undergoing a subtotal thyroidectomy?
○ 1. A dressing change kit
○ 2. A tracheostomy tray

○ 3. An ampule of epinephrine
○ 4. A mechanical ventilator

The client returns in stable condition to the nursing unit after having a subtotal thyroidectomy.

25 In which position is it *most appropriate* to maintain the client following a subtotal thyroidectomy?
○ 1. Supine
○ 2. Sims
○ 3. Fowler's
○ 4. Recumbent

26 Postoperatively, it is *most important* for the nurse to consult with the physician before encouraging the client with the subtotal thyroidectomy to
○ 1. Routinely cough
○ 2. Deep breathe
○ 3. Ambulate
○ 4. Dangle

27 Which nursing order is *best* to add to the plan of care for monitoring incisional bleeding on the client who had a subtotal thyroidectomy?
○ 1. Pass a flashlight across the incisional dressing.
○ 2. Feel for dampness at the back of the client's neck.
○ 3. Remove the dressing to directly inspect the wound.
○ 4. Weigh all gauze dressings before and after changing.

28 Which assessment technique is *best* for checking the postoperative thyroidectomy client for laryngeal nerve damage?
○ 1. Auscultate lung sounds.
○ 2. Observe the client swallow.
○ 3. Look for tracheal deviation.
○ 4. Ask the client to say "ah."

29 Which one of the following statements made by the client following a subtotal thyroidectomy is *most indicative* that the client is experiencing hypocalcemia?
○ 1. "I don't have much of an appetite."
○ 2. "My lips feel numb and tingly."
○ 3. "Light seems to bother my eyes."
○ 4. "I feel so weak when I ambulate."

The care plan indicates that the nurse should assess for Chvostek's sign if hypocalcemia is suspected.

30 Which technique *best describes* how Chvostek's sign is elicited?
○ 1. The nurse lightly taps over the client's facial nerve.
○ 2. The nurse strokes the sole of the client's foot.
○ 3. The nurse dorsiflexes each of the client's feet.
○ 4. The nurse asks the client to touch her nose.

31 Which sign, if manifested, is *most indicative* that the postoperative thyroidectomy client is developing thyroid crisis (thyrotoxic crisis or thyroid storm)?
- ○ 1. The client develops a very high fever.
- ● 2. The client's blood pressure falls severely.
- ○ 3. The client's respirations become noisy.
- ○ 4. The client experiences hand spasms.

NURSING CARE OF CLIENTS WITH DISORDERS OF THE PARATHYROID GLANDS

A client who develops a benign parathyroid tumor manifests signs of hyperparathyroidism.

32 When the nurse completes the nursing history, which one of the following data is most associated with the client's diagnosis?
- ○ 1. The client experiences nightly leg cramps.
- ● 2. The client recently passed a kidney stone.
- ○ 3. The client usually has loose bowel movements.
- ○ 4. The client has difficulty falling asleep.

The nursing assistant assigned to care for the client with the parathyroid tumor asks why the care plan indicates that the client is at risk for injury.

33 The *best explanation* from the nurse is that a consequence of hyperparathyroidism is
- ○ 1. inability to maintain balance.
- ○ 2. the risk of developing seizures.
- ○ 3. fainting when changing positions.
- ● 4. pathologic bone fractures.

The client with the parathyroid tumor has three of the four lobes of the parathyroid gland surgically removed.

34 After the client with the parathyroid tumor returns from surgery and resumes eating, which one of the following food groups is it *most appropriate* for the nurse to encourage?
- ○ 1. Bread and cereals
- ● 2. Milk and cheese
- ○ 3. Meat and seafood
- ○ 4. Fruit and vegetables

A client with hypoparathyroidism develops tetany.

35 If all of the following emergency drugs are available, which one can the nurse expect the physician will order for intravenous administration?
- ● 1. Calcium gluconate
- ○ 2. Ferrous sulfate
- ○ 3. Potassium chloride
- ○ 4. Sodium bicarbonate

NURSING CARE OF CLIENTS WITH DISORDERS OF THE ADRENAL GLANDS

The nurse cares for a client with Addison's disease.

36 When the nurse assesses the client with Addison's disease, which finding is *most characteristic* of this adrenal disorder?
- ○ 1. Enlarged abdomen
- ○ 2. Skin blemishes
- ○ 3. Moon-shaped face
- ● 4. Bronzed skin

37 Which one of the following nursing assessments is most helpful in evaluating the status of a client with Addison's disease?
- ● 1. Blood pressure
- ○ 2. Bowel sounds
- ○ 3. Lung sounds
- ○ 4. Heart sounds

The care plan of the client with Addison's disease indicates that the client should be assisted to select foods that are good sources of sodium.

38 If all the following are available, it is *best* for the nurse to recommend that the client select
- ○ 1. graham crackers.
- ● 2. cheddar cheese.
- ○ 3. raw carrots.
- ○ 4. canned peaches.

The client with Addison's disease has recurrent episodes of hypoglycemia.

39 If a regular diet is ordered, which between-meal snack is *best* for the nurse to provide to regulate the client's blood sugar?
- ● 1. Lemonade and peanuts
- ○ 2. Cola and potato chips
- ○ 3. Coffee and a muffin
- ○ 4. Milk and crackers

40 Which of the following is the nurse *most accurate* in teaching the client to avoid since it predisposes to the development of a life-threatening condition called Addisonian crisis?
- ● 1. Stress-producing situations
- ○ 2. Consuming alcoholic beverages
- ○ 3. Eating complex carbohydrates
- ○ 4. Getting too little sleep

A 38-year-old female client develops signs and symptoms that resemble Cushing's syndrome.

41 When the initial physical assessment is performed, which one of the following is the nurse *most likely* to observe?

1. The client has very thin legs.
2. The client looks emaciated.
3. The client has bulging eyes.
4. The client's skin is pale.

The physician orders a 24-hour urine collection to aid in the diagnosis.

42 The nurse is *most accurate* in instructing the client that the urine collection will begin
    1. with the client's next voiding.
    2. after the client's next voiding.
    3. at midnight.
    4. at noontime.

43 When the nurse collects the urine for the 24-hour specimen, which action is *most correct?*
    1. The volume of each voiding is measured and recorded.
    2. The urine is placed in a container of preservative.
    3. Each voiding is taken immediately to the laboratory.
    4. The client voids directly into the specimen container.

The nursing team discusses the nursing problems of the client with Cushing's syndrome and adds **Possible Disturbance in Body Image** *to the list.*

44 The *best rationale* for adding this nursing diagnosis to the care plan is that female clients with Cushing's syndrome
    1. develop masculine characteristics.
    2. experience heavy menstrual flow.
    3. suffer from severe dysmenorrhea.
    4. develop large pendulous breasts.

Diagnostic tests confirm that the client's adrenal glands are producing excessive amounts of adrenocortical hormones.

45 When the nurse reinforces the physician's explanation of the disorder to the client's spouse, it is *accurate* to stress that the client also is likely to experience
    1. anxiety and occasional panic attacks.
    2. depression and suicidal tendencies.
    3. impulsivity and poor self-control.
    4. forgetfulness and memory changes.

The client with Cushing's syndrome is placed on a low-sodium diet.

46 Which daily nursing assessment will provide the *best data* for monitoring the client's therapeutic response to restricting dietary sodium?

1. Monitoring percent eaten
2. Measuring abdominal girth
3. Assessing skin integrity
4. Weighing the client

47 Which nursing intervention is *most appropriate* for managing the basic care of the client with Cushing's syndrome?
    1. Applying an egg-crate mattress to the bed.
    2. Ambulating the client at frequent intervals.
    3. Reducing environmental stimuli like noise.
    4. Offering high carbohydrate nourishment.

Eventually the client with Cushing's syndrome undergoes bilateral adrenalectomy.

48 Which one of the following is the *best indication* that an adrenal (Addisonian) crisis is *not* occurring postoperatively?
    1. Urinary output is approximately 2000 mL/day.
    2. Pain is controlled at a tolerable level.
    3. Capillary blood sugar is within normal limits.
    4. Vital signs are within preoperative ranges.

49 Based on the fact that clients with Cushing's syndrome heal slowly, which one of the following nursing measures is *most appropriate* when caring for the client postoperatively?
    1. Ambulate with assistance.
    2. Remove tape toward incision.
    3. Increase dietary protein.
    4. Cover the wound with gauze.

50 Which one of the following statements is the *best evidence* that the client understands her postoperative course?
    1. "I should avoid people with infectious disorders."
    2. "I need to limit my fluid intake to 1 quart per day."
    3. "My appearance will never be the same as it was before."
    4. "No other treatment is necessary after I recover from surgery."

A client with pheochromocytoma, a tumor of the adrenal medulla, is scheduled to have the tumor surgically removed.

51 At the time of the admission assessment, which one of the following is the *most outstanding* sign that the nurse is likely to find?
    1. Hyperkalemia
    2. Hypertension
    3. Hyperinsulinism
    4. Hyperthermia

52 If all of the following are served on the dietary tray of the client with a pheochromocytoma, which one is *most appropriate* for the nurse to remove?
- ○ 1. Hot tea
- ○ 2. Ice water
- ○ 3. Skim milk
- ○ 4. Apple juice

NURSING CARE OF CLIENTS WITH PANCREATIC ENDOCRINE DISORDERS

A 23-year-old female manifests symptoms of hyperinsulinism, sometimes referred to as functional or reactive hypoglycemia.

53 When the nurse obtains a nursing history, the client is most likely to describe experiencing her symptoms
- ○ 1. when fasting more than 6 hours.
- ○ 2. 2 hours after eating a meal.
- ○ 3. late in the evening, before bedtime.
- ○ 4. early in the morning, before breakfast.

A 5-hour glucose tolerance test is ordered to determine if the client has functional hypoglycemia.

54 Which one of the following nursing statements concerning the test procedure is *most accurate*?
- ○ 1. You need to eat a large meal just before the test.
- ○ 2. Bring a voided urine specimen to the laboratory.
- ○ 3. You can have liquids, like coffee, before the test.
- ○ 4. You will be given a sweetened drink before the test.

55 To reduce or eliminate the symptoms the client with functional hypoglycemia experiences, it is *best* for the nurse to recommend eating five or six small meals containing
- ○ 1. simple sugars.
- ○ 2. complete proteins.
- ○ 3. complex carbohydrates.
- ○ 4. unsaturated fats.

56 The *best evidence* that the dietary measures to control functional hypoglycemia are therapeutic is that the client experiences fewer incidences of
- ○ 1. weakness and tremors.
- ○ 2. thirst and dry mouth.
- ○ 3. muscle spasms and fatigue.
- ○ 4. hunger and abdominal cramps.

A nurse participates in a community-wide screening to identify adults who may have undiagnosed diabetes mellitus.

57 If the screening includes a measurement of postprandial blood sugar, the nurse is *correct* in explaining that blood will be drawn approximately two hours

- ○ 1. before breakfast.
- ○ 2. after a meal.
- ○ 3. before bedtime.
- ○ 4. after a fast.

58 Which statement indicates that a client with an elevated 2-hour postprandial blood sugar understands the significance of the screening test?
- ○ 1. "I need to eat less frequently."
- ○ 2. "I need to stop eating candy."
- ○ 3. "I need to consult my physician."
- ○ 4. "I need to begin taking insulin."

59 Which signs and symptoms are *most appropriate* for the nurse to inquire about when screening adults who have come to have their blood sugar tested?
- ○ 1. Diarrhea, anorexia, and weight gain
- ○ 2. Constipation, weight loss, and thirst
- ○ 3. Polycholia, polyemia, and polyplegia
- ○ 4. Polyuria, polydipsia, and polyphagia

Further diagnostic tests confirm that one of the screened adults has Type II diabetes mellitus.

60 When the client demonstrates a shocked response to the news of her diagnosis, which nursing action is *best* at this time?
- ○ 1. Emphasize the importance of treatment.
- ○ 2. Offer assurance that injections are easy.
- ○ 3. Explain that many people live with diabetes.
- ○ 4. Listen as she expresses her current feelings.

The newly diagnosed client with Type II diabetes mellitus is referred to the diabetic clinic for teaching.

61 When the client asks the nurse why regular exercise is recommended for diabetics, the *best answer* in this client's case is that exercise tends to
- ○ 1. control weight gain.
- ○ 2. decrease the appetite.
- ○ 3. reduce the blood sugar.
- ○ 4. lower the heart rate.

A dietitian explains how to use the American Diabetes Association exchange list.

62 Which statement is the *best evidence* that the client understands the principle of an exchange list?
- ○ 1. The client says she can eat one serving from each category on the exchange list per day.
- ○ 2. The client says that measured amounts of food in each category are equal to one another.
- ○ 3. The client says that the number of servings from the exchange list are unlimited.
- ○ 4. The client says that she must use the exchange list to determine the nutrition in food.

63 When discussing *free foods*, those foods or beverages that can be consumed as often as the diabetic client wants, the client's understanding is accurate if he *excludes*
○ 1. Iced tea
○ 2. Mineral water
○ 3. Light beer
○ 4. Club soda

The physician prescribes glyburide (Diabeta) orally for the client with Type II diabetes mellitus.

64 When the client asks why his diabetic relative cannot take his insulin orally, the *best answer* is that insulin is
○ 1. inactivated by digestive enzymes.
○ 2. absorbed too quickly in the stomach.
○ 3. irritating to the gastric mucosa.
○ 4. incompatible with many foods.

65 Which one of the following is the nurse correct in telling the client who takes glyburide to avoid because it causes a drug-food interaction?
○ 1. Chocolate
○ 2. Pecans
○ 3. Yogurt
○ 4. Alcohol

66 When the client with Type II diabetes mellitus says he never eats breakfast, the *best* nursing response is
○ 1. "If you drink a glass of milk, it will be sufficient for breakfast."
○ 2. "You should eat each meal and between-meal snacks at a consistent time."
○ 3. "If you omit breakfast, eat a high-calorie snack at mid-morning."
○ 4. "Wait to take your medication until you eat your first meal of the day."

The physician wants the client with Type II diabetes mellitus to monitor his response to the therapeutic regimen.

67 If the client lives on a very limited income, which monitoring technique is the most economical for the nurse to recommend?
○ 1. Testing his urine with a chemical reagent strip.
○ 2. Using a glucometer to check capillary blood glucose.
○ 3. Having laboratory personnel draw venous blood samples.
○ 4. Arranging for testing by a home health agency nurse.

A lethargic and confused adult is brought to the emergency department by emergency medical personnel. The tentative diagnosis is insulin-dependent diabetes mellitus and diabetic ketoacidosis (DKA).

68 When the nurse assesses the client with DKA, which data are *most likely* to be found?
○ 1. The client is hypertensive and tachycardic.
○ 2. The client is dyspneic and hypotensive.
○ 3. The client breathes noisily and smells of acetone.
○ 4. The client stares blankly and smells of alcohol.

The nurse plans to monitor the client's response to insulin therapy closely with an electronic glucometer.

69 When the nurse monitors the client's blood sugar using an electronic glucometer, which action is *correct*?
○ 1. The nurse cleans the client's finger with povidone iodine (Betadine).
○ 2. The nurse applies a rubber band around the test finger.
○ 3. The nurse pierces the central pad of the client's finger.
○ 4. The nurse applies a large drop of blood to a test strip or area.

70 If the electronic glucometer indicates that the client's blood sugar is 58 mg/dL and he is shaky and dizzy, the best nursing action to take *next* is to
○ 1. administer the next scheduled dose of insulin.
○ 2. give the client some sweetened fruit juice.
○ 3. report the client's symptoms to the physician.
○ 4. perform a complete head-to-toe assessment.

The physician orders a sliding scale of regular insulin that is rapid-acting and has a short duration. The insulin dose varies according to the client's capillary blood sugar levels.

71 When the client receives a dose of regular insulin, the nurse is correct in *initially* assessing for signs of hypoglycemia approximately
○ 1. 5 minutes later.
○ 2. 30 minutes later.
○ 3. 6 hours later.
○ 4. 10 hours later.

The insulin-dependent diabetic must learn to combine two insulins, regular- and intermediate-acting, and self-administer the injection before being discharged.

72 Which of the following actions *best indicates* that the client needs more practice in combining two insulins in one syringe?
○ 1. The client rolls the vial of intermediate-acting insulin to mix it with its additive.
○ 2. The client instills air into both the fast-acting and intermediate-acting insulin vials.
○ 3. The client instills the intermediate-acting insulin into the vial of rapid-acting insulin.
○ 4. The client inverts each vial prior to withdrawing the specified amount of insulin.

73 When the client practices self-administration of the insulin, which action is *correct*?
○ 1. The client pierces the skin at a 30-degree angle.
○ 2. The client uses a syringe calibrated in minims.
○ 3. The client uses a 2-inch needle on the syringe.
● 4. The client rotates the sites of each injection.

The nurse implements a diabetic teaching plan in anticipation of the client's future discharge.

74 Which statement indicates that the client has *misunderstood* the nurse's teaching?
○ 1. The client says he may need more insulin during times of stress.
○ 2. The client says he may need more food when exercising strenuously.
○ 3. The client says his insulin needs may change as he gets older.
● 4. The client says his dependence on insulin may cease eventually.

75 When asked how to store insulin, the best answer the nurse can give is that insulin is always administered at room temperature, but it can be stored
○ 1. in an unheated oven close to body temperature.
● 2. in any cool place or in the refrigerator.
○ 3. at any temperature.
○ 4. in a home freezer.

The nurse stresses foot care as a component of the diabetic teaching.

76 If the nurse provides all of the following information, which one is *least correct*?
○ 1. "Inspect your feet daily."
● 2. "Soak your feet each day."
○ 3. "Wear shoes when not sleeping."
○ 4. "See a podiatrist for foot care."

After three months, the client returns for a follow-up appointment with his physician to evaluate his self-care.

77 Which of the following data is *best* for evaluating the client's compliance with the prescribed therapy?
○ 1. The client is asked to identify his dose and frequency of insulin administration.
● 2. The client is asked to share his glucose monitoring records for the past week.

○ 3. The client is weighed and his vital signs are taken before the office interview.
○ 4. The client is asked to share symptoms that he has experienced in the past month.

78 Which one of the following laboratory test results is *best* for the nurse to monitor to determine how effectively the client's diabetes is being managed?
○ 1. Fasting blood sugar
○ 2. Blood chemistry profile
○ 3. Complete blood count
● 4. Glycosylated hemoglobin

An insulin-dependent diabetic client discusses managing his disorder with a continuous insulin infusion pump.

79 If asked where the insulin infusion is administered, the nurse is *most accurate* in telling the client that the infusion site is generally
○ 1. in a vein within the nondominant hand.
○ 2. in the muscular tissue of the thigh.
● 3. in the subcutaneous tissue of the abdomen below the belt line.
○ 4. in an implanted intravenous catheter threaded into the neck.

The nurse cares for an older male client who is insulin-dependent and in a nursing home.

80 When developing the client's plan of care, which nursing order is *most appropriate* to add?
○ 1. Encourage use of electric razor.
● 2. File rather than cut toenails.
○ 3. Provide mouth care twice a day.
○ 4. Use deodorant soap for bathing.

81 Which one of the following signs is *most suggestive* that a Type II non–insulin-dependent diabetic is developing hyperglycemic hyperosmolar nonketotic syndrome (HHNS)?
○ 1. The client's blood sugar is 200 mg/dL.
● 2. The client urinates copious amounts.
○ 3. The client's skin is warm and dry.
○ 4. The client's urine contains acetone.

82 When the client asks about the long-term effects of diabetes mellitus, the nurse is accurate in mentioning all of the following complications *except*
○ 1. blindness.
● 2. stroke.
○ 3. renal failure.
○ 4. liver failure.

Directions: Two numbers appear in parentheses following each rationale. The first number identifies the textbook listed in the references, page 512, and the second number identifies the page(s) in that textbook on which the correct answer can be verified. Occasionally two or more textbooks are given to verify the correct answer.

NURSING CARE OF CLIENTS WITH DISORDERS OF THE PITUITARY GLAND

1 2. Clients with diabetes insipidus may excrete as much as 20 L of urine a day. They also experience polydipsia, or intense thirst. Polyphagia (increased appetite) is not a characteristic of this disorder, nor is glycosuria or hyperglycemia. (18:1057; 21:776)
Nursing Process—Data collection
Client Need—Physiological integrity

2 3. The urine of someone with diabetes insipidus is so dilute that it appears colorless. Dark urine indicates that the urine contains a large amount of urobilin in relation to the volume of water. Normal urine appears pale yellow. Light green urine might be caused by the excretion of chemical dyes that are used as urinary antiseptics or that are present in the coating of certain drugs. (21:776)
Nursing Process—Data collection
Client Need—Physiological integrity

3 1. To prevent dehydration, it is essential to replace fluids according to the deficit that exists between the client's intake and output. Glucose metabolism is unaffected in diabetes insipidus. Clients with diabetes insipidus might not eat well because they are constantly drinking, but maintaining an adequate fluid volume is the primary concern. Vital signs are important to assess, but nursing care is inadequate if intake and output is not monitored. (4:948; 21:776)
Nursing Process—Planning
Client Need—Physiological integrity

4 2. For the sake of comparison, clients are weighed at the same time each day, on the same scale, and wearing similar clothing each time. In this situation, the data does not indicate that a standing scale has been used nor that the client did not wear slippers during previous weight assessments. The predisease weight has no relationship to this client's pres-

ent condition except as a point of reference. (18:447; 21:341)
Nursing Process—Implementation
Client Need—Safe, effective care environment

5 4. When lypressin is administered, the client's head and body should be upright. The tip of the container is inserted upright into a nostril. The client then inhales as the container is compressed. (20:347; 28:659)
Nursing Process—Evaluation
Client Need—Health promotion/maintenance

6 1. The need to administer additional doses of lypressin is based on increased thirst and frequency of urination. If more than the prescribed number of doses is required, the intervals between the routinely scheduled drugs are decreased rather than altering the number of sprays. (20:347; 28:659)
Nursing Process—Data collection
Client Need—Physiological integrity

7 2. Acromegaly results from an overproduction of growth hormone. When the pathology occurs in adults, the bones of the hands, jaw, feet, and forehead enlarge, but they do not lengthen. If the condition occurs at or before puberty, it generally causes gigantism. Males with acromegaly are likely to experience impotence, but their testes are not unusually small. There may be wide spaces between the teeth due to the jaw changes, but acromegaly is not known to cause tooth loss. (4:945; 21:775)
Nursing Process—Data collection
Client Need—Physiological integrity

8 1. Despite the client's size, he or she is likely to experience muscle weakness, joint pain, and joint stiffness. Cognitive functions are not affected unless there is metastatic disease involving the cortex. Pulmonary functions remain adequate. Clients with acromegaly have difficulty chewing due to the malformations in their jaw and teeth, but swallowing is unaffected. (4:946)

> Nursing Process—Planning
> Client Need—Physiological integrity

9 3. Dizziness may be experienced when the blood pressure falls due to rapid positional changes. Lying down after taking the medication and avoiding heights will not prevent postural hypotension. It is appropriate to have the blood pressure monitored, but the assessment is performed first in a supine position and then in an upright position, which this option does not specify. (28:184)

> Nursing Process—Implementation
> Client Need—Health promotion/maintenance

10 1. Unfortunately, the client's appearance will never change despite successful treatment of the disease. Hormone replacement therapy is necessary following surgery or irradiation of the anterior pituitary gland. The client should wear a medical alert tag and see his or her physician regularly. The surgical incision is made through the nose and is not visible. (4:945; 18:1057)

> Nursing Process—Evaluation
> Client Need—Health promotion/maintenance

11 2. The surgical incision is made through the upper gingival mucosa, along one side of the nasal septum, and through the sphenoid sinus. The nose is packed with gauze postoperatively. In addition to checking the saturation and appearance of the gauze packing, the nurse inspects the pharynx where blood or cerebrospinal fluid may drain posteriorly. (27:493)

> Nursing Process—Data collection
> Client Need—Physiological integrity

NURSING CARE OF CLIENTS WITH DISORDERS OF THE THYROID GLAND

12 2. The amount of radiation that is used in a radioactive iodine uptake test is minute and harmless. There is no justification for isolating the client. There is no antidote for the radioactive iodine. Despite the fact that the urine may emit radioactivity, special urine precautions are unnecessary. (7:680)

> Nursing Process—Implementation
> Client Need—Health promotion/maintenance

13 1. Signs of myxedema include a hoarse voice, slow speech, lethargy, expressionless face, protruding tongue, coarse and sparse hair, weight gain, and dry skin. (21:779)

> Nursing Process—Data collection
> Client Need—Physiological integrity

14 2. Due to the lowered rate of metabolism, individuals with myxedema are not able to produce the same amount of energy and body heat as others with normal metabolism. The disorder is not associated with difficulty in urination, profuse perspiration, or an excessive appetite. (21:779)

> Nursing Process—Data collection
> Client Need—Physiological integrity

15 3. Thyroid replacement therapy is maintained during the course of a client's lifetime. The drug is prescribed once a day. Consequently, it is incorrect to take a dose before each meal. Levothyroxine is more likely to cause insomnia that fatigue or sleepiness. The physician is consulted before the medication is omitted or discontinued for any reason. (28:636)

> Nursing Process—Evaluation
> Client Need—Health promotion/maintenance

16 2. One of the causes of endemic (colloid or simple) goiter is a deficiency of iodine in the diet. One method of ensuring an adequate supply of iodine is to use iodized rather than plain table salt. Leafy vegetables, whole grains, or citrus fruits are not good sources of iodine. (18:1062; 21:781)

> Nursing Process—Implementation
> Client Need—Health promotion/maintenance

17 3. An endemic (colloid or simple) goiter is not likely to cause any symptoms unless it becomes so large as to create pressure on the airway or esophagus. Weight is not affected by the disorder. Hand tremors are a sign of toxic goiter (Graves disease). Sparse loss of hair is a characteristic of myxedema. (18:1062; 21:781)

> Nursing Process—Data collection
> Client Need—Physiological integrity

18 1. Exophthalmos, enlarged eyes, is a common assessment finding among clients with Graves disease (toxic diffuse goiter). The facial features described in the other options, if they are present, are not directly related to this thyroid disorder. (18:1058; 21:778)

> Nursing Process—Data collection
> Client Need—Physiological integrity

19 4. Antithyroid drugs, like propylthiouracil, can cause cretinism (hypothyroidism) in a developing fetus. Although the client may have trouble swallowing and the drug may cause gastrointestinal side effects, the information is not more essential to the safety of client or fetus. Propylthiouracil is not available in a liquid form, but the client may be instructed to crush the tablet and mix it with food. (17:556; 28:950–951)

Nursing Process—Data collection
Client Need—Physiological integrity

20 1. A sore throat, fever, and malaise may indicate that the client has insufficient white blood cells to prevent infections. Heart palpitations, a symptom of Graves disease, becomes infrequent as treatment with propylthiouracil continues. The client may experience nausea, vomiting, and epigastric distress, but these symptoms may occur regardless of ingesting any particular food. Thrombocytopenia is evidenced by prolonged bleeding, but this is not a sign of agranulocytosis. (17:556; 20:360)

Nursing Process—Implementation
Client Need—Health promotion/maintenance

21 3. Diluting the strong iodine solution in fruit juice or water tends to disguise its unpleasant taste. Although swallowing the drug quickly may ensure that all of the drug is taken, it is not the best instruction. There is no real reason to recommend chilling the drug or taking it before meals. (20:362)

Nursing Process—Implementation
Client Need—Health promotion/maintenance

22 3. Preoperative therapy with antithyroid drugs reduces the potential for postoperative bleeding and developing thyroid crisis or storm. The size of the gland is reduced, but that is not the underlying purpose for antithyroid drug therapy. The postoperative recovery period is shortened if complications are prevented, but reducing the potential for bleeding is a more specific answer. Thyroid replacement therapy may still be required after a subtotal thyroidectomy despite preoperative antithyroid drug therapy. (20:362)

Nursing Process—Implementation
Client Need—Health promotion/maintenance

23 1. Preoperative instructions must include how to support the head and neck when turning or rising to a sitting or standing position. The other information is important to include, but it is not information that will necessarily affect the client's comfort or safety as much as learning how to support the head and neck. (4:952)

Nursing Process—Implementation
Client Need—Health promotion/maintenance

24 2. Airway obstruction is a potential postoperative complication for clients who undergo thyroidectomy. Therefore, a common standard of practice is to keep a tracheostomy tray in the client's room. A mechanical ventilator probably will be unnecessary once airway patency is reestablished. A dressing change kit can be easily obtained and is not an emergency item. Epinephrine may be necessary if the client develops a life-threatening cardiac dysrhythmia, but this drug is usually stocked in emergency carts. (26:488)

Nursing Process—Planning
Client Need—Physiological integrity

25 3. A semi-Fowler's position with the head elevated 30 to 45 degrees is best for reducing postoperative incisional edema and facilitating ventilation. None of the other identified positions are therapeutic for accomplishing this goal. (4:953; 26:488)

Nursing Process—Planning
Client Need—Physiological integrity

26 1. Coughing may precipitate bleeding in and around the surgical area and increase the risk for airway obstruction. Therefore, if the physician has not specified otherwise, it is best to consult before encouraging the client to cough postoperatively. (4:952; 21:784)

Nursing Process—Implementation
Client Need—Physiological integrity

27 2. Gently passing the hand behind the client's neck and feeling for dampness determines if blood is oozing around to the back of the client's neck. The bed linen also is inspected for drainage each time the client is turned. (21:785)

Nursing Process—Planning
Client Need—Physiological integrity

28 4. Although hoarseness may be temporary after a subtotal thyroidectomy, laryngeal nerve damage is manifested by persistent voice changes or the inability to make vocal sound. None of the other assessment techniques are appropriate for assessing laryngeal nerve function. (4:953; 26:489)

Nursing Process—Planning
Client Need—Physiological integrity

29 2. Tingling and numbness around the mouth and extremities are symptoms of hypocalcemia. This often is the first symptom noted by the client. The remaining complaints listed in this question normally are not associated with hypocalcemia. (4:953; 21:784)

Nursing Process—Data collection
Client Need—Physiological integrity

30 1. If a client is hypocalcemic, the client will manifest Chvostek's sign, which consists of facial muscle spasms when the cheek over the facial nerve is tapped gently. Stroking the sole of the foot is a means of assessing the Babinski response. Homans' sign is assessed by dorsiflexing the foot. Closing the eyes and touching the nose is a method for testing proprioception, the ability to identify the location of a body part without looking at it. (4:953)

Nursing Process—Implementation
Client Need—Physiological integrity

31   1. Thyroid crisis is manifested by exaggerated signs of increased metabolism. Some signs include hyperpyrexia (fever), hypertension, and severe tachycardia. Carpal spasms are a sign of hypocalcemia. Noisy respirations may indicate laryngospasm due to hypocalcemia or a partial airway obstruction. Hypotension is not a sign of thyroid crisis. (4:953; 21:784)

Nursing Process—Data collection
Client Need—Physiological integrity

NURSING CARE OF CLIENTS WITH DISORDERS OF THE PARATHYROID GLANDS

32   2. A parathyroid tumor usually causes a loss of calcium from the bones to the blood. Hypercalcemia leads to the formation of kidney stones and other renal complications. Leg cramps are caused by hypocalcemia or other etiologies. Constipation is more common among clients with hyperparathyroidism. Insomnia is not commonly associated with hyperparathyroidism. (21:786)

Nursing Process—Data collection
Client Need—Physiological integrity

33   4. Loss of calcium from the bones weakens the skeletal system, which potentiates the risk of pathologic fractures. Impaired equilibrium, seizures, and syncope are not common among clients with hyperparathyroidism. (18:1062; 21:786)

Nursing Process—Implementation
Client Need—Safe, effective care environment

34   2. Postoperatively it is therapeutic to include sources of calcium in the diet because the function of the parathyroid gland is suddenly and severely compromised. Calcium gluconate for intravenous administration is given for hypocalcemia. (18:1062)

Nursing Process—Implementation
Client Need—Physiological integrity

35   1. Calcium gluconate or calcium chloride are the drugs of choice for intravenous administration when tetany occurs. Ferrous sulfate is a source of iron; it is administered orally. Potassium chloride is given to prevent or relieve hypokalemia. Sodium bicarbonate is administered to maintain normal acid-base balance. (4:959)

Nursing Process—Planning
Client Need—Physiological integrity

NURSING CARE OF CLIENTS WITH DISORDERS OF THE ADRENAL GLANDS

36   4. Clients with Addison's disease, which develops from adrenal insufficiency, appear unusually tan or darkly pigmented. A moon-shaped face, skin blemishes, and obesity are more characteristic of hyperfunction of the adrenal cortex or endogenous steroid therapy. (18:1063; 21:788)

Nursing Process—Data collection
Client Need—Physiological integrity

37   1. Addison's disease, if not adequately treated, leads to dehydration and hypotension. Monitoring the blood pressure and its subsequent trends provides one of the best data for evaluating the client's health status. Bowel, lung, and heart sounds are not generally abnormal in Addison's disease. (18:1063; 21:788)

Nursing Process—Data collection
Client Need—Physiological integrity

38   2. Milk products and other sources of animal protein are high in natural sodium content. Although baked goods also contain hidden sodium, 2 graham crackers have half the amount of sodium as 1 ounce of cheddar cheese. Fruits and vegetables are considered low in sodium when compared to other food sources. (6:203, 642, 660)

Nursing Process—Implementation
Client Need—Physiological integrity

39   4. Snacks like milk and crackers contain complex carbohydrates that take longer to metabolize than simple sugars. Therefore, they are more likely to help maintain a stable blood sugar level. To reduce episodes of hypoglycemia, it is appropriate to request at least six meals a day or between-meal snacks. Although the other choices do contain some complex carbohydrate, they also contain sources of quickly metabolized sugars. (21:790)

Nursing Process—Implementation
Client Need—Physiological integrity

40   1. Any of the following factors can overwhelm the ability of the client with Addison's disease to maintain homeostasis: extreme stress, salt deprivation, infection, trauma, exposure to cold, and overexertion. (21:789)

Nursing Process—Implementation
Client Need—Health promotion/maintenance

41   1. Muscle wasting and weakness; moon face; buffalo hump; ruddy face; thin, fragile skin; bruising; striae; peripheral edema; hypertension; hirsutism (females); mood changes; depression; and psychosis are examples of the signs and symptoms of Cush-

ing's syndrome. The remaining options usually are not associated with this disorder. (21:791)
Nursing Process—Data collection
Client Need—Physiological integrity

42 2. To be precise, a 24-hour urine collection begins after a client empties his or her bladder and ends with a final voiding at the same time a day later. (25:635)
Nursing Process—Implementation
Client Need—Safe, effective care environment

43 2. To avoid chemical changes in the contents of the urine, a 24-hour specimen is deposited in a container with preservative. The urine is generally stored under refrigeration or on ice during the collection period. It is not necessary to measure each voided volume; if this is done, it is for reasons other than specimen collection. Clients generally void into a urinal or bowl suspended in the toilet; the urine is then added to the collection container. (7:488; 25:635)
Nursing Process—Implementation
Client Need—Safe, effective care environment

44 1. Females with Cushing's syndrome acquire masculine characteristics such as excessive growth of body hair including facial hair. If premenopausal, they also may develop amenorrhea. Large breasts, heavy menstruation, and severe dysmenorrhea are not characteristics of Cushing's syndrome. (21:791)
Nursing Process—Implementation
Client Need—Safe, effective care environment

45 2. Depression is very common among clients with Cushing's syndrome and there is an accompanying potential for suicide. The other emotional symptoms are not associated with this endocrine disorder, although they may occur randomly in clients with this disorder for other psychophysiological reasons. (4:961; 21:791)
Nursing Process—Implementation
Client Need—Health promotion/maintenance

46 4. A sodium-restricted diet is prescribed to reduce the potential for fluid volume excess and increased serum sodium levels. One of the best data to monitor is the client's trend in daily weight. Skin turgor and abdominal girth are not likely to change as much as the client's weight from one day to the next. Monitoring the percent the client consumes from the dietary tray is appropriate to document, but it is not as objective an assessment as the daily weight. (4:962; 21:792)
Nursing Process—Evaluation
Client Need—Physiological integrity

47 1. Clients with Cushing's syndrome have thin, fragile skin that is susceptible to the effects of prolonged pressure. Therefore, it is appropriate to exercise gentleness when turning and repositioning the client and to use pressure-relieving devices like an egg-crate mattress. The client needs rest more than activity to accommodate for weakness and fatigue. Controlling environmental stimuli is not more important for this client than for any other. Carbohydrate intake is limited due to the tendency for clients with Cushing's syndrome to be hyperglycemic. (4:961–962)
Nursing Process—Implementation
Client Need—Physiological integrity

48 4. Addisonian crisis, which occurs from a sudden drop in adrenocortical hormones, is evidenced by extreme hypotension, fever, vomiting, diarrhea, abdominal pain, profound weakness, headache, and restlessness. An adequate urinary output, normal blood sugar, and comfort are all positive outcomes of nursing care, but they are not the best evidence that Addisonian crisis has been prevented. (21:789; 26:491)
Nursing Process—Evaluation
Client Need—Physiological integrity

49 2. To prevent separation of the incision, tape is pulled toward the suture line rather than away from it. Protein promotes healing, but this dietary measure, ambulating the client with assistance, and covering the wound are not as important to healing as is preventing physical trauma. (25:272; 26:491)
Nursing Process—Implementation
Client Need—Physiological integrity

50 1. Preoperatively and postoperatively, clients are at risk for acquiring infections due to the effects of corticosteroid hormones. Clients are at risk for fluid volume deficit and should maintain an adequate fluid intake. The client's Cushingoid appearance slowly recedes as hormone levels are reestablished at lower than preoperative levels. After a bilateral adrenalectomy, hormone replacement therapy is a lifelong necessity. In fact, a medical alert tag should be worn at all times. (26:492)
Nursing Process—Evaluation
Client Need—Health promotion/maintenance

51 2. The adrenal medulla secretes epinephrine and norepinephrine. A tumor involving the adrenal medulla produces signs of sympathetic nervous system stimulation such as severe hypertension, tachycardia, anxiety, insomnia, tremors, headache, and sweating. Hyperglycemia is more apt to occur than hyperinsulinism. There may be an intolerance to heat and diaphoresis, but body temperature is not extremely increased. Hyperkalemia is not associated with pheochromocytoma. (4:964; 21:790)

Nursing Process—Data collection
Client Need—Physiological integrity

52 1. Caffeine in any form—tea, coffee, cola—compounds systemic stimulation already manifested as a result of the pheochromocytoma. Ice water, skim milk, or apple juice are not as potentially dangerous for this client as caffeine. (4:964)

Nursing Process—Implementation
Client Need—Physiological integrity

NURSING CARE OF CLIENTS WITH PANCREATIC ENDOCRINE DISORDERS

53 2. Functional hypoglycemia is caused by an overproduction of insulin, which occurs about 2 hours after eating a meal, especially one that contains refined sugar or simple carbohydrates. (6:627)

Nursing Process—Data collection
Client Need—Physiological integrity

54 4. A container of 75 to 100 g of glucose is consumed orally, or administered intravenously, before the glucose tolerance test begins. The client fasts before and during the test. Only water is allowed during the test. Urine specimens are collected before the glucose is administered and when subsequent blood samples are taken. An adequate diet containing carbohydrates is eaten for at least 3 days before the diagnostic test, but the client fasts for 12 hours before the test. (7:424)

Nursing Process—Implementation
Client Need—Safe, effective care environment

55 3. To maintain stable blood sugar levels, it is best for clients with functional hypoglycemia to consume small, frequent meals that contain high-fiber complex carbohydrates. Some examples include fruits, vegetables, legumes, and whole grains. Simple sugars like glucose, fructose, and galactose tend to stimulate the release of insulin and lower the blood sugar drastically. Complete proteins and unsaturated fats in moderate amounts are components of a healthy diet, but they are not as therapeutic for stabilizing the blood sugar. (6:627)

Nursing Process—Implementation
Client Need—Health promotion/maintenance

56 1. If dietary measures are appropriate, clients experience fewer symptoms of hypoglycemia such as

weakness, tremors, headache, nausea, hunger, malaise, excess perspiration, confusion, and personality changes. (6:626; 21:805)

Nursing Process—Evaluation
Client Need—Health promotion/maintenance

57 2. The term *postprandial* means after eating a meal. The meal acts as a glucose challenge. There is normally an elevation in blood sugar in response to the intake of carbohydrate. Two hours later, the blood sugar of nondiabetics ought to have returned to normal. If the blood sugar is elevated two hours after eating, it suggests a metabolic disorder like diabetes mellitus. (7:416)

Nursing Process—Implementation
Client Need—Health promotion/maintenance

58 3. Positive screening test results are an indication that a person needs further evaluation by a physician. Several factors and disease pathologies can cause hyperglycemia. It is best to refer hyperglycemic individuals to a physician. (4:976)

Nursing Process—Evaluation
Client Need—Health promotion/maintenance

59 4. Polyuria (excessive secretion and voiding of urine), polydipsia (excessive thirst), and polyphagia (increased appetite) are the classic signs and symptoms of diabetes mellitus. Polycholia (increased secretion of bile), polyemia (increased amount of circulating blood), polyplegia (paralysis of several muscles), diarrhea, constipation, and anorexia are not considered signs and symptoms of this endocrine disorder. Weight gain or loss is seen in some people. (4:966; 21:800)

Nursing Process—Data collection
Client Need—Physiological integrity

60 4. Clients need time to accept their diagnosis and to talk about their fears and concerns. Stressing the importance of treatment is likely to increase a client's fears. The client with Type II diabetes may or may not be required to self-administer injections. Telling the client that others manage their diabetes ignores the fact that this disorder is unique to the newly diagnosed diabetic. (21:808)

Nursing Process—Implementation
Client Need—Psychosocial integrity

61 3. Exercise has many beneficial effects like controlling weight, reducing appetite, and lowering the heart rate, regardless of a person's health status. For the diabetic, one of the primary benefits is that the blood sugar is reduced. If the blood sugar is lowered with exercise, drug treatment with oral hypo-glycemic agents or insulin may be delayed, re-duced, or eliminated. (4:969; 18:1067)

Nursing Process—Implementation
Client Need—Health promotion/maintenance

62 2. The advantage of using an exchange list is that it eliminates the need to count calories. Instead, cli-ents are prescribed the number of exchanges they may use in particular categories. They can pick from among the items of equal nutritional value, provided they consume the size serving that the list specifies. (6:431)

Nursing Process—Evaluation
Client Need—Health promotion/maintenance

63 3. "Lite" or "light" is a food labeling term that means the product contains one-third fewer calories than a similar unaltered item. Thus, light beer does contain calories or grams of nutrients that must be calcu-lated in the diabetic's diet and exchange list. (6:441)

Nursing Process—Evaluation
Client Need—Health promotion/maintenance

64 1. Insulin is administered parenterally because it is a protein substance that is readily destroyed in the gastrointestinal tract. None of the other choices are accurate in describing the rationale for excluding insulin administration by the oral route. (20:328)

Nursing Process—Implementation
Client Need—Health promotion/maintenance

65 4. Clients who take glyburide and consume alcohol may have a "disulfiram (Antabuse) reaction." A re-action includes flushing, throbbing head pain, re-spiratory difficulty, nausea, vomiting, sweating, thirst, chest pain, palpitations, tachycardia, hypo-tension, syncope, blurred vision, and confusion. (17:567; 28:403)

Nursing Process—Implementation
Client Need—Health promotion/maintenance

66 2. To maintain stable control of blood sugar levels, it is essential to take medication, eat, and exercise at regular, consistent times each day. Implying that the therapeutic regimen is flexible predisposes cli-ents to develop unstable blood sugar levels and metabolic complications. (20:337)

Nursing Process—Implementation
Client Need—Health promotion/maintenance

67 1. Urine testing using reagent tablets or strips is the most economical of diabetic monitoring tech-niques. A home glucometer is more accurate and preferred for poorly controlled diabetics. Self-moni-toring with a glucometer is costly, but less expen-sive than the added charges for the services of labo-ratory personnel or a home health nurse. (4:969; 18:1075; 21:802)

Nursing Process—Implementation
Client Need—Safe, effective care environment

68 3. An acetone, sometimes described as sweet or "fruity," odor to the breath, weakness, thirst, an-orexia, vomiting, drowsiness, abdominal pain, rapid and weak pulse, hypotension, flushed skin, and Kussmaul respirations, which are rapid, deep, and noisy, are manifested by persons in DKA. In severe cases, the client may be comatose or semico-matose. (18:1071; 21:804)

Nursing Process—Data collection
Client Need—Physiological integrity

69 4. It is best to let the blood flow passively by gravity onto the test strip or reflecting area of the electronic glucometer. The skin usually is cleaned with soap and water. If alcohol is used, it is allowed to totally evaporate before obtaining the specimen. A rubber band is not applied. In fact, some recommend that the nurse avoid squeezing the tissue to promote bleeding. Piercing the central pad of a finger is avoided; the margin around the digit produces less pain. (25:216–220)

Nursing Process—Implementation
Client Need—Safe, effective care environment

70 2. A blood sugar below 70 mg/dL is a sign of hypogly-cemia. Assuming the glucometer reading is accurate and the client is symptomatic, the best action is to implement some means of increasing the client's blood sugar. This may be done with a variety of substances such as sweetened fruit juice, honey, hard candy, cake icing, and packets of granulated sugar. Parenterally administered glucose or gluca-gon is prescribed by the physician if the client is unresponsive. (20:338)

Nursing Process—Implementation
Client Need—Physiological integrity

71 2. Most rapid acting insulins, and regular in particular, have the onset of their action in 30 to 90 minutes after they have been administered. Hypoglycemia is even more likely to occur when insulin reaches its peak effect. For regular insulin, this is approxi-mately 2 to 5 hours later. The duration of regular insulin is approximately 8 hours. (18:1068; 20:327)

Nursing Process—Data collection
Client Need—Physiological integrity

72 3. Care is taken to avoid mixing the intermediate-acting insulin that contains an additive with the

additive-free insulin. The additive-free insulin is always withdrawn first. The actions described in the other options are safe and appropriate for mixing two different types of insulins. (17:570; 25:738)
Nursing Process—Evaluation
Client Need—Health promotion/maintenance

73 4. To prevent lipodystrophy and lipoatrophy and promote appropriate absorption of insulin, it is correct to rotate insulin injection sites. Insulin is prepared in an insulin syringe that is calibrated in units. The needle length is ½ to ⅝ inch. Insulin is injected at a 45-degree or 90-degree angle, depending on the size of the client. (4:971; 21:803)
Nursing Process—Evaluation
Client Need—Health promotion/maintenance

74 4. Insulin-dependent clients are likely to remain so for the rest of their lives. Even some Type II diabetics eventually become insulin-dependent. The client is correct in the fact that insulin needs increase during time of stress, such as during infections and emotional crises. Although exercise is beneficial, clients may need additional calories to prevent symptoms of hypoglycemia. (4:978; 18:1074–1077; 21:810)
Nursing Process—Evaluation
Client Need—Health promotion/maintenance

75 2. Insulin deteriorates if exposed to excessive heat or light. Insulin is kept at room temperature or stored in a cool area. Unopened vials may be kept refrigerated. Insulin is never frozen. (18:1067; 20:333)
Nursing Process—Implementation
Client Need—Health promotion/maintenance

76 2. Soaking the feet tends to soften the skin and predisposes to trauma. The feet are washed daily with soap and water, then dried thoroughly before donning clean socks and supportive shoes. Diabetics should inspect their feet daily for signs of injury or poor circulation. Going barefoot is contraindicated because it predisposes the client to foot injuries. (4:972; 18:1076)
Nursing Process—Implementation
Client Need—Health promotion/maintenance

77 2. The most objective evidence for evaluating how well the client is managing his therapy is a record of glucose monitoring values. Some glucometers store the data so that it can be retrieved and evaluated. Otherwise, clients keep a written record of their monitoring results. Identifying the dose and frequency of insulin administration does not indicate that the client is actually self-administering the insulin. Maintaining or gradually losing weight is

good evaluative data, but it is not as specific as glucose monitoring values. Some clients are not as self-aware of symptoms and some have an exaggerated awareness of their body functions. Therefore, subjective symptoms are valuable, but they are not as objective as hard data. (18:1074)
Nursing Process—Evaluation
Client Need—Health promotion/maintenance

78 4. A glycosylated hemoglobin test reveals the effectiveness of diabetic therapy for the preceding 8 to 12 weeks. A fasting blood sugar provides information on the blood sugar status for the immediate period of time. A blood chemistry includes a blood sugar measurement, but there are several additional diagnostic test results. A complete blood count indicates the status of the client's hematopoeitic functions. (4:976; 7:426–427)
Nursing Process—Evaluation
Client Need—Health promotion/maintenance

79 3. Continuous insulin infusions are administered by the subcutaneous route usually in tissue of the abdomen. However, any of the subcutaneous sites such as the buttocks, thighs, arms, and sections of the back may be used. An insulin infusion pump delivers regular insulin at a carefully regulated rate. Insulin is absorbed too quickly when instilled intravenously or intramuscularly. (4:971; 17:572–573)
Nursing Process—Implementation
Client Need—Health promotion/maintenance

80 2. The physician is consulted about trimming or cutting the toenails of diabetic clients. An abrasive file is used to keep the nails short, but it is best to refer diabetic clients to a podiatrist for nail maintenance or other foot problems. The other hygiene measures are good to implement, but they are not as pertinent to a diabetic's care. (4:972)
Nursing Process—Planning
Client Need—Physiological integrity

81 2. Hyperglycemic hyperosmolar nonketotic syndrome (HHNS) is characterized by extremely high blood sugar levels between 600 to 1000 mg/dL without signs of ketoacidosis. The severe hyperglycemia causes fluid to shift from the intracellular space to the extracellular space and copious amounts of urine are excreted. Warm dry skin is a normal finding. In HHNS, the skin is hot and dry from dehydration. Acetone is not present in the urine of clients experiencing HHNS as it is in ketoacidosis. (4:973; 18:1073)
Nursing Process—Data collection
Client Need—Physiological integrity

82 4. Diabetics are prone to many systemic vascular and neurological complications. They include a higher incidence for premature cataract formation, retinal hemorrhage and blindness, cerebrovascular accidents, myocardial infarctions, renal failure, peripheral neurovascular disease and amputations, and sexual dysfunction. Liver disease is atypical among clients with diabetes mellitus. (4:977)
   Nursing Process—Implementation
   Client Need—Health promotion/maintenance

Classification of Test Items

Unit I   Review Test 8

The Nursing Care of Clients with Endocrine Disorders

Directions: After each question, the correct answer is given as well as a classification of each test question. Compare the correct answer with your answer. If a question has been answered *incorrectly*, draw a line to the end of all the columns. When finished, add up the number of your correct answers in each column and place that number in the respective box at the end in the area identified as *Number Correct*.

To determine the percentage of questions you answered correctly and your performance in each of the test plan categories, divide the *Number Correct* in each column by the *Number Possible* in each column. Then multiply the decimal by 100. For example:

$$\frac{\text{Number Correct: } 65}{\text{Number Possible: } 82} = 0.792 \times 100 = 79\%$$

Any score that is less than 75% indicates an area where further review would be beneficial.

NURSING PROCESS

D = Data collection
P = Planning
I = Implementation
E = Evaluation

CLIENT NEEDS

S = Safe, effective care environment
P = Physiological integrity
M = Psychosocial integrity
H = Health promotion/maintenance

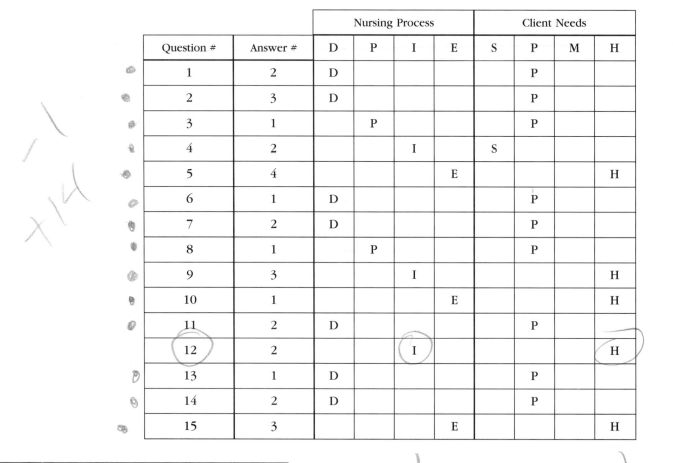

Question #	Answer #	Nursing Process				Client Needs			
		D	P	I	E	S	P	M	H
1	2	D					P		
2	3	D					P		
3	1		P				P		
4	2			I		S			
5	4				E				H
6	1	D					P		
7	2	D					P		
8	1		P				P		
9	3			I					H
10	1				E				H
11	2	D					P		
12	2			I					H
13	1	D					P		
14	2	D					P		
15	3				E				H

Parathyroid, Adrenal

Question #	Answer #	Nursing Process				Client Needs			
		D	P	I	E	S	P	M	H
16	2			I					H
17	3	D					P		
18	1	D					P		
19	4	D					P		
20	1			I					H
21	3			I					H
22	3			I					H
23	1			I					H
24	2		P				P		
25	3		P				P		
26	1			I			P		
27	2		P				P		
28	4		P				P		
29	2	D					P		
30	1			I			P		
31	1	D					P		
32	2	D					P		
33	4			I		S			
34	2			I			P		
35	1		P				P		
36	4	D					P		
37	1	D					P		
38	2			I			P		
39	4			I			P		
40	1			I					H
41	1	D					P		
42	2			I		S			
43	2			I		S			
44	1			I		S			
45	2			I					H
46	4				E		P		
47	1			I			P		

Question #	Answer #	Nursing Process				Client Needs			
		D	P	I	E	S	P	M	H
48	4				E		P		
49	2			I			P		
50	1				E				H
51	2	D					P		
52	1			I			P		
53	2	D					P		
54	4			I		S			
55	3			I					H
56	1				E				H
57	2			I					H
58	3				E				H
59	4	D					P		
60	4			I				M	
61	3			I					H
62	2				E				H
63	3				E				H
64	1			I					H
65	4			I					H
66	2			I					H
67	1			I		S			
68	3	D					P		
69	4			I		S			
70	2			I			P		
71	2	D					P		
72	3				E				H
73	4				E				H
74	4				E				H
75	2			I					H
76	2			I					H
77	2				E				H
78	4				E				H
79	3			I					H

Question #	Answer #	Nursing Process				Client Needs			
		D	P	I	E	S	P	M	H
80	2		P				P		
81	2	D					P		
82	4			I					H
Number Correct	67	19	8	27	13	5	36	1	25
Number Possible	82	22	8	37	15	8	41	1	32
Percentage Correct	82	86	100	73	87	63	88	100	78

−1

−15
+67

3   10   2   3   5   7

Directions: With a pencil, blacken the circle in front of the option you have chosen for your correct answer.

NURSING CARE OF CLIENTS WITH URINARY INCONTINENCE

1 The most important nursing assessment before beginning bladder retraining with an incontinent person is
- 1. recording the times at which he or she is incontinent.
- ○ 2. checking the specific gravity of the urine.
- ○ 3. monitoring the extent of bladder distention.
- ○ 4. observing the color of the client's urine.

Postpartum clients who have had vaginal deliveries are taught how to perform Kegel exercises to prevent future problems with urinary stress incontinence.

2 Which one of the following instructions is *correct* when the nurse teaches a client to perform Kegel exercises?
- 1. Contract and relax the muscles in the vagina.
- ○ 2. Stand and rock the pelvis back and forth.
- ○ 3. Push down with the feet and elevate the hips.
- ○ 4. Pull the abdominal muscles inward and ease off.

During bladder retraining, a client tells the nurse that he intends to restrict his intake of fluid to remain dry for longer periods of time.

3 The *best* response from the nurse in this situation is to
- ○ 1. encourage the practice because it shows evidence of client cooperation.
- ○ 2. encourage the practice because it leads to accomplishing the goal.
- ○ 3. discourage the practice because it contributes to constipation.
- 4. discourage the practice because it potentiates fluid imbalance.

An elderly nursing home resident who is incontinent of urine says, "What's the sense in living? I'm just a baby nowadays."

4 The *best* response the nurse can offer at this time is to say
- ○ 1. "You're a very nice gentleman."
- ○ 2. "Cheer up. You can't be serious."
- ○ 3. "You should expect this at your age."
- 4. "You're discouraged right now."

Following a stroke, the nursing team has been using an external catheter to prevent skin breakdown on an incontinent male client.

5 When applying an external catheter, which nursing action is *correct*?
- ○ 1. Lubricate the penis before applying the catheter.
- ○ 2. Measure the length and circumference of the penis.
- ○ 3. Leave space between the end of the penis and drainage end of the catheter.
- 4. Retract the foreskin before rolling the catheter sheath over the penis.

6 After inserting an indwelling catheter into a male client, which one of the following describes an appropriate technique for stabilizing the catheter to avoid a penoscrotal fistula?
- ○ 1. Tape the catheter to the abdomen.
- ○ 2. Pass the catheter under the client's leg.
- 3. Fasten the drainage tubing to the bed with a safety pin.
- ○ 4. Insert the catheter into the tubing of a collecting bag.

NURSING CARE OF CLIENTS WITH INFECTIOUS AND INFLAMMATORY UROLOGIC DISORDERS

A female with Type I diabetes mellitus consults a physician because she has been experiencing urinary symptoms.

7 When the nurse interviews the client, which symptom is the client *most likely* to report if she has a bladder infection?
   ○ 1. Sharp flank pain
   ○ 2. Urethral discharge
   ○ 3. Strong-smelling urine
   ◉ 4. Burning on urination

8 When the nurse instructs the client on the technique for collecting a clean-catch midstream urine specimen for routine urinalysis, which statement is *accurate*?
   ○ 1. Cleanse the urethral area using several circular motions.
   ○ 2. Void into the plastic liner that is under the toilet seat.
   ◉ 3. After voiding a small amount, collect a sample of urine.
   ○ 4. Mix the antiseptic solution with the collected urine specimen.

9 When the nurse reviews the results of the urinalysis, which finding is *most suggestive* that the client has a bladder infection?
   ○ 1. The urine contains glucose.
   ◉ 2. The urine contains blood.
   ○ 3. The urine contains bilirubin.
   ○ 4. The urine contains protein.

To relieve the client's symptoms, the physician orders phenazopyridine (Pyridium), a urinary analgesic.

10 It is *most appropriate* for the nurse to inform the client that this drug will cause the urine to
   ○ 1. look cloudy.
   ◉ 2. appear orange.
   ○ 3. become scant.
   ○ 4. smell strong.

11 Which of the following is the *best evidence* that the phenazopyridine (Pyridium) is achieving its intended therapeutic effect?
   ○ 1. The client indicates that her urinary frequency is decreased.
   ◉ 2. The client indicates that her urinary urgency is decreased.
   ○ 3. The client indicates that it burns less when she urinates.
   ○ 4. The client indicates that she is urinating greater volumes.

In addition to the phenazopyridine (Pyridium), the physician prescribes methenamine mandelate (Mandelamine).

12 It is *most appropriate* for the nurse to monitor the client for which *common* side effect while the client takes methenamine (Mandelamine)?
   ○ 1. Sensitivity to sunlight
   ○ 2. Shortness of breath
   ○ 3. Unusual thirst
   ◉ 4. Persistent nausea

13 Which nursing action is *best* for potentiating the therapeutic effect of methenamine mandelate (Mandelamine)?
   ○ 1. Encourage drinking citrus juices.
   ◉ 2. Encourage drinking cranberry juice.
   ○ 3. Encourage a diet high in dairy products.
   ○ 4. Encourage a diet high in whole grains.

14 When the client asks the nurse why women have so many more bladder infections than men, the *most accurate* answer is that
   ○ 1. the male urethra is straighter, which facilitates the elimination of pathogens.
   ○ 2. the male urethra is lined with a layer of mucous membrane, which traps microorganisms.
   ◉ 3. the female urethra is shorter, and pathogens enter the bladder more quickly.
   ○ 4. the female urethra has a larger diameter and is more easily contaminated.

15 Since this client also has diabetes mellitus, the nurse is *correct* in explaining that the client is at higher risk for acquiring a bladder infection because
   ◉ 1. glucose in urine supports bacterial growth.
   ○ 2. diabetes suppresses white blood cell activity.
   ○ 3. diet therapy may cause a deficiency of nutrients.
   ○ 4. there is less energy for attending to hygiene.

16 Which one of the following nursing instructions is *most effective* for this client to reduce the growth of bacteria in the bladder?
   ◉ 1. Drink a large quantity of fluid.
   ○ 2. Change underclothing each day.
   ○ 3. Avoid using public restrooms.
   ○ 4. Use only white toilet tissue.

17 If the client says she does all of the following, which one indicates the *best measure* for preventing cystitis?
   ◉ 1. She wipes away from the urinary meatus after bowel elimination.
   ○ 2. She performs appropriate handwashing after bowel elimination.
   ○ 3. She uses a feminine hygiene spray after bowel elimination.
   ○ 4. She dries the perineum thoroughly after bowel elimination.

A nurse makes an office appointment for a male client who describes having a slight tickling sensation during urination and a urethral discharge.

18 To facilitate obtaining truthful information regarding this client's sexual history, which one of the following attitudes is *most important* for the nurse to convey?
- ○ 1. Sympathetic
- ◉ 2. Nonjudgmental
- ○ 3. Encouraging
- ○ 4. Optimistic

19 When obtaining a sexual history from this client, which question is *most important* for the nurse to ask?
- ◉ 1. Have you ever had a painless sore on your penis?
- ○ 2. Does any sexual partner have similar symptoms?
- ○ 3. At what age did you first have intercourse?
- ○ 4. When did you last have sexual intercourse?

The physician informs the nurse that during the examination he will need to obtain a culture of urethral secretions.

20 While assisting the physician, in addition to furnishing a sterile swab and culture tube, it is *most important* for the nurse to provide the physician with
- ○ 1. antiseptic.
- ○ 2. lubricant.
- ○ 3. a mask.
- ◉ 4. gloves.

The culture indicates the client has nonspecific urethritis from a nongonococcal organism, Chlamydia trachomatis. *The physician prescribes doxycycline (Vibramycin) 100 mg b.i.d. with a sufficient number of capsules for 7 days of treatment.*

21 After the nurse calls the pharmacist, which of the following information is *most appropriate* to provide to the client?
- ○ 1. Take the medication until the symptoms clear.
- ○ 2. Refill the prescription if symptoms persist.
- ◉ 3. Take the medication for the full amount of time.
- ○ 4. Treatment of this infection is likely to be lifelong.

22 One of the *best methods* the nurse can stress to prevent a recurrence of the chlamydial infection is
- ○ 1. showering or bathing after intercourse.
- ○ 2. good handwashing with an antiseptic soap.
- ◉ 3. testing and treating sexual partners.
- ○ 4. adequate nutrition and fluid intake.

A female client becomes acutely ill with flank pain, fever, and chills. The physician makes a tentative diagnosis of acute pyelonephritis and orders a catheterized urine specimen for culture.

23 When preparing the client for catheterization, the *best plan* is to position the client in
- ○ 1. lithotomy position.
- ◉ 2. recumbent position.
- ○ 3. knee-chest position.
- ○ 4. prone position.

24 When the nurse inserts the catheter into the client's vagina rather than the urinary meatus, which action is *best* to take *next*?
- ○ 1. Wipe the catheter tip with an alcohol swab.
- ○ 2. Cleanse the catheter tip with Betadine solution.
- ◉ 3. Discard the catheter and use another sterile one.
- ○ 4. Withdraw the catheter and insert it in the urethra.

The physician prescribes a urinary anti-infective combination of trimethoprim and sulfamethoxazole (Bactrim) twice a day.

25 Which nursing instruction is *most appropriate* for preventing crystal formation in the urine?
- ○ 1. Eat more citrus fruits.
- ○ 2. Avoid carbonated drinks.
- ◉ 3. Drink 3 quarts of water per day.
- ○ 4. Take the drug with food.

The client who is being treated for pyelonephritis is scheduled for an intravenous pyelogram (IVP).

26 When the nurse prepares the client for the IVP, the *best explanation* for administering a laxative is that emptying the bowel
- ○ 1. also aids in examining the lower gastrointestinal tract.
- ○ 2. prevents accidental stool incontinence during the x-ray.
- ○ 3. reduces the potential for constipation or impaction.
- ◉ 4. improves the ability to visualize the urinary structures.

27 If the client mentions all of the following, which one is *most important* to report before the client has the intravenous pyelogram?
- ○ 1. "Strong laxatives cause me to have diarrhea."
- ○ 2. "I have a low pain tolerance during procedures."
- ◉ 3. "I had a reaction when my gallbladder was x-rayed."
- ○ 4. "My insurance company may require a second opinion."

Despite the fact that a middle-aged female's symptoms of malaise and headache are rather unremarkable, she is diagnosed with acute glomerulonephritis.

28 Which statement from the spouse correlates most with the client's diagnosis of acute glomerulonephritis?
- ● 1. "My wife's face looks rather puffy lately."
- ○ 2. "Recently my wife has been quite forgetful."
- ○ 3. "My wife has been salting her food heavily."
- ○ 4. "It seems that my wife sleeps quite poorly."

29 When the nurse reviews the medical history of the client with acute glomerulonephritis, which is *most likely* to have precipitated her present illness?
- ○ 1. Trauma to the lower abdomen
- ● 2. An upper respiratory infection
- ○ 3. Treatment with an antibiotic
- ○ 4. An allergic reaction to x-ray dye

30 If this client is similar to others with glomerulonephritis, which one of the following is the nurse *most likely* to observe when conducting a head-to-toe physical assessment?
- ○ 1. Skin hemorrhages
- ○ 2. Absence of body hair
- ○ 3. Flushed appearance
- ● 4. Peripheral edema

31 Which one of the following laboratory tests is *best* for the nurse to monitor when caring for a person with glomerulonephritis?
- ○ 1. Serum amylase
- ○ 2. Blood glucose
- ● 3. Blood urea nitrogen (BUN)
- ○ 4. Complete blood count (CBC)

32 Which one of the following nursing actions is *most important* when planning the care of a person with acute glomerulonephritis?
- ○ 1. Ambulate twice daily.
- ○ 2. Assist with mouth care.
- ● 3. Monitor weight daily.
- ○ 4. Encourage fluid intake.

33 When a client with glomerulonephritis complains of a headache, which nursing action is performed *first*?
- ○ 1. Administer a prescribed analgesic.
- ● 2. Assess the client's blood pressure.
- ○ 3. Reduce environmental stimuli.
- ○ 4. Change the client's position.

The nurse caring for the client with glomerulonephritis is told during the shift report that a 24-hour urine collection for creatinine clearance is to begin at 8 AM.

34 Which of the following actions is *correct* in relation to collecting the urine specimen?

- ○ 1. The nurse has the client void at 8 AM and refrigerates the specimen.
- ○ 2. The nurse has the client void at 8 AM and disposes of the specimen.
- ○ 3. The nurse has the client void at 8 AM and sends the specimen to the laboratory.
- ● 4. The nurse has the client void at 8 AM and places the specimen in preservative.

The nurse uses a color reagent strip (dipstick) to test a voided urine specimen.

35 If the reagent strip can detect all of the following, which one can the nurse expect to be present in the urine of a client with glomerulonephritis?
- ○ 1. Glucose
- ● 2. Bilirubin
- ○ 3. Albumin
- ○ 4. Acetone

36 When the nurse inspects the urine of a client with glomerulonephritis, which one of the following is *most suggestive* that the urine contains red blood cells?
- ○ 1. The urine appears cloudy.
- ○ 2. The urine appears smoky.
- ○ 3. The urine appears bright orange.
- ● 4. The urine appears dark yellow.

The client with glomerulonephritis is on a low-sodium diet.

37 Which one of the following menu choices is *best* for the nurse to recommend?
- ○ 1. Hot dog with potato salad
- ○ 2. Beef bouillon and crackers
- ● 3. Chicken breast on lettuce
- ○ 4. Cheese pizza with thin crust

The client with glomerulonephritis is being treated with the steroid methylprednisolone (Medrol) on alternate days by oral administration.

38 The *best* response when the client asks the nurse why this drug is not taken daily is that
- ○ 1. it is too toxic if taken on a daily basis.
- ○ 2. this schedule maintains adrenal function.
- ● 3. the drug has a prolonged period of action.
- ○ 4. most people cannot tolerate its side effects.

NURSING CARE OF CLIENTS WITH RENAL FAILURE

A client who has chronic glomerulonephritis has deteriorated to the point of being in the early stages of renal failure.

39 If this client is similar to others in the *oliguric phase* of renal failure, the nurse is *most likely* to find that the urine output is
- 1. between 50 and 100 mL per hour.
- 2. between 100 and 150 mL per hour.
- 3. between 500 and 1000 mL per day.
- 4. between 100 and 500 mL per day.

A team conference is held to discuss the care of the client in early renal failure.

40 Which one of the following nursing assessments is *essential* to add to this client's plan of care?
- 1. Monitoring body temperature
- 2. Measuring intake and output
- 3. Checking for urinary retention
- 4. Listening for bowel sounds

The physician orders a fluid challenge of 500 mL of intravenous fluid to be infused at a rapid rate, followed by the administration of a loop diuretic intravenously to sustain or improve renal function.

41 While the fluid is being administered, which one of the following is *most important* for the nurse to assess?
- 1. Pedal edema
- 2. Skin integrity
- 3. Oral mucosa
- 4. Lung sounds

42 Because of impaired urine elimination, which one of the following potential skin problems will require *additional* team planning?
- 1. Reduced perspiration
- 2. Extreme oiliness
- 3. Loss of skin turgor
- 4. Pronounced itching

The client in renal failure is on a sodium-restricted diet.

43 When the client complains about the bland taste of the food, which one of the following is *best* for the nurse to recommend *instead* of salt?
- 1. Catsup
- 2. Mustard
- 3. Soy sauce
- 4. Lemon juice

44 Which one of the following nursing actions is *most appropriate* when the client in renal failure complains about being thirsty due to fluid restrictions?
- 1. Give the client hard candy to suck.
- 2. Provide the client with ice chips.
- 3. Offer the client an ice cream bar.
- 4. Supply the client with fresh fruit.

The care plan indicates that the client in renal failure is to be weighed regularly.

45 Which one of the following factors in *most important* to consider when planning to weigh this client?
- 1. When the client has been weighed before
- 2. When the client last took a drink of fluid
- 3. How much the client has eaten so far today
- 4. Whether the client feels like being weighed

When it becomes evident that the client in renal failure will need long-term hemodialysis, an internal arteriovenous fistula is created.

46 Which one of the following assessments is *most important* for the nurse to perform regularly on the client with an arteriovenous fistula?
- 1. Check the color and temperature of the hand.
- 2. Monitor wrist and finger range of motion.
- 3. Observe tone and coordination of arm muscles.
- 4. Inspect forearm skin integrity and turgor.

47 Which nursing intervention is *most helpful* in assisting the client who undergoes hemodialysis cope with his chronic health condition?
- 1. Give the client literature to read about renal failure.
- 2. Advise the client's spouse to spend more time with him.
- 3. Keep the client informed of the latest research findings.
- 4. Explore with the client how this disorder has affected his life.

Another person with renal failure is treated with peritoneal dialysis.

48 Which pre- and post-assessment data is *most valuable* for evaluating the outcome of peritoneal dialysis?
- 1. Pulse rate
- 2. Body weight
- 3. Skin turgor
- 4. Urine output

49 Immediately after the dialysate solution has been instilled, which one of the following nursing actions is *correct*?
- 1. Clamp the tubing from the infusion.
- 2. Drain the infused dialysate solution.
- 3. Restrict movement as much as possible.
- 4. Encourage the client to drink fluids.

50 Which one of the following is the *most significant* information to report when caring for a client undergoing peritoneal dialysis?
   ○ 1. Loss of body weight
   ○ 2. Regular, deep breathing
   ● 3. Elevated body temperature
   ○ 4. Output that exceeds intake

51 Which one of the following findings is the *best evidence* that peritoneal dialysis is achieving a therapeutic effect?
   ○ 1. The client's urine output increases.
   ● 2. The client's appetite improves.
   ○ 3. The client's potassium level falls.
   ○ 4. The client's red cell count is lower.

A client with renal failure is a candidate for a kidney transplant.

52 When the client asks the source of donated kidneys, the nurse is most accurate in telling the client that the *preferred* donor is a(n)
   ○ 1. recently deceased human.
   ● 2. sibling or living relative.
   ○ 3. unrelated living human.
   ○ 4. chimpanzee or research animal.

NURSING CARE OF CLIENTS WITH UROLOGIC OBSTRUCTIONS

53 Which one of the following assessment findings is *most suggestive* that the etiology for a reduced volume of voided urine is due to an obstructive disorder?
   ● 1. The client feels a continued need to void.
   ○ 2. The client's urine appears dark amber.
   ○ 3. The client's bladder is below the pubis.
   ○ 4. The client experiences abdominal cramps.

54 If the physician inserts a suprapubic cystostomy tube to drain the accumulating urine, the nurse assesses the characteristics of urine from a catheter that exits from the
   ○ 1. urethra.
   ● 2. abdomen.
   ○ 3. ureter.
   ○ 4. flank.

55 If the written plan for managing the care of the client with a suprapubic catheter includes all of the following instructions, which one is *essential* for evaluating the patency of the catheter?
   ○ 1. Inspect the skin around the insertion site.
   ● 2. Monitor the urinary output every 2 hours.
   ○ 3. Attach the catheter to a leg bag when up.
   ○ 4. Encourage 100 mL of oral fluid hourly.

A client comes to the emergency department for relief from severe, stabbing, colicky flank pain. The physician makes a tentative diagnosis of urolithiasis.

56 When the nurse examines the voided urine specimen, which finding is *most supportive* of the diagnosis of urolithiasis?
   ○ 1. The urine appears cloudy.
   ● 2. The urine contains blood.
   ○ 3. The urine is light yellow.
   ○ 4. The urine has a strong odor.

A cystoscopy is scheduled for the client with possible urolithiasis.

57 After the cystoscopy, the nurse can expect the client to experience
   ○ 1. polyuria.
   ● 2. dysuria.
   ○ 3. anuria.
   ○ 4. pyuria.

58 Which one of the following nursing interventions is *most appropriate* to add to the care plan of the client with urolithiasis?
   ○ 1. Restrict fluids to 1000 mL/day.
   ○ 2. Maintain a Fowler's position.
   ○ 3. Limit activity to bed rest.
   ● 4. Strain all voided urine.

The client with urolithiasis is scheduled for extracorporeal shock wave lithotripsy (ESWL) to pulverize the stone.

59 Which statement is the *best evidence* that the client who will undergo ESWL understands the prospective procedure?
   ● 1. "I will be submerged in a tank of water."
   ○ 2. "Radiation will be blasted through my body."
   ○ 3. "A laser beam will be aimed at my kidneys."
   ○ 4. "I will experience a tingling sensation."

An older adult male makes an appointment with a physician concerning urinary symptoms he is experiencing.

60 When the office nurse obtains the client's history, which statement is the *best indication* that the client has benign prostatic hypertrophy (BPH)?
   ○ 1. "There is some burning when I urinate."
   ● 2. "I wake up nightly needing to urinate."
   ○ 3. "I feel pressure in my back before voiding."
   ○ 4. "My urine is almost colorless, like water."

61 To gather more information about symptoms associated with benign prostatic hypertrophy, which one of the following questions is *most important* for the nurse to ask *next*?
○ 1. "Have you noticed any changes in sexual function?"
○ 2. "Have you felt any lumps in your scrotum recently?"
◉ 3. "Do you have difficulty starting to void?"
○ 4. "Do you have problems controlling urination?"

An older male with a history of benign prostatic hypertrophy has been unable to urinate in 18 hours. The physician instructs the nurse to insert a urethral catheter.

62 Which one of the following techniques is *best* for helping the nurse insert the tip of the catheter past the enlarged prostate gland?
◉ 1. Angle the penis in the direction of the toes.
○ 2. Massage the tissue below the base of the penis.
○ 3. Push the catheter with additional force.
○ 4. Grasp the penis firmly within the hand.

The client with benign prostatic hypertrophy is scheduled to undergo a transurethral resection of the prostate (TURP).

63 Following the TURP, which one of the following findings can the nurse *most expect* to observe during the *immediate* postoperative period?
○ 1. The urine is light pink to clear.
○ 2. The urine contains mucoid sediment.
○ 3. The urine volume is decreased.
◉ 4. The urine appears grossly bloody.

The nurse is told in report that the client who had the TURP is to receive a continuous bladder irrigation through a three-way catheter.

64 Which one of the following will the nurse need to obtain when planning to implement this procedure?
◉ 1. An intravenous pole
○ 2. An Asepto (bulb) syringe
○ 3. A round sterile basin
○ 4. Antiseptic solution

Postoperatively, the client who is receiving continuous bladder irrigations tells the nurse that he is having a great deal of discomfort in the area of his bladder.

65 Before administering an analgesic, it is *most appropriate* for the nurse to assess that the
○ 1. client's pulse rate is normal.
○ 2. dressing is dry and intact.
◉ 3. catheter is draining well.
○ 4. client is coughing adequately.

The physician has written several analgesic drug orders for the client who has undergone a TURP.

66 Which one of the physician's drug orders is *most appropriate* for the nurse to implement if the client is having bladder spasms?
○ 1. Acetylsalicylic acid (aspirin) by mouth
○ 2. Propoxyphene napsylate (Darvocet) by mouth
○ 3. Meperidine hydrochloride (Demerol) intramuscularly
◉ 4. Belladonna and opium (B&O) rectal suppository

A nurse is assigned to care for a client following a suprapubic prostatectomy. The client has a catheter in the urethra and another in an abdominal incision.

67 When documenting the urinary output in the medical record, it is *most correct* for the nurse to record
○ 1. only the output from the urethral catheter.
○ 2. only the output from the wound catheter.
◉ 3. the output from each catheter separately.
○ 4. the combined output from both catheters.

Several days after a client has had a suprapubic prostatectomy, the physician removes the catheter from the abdominal incision.

68 Which one of the following nursing interventions is *most important* to add to the plan for care following the removal of the suprapubic catheter?
○ 1. Reposition the client every 2 hours.
○ 2. Ambulate the client with assistance.
◉ 3. Change abdominal dressing when wet.
○ 4. Encourage deep breathing hourly.

NURSING CARE OF CLIENTS WITH UROLOGIC TUMORS

A physician asks the office nurse to schedule a series of examinations and tests for a client to determine if he has cancer of the prostate gland.

69 If all of the following are ordered, which one should the nurse schedule *before* any manipulation of the prostate tissue to avoid erroneous test results?
○ 1. Kidneys, ureters, bladder (KUB) x-ray
○ 2. Needle biopsy of the prostate gland
◉ 3. Prostatic-specific antigen (PSA) test
○ 4. Transrectal ultrasound examination

The client who is diagnosed with prostatic cancer undergoes a radical perineal prostatectomy. Postoperatively the client has a Foley catheter.

70 When managing the care of the catheter, which nursing action is *most important* for promoting wound healing?
   ○ 1. Avoid tension on the catheter.
   ◉ 2. Encourage oral fluid intake.
   ○ 3. Cleanse the urethral meatus daily.
   ○ 4. Clamp and release the catheter q2h.

Postoperatively, the physician prescribes estradiol (Estrace) for the client with prostatic cancer.

71 Which statement is the *best evidence* that this client understands a potential side effect associated with his hormonal therapy?
   ◉ 1. The client says both of his breasts may enlarge.
   ○ 2. The client says he may have spontaneous erections.
   ○ 3. The client says his sperm count will be higher.
   ○ 4. The client says he will have strong sexual urges.

A nephrectomy is performed on a client with a kidney tumor.

72 Postoperatively, which assessment finding is *most suggestive* that the client with a nephrectomy is hemorrhaging?
   ◉ 1. The client develops sudden flank pain.
   ○ 2. The client's abdomen becomes distended.
   ○ 3. The client's skin is warm and flushed.
   ○ 4. The client becomes nauseated and vomits.

A nurse cares for a client with bladder cancer.

73 If this client is similar to others who acquire bladder cancer, which symptom is the client *most likely* to have manifested in the *early stage* of this disease?
   ○ 1. Difficulty voiding
   ○ 2. Persistent oliguria
   ◉ 3. Painless hematuria
   ○ 4. Urethral discharge

74 When asked about factors that are linked to causing cancerous changes in the bladder, the nurse is *most correct* in identifying which one of the following?
   ○ 1. Stress incontinence
   ○ 2. Frequent intercourse
   ○ 3. Sexual promiscuity
   ◉ 4. Cigarette smoking

The physician recommends that the client's bladder cancer be treated conservatively by instilling an antineoplastic drug within the bladder.

75 When administering the bladder instillation containing the chemotherapeutic drug, it is *most important*, in the interest of safety, for the nurse to
   ◉ 1. wear a double pair of latex gloves.
   ○ 2. use a glass syringe for the drug.
   ○ 3. avoid clothing with long sleeves.
   ○ 4. limit contact time with the client.

NURSING CARE OF CLIENTS WITH URINARY DIVERSIONS

A client whose bladder cancer has been unresponsive to treatment will have his bladder surgically removed and an ileal conduit will be created to facilitate urinary elimination.

76 When the client asks the nurse to clarify the surgeon's explanation of the procedure, which one of the following is *most correct*?
   ○ 1. Your urine will be deposited in your small intestine.
   ○ 2. Urine will be eliminated with stool from the rectum.
   ◉ 3. Urine will drain from an abdominal opening.
   ○ 4. Your urine will empty from a special catheter.

The night nurse reports that the preoperative client who will have the cystectomy and ileal conduit was awake much of the time. When he slept, he was restless.

77 Which one of the following assessments *most supports* that the client's sleep disturbance is due to anxiety?
   ○ 1. The client's temperature is 98.9°F (37.1°C).
   ○ 2. The client's blood pressure is 132/88 mm Hg.
   ◉ 3. The client's pulse is 106 beats per minute at rest.
   ○ 4. The client's pulse pressure is 44 mm Hg.

78 To facilitate coping, which nursing statement is the *most therapeutic* form of communication at this time?
   ◉ 1. "It must be difficult facing this type of surgery."
   ○ 2. "You have one of the best surgeons at this hospital."
   ○ 3. "You'll see; everything will turn out OK for you."
   ○ 4. "Others with your diagnosis have done just fine."

The client who will have the urinary diversion says, "Imagine being unable to control urination."

79 The *most therapeutic* response from the nurse is
- ● 1. "Tell me what that means to you."
- ○ 2. "I know just how you're feeling."
- ○ 3. "Well, it's not quite as bad as that."
- ○ 4. "You need to think more positively."

Postoperatively, the client with the ileal conduit wears an appliance that collects his urine. He tells the nurse that his skin feels raw and irritated near the stoma.

80 Which nursing action is *most appropriate* at this time?
- ● 1. Increase oral fluids to dilute the urine.
- ○ 2. Remove the appliance and inspect the skin.
- ○ 3. Empty the appliance at more frequent intervals.
- ○ 4. Leave the appliance off for 1 or 2 days.

The nurse teaches the client how to change his ostomy appliance before being discharged.

81 Which of the following suggestions is *most helpful* to control leaking urine during the time the appliance is being changed?
- ○ 1. When the appliance is removed, let the urine drip into the toilet.
- ○ 2. When the appliance is removed, insert a tampon into the stoma.
- ● 3. When the appliance is removed, press a gloved finger over the stoma.
- ○ 4. When the appliance is removed, pinch the stoma with two fingers.

82 Which of the following suggestions is *most helpful* for ensuring that the appliance remains attached?
- ● 1. Empty the collection bag frequently.
- ○ 2. Limit fluid intake throughout the day.
- ○ 3. Change the appliance each morning.
- ○ 4. Avoid eating gas-forming vegetables.

Correct Answers and Rationale

The Nursing Care of Clients with Urologic Disorders

Directions: Two numbers appear in parentheses following each rationale. The first number identifies the textbook listed in the references, page 512, and the second number identifies the page(s) in that textbook on which the correct answer can be verified. Occasionally two or more textbooks are given for verifying the correct answer.

NURSING CARE OF CLIENTS WITH URINARY INCONTINENCE

1 1. Keeping a log of incontinence helps the nurse identify patterns in the frequency of urination. The data are then used to schedule toilet activities to correspond to the filling and emptying patterns demonstrated by the client. Checking the urine's specific gravity, monitoring bladder distention, and observing the color of urine are all appropriate assessments when caring for clients having problems with urinary elimination. However, these assessments are not necessarily as pertinent to planning a successful bladder retraining program as identifying urinary elimination patterns. (18:541, 1287; 25:640)
   Nursing Process—Data collection
   Client Need—Physiological integrity

2 1. Kegel exercises are performed by contracting and relaxing the muscles in the vagina. Pelvic rocking helps to relieve backache associated with dysmenorrhea and is considered a good conditioning exercise during the prenatal period. The other options describe exercises for improving muscle tone but are not specific to the pubococcygeal muscles. (18:1330; 25:642)
   Nursing Process—Implementation
   Client Need—Health promotion/maintenance

3 4. Restricting fluid intake is discouraged because it potentially can lead to fluid imbalance. Concentrated urine also is more likely to foster stone formation. Inadequate fluid intake does contribute to constipation, but that is not the main reason for discouraging the client from limiting his fluid intake. Although the client is invested in the plan, it is unsafe to encourage him in his plan to restrict his fluid intake. (18:542; 21:591)
   Nursing Process—Implementation
   Client Need—Health promotion/maintenance

4 4. Reflecting feelings demonstrates empathy. It is a useful therapeutic communication technique. It lets the client know that the nurse has recognized the emotion underlying the spoken words in the verbal statement. Disagreeing with the client by saying that he is a "nice gentleman" often blocks further communication. Belittling the client's feelings by challenging the seriousness of his statement also interferes with communication. Giving advice is a nontherapeutic form of interaction; it is demonstrated in the examples in which the nurse says "Cheer up" and "You should expect this at your age." (9:139; 25:79–80)
   Nursing Process—Implementation
   Client Need—Psychosocial integrity

5 3. Space is provided between the end of the penis and the drainage end of the catheter. This prevents irritation to the urinary meatus and promotes drainage of urine. Lubrication is not appropriate because it interferes with maintaining the catheter in place. External catheters are similar to latex condoms. They stretch to fit. Therefore measuring the penis is unnecessary. The foreskin of an uncircumcised male is never left in a retracted position because it could have a tourniquet effect and interfere with circulation of blood to the tissue. (25:646)
   Nursing Process—Implementation
   Client Need—Physiological integrity

6 1. Anchoring the indwelling catheter to the abdomen eliminates pressure and irritation at the penoscrotal angle. Pressure in this area predisposes to fistula formation. The catheter and tubing are passed over a client's leg to prevent obstruction of drainage from body weight. It is appropriate to fasten the drainage tubing to the bed so that there is a straight line from the bed to the collection bag, and to insert the catheter into the tubing of the collection bag. However, neither of these nursing actions will prevent a penoscrotal fistula from forming. (25:657)
   Nursing Process—Implementation
   Client Need—Physiological integrity

NURSING CARE OF CLIENTS WITH INFECTIOUS AND INFLAMMATORY UROLOGIC DISORDERS

7 4. One of the classic symptoms of cystitis is pain or burning on urination. Other symptoms include frequency and urgency. Flank pain is more often experienced by people who have pyelonephritis. The urine may contain white blood cells, causing it to appear cloudy, but a purulent discharge is not a common complaint. Concentrated urine has a strong odor, but this is not usually the case among people who develop cystitis. Although the urine may develop an odor depending on how much urine is retained and the amount of bacterial growth, it is not a commonly reported symptom. (4:843; 21:944)
   Nursing Process—Data collection
   Client Need—Physiological integrity

8 3. The initial voided stream is discarded and a portion of what follows is collected as the specimen. A female is instructed to cleanse the urethral area from front to back; males cleanse the penis using a circular motion. The specimen is collected in a sterile container. The substance used for cleansing is not mixed with the urine specimen. (18:555–556; 25:634)
   Nursing Process—Implementation
   Client Need—Safe, effective care environment

9 2. Infectious and inflammatory conditions affecting the urinary tract are accompanied by blood and pus in the urine which may be grossly visible or microscopic. Glucose in the urine may be caused by a metabolic problem like diabetes mellitus. Liver and gallbladder disorders are evidenced by the presence of bilirubin in the urine. Protein in the urine suggests pathology within the nephrons of the kidneys. (18:1288; 20:905, 944)
   Nursing Process—Data collection
   Client Need—Physiological integrity

10 2. Phenazopyridine changes the color of the urine to orange. Phenazopyridine does not cause the urine to look cloudy, decrease in volume, or smell strong. (17:149; 20:318)
   Nursing Process—Implementation
   Client Need—Health promotion/maintenance

11 3. Phenazopyridine is a urinary analgesic agent that rapidly decreases the burning associated with urinary tract infections. Reducing discomfort eventually results in less frequent and urgent urination, but these are secondary effects. Emptying the bladder at less frequent intervals may increase the volume that

is eliminated, but this is also a secondary effect of phenazopyridine therapy. (17:1430; 20:319)
   Nursing Process—Evaluation
   Client Need—Physiological integrity

12 4. Clients who take methenamine (Mandelamine) are likely to experience gastrointestinal symptoms such as nausea, abdominal cramps, vomiting, and diarrhea. Offering small, frequent meals assists in meeting the client's nutritional needs. Administering the drug with milk is contraindicated since it tends to alkalinize the urine, which reduces the drug's effectiveness. Dyspnea is not a common side effect, but if it occurs, it may be a sign of drug sensitivity or drug allergy. Photosensitivity and polydipsia are not common side effects of this drug. (20:319; 28:708–709)
   Nursing Process—Data collection
   Client Need—Physiological integrity

13 2. Clients for whom methenamine madelate (Mandelamine) is prescribed are advised to avoid foods and drugs that alkalinize urine. Some items to avoid include milk, fruit juices other than cranberry, prune, and plum juice, sodium bicarbonate, and Alka-Seltzer. (17:144; 28:708–709)
   Nursing Process—Implementation
   Client Need—Physiological integrity

14 3. Because the female urethra is shorter than the male's, pathogens travel to the bladder at a much faster rate. Also, the female urethra is more easily contaminated with organisms about the rectum if hygiene is not adequate. Pathogens have to travel further in the longer male urethra. The male urethra is more curved, which tends to act as a barrier to the progression of pathogens toward the bladder. Both the male and female urethra are lined with mucous membrane. The diameter of the urethra is similar in both sexes. (21:944)
   Nursing Process—Implementation
   Client Need—Health promotion/maintenance

15 1. Many chronic health states such as diabetes mellitus, multiple sclerosis, and spinal cord injuries predispose affected clients to urinary tract infections. Diabetes mellitus does not suppress white blood cell activity. Diet therapy to control diabetes is adequate in providing all the essential nutrients in sufficient amounts to maintain health. If diabetes mellitus is controlled, there should be no reduction in energy. (4:842)
   Nursing Process—Implementation
   Client Need—Health promotion/maintenance

16 1. A large intake of fluids promotes frequent urinary elimination. Frequent voiding causes pathogens to pass out of the bladder with the urine. Decreasing the numbers of pathogens present in the urinary tract reduces the rate of growth. Changing underclothing regularly is an appropriate hygiene measure; however, it is not the most effective measure for reducing bacteria in the bladder. Personal hygiene measures rather than the sanitary conditions of a restroom, regardless of whether it is public or private, are more important in reducing bladder infections. The color of toilet tissue does not contribute to or prevent cystitis. (18:1289; 21:945)

Nursing Process—Implementation
Client Need—Health promotion/maintenance

17 1. The most important technique for preventing future urinary tract infections is to eliminate introduction of organisms from the rectum or vagina through improper wiping. Handwashing following elimination assists in reducing the transmission of pathogens to other body structures such as the eyes and mouth. However, handwashing is not as likely to reduce the risk of cystitis as much as correct wiping. The use of chemicals like those in feminine hygiene sprays are avoided because they often contain substances to which many people are sensitive. Drying the perineum is a comfort measure and is appropriate in eliminating moisture that facilitates bacterial growth, but it is not as significant as the manner in which the perineum is wiped. (18:1318)

Nursing Process—Evaluation
Client Need—Health promotion/maintenance

18 2. Conveying a nonjudgmental attitude facilitates obtaining truthful information from the person who feels uncomfortable discussing sexual information. Being sympathetic, encouraging, and optimistic are all positive attributes, but none of these is as important as being nonjudgmental. (21:893)

Nursing Process—Planning
Client Need—Psychosocial integrity

19 2. Asking a person if any sexual partner has similar symptoms helps to determine if the cause is due to a sexually transmitted disease. A painless sore is more likely a symptom of syphilis infection, which does not commonly cause the symptoms this patient describes. The age at which a person first had sexual intercourse is unrelated to the present symptoms. Incubation periods vary among sexually transmitted diseases; identifying the most recent date of intercourse does not provide significant information. (21:946)

Nursing Process—Data collection
Client Need—Health promotion/maintenance

20 4. Because body secretions potentially contain microorganisms that can be transmitted to caregivers, it is important to wear gloves as a barrier against direct contact with infectious material. The use of an antiseptic or lubricant interferes with obtaining an adequate specimen. Wearing a mask is not as important as wearing gloves, because the urethral secretions are not apt to splash or spray areas such as the nose or mouth. Sexually transmitted diseases are spread by direct contact rather than droplet or air transmission. (25:452)

Nursing Process—Implementation
Client Need—Safe, effective care environment

21 3. To ensure adequate treatment, the client with a sexually transmitted disease is told to continue taking the prescribed medication for the full amount of time. Symptoms may clear in a short time after initial treatment, but the organisms might not be totally destroyed. The infection may persist without adequate treatment. The need for a refill is at the discretion of the health professional. Long-term or repeated use of an antibiotic can cause an organism to develop resistance. Aggressive and appropriate short-term treatment is adequate for the present infection. Further treatment is not required unless reinfection occurs. (21:946)

Nursing Process—Implementation
Client Need—Health promotion/maintenance

22 3. Although all of the measures listed are important health practices for preventing infections, the most important method for preventing a recurrence of a sexually transmitted disease is to eliminate the infection in other sex partners. Unless this occurs, the pathogenic organism is transmitted again. (21:888)

Nursing Process—Implementation
Client Need—Health promotion/maintenance

23 2. When it is necessary to insert a catheter, the recumbent position is best for the majority of female clients. This position involves placing the client on the back with the knees flexed and the soles of the feet flat on the bed. For females who have arthritis of the hips or another condition that interferes with recumbent positioning, a side-lying position is used as an alternative. The lithotomy position involves supporting the feet in stirrups. It is used when a female undergoes a pelvic examination. The knee-chest position is used for rectal or lower bowel examinations. The prone position is used when examining the spine and back. (18:650; 25:649)

Nursing Process — Planning
Client Need — Safe, effective care environment

24 3. A contaminated catheter is discarded. Before proceeding, the nurse obtains a second, sterile catheter. Sterility is not ensured by wiping the contaminated catheter with an alcohol swab or cleansing with Betadine solution. If the contaminated catheter is reinserted from the vagina into the urethra, there is a potential for transferring pathogens to the urinary tract. (25:652)

Nursing Process — Implementation
Client Need — Safe, effective care environment

25 3. Clients who take sulfonamides such as sulfamethoxazole reduce the risk of developing crystalluria by consuming 3 to 4 quarts of fluid per day. Water is preferable for a diabetic client since it is calorie-free. Sulfonamides are best taken on an empty stomach unless gastric irritation occurs. Carbonated drinks and citrus fruits do not reduce the risk of crystalluria. (18:1289; 20:87–89)

Nursing Process — Implementation
Client Need — Health promotion/maintenance

26 4. A laxative is given the evening before an IVP to empty the bowel of gas and stool, which, if present, could obstruct the view of the urinary structures during the x-ray. An IVP is not used to examine the lower gastrointestinal tract. Stool incontinence is not generally a problem with an IVP. Laxatives are generally given to treat constipation, not to prevent it. (4:827; 21:903)

Nursing Process — Implementation
Client Need — Health promotion/maintenance

27 3. A history of a previous allergic reaction to radiopaque dye indicates the client is at risk for a similar episode. The physician may prescribe a corticosteroid or antihistamine drug prior to the test to reduce the potential for an allergic reaction. The other information has value, but reporting the previous reaction has the greatest potential for preserving the client's safety. (4:826)

Nursing Process — Implementation
Client Need — Physiological integrity

28 1. Family members often notice that the face of a person with glomerulonephritis appears pale and puffy. Mentation usually is unaffected in the early stages of the disease. Salting food and sleeping poorly are atypical signs of glomerulonephritis. (4:856; 20:916)

Nursing Process — Data collection
Client Need — Physiological integrity

29 2. Although definite evidence linking a streptococcal infection with glomerulonephritis has not been established, many identify that they experienced an upper respiratory infection or sore throat 2 to 3 weeks before the onset of glomerulonephritis. There is no correlation between acute glomerulonephritis and trauma, antibiotic therapy, or an allergy specific to x-ray dye. (4:856; 21:916)

Nursing Process — Data collection
Client Need — Safe, effective care environment

30 4. A common sign associated with glomerulonephritis is peripheral edema that ranges from slight ankle edema in the evening to generalized fluid retention that may compromise cardiac function. The skin is pale, not flushed. Skin hemorrhages are a common finding in liver disease and blood dyscrasias. The distribution of body hair is not directly related to glomerulonephritis. (4:856; 21:916)

Nursing Process — Data collection
Client Need — Physiological integrity

31 3. The results of a BUN test indicate how efficiently the glomeruli are removing nitrogen wastes from the blood. An elevation indicates glomerular dysfunction. Serum amylase levels aid in diagnosing and monitoring pancreatitis. A blood glucose test is used for monitoring diabetes mellitus. A complete blood count is helpful for baseline information, but it is not as essential in evaluating the course of glomerulonephritis as the BUN. (4:856; 21:916)

Nursing Process — Data collection
Client Need — Physiological integrity

32 3. Because glomerulonephritis impairs renal function, monitoring weight on a daily basis is essential for evaluating how much fluid the person is retaining. Ambulation is not usually impaired; however, if the client is hypertensive or has other circulatory complications, activity may be restricted. Mouth care is important for all who cannot attend to their own self-care; it is not a common problem among people with glomerulonephritis. Owing to fluid retention, many people who have glomerulonephritis are on fluid restrictions. (18:1290; 21:918)

Nursing Process — Planning
Client Need — Physiological integrity

33 2. It is important for the nurse to first assess the client's blood pressure. People with glomerulonephritis often are hypertensive; hypertension can be accompanied by a headache. Hypertension also is an indication of increased intracranial pressure. If the headache is caused by hypertension, a priority intervention is to reduce the blood pressure and treat the cause. Implementing comfort measures, such as reducing environmental stimuli, administering a prescribed analgesic, and changing the client's position are appropriate, but assessing the client takes place first. (4:856)

Nursing Process—Implementation
Client Need—Physiological integrity

34 2. Urine that formed before the time a 24-hour urine collection starts is not included with the collected urine. Valid results require that the urine collected be produced within the 24-hour period. Properly collected urine is refrigerated in a large container, or the container is kept in a basin of ice. After all of the urine from the 24-hour period is collected, the entire specimen is sent to the laboratory. Laboratory policy is consulted as to whether urine from a 24-hour collection is mixed with a preservative rather than refrigerated. (18:556; 25:635)

Nursing Process—Implementation
Client Need—Safe, effective care environment

35 3. People with glomerulonephritis generally manifest albuminuria. Glucose and acetone are expected in a person with uncontrolled diabetes mellitus. Bilirubin is present in the urine of a person with liver or gallbladder disease. (18:1290; 21:916)

Nursing Process—Data collection
Client Need—Physiological integrity

36 2. The presence of blood gives a smoky appearance to urine. Cloudy urine suggests the presence of white blood cells. If the urine appears bright orange, the nurse might investigate whether the client has ingested a substance containing a water-soluble dye. Concentrated urine is likely to appear dark yellow. (18:1290)

Nursing Process—Data collection
Client Need—Physiological integrity

37 3. Chicken breast on lettuce is the menu item that contains the least amount of sodium among the options provided. Processed meats are highly salted. Bouillon and other canned soups generally contain a great deal of salt. Dairy products are high in sodium. Baked goods, such as crackers and pizza crust, also contain sodium bicarbonate or salt. (6:539)

Nursing Process—Implementation
Client Need—Health promotion/maintenance

38 2. Alternate-day therapy is used when administering glucocorticoid drugs to prevent adrenal suppression. By alternating exogenous hormone therapy on one day, it allows the adrenal cortex to produce endogenous hormone as the blood level drops the

following day. Steroids have many undesirable side effects, but most are tolerable. Steroids can and are administered on a daily basis when clients require short-term therapy. The duration of action is generally 24 hours. (20:350)

Nursing Process—Implementation
Client Need—Health promotion/maintenance

NURSING CARE OF CLIENTS WITH RENAL FAILURE

39 4. The first stage of renal failure generally is characterized by oliguria; that is, a urine output of less than 400 to 500 mL in 24 hours. The nurse observes a diuretic phase following a period of oliguria or anuria as the client's condition improves. People in renal failure do not experience pain or discomfort with urination. The urine of a person in renal failure does not contain abnormal amounts of ketones or red blood cells. (4:858; 21:928)

Nursing Process—Data collection
Client Need—Physiological integrity

40 2. Measuring intake and output accurately is a priority when planning the care of a client with renal failure. This information aids in evaluating fluid balance and adjusting fluid restrictions. Urinary retention is not common in renal failure because the client is not producing much urine. Generally, a urinary catheter is inserted to aid in monitoring the output of a person in renal failure. The body temperature is monitored to assess for signs of infection or other complications; however, it is not likely to be affected by the primary condition. The nurse would not expect any abnormalities in bowel sounds in clients with renal failure. (21:931)

Nursing Process—Planning
Client Need—Physiological integrity

41 4. It is most important to assess lung sounds because administering fluid in the presence of oliguria or anuria may lead to congestive heart failure and pulmonary edema. Fluid overload is manifested by pedal edema, but that is not a life-threatening consequence. Skin integrity becomes impaired due to inactivity, edema, and elimination of nitrogenous wastes through the skin. Skin impairment is not an immediate problem with fluid therapy. The oral mucosa does not undergo adverse changes with the administration of fluid. (21:931)

Nursing Process—Data collection
Client Need—Physiological integrity

42 4. The skin of a client in renal failure becomes dry and intensely itchy due to the excretion and evaporation of nitrogenous wastes through the skin. Skin care involves frequent cleaning with plain, warm water and then patting the skin dry. The nurse may choose to apply a lubricating skin cream or lotion. Edema causes taut and puffy skin. (21:931)

    Nursing Process—Planning
    Client Need—Physiological integrity

43 4. Lemon juice is used to enhance the flavor of fish, eggs, and some vegetables. Other seasonings that are recommended include fresh herbs such as parsley, dill, oregano, and so forth. Fresh onion also is acceptable. Catsup, prepared mustard, and soy sauce are high in sodium and are avoided. (6:544)

    Nursing Process—Implementation
    Client Need—Health promotion/maintenance

44 1. Hard candy, especially if it is sour or tart-flavored, increases salivation and reduces the sensation of thirst without increasing fluid intake. People in renal failure, unless they are diabetic, are not generally restricted in the amount of carbohydrate they may consume. Ice chips, ice cream, and fresh fruit all contain fluid, which must be considered in the fluid restriction. Fruit contains potassium, which also is contraindicated for renal failure clients. (4:860)

    Nursing Process—Implementation
    Client Need—Physiological integrity

45 1. To evaluate trends in weight, the nurse weighs the client at the same time daily using the same scale each time. The amount of clothing is similar at each weighing. If the time of weighing is consistent, the amount of food or liquids that the client has been consuming is not likely to vary considerably. It is important to collaborate with the client, but obtaining the weight is not omitted or postponed for frivolous reasons. (4:164)

    Nursing Process—Planning
    Client Need—Physiological integrity

46 1. The color and temperature of the hands are assessed regularly for signs of inadequate circulation. Blood clots may form in the joined vessels and occlude tissue perfusion. Joint range of motion, muscle tone and coordination, and skin integrity are not likely to be affected. (26:691)

    Nursing Process—Data collection
    Client Need—Physiological integrity

47 4. Discussing an actual or potential stressor helps to place the event in more realistic perspective. Giving a client an opportunity for discussion empowers

the client to confront the issues and acquire support in the process. (2:137, 139, 143)

    Nursing Process—Implementation
    Client Need—Psychosocial integrity

48 2. Along with measuring the volume of infused and drained dialysis solution, comparing the client's pre- and post-dialysis weight provides objective data for evaluating the outcome of peritoneal dialysis. (26:695)

    Nursing Process—Planning
    Client Need—Safe, effective care environment

49 1. The dialysate infusion tubing is clamped, usually for 15 to 45 minutes, to allow osmosis and diffusion to take place between the dialysate and the peritoneum. The peritoneal cavity is drained after the dwell time. The client is free to ambulate, change positions, or remain in bed during peritoneal dialysis. The amount of activity depends on the safety needs of each client. The client may eat and drink during peritoneal dialysis; however, oral fluids continue to be restricted throughout dialysis and for as long as the client is in renal failure. (4:864; 26:693)

    Nursing Process—Implementation
    Client Need—Safe, effective care environment

50 3. An elevated temperature is unexpected. Its presence indicates that an infection is occurring. It is expected that a client undergoing peritoneal dialysis will lose weight and have an output that exceeds intake. Regular, deep breathing generally indicates that ventilation is adequate. (26:695)

    Nursing Process—Implementation
    Client Need—Physiological integrity

51 3. One of the beneficial effects of dialysis is the lowering of the elevated serum potassium. A lower red cell count is not a desired effect. Most people with renal failure become anemic because the kidney's ability to produce erythropoietin is impaired. Blood transfusions or injections of genetically engineered erythropoietin often are necessary. Peritoneal dialysis is not expected to improve renal output. If renal function improves, it is rather due to accompanying therapy or healing on the cellular level. Improvement of appetite is far too subjective to be used as an indicator of a therapeutic response to peritoneal dialysis. (26:695)

    Nursing Process—Evaluation
    Client Need—Physiological integrity

52 2. Relatives, especially siblings who were conceived by the same father and mother, prove to be the most compatible genetic matches for clients who receive transplanted organs. Immunosuppressant drugs make it possible to reduce the potential for rejection regardless of the source of human organs. Kidneys from other species are not successfully transplanted. (18:1281; 21:936)

> Nursing Process—Implementation
> Client Need—Health promotion/maintenance

NURSING CARE OF CLIENTS WITH UROLOGIC OBSTRUCTIONS

53 1. Subjective data that are associated with obstructive urinary disorders include a persistent feeling of needing to void and dull flank pain. Feeling the urge to void is related to urine accumulating in the bladder secondary to incomplete emptying. A palpable bladder above the pubis is an objective sign that urine is being retained. Dark urine is associated with fluid volume deficit. (4:846)

> Nursing Process—Data collection
> Client Need—Physiological integrity

54 2. A cystostomy tube is surgically inserted directly into the bladder through the abdominal wall. A ureterostomy tube is inserted into one of the ureters through a flank incision. A retention catheter, such as a Foley catheter, is inserted through the urethra. (4:846)

> Nursing Process—Data collection
> Client Need—Physiological integrity

55 2. Ensuring that there is adequate urinary output from the suprapubic catheter is the best evidence that the catheter is patent. Inspecting the skin is essential for detecting skin breakdown or infection. Attaching the catheter to a leg bag promotes the ability of the client to move about. Encouraging oral intake promotes the formation of urine, but an increased fluid intake is not a measure of catheter patency. (4:832; 21:953)

> Nursing Process—Evaluation
> Client Need—Physiological integrity

56 2. Gross or microscopic hematuria is more characteristic of trauma from a moving urinary stone than cloudy, light yellow, or strong-smelling urine. (4:846)

> Nursing Process—Data collection
> Client Need—Physiological integrity

57 2. Due to the instrumentation and dilation of the urethra, it is common for people to complain of burning when urinating following a cystoscopy. The nurse can reduce or relieve the discomfort by promoting a liberal fluid intake, providing sitz baths, and administering a prescribed mild analgesic. Polyuria, anuria, and pyuria indicate other complications or conditions affecting the renal system. (4:827)

> Nursing Process—Data collection
> Client Need—Safe, effective care environment

58 4. Urine is strained to assess for evidence that the urinary stone or stones have been passed. Fluids are encouraged rather than restricted. Activity promotes movement of urinary stones. A Fowler's position is not likely to benefit nor to interfere with the passage of a urinary stone. (4:848; 18:1284)

> Nursing Process—Planning
> Client Need—Physiological integrity

59 1. Extracorporeal shock wave lithotripsy is a procedure that is performed while the client's lower body is submerged in a tank of water or surrounded by a fluid-filled bag. Ultrasound is the mechanism that is used to pulverize the stone(s), not radiation or a laser beam. Clients are sedated and given preprocedural analgesic medication to reduce the discomfort that is described as blows to the body. It is common for bruises to appear as a consequence of the ultrasonic energy. (4:848; 18:1285)

> Nursing Process—Evaluation
> Client Need—Health promotion/maintenance

60 2. Nocturia, being awakened by a need to urinate, is a common finding among people with benign prostatic hypertrophy. Burning on urination is more likely a sign of a bladder infection, which could be secondary to benign prostatic hypertrophy. Feeling pressure in the back is more indicative of pathology involving the kidney. Colorless or very light yellow urine indicates that the urine is dilute. This could be caused from an endocrine disturbance, such as diabetes insipidus, or from some other dysfunction in renal tubular reabsorption. (4:851; 21:872)

> Nursing Process—Data collection
> Client Need—Physiological integrity

61 3. Due to obstruction of the urethra from an enlarging prostate gland, men with benign prostatic hypertrophy often describe hesitancy when initiating urination. That is, they feel the need to urinate, but it takes some time before urine is released. The stream of urine also is diminished. Benign prostatic hypertrophy usually does not cause sexual dysfunction or incontinence. The prostate gland is not located in the scrotum. It is palpated by rectal examination. (4:851; 21:872)

> Nursing Process—Data collection
> Client Need—Physiological integrity

62 1. Lowering the penis from an upright position to one in which the penis is pointed in the direction of the toes sometimes helps to pass a catheter beyond the narrowing caused by an enlarged prostate gland. The penis is grasped firmly whenever a catheter is inserted. If resistance is met when inserting a catheter, it is never forced. Massaging the tissue below the base of the penis is not a technique that facilitates passage through an enlarged prostate gland. (25:657)

Nursing Process—Implementation
Client Need—Physiological integrity

63 4. Hematuria generally is present for at least 24 hours following a TURP. Vital signs are monitored to evaluate if the volume of blood loss is causing shock. It may take 24 to 48 hours for the urine to become light pink and transparent. The volume of urine is within normal range unless complications, such as hypovolemic shock or obstruction of the catheter, occur. Sediment, if present is due to the remnants of prostatic tissue; however, the blood that is mixed with the urine initially obscures the ability of the nurse to identify the presence of tissue or mucoid debris. (4:851)

Nursing Process—Data collection
Client Need—Physiological integrity

64 1. A continuous bladder irrigation is performed by instilling normal saline solution through one lumen of the urinary catheter. The solution flows into the bladder, dilutes the urine and sediment, and drains out of the catheter into a gravity drainage bag. An Asepto syringe and sterile container for irrigation solution are used for performing an intermittent catheter irrigation. Sterile normal saline, not an antiseptic solution, is used for a continuous bladder irrigation and intermittent catheter irrigation. (25:662)

Nursing Process—Planning
Client Need—Safe, effective care environment

65 3. The nurse assesses if the catheter is draining well before administering an analgesic for bladder discomfort. Obstruction of the catheter causes bladder spasms. Restoring patency is more appropriate in the case of catheter obstruction than administering an analgesic. Administering an analgesic is not necessarily contingent on a normal pulse rate. There is no dressing following a TURP; the surgery is performed through the urethra. A narcotic analgesic may depress the respiratory center, but assessing the client's ability to cough does not affect the decision to withhold or administer an analgesic. (4:851; 21:876)

Nursing Process—Data collection
Client Need—Physiological integrity

66 4. Belladonna and opium rectal suppositories are considered the most effective drugs for relieving blad-

der spasms following a TURP. Aspirin is avoided because it increases the tendency to bleed. Darvocet and Demerol are synthetic narcotic analgesics. Narcotics alone do not seem to lessen the spasms; they may decrease the pain. (4:851)

Nursing Process—Implementation
Client Need—Physiological integrity

67 3. The best method for recording output when a client has more than one catheter is to record the volume that drained from each catheter as a separate entry in the medical record. Recording only the output from the urethral catheter or the output from the wound catheter does not provide accurate data on total output. If the two volumes are added together and recorded as a single entry, it is difficult to evaluate the status of urinary drainage from each catheter. (18:1302; 21:926)

Nursing Process—Implementation
Client Need—Safe, effective care environment

68 3. After a suprapubic catheter is removed, urine may leak from the incisional area and saturate the sterile dressing. A wet dressing provides a "wicking" action by which microorganisms are attracted in the direction of the impaired tissue. A dressing saturated with urine also leads to skin breakdown. If standards of care are being followed, the postoperative care plan already indicates nursing orders for repositioning the client, ambulating with assistance, and encouraging deep breathing. (18:1303; 25:570)

Nursing Process—Planning
Client Need—Physiological integrity

NURSING CARE OF CLIENTS WITH UROLOGIC TUMORS

69 3. There are falsely high levels of prostatic-specific antigen (PSA) for up to 12 days after a rectal examination or instrumentation around the prostate gland as may occur with a cystoscopy. The other examinations and tests are not influenced by physical manipulation of the prostate gland. (4:853)

Nursing Process—Planning
Client Need—Safe, effective care environment

70 1. Tension on the catheter may disrupt the healing where the bladder and the urethra have been surgically reconnected following removal of the prostate gland and its capsule. Encouraging oral fluids and cleansing the meatus are appropriate postoperative nursing measures, but they are not likely to have as significant an effect on wound healing. Clients who undergo a radical prostatectomy have a high potential for urinary incontinence as a consequence of the surgical procedure. Clamping and releasing the catheter is not likely to promote bladder control. (4:853)

> Nursing Process—Implementation
> Client Need—Physiological integrity

71 1. Males who receive estrogen therapy are prone to developing feminizing characteristics such as breast enlargement, breast tenderness, and testicular atrophy. An alternative approach is to remove both testicles to reduce the production of testosterone. (4:853; 20:442)

> Nursing Process—Evaluation
> Client Need—Health promotion/maintenance

72 1. The sudden onset of flank pain along with other signs of shock such as hypotension, restlessness, and tachycardia are suggestive of hemorrhage. The skin generally is pale and cool in shock. A distended abdomen generally is caused by the accumulation of intestinal gas. Pain sometimes causes nausea and vomiting, but these signs and symptoms may be due to multiple etiologies. (21:926)

> Nursing Process—Data collection
> Client Need—Physiological integrity

73 3. The most common symptom of bladder cancer is painless hematuria. Dysuria, if present, generally is due to a concurrent urinary tract infection secondary to obstruction of urine. Oliguria occurs later as the disease becomes more advanced and obstruction occurs. Bladder cancer, which has not spread to adjacent pelvic structures, usually is not associated with an unusual discharge from any body orifice. (21:950)

> Nursing Process—Data collection
> Client Need—Physiological integrity

74 4. There is a correlation between cigarette smoking, even passive exposure to cigarette smoke, and the development of bladder cancer. Other carcinogenic factors include long-term exposure to chemical solvents and dyes. Neither stress incontinence nor sexual activities are implicated as a causal agent in bladder cancer. (4:849; 21:949)

> Nursing Process—Implementation
> Client Need—Health promotion/maintenance

75 1. Recommendations for promoting safety when handling toxic chemotherapeutic agents include wearing two pairs of surgical latex gloves, which are less permeable than polyvinyl gloves. A gown with cuffs and a mask or goggles also are worn to prevent direct contact with the drug. There is no particular advantage in using a glass syringe. In fact, there is a greater potential hazard if a glass syringe is dropped and broken. The uncontained drug is considered

a toxic spill. Time in contact with the client is not a safety hazard with chemotherapy, but it is a factor in radiation therapy involving sealed and unsealed implants. (25:768)

> Nursing Process—Implementation
> Client Need—Safe, effective care environment

NURSING CARE OF CLIENTS WITH URINARY DIVERSIONS

76 3. An ileal conduit, or ileal loop procedure, involves implanting the ureters into a section of the ileum that has been removed from the rest of the small intestine. The section of ileum is fashioned into a stoma that opens onto the abdomen. When a ureterosigmoidostomy is performed, the ureters are attached to the sigmoid colon, and urine is eliminated with stool by way of the rectum. Currently, there are no procedures in which the ureters are implanted directly into the small intestine. If a Koch pouch, or continent urostomy, is performed, urine is siphoned with a catheter from an internal collection pouch. (21:950–951)

> Nursing Process—Implementation
> Client Need—Health promotion/maintenance

77 3. A pulse rate of more than 100 in the absence of activity or some accompanying pathology suggests that the sympathetic nervous system is stimulated. The sympathetic nervous system responds when a person is experiencing a real or perceived threat to his well-being. The data in the other options are generally within normal limits. (2:138; 25:103)

> Nursing Process—Data collection
> Client Need—Physiological integrity

78 1. Sharing perceptions with the client by stating that "it must be difficult" shows empathy. It gives the person permission to unburden himself. Telling the client that he has one of the best surgeons does not encourage the client to verbalize further because it is unlikely that he will disagree. The reassuring cliché that "everything will turn out OK" cannot be guaranteed. It indicates that the nursing assistant feels uncomfortable discussing the client's feelings. Saying that "others have done just fine" minimizes and belittles the uniqueness of the situation from the client's perspective. (9:138–139; 23:94–95)

> Nursing Process—Implementation
> Client Need—Psychosocial integrity

79 1. Encouraging the client to verbalize more and express his feelings is a therapeutic communication technique. Because it is impossible for a nurse to know how a client is feeling, this statement diminishes the nurse's credibility. The client may lose faith in the ability of the nurse to be truly empathetic. Minimizing the despair that he is feeling by saying "It's not as bad as that" is likely to interfere with any further discussion. Advising the client to "think more positively" is likely to be interpreted as disapproval of the way the client currently is feeling. (9:138–139; 25:79–80)

    Nursing Process—Implementation
    Client Need—Psychosocial integrity

80 2. It is important for the nurse to assess the condition of the skin to plan appropriate interventions. If the skin is excoriated, it probably will take more than just diluting the urine or emptying the appliance more frequently to restore skin integrity. It is impossible to leave the appliance off because urine is released constantly. (25:684)

    Nursing Process—Implementation
    Client Need—Physiological integrity

81 2. Inserting a tampon or a gauze square into the stoma momentarily absorbs the urine and keeps the skin dry. Leaning over the toilet puts the client in an awkward position during the time the appliance is being changed. It generally takes two hands to manipulate the appliance during its application; therefore, pressing a finger over the stoma or pinching the stoma interferes with the coordination that is needed. (4:467; 25:663)

    Nursing Process—Implementation
    Client Need—Health promotion/maintenance

82 1. Emptying the collection bag decreases the weight and pull on the skin to which the appliance is attached. Fluids are not restricted; this concentrates the urine and increases the risk for dehydration, skin irritation, and infection. To avoid skin impairment, an appliance generally is not changed on a daily basis. However, it must be changed if it becomes loose or uncomfortable. It is unlikely that avoiding gas-forming food would have any effect at all on a person with a urostomy. (4:867; 25:663)

    Nursing Process—Implementation
    Client Need—Health promotion/maintenance

Classification of Test Items

Unit I Review Test **9**

The Nursing Care of Clients with Urologic Disorders

Directions: After each question, the correct answer is given, as well as a classification of each test question. Compare the correct answer with your answer. If a question has been answered *incorrectly*, draw a line to the end of all the columns. When finished, add up the number of your correct answers in each column and place that number in the respective box at the end in the area identified as *Number Correct*.

To determine the percentage of questions you answered correctly and your performance in each of the test plan categories, divide the *Number Correct* in each column by the *Number Possible* in each column. Then multiply the decimal by 100. For example:

$$\frac{\text{Number Correct: 65}}{\text{Number Possible: 82}} = 0.792 \times 100 = 79\%$$

Any score that is less than 75% indicates an area where further review would be beneficial.

KEY TO ITEM CLASSIFICATION:

NURSING PROCESS	CLIENT NEEDS
D = Data collection	S = Safe, effective care environment
P = Planning	P = Physiological integrity
I = Implementation	M = Psychosocial integrity
E = Evaluation	H = Health promotion/maintenance

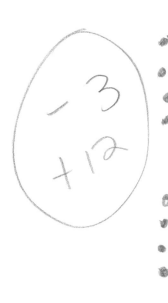

Question #	Answer #	Nursing Process				Client Needs			
		D	P	I	E	S	P	M	H
1	1	D					P		
2	1			I					H
3	4			I					H
4	4			I					M
5	3			I			P		
6	1			I			P		
7	4	D					P		
8	3			I		S			
9	2	D					P		
10	2			I					H
11	3				E		P		
12	4	D					P		
13	2			I			P		
14	3			I					H
15	1			I					H

2 1 3

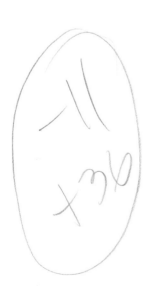

Question #	Answer #	Nursing Process				Client Needs			
		D	P	I	E	S	P	M	H
16	1			I					H
17	1				E				H
18	2		P				P		
19	2	D							H
20	4			I		S			
21	3			I					H
22	3			I					H
23	2		P			S			
24	3			I		S			
25	3			I					H
26	4			I					H
27	3			I			P		
28	1	D					P		
29	2	D				S			
30	4	D					P		
31	3	D					P		
32	3		P				P		
33	2			I			P		
34	2			I		S			
35	3	D					P		
36	2	D					P		
37	3			I					H
38	2			I					H
39	4	D					P		
40	2		P				P		
41	4	D					P		
42	4		P				P		
43	4			I					H
44	1			I			P		
45	1		P				P		
46	1	D					P		
47	4			I				M	

Question #	Answer #	Nursing Process				Client Needs			
		D	P	I	E	S	P	M	H
48	2		P			S			
49	1			I		S			
50	3			I			P		
51	3				E		P		
52	2			I					H
53	1	D					P		
54	2	D					P		
55	2				E		P		
56	2	D					P		
57	2	D				S			
58	4		P				P		
59	1				E				H
60	2	D					P		
61	3	D					P		
62	1			I			P		
63	4	D					P		
64	1		P			S			
65	3	D					P		
66	4			I			P		
67	3			I		S			
68	3		P				P		
69	3		P			S			
70	1			I			P		
71	1				E				H
72	1	D					P		
73	3	D					P		
74	4			I					H
75	1			I		S			
76	3			I					H
77	3	D					P		
78	1			I				M	
79	1			I				M	

Question #	Answer #	Nursing Process				Client Needs			
		D	P	I	E	S	P	M	H
80	2			I			P		
81	2			I					H
82	1			I					H
Number Correct	6	21	10	31	4	11	33	3	19
Number Possible	82	25	11	40	6	13	43	4	22
Percentage Correct	80%	94	91	78	67	85	77%	75	86

The Nursing Care of Clients with Disorders of Sensory Organs and the Integument

Nursing Care of Clients with Eye Disorders

Nursing Care of Clients with Disorders of Accessory Eye Structures

Nursing Care of Clients with Ear Disorders

Nursing Care of Clients with Nasal Disorders

Nursing Care of Clients with Disorders of the Skin and Related Structures

Correct Answers and Rationale

Classification of Test Items

Directions: With a pencil, blacken the circle in front of the option you have chosen for your correct answer.

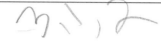

NURSING CARE OF CLIENTS WITH EYE DISORDERS

A chemistry student is sent to the school nurse after having been splashed in the eyes with a chemical.

1 Which one of the following is the *most important* information for the nurse to obtain at this time?
- ○ 1. If safety glasses were worn
- ● 2. The names of the chemicals
- ○ 3. The treatment already given
- ○ 4. If the client's vision is impaired

The nurse prepares to irrigate the student's irritated eye.

2 Assuming all of the following solutions are available, which one is *best* for the nurse to use at this time?
- ○ 1. Tap water
- ● 2. Sodium bicarbonate
- ○ 3. Acetic acid
- ○ 4. Magnesium sulfate

3 The *best technique* when irrigating the eyes is to direct the flow of the irrigating solution
- ○ 1. directly onto the cornea.
- ● 2. away from the inner canthus.
- ○ 3. within the anterior chamber.
- ○ 4. toward the nasolacrimal duct.

4 After providing emergency treatment of an eye injury, it is *best* to refer the client to a(n)
- ○ 1. optician.
- ○ 2. ophthalmologist.
- ● 3. optometrist.
- ○ 4. podiatrist.

5 When a foreign body becomes embedded in a person's eye, the *first action* to take before referring the person for medical treatment is to
- ○ 1. remove the object with a forceps.
- ○ 2. ask the person to blink rapidly.
- ○ 3. instill antibiotic ointment.
- ● 4. loosely patch both eyes.

A nurse uses a Snellen chart to assess the visual acuity of clients before they are examined by the physician.

6 Before this examination, the nurse is *most correct* in explaining to clients that they must
- ○ 1. read words that are the size of newsprint.
- ● 2. read letters from a distance of 20 feet.
- ○ 3. look at a colored picture and identify an image.
- ○ 4. look at a screen and say when an object is seen.

7 When a client asks the nurse to tell her the technical name for nearsightedness, the *most accurate* response is
- ○ 1. presbyopia.
- ○ 2. amblyopia.
- ○ 3. hyperopia.
- ● 4 myopia.

A nursing assistant confides to the nurse that her father is in need of eyeglasses, but he cannot afford them.

8 Which is the *most appropriate* organization to which the nurse can refer the nursing assistant and her father?
- ○ 1. The Loyal Order of Moose
- ○ 2. The American Legion
- ● 3. Lions International
- ○ 4. The Knights of Columbus

The nurse reads in the medical record that a client has astigmatism.

9 Based on the recorded data, the nurse expects that when the client looks at an object while not wearing corrective glasses or contact lenses, the client
○ 1. sees near objects more clearly.
● 2. finds a blurred area in his visual field.
○ 3. sees far objects more clearly.
○ 4. finds that he sees two of the same object.

10 When instructing a nursing assistant on the technique for cleaning a client's prescription glasses, the *best recommendation* is to wash the lenses with soap and warm water or commercial glass cleaner and dry them
○ 1. with a paper tissue.
● 2. with a soft cloth.
○ 3. using a paper towel.
○ 4. by air evaporation.

11 When caring for a client who is blind or has both eyes patched, which addition to the care plan is the *best method* for reducing the client's anxiety?
○ 1. Touch the client before speaking.
● 2. Explain what you plan to do beforehand.
○ 3. Shut the room door to decrease noise.
○ 4. Leave the room lights on at all times.

The nurse observes the nursing assistant ambulating a blind client.

12 Which of the following instructions is *best* for maintaining the client's safety and security?
● 1. Let the client take your arm while walking.
○ 2. Take the client's arm while walking with him.
○ 3. Position the client in front and to your side.
○ 4. Have the client walk independently by your side.

13 Which of the following is the *best plan* for promoting a blind client's feeling of self-reliance when eating?
● 1. Help the client locate his food by comparing its placement to clock positions.
○ 2. Ask a hospital volunteer to feed the client so he does not have to ask for help.
○ 3. Order food that can be sipped from containers rather than those that require eating utensils.
○ 4. Ask the dietary department to serve the client's food on paper plates and in cups.

The nurse is assigned to care for an older adult who has bilateral senile cataracts.

14 When assessing the client with cataracts, which symptom is the client *most likely* to manifest as a result of his medical condition?

● 1. Gradual loss of vision
○ 2. Fullness within the eye
○ 3. Ocular pain or discomfort
○ 4. Flashes of light

15 When the nurse inspects the eyes of the client with cataracts, the sign that is *most indicative* of cataracts is
○ 1. ruptured blood vessels on the eye.
○ 2. an irregularly shaped iris.
● 3. a white spot behind the pupil.
○ 4. a painless corneal lesion.

16 Which of the statements made by the client with cataracts is the *best indication* that the client understands when surgical treatment to remove the cataracts is appropriate?
● 1. Surgery is indicated when the loss of vision interferes with activities of daily living.
○ 2. Surgery is indicated when the pain can no longer be controlled through the use of eye drops.
○ 3. Surgery is indicated when his appearance makes him feel self-conscious.
○ 4. Surgery is indicated when the cataracts reach maximum maturity, and no further changes are observed.

The client with bilateral cataracts is scheduled to have a cataract removed from his right eye. Preoperative orders include the following: (1) Scrub face with povidone iodine (Betadine) for 10 minutes on the morning of surgery; (2) Clip eyelashes on the right eye after admission; (3) Instill 2 gtt of tropicamide (Mydriacil) o.s. 30 minutes before surgery.

17 After reviewing the medical orders, it is *essential* that the nurse
● 1. carry out the physician's orders as written.
○ 2. question the directions for giving eye drops.
○ 3. let the operating room nurse clip the lashes.
○ 4. encourage the client to scrub his own face.

18 The *best technique* for instilling eye drops is for the nurse to dispense the medication
○ 1. onto the cornea.
○ 2. at the inner canthus.
○ 3. at the outer canthus.
● 4. in the lower conjunctival sac.

The nursing team meets to individualize a standardized postoperative nursing care plan for the client who will undergo a cataract extraction.

19 Which nursing order is *most appropriate* to *eliminate* from the plan of care?

○ 1. Keep bed in low position at all times.
○ 2. Reapply antiembolic stockings b.i.d.
● 3. Urge to cough every 2 hours while awake.
○ 4. Assist when ambulating in hall or room.

20 Postoperatively, when the client who has had a cataract extraction tells the nurse that he is experiencing severe pain in his operative eye, which nursing action is *most appropriate*?
● 1. Report the finding to the nurse in charge.
○ 2. Give the client a prescribed analgesic.
○ 3. Assess his pupil response with a penlight.
○ 4. Reposition him on his operative side.

Before discharging the client who had a cataract extraction, the physician instructs him to wear a metal shield over the operative eye while sleeping.

21 When the client asks the nurse about the purpose for the eye shield, the *best explanation* is that it is used to
○ 1. keep foreign substances out of the eye.
● 2. protect the eye from accidental trauma.
○ 3. reduce rapid eye movement when dreaming.
○ 4. promote dilation of the pupil at night.

22 Which of the following is *correct information* to include when providing discharge instructions for the client who has undergone a cataract extraction?
○ 1. Avoid bending over from the waist.
○ 2. Keep both eyes patched at all times.
● 3. Sleep with the head slightly elevated.
○ 4. Bleeding will decrease in one week.

A nurse is assigned to care for an older adult female with chronic open-angle glaucoma.

23 A common characteristic of open-angle glaucoma that the client is *most likely* to report is
○ 1. itching and burning eyes.
○ 2. headaches while reading.
○ 3. seeing halos around lights.
● 4. loss of central vision.

The nurse prepares to assist the physician while he examines the client with open-angle glaucoma.

24 If the physician wants to check the client's intraocular pressure, which instrument is *most appropriate* for the nurse to have available?
○ 1. Ophthalmoscope
● 2. Tonometer
○ 3. Retinoscope
○ 4. Speculum

25 Which of the following is the client with untreated glaucoma *most likely* to report to the nurse as a result of the chronic progression of the disease?

○ 1. Tunnel vision
○ 2. Double vision
○ 3. Bulging eyes
○ 4. Bloodshot eyes

The client with chronic open-angle glaucoma is to administer timolol maleate (Timoptic) 1 gtt in each eye daily.

26 Which comment is *most indicative* that the client needs more teaching?
○ 1. "I must wash my hands before instilling the drops."
○ 2. "This drug decreases the formation of fluid in my eye."
● 3. "I'll need to take this until my eye pressure is normal."
○ 4. "The cap on the container should be replaced immediately."

27 It is *essential* that the nurse withhold medication administration and notify the physician if which of the following drugs is ordered for a client with glaucoma?
● 1. Atropine sulfate
○ 2. Morphine sulfate
○ 3. Magnesium sulfate
○ 4. Ferrous sulfate

28 Which of the following is *common* when the intraocular pressure of a client with closed-angle (narrow angle) glaucoma becomes dangerously high?
● 1. The client sees "spots" in the visual field.
○ 2. The client experiences severe eye pain.
○ 3. The client's pupils appear pinpoint.
○ 4. The client's eyes bulge from the orbit.

Once the intraocular pressure has been temporarily reduced, the physician performs an iridectomy on a client with closed-angle (narrow angle) glaucoma.

29 When the nurse assesses the client's operative eye following surgery, which finding is *most expected*?
○ 1. The pupil appears cloudy and gray.
○ 2. The pupil is a fixed size and shape.
○ 3. The colored area of the iris is gone.
● 4. A section of the iris appears black.

The nurse takes a health history from a client with a retinal detachment.

30 If the client provides all of the following information, which is the *most likely* factor for causing a retinal detachment?
○ 1. The client is younger than 40 years old.
● 2. The client fell within the last day.
○ 3. The client has multiple allergies.
○ 4. The client is recovering from pneumonia.

The physician orders that the nurse patch both the eyes of the client with the retinal detachment.

31 When applying the eye patches, the nurse is *most correct* in
○ 1. occluding all sources of room light.
○ 2. ensuring that tight pressure is exerted.
◉ 3. keeping the eyelids in a closed position.
○ 4. promoting some ability for the client to see.

The nurse delivers a phone message to the client with the retinal detachment whose eyes are patched.

32 To maintain the client's dignity, the *most important* nursing action before leaving the room is to
○ 1. straighten the client's linen.
◉ 2. tell the client you are going.
○ 3. offer to give the client a back rub.
○ 4. share some current events with her.

The client with the retinal detachment is on strict bed rest with the head of her bed slightly elevated. One day the client says, "I'm not having any pain, and I'm not dying. Why can't I just get up once to go to the bathroom?"

33 The *best response* from the nurse is
◉ 1. "Gravity helps to reattach the separated retina."
○ 2. "You don't want to be permanently blind, do you?"
○ 3. "I can get you a sedative if it's hard to lay still."
○ 4. "It sounds like you got up on the wrong side of the bed."

The client with the detached retina undergoes a scleral buckling procedure.

34 Postoperatively, if the client experiences all of the following problems, which one has the *highest priority* for the nurse's attention at this time?
○ 1. Pain
◉ 2. Vomiting
○ 3. Anxiety
○ 4. Boredom

A client with myopia has a radial keratotomy (RK) procedure.

35 The *best evidence* that the client understands the *anticipated outcome* of this procedure is that the client indicates the procedure will help him
○ 1. have better night vision.
○ 2. identify colors correctly.
◉ 3. see well without glasses.
○ 4. use both eyes when reading.

A nurse is asked to assess a person who says he has "pinkeye."

36 If the client has conjunctivitis, upon inspecting the affected eye the nurse is *most likely* to observe erythema and
◉ 1. dried secretions along the lid.
○ 2. lack of pupil response to light.
○ 3. bulging of the eye from the orbit.
○ 4. loss of moisture on the cornea.

37 The *most important* health teaching the nurse can provide the client with conjunctivitis is to
○ 1. eat a well-balanced, nutritious diet.
○ 2. wear sunglasses in bright light.
◉ 3. cease sharing towels and washcloths.
○ 4. avoid products containing aspirin.

The physician seeks assistance from the nurse to apply a stain to the eye for the purposes of looking for a foreign body or injury to the cornea.

38 The nurse is *most correct* in providing the physician a solution containing
○ 1. povidone iodine.
○ 2. gentian violet.
◉ 3. methylene blue.
○ 4. fluorescein.

39 If a client develops macular degeneration, he or she is *most likely* to describe having an ability to see images only
○ 1. if they are close to the face.
○ 2. if they are at far distances.
◉ 3. in the outer peripheral fields.
○ 4. in the central field of vision.

A nurse makes home visits to several older adult clients with chronic health problems.

40 To which client is it *most important* that the nurse recommend regular eye examinations by an ophthalmologist so as to identify problems that may compromise the client's vision?
○ 1. Client A who takes aspirin daily.
◉ 2. Client B who has diabetes mellitus.
○ 3. Client C who has lactose intolerance.
○ 4. Client D who uses a potassium supplement.

A client with a malignant eye tumor has consented to have an enucleation of the eye.

41 Which statement is the *best evidence* that the client understands the postoperative outcome of this surgery.

1. "My vision will be restored with a plastic prosthesis."
2. "The prosthetic eye will be inserted during surgery."
3. "I will have to remove my prosthesis for cleaning."
4. "I will have a permanently empty eye socket."

42 Which sign or symptom is *most suggestive* that a client who had a corneal transplant is experiencing rejection of the donor tissue?
1. Excessive tearing
2. Change in vision
3. Itching of the eye
4. Frequent blinking

NURSING CARE OF CLIENTS WITH DISORDERS OF ACCESSORY EYE STRUCTURES

An older client's lower eyelid margins droop outward, exposing the conjunctival membrane and lower portion of the eyeball.

43 Based on the anatomical changes in the tone of the eyelid, the nurse is *most likely* to find that the client will experience
1. double vision.
2. photophobia.
3. lid spasms.
4. dry eyes.

The nurse observes that a client has inflamed eyelid margins and patchy dandruff-like flakes that cling to the eyelids and eyelashes.

44 If the etiology of the client's blepharitis is hypersecretion of sebaceous glands, it is *most appropriate* for the nurse to recommend
1. increasing attention to hygiene.
2. limiting oral fluid intake.
3. eating more deep yellow vegetables.
4. reducing time watching television.

45 When a person with a stye (hordeolum) asks a nurse to suggest measures to relieve his discomfort, the *best advice* the nurse can offer is to
1. squeeze the lesion to express the exudate.
2. apply warm, moist compresses to the area.
3. pierce the lesion with the tip of a pin.
4. cover the lesion with a dry, gauze dressing.

A physician has diagnosed the swelling within the inner surface of a client's eyelid as a chalazion, a gland obstructed with sebum.

46 The nurse is *correct* in telling the client that if the tissue continues to proliferate
1. it may lead to blindness.
2. the lashes may fall out.
3. surgery may be necessary.
4. it may cause severe pain.

NURSING CARE OF CLIENTS WITH EAR DISORDERS

A nurse notes that a client asks that questions be repeated during the nursing admission interview.

47 If the client worked at all of the following occupations, which one is *most likely* to have contributed to the hearing loss?
1. Telephone operator
2. Computer programmer
3. Musician
4. Accountant

A client is embarrassed when the nurse inspects his ear canal. He says, "Please bring me something so I can clean the earwax from my ears."

48 The *best response* for the purpose of health teaching is:
1. "It is best to use the corner of a soapy wash cloth."
2. "Do you prefer a short or long cotton applicator?"
3. "Have you ever tried removing earwax with a hairpin?"
4. "I can refer you to a doctor who will clean them."

49 Which one of the following instruments is *most appropriate* for the nurse to use for the purpose of testing the client's hearing acuity?
1. Otoscope
2. Tuning fork
3. Reflex hammer
4. Stethoscope

A client tells a nurse that he experiences continuous ringing in his ears.

50 Which question is *most appropriate* for the nurse to ask at this time?
1. "What childhood diseases have you had?"
2. "Were you born prematurely?"
3. "Do you eat a well-balanced diet?"
4. "How much aspirin do you take?"

A client who wears a hearing aid is frustrated by the loud, shrill noise, called feedback, that he hears occasionally.

51   Which of the following nursing actions is *most helpful* for reducing or eliminating feedback?
   ○ 1.   Repositioning the hearing aid within the ear
   ○ 2.   Cleaning the hearing aid with a soft cloth
   ○ 3.   Replacing the battery in the hearing aid
   ● 4.   Turning down the volume in the hearing aid

52   If a client who has recently experienced diminished hearing takes drugs from each of the following drug categories, which one is *most likely* to have affected the client's hearing?
   ○ 1.   Nonsteroidal anti-inflammatory drug
   ○ 2.   Beta adrenergic blocking agent
   ● 3.   Aminoglycoside antibiotic
   ○ 4.   Histamine (H$_2$) antagonist

53   When instilling prescribed medication into the ear of an adult, which is the *correct technique* for the nurse to use to straighten the ear canal?
   ● 1.   Pull the ear upward and backward.
   ○ 2.   Pull the ear downward and forward.
   ○ 3.   Pull the ear upward and forward.
   ○ 4.   Pull the ear downward and backward.

54   After instilling medication within the ear, what instruction is *most appropriate* for the nurse to give the client?
   ● 1.   Remain in position for at least 5 minutes.
   ○ 2.   Pack a cotton pledget tightly in the ear.
   ○ 3.   Don't blow your nose for at least 1 hour.
   ○ 4.   Avoid drinking very warm or cold beverages.

A person who is considering having her earlobes pierced consults a nurse on self-care techniques if the procedure is performed.

55   If the nurse provides the following information, which is *most important* for reducing the potential for infection?
   ○ 1.   Use earrings made of 14-kt gold.
   ○ 2.   Leave the earrings in place for 2 weeks.
   ○ 3.   Turn the earrings frequently.
   ● 4.   Swab the earlobes with alcohol daily.

When inspecting a client's ear, the nurse finds that the ear canal is red, swollen, and tender. The tympanic membrane is intact.

56   Which other assessment data is *most indicative* that the client has an infection in the *external* ear?
   ● 1.   There is a foul-smelling drainage.
   ○ 2.   The nurse notes the presence of dandruff.
   ○ 3.   The client's hearing is diminished in that ear.
   ○ 4.   The client hurt his head in a fall from a bicycle.

A client asks the nurse why adults do not experience middle ear infections as frequently as children.

57   The nurse is *most correct* in explaining that, in a child, organisms travel more easily from the nasopharynx to the middle ear because the eustachian tube is
   ● 1.   shorter and straighter.
   ○ 2.   longer and straighter.
   ○ 3.   shorter and more curved.
   ○ 4.   longer and more curved.

58   Which is the *best evidence* that the antibiotic the nurse is administering for the treatment of acute otitis media is having a therapeutic effect?
   ○ 1.   The ear feels less warm to the touch.
   ○ 2.   Ringing sounds within the ear stop.
   ○ 3.   Ear drainage is watery.
   ● 4.   Ear discomfort is relieved.

59   If a client with a middle ear infection described all of the following, which one is *most indicative* that the infection has spread to the inner ear?
   ○ 1.   The client indicates that he is experiencing headaches.
   ○ 2.   The client indicates that he is experiencing sore throat.
   ○ 3.   The client indicates that he is experiencing nasal congestion.
   ● 4.   The client indicates that he is experiencing dizziness.

A physician intends to perform a myringotomy on a client with a middle ear infection.

60   When the nurse prepares the client for the myringotomy, the *best explanation* as to the purpose for the procedure is that it will
   ○ 1.   prevent permanent hearing loss.
   ● 2.   provide a pathway for drainage.
   ○ 3.   aid in administering medications.
   ○ 4.   maintain motion of the ear bones.

61   When planning the discharge instructions for the client following a myringotomy, it is *best* for the nurse to tell the client that the cotton pledget in his ear canal should be
   ○ 1.   left in place until it is saturated.
   ● 2.   loosely placed within the ear canal.
   ○ 3.   soaked in peroxide before insertion.
   ○ 4.   removed when the cotton becomes dry.

A middle-aged female is seen in the physician's office for diminished hearing due to otosclerosis.

62   In acquiring the client's health history, which one of the following is *common* among people with otosclerosis?

○ 1. The onset of hearing loss started in childhood.

○ 2. High fevers accompanied upper respiratory infections.

○ 3. The tonsils and adenoids have usually been removed.

◉ 4. One or more relatives have been similarly diagnosed.

The client with otosclerosis asks the nurse to explain what the doctor meant by saying that she had a conductive hearing loss.

63 The nurse is *most correct* in explaining that a conductive hearing loss results when

◉ 1. sound waves do not travel to the inner ear.

○ 2. the structures in the inner ear malfunction.

○ 3. the eighth cranial nerve is permanently damaged.

○ 4. electric conversion of sound is not produced.

*The team leader who is responsible for the initial nursing care plan on the client with otosclerosis makes a nursing diagnosis of "**Risk for Impaired Verbal Communication Related to Hearing Loss.**"*

64 When the team leader asks the admitting nurse to assist with developing a goal for the identified diagnosis, the *best goal* is that

◉ 1. the client will state she can understand staff communication.

○ 2. the staff will improve verbal communication techniques.

○ 3. the client will demonstrate the ability to express herself.

○ 4. the client will be able to communicate basic needs.

The nurse helps the team leader plan interventions to promote effective communication with the client with otosclerosis.

65 Which is the *most appropriate* nursing order to include in the care plan of this client?

○ 1. Speak directly into the client's ear.

◉ 2. Face the client when speaking to her.

○ 3. Drop voice at the end of each sentence.

○ 4. Raise pitch of voice one octave higher.

The client with otosclerosis is scheduled for a stapedectomy, but she does not seem to understand the verbal information the doctor provided about the surgery.

66 The next *best alternative* for helping the client comprehend the details of the procedure at this time is to

◉ 1. provide her with a printed pamphlet on the topic.

○ 2. ask another stapedectomy client to talk with her.

○ 3. refer the communication to someone who can sign.

○ 4. write all of the information out in longhand.

The client who will undergo a stapedectomy says to the nurse, "There are so many awful complications that can happen with this surgery."

67 The *best* response from the nurse is

○ 1. "You've got the best surgeon on the staff."

◉ 2. "Tell me more about how you're feeling."

○ 3. "Don't worry. Those things hardly ever happen."

○ 4. "Let's think about something more pleasant."

68 After the stapedectomy, which is the *most appropriate technique* for assessing if the client's facial nerve function is intact?

○ 1. Ask the client to identify familiar odors.

◉ 2. Ask the client to smile or raise the eyebrows.

○ 3. Ask the client to stick out his or her tongue.

○ 4. Ask the client to read printed information.

69 For the first 24 hours after a stapedectomy, the nurse is *correct* to specify on the plan of care to position the client

◉ 1. flat with the operative ear uppermost.

○ 2. with the head raised and the knees flexed.

○ 3. supine with the head of the bed elevated.

○ 4. prone with the head on the operated side.

The day after the stapedectomy, the client is discouraged because her hearing is more impaired than it was preoperatively.

70 Which one of the following is the *most accurate explanation* for the client's hearing loss?

◉ 1. The hearing loss is temporary until edema and packing in the operative area are gone.

○ 2. The hearing loss is temporary until the nerve regenerates after the operative procedure.

○ 3. The hearing loss is temporary until being fitted with a molded plastic hearing aid.

○ 4. The hearing loss is temporary until the prosthesis becomes stabilized with new bone.

71 Which nursing instruction is *best* following a stapedectomy to prevent dislodging the internal prosthesis?

○ 1. When chewing food, keep your mouth closed.

○ 2. When blowing the nose, use a paper tissue.

◉ 3. When sneezing, keep your mouth wide open.

○ 4. When coughing, turn your head.

72 The nurse is *most accurate* in advising the staff person assigned to the client who had a stapedectomy that the client is at risk for injury due to the possibility of manifesting
○ 1. fatigue.
○ 2. diplopia.
● 3. vertigo.
○ 4. pain.

73 The *best evidence* that the client who has had a stapedectomy understands the activity restrictions after discharge is the client states that for the next 6 months he or she must avoid
○ 1. listening to music.
● 2. flying in an airplane.
○ 3. driving an automobile.
○ 4. singing in the choir.

A client is admitted to the hospital for possible Ménière's disease.

74 The subjective symptom this client is *most likely* to describe to the nurse is
○ 1. burning.
○ 2. pressure.
● 3. vertigo.
○ 4. pain.

The client with possible Ménière's disease will undergo a caloric test.

75 The teaching plan for preparing the client for this diagnostic test includes the explanation that
● 1. cold and warm water is instilled within each of the ears.
○ 2. earphones are worn through which sounds are transmitted.
○ 3. scalp electrodes are attached to the head in a darkened room.
○ 4. blood is drawn from a vein and examined microscopically.

76 During the caloric test, if the client has Ménière's disease, the nurse is *most likely* to observe
● 1. the onset of severe symptoms.
○ 2. no response or change in symptoms.
○ 3. nystagmus and slight dizziness.
○ 4. aphasia and loss of consciousness.

The nurse observes that the client with symptoms of Ménière's disease seems anxious whenever a member of the nursing staff enters the room.

77 If the client's anxiety is due to fear that nursing care will intensify his symptoms, which nursing intervention is *most appropriate* to add to the plan for care?

● 1. Let the client suggest ways to carry out his care.
○ 2. Discontinue all nursing care measures at this time.
○ 3. Restrict care to just nutrition and elimination needs.
○ 4. Carry out nursing activities quickly and efficiently.

The client asks the nurse to clarify the physician's explanation about the cause of Ménière's disease.

78 The nurse is *most accurate* in stating that the cause of Ménière's disease is unknown but that the symptoms are related to a(n)
○ 1. electrolyte deficit.
● 2. excess of fluid.
○ 3. vitamin deficiency.
○ 4. genetic defect.

79 While caring for a client with Ménière's disease, which nursing action is *most helpful* in preventing nausea and vomiting?
○ 1. Increasing oral fluids.
○ 2. Changing positions often.
○ 3. Keeping room lights dim.
● 4. Avoiding jarring the bed.

The client with Ménière's disease responds to conservative treatment and will be discharged.

80 Which statement indicates that the client needs additional teaching?
○ 1. The client says, "I must stop salting my food so much."
○ 2. The client says, "Future attacks may last minutes or days."
● 3. The client says, "My hearing will gradually improve."
○ 4. The client says, "Ménière's disease is not curable."

NURSING CARE OF CLIENTS WITH NASAL DISORDERS

81 When the nurse assesses a newly admitted client, which finding is *most suggestive* that the client may have had a fractured nose in the past?
○ 1. Multiple polyps are noted on the nasal mucous membranes.
○ 2. The client's nose is red, unusually large, and bulbous.
● 3. The septum deviates to the side, narrowing one naris.
○ 4. Serous drainage is noted within the nares and pharynx.

An older adult male comes to the emergency department with a nosebleed.

82 Based on the nurse's assessment findings, which is *most likely* to have been a *causative* factor in the client's nosebleed?
○ 1. The client's pulse rate is 110 beats per minute.
● 2. The client's blood pressure is 200/104 lying down.
○ 3. The client's temperature is 97.6°F (36.7°C) orally.
○ 4. The client's respirations are 24 per minute.

The client with the nosebleed is frightened by seeing the amount of blood that has collected on his shirt.

83 Which nursing action is *best* for relieving the client's fear and anxiety at this time?
○ 1. Lay the client down so he won't see his clothes.
○ 2. Give the client a popular magazine to read.
● 3. Replace the client's clothing with a hospital gown.
○ 4. Cover the client's eyes with a bath towel.

84 Which nursing action is *best* for controlling the client's nosebleed?
○ 1. Have the client lie down and swallow frequently.
○ 2. Have the client lie down and breathe through his mouth.
● 3. Have the client lean forward and apply direct pressure.
○ 4. Have the client lean forward and clench his teeth.

The nasal area from which the nosebleed is occurring is chemically cauterized with silver nitrate.

85 Before the client leaves the emergency department it is *essential* that the nurse tell the client to
○ 1. limit his dietary intake to just fluids.
○ 2. sleep in a recliner or with his head up.
○ 3. take his carotid pulse at hourly intervals.
● 4. avoid blowing his nose for several hours.

A client consults a physician concerning nasal polyps.

86 To assist the physician in identifying the etiology of the client's condition, it is *most important* for the nurse to inquire as to whether the client
○ 1. has had a recent nasal injury.
○ 2. has respiratory allergies.
● 3. has had previous nasal surgery.
○ 4. has ever had his tonsils removed.

A nasal polypectomy is performed and nasal packing is in place when the client returns from surgery.

87 Besides monitoring for blood on the anterior end of the packing, which other sign is *most indicative* that the client is bleeding from the operative site?
● 1. The client swallows frequently.
○ 2. The client's appetite is impaired.
○ 3. The client's voice sounds hoarse.
○ 4. The client has diminished hearing.

A middle-aged female is having a rhinoplasty procedure to improve the appearance of her nose.

88 When the nurse collects the following postoperative data, which finding is *most indicative* that the client with the rhinoplasty needs frequent oral care?
○ 1. The client says her throat is sore.
○ 2. The client's dressing is bloody.
○ 3. The client is slightly nauseated.
● 4. The client is mouth-breathing.

The client who has had a rhinoplasty asks the nurse postoperatively what she looks like.

89 The *best* response from the nurse at this time is,
○ 1. "I'm sure you will look absolutely gorgeous."
○ 2. "I didn't think you were unattractive before."
● 3. "Your face is swollen with bruises around the eyes."
○ 4. "Your personality is more important than your looks."

NURSING CARE OF CLIENTS WITH DISORDERS OF THE SKIN AND RELATED STRUCTURES

A nurse stops to give first aid to a female burn victim who has run from her home. The victim's clothing is on fire.

90 The *most appropriate* nursing action to take *first* is to
○ 1. rub petroleum jelly into the burned areas.
○ 2. wrap the affected areas with clean cloth.
○ 3. apply ice to the affected burned areas.
● 4. roll the victim to smother the flames.

The chest and neck of the victim are burned.

91 The *next priority* for the nurse is to
○ 1. obtain the victim's pulse and blood pressure.
● 2. monitor the victim for respiratory distress.
○ 3. identify the victim's next of kin.
○ 4. determine the extent of the burn.

In the emergency department, it is determined that the burn victim has deep partial- and full-thickness burns over 35% of her upper body.

92   The nurse who documents the burn injury is accurate in identifying the initial appearance of the full-thickness burns as those areas that are
○ 1. white and leathery.
○ 2. pink and blistered.
○ 3. red and painful.
○ 4. mottled and wet.

93   Once the blood pressure is stabilized, the *best assessment* for determining the client's response to the *initial* burn treatment is the client's
○ 1. body temperature.
○ 2. level of pain.
○ 3. urinary output.
○ 4. range of motion.

The client's treatment plan includes using the open method of burn wound management.

94   It is *most appropriate* for the nurse to monitor a client being treated by the open method for
○ 1. infection.
○ 2. hyperthermia.
○ 3. depression.
○ 4. malnutrition.

The physician orders the application of mafenide (Sulfamylon) to the burn wound.

95   The nurse who applies the Sulfamylon is accurate in the knowledge that its *chief disadvantage* is
○ 1. skin discoloration.
○ 2. pain on application.
○ 3. fluid volume deficit.
○ 4. contact dermatitis.

The burn wound periodically is debrided using hydrotherapy.

96   Shortly before each debridement, it is *essential* that the nurse
○ 1. keep the client in a fasting state.
○ 2. witness a signed consent form.
○ 3. administer a prescribed analgesic.
○ 4. weigh the client on a bed scale.

The health care team is informed that skin autografting is planned for the burn victim.

97   Which one of the following is *most appropriate* for the postoperative plan of care when the client has skin grafts?

○ 1. Minimizing movement to prevent graft disruption
○ 2. Changing the dressing over the graft every 8 hours
○ 3. Reinforcing the graft dressing if drainage occurs
○ 4. Applying wet soaks to the graft every 4 hours

Before the burn victim is discharged, she is fitted for an elasticized pressure garment that covers the burned areas of skin.

98   The *best evidence* that the client understands the purpose for wearing the pressure garment is the statement that it will
○ 1. prevent subsequent wound infection.
○ 2. prevent exposure to the sun.
○ 3. reduce the severity of scar formation.
○ 4. reduce the potential for social rejection.

When a nurse performs an initial physical assessment on an older adult transferred from a nursing home, it is noted that the client has a Stage III pressure sore on his left hip and sacrum.

99   Based on the etiology of a pressure sore, the *best nursing intervention* for promoting skin integrity is to
○ 1. apply a skin-toughening agent to susceptible areas.
○ 2. massage skin areas that remain persistently red.
○ 3. keep the head of the bed elevated 30 degrees.
○ 4. reposition the client every 2 hours.

A health nurse visits the home of a family being treated for pediculosis (head lice).

100   Which of the mother's statements indicates she needs more teaching?
○ 1. "One use of medicated shampoo eliminated the lice."
○ 2. "I've washed all the bed linen in soap and hot water."
○ 3. "None of the children share each other's combs."
○ 4. "I hope no other classmates have acquired lice."

101   Which of the following nursing interventions is *best* to add to the plan of care for a client with a venous stasis ulcer to promote wound healing?
○ 1. Elevate the lower extremities at all times.
○ 2. Keep the legs covered with warm blankets.
○ 3. Assess peripheral pulse sites every shift.
○ 4. Assist to sit in a chair three times a day.

A biopsy reveals that an Anglo-American client's scalp lesion is a basal cell carcinoma.

102 If all of the following data is obtained, which is the *most likely* contributing factor for developing skin cancer?
- ○ 1. The client is a chronic cigarette smoker.
- ● 2. The client has male pattern baldness.
- ○ 3. The client eats very few vegetables.
- ○ 4. The client bathes with a deodorant soap.

103 Which area of health teaching is *essential* when a female client is prescribed isotretinoin (Accutane) for treating acne vulgaris?
- ○ 1. Breast self-examination techniques
- ● 2. Techniques for avoiding pregnancy
- ○ 3. Methods for predicting ovulation
- ○ 4. Information on preventing sexual transmission

104 What is the *best nursing advice* for individuals who have frequent outbreaks of tinea pedis (athlete's foot)?
- ○ 1. "Never go barefoot when outdoors."
- ○ 2. "Cut your nails straight across."
- ● 3. "Wear different shoes each day."
- ○ 4. "Avoid wearing white cotton socks."

A client with shingles (herpes zoster) takes acyclovir (Zovirax).

105 When the client asks what causes shingles, the *most correct* reply is that shingles is caused by
- ● 1. the reactivation of a dormant virus.
- ○ 2. a vector-borne insect, like a tick.
- ○ 3. a toxin from a previous bacterial infection.
- ○ 4. an antibody response to a drug allergen.

106 Which information is *best* when providing health teaching to a client with a herpes simplex virus type 1 infection?
- ○ 1. Apply petroleum jelly to the lesions to prevent spread to adjacent areas.
- ● 2. Use good personal hygiene to prevent spreading the virus to other body parts.
- ○ 3. Avoid the use of soap and water on any open lesions.
- ○ 4. Remove the scabs daily by soaking with hot compresses.

A nurse assesses a client with psoriasis at a skin disorder clinic.

107 When examining the skin of the client with psoriasis, the nurse is *most likely* to observe
- ○ 1. weeping skin lesions on the trunk of the body.
- ● 2. red skin patches covered with silvery scales.
- ○ 3. fluid-filled blisters surrounded by crusts.
- ○ 4. a red rash containing raised pustules.

A nursing assistant with an allergy to latex asks the nurse for advice on carrying out standard precautions for preventing the transmission of blood-borne viruses.

108 The *best advice* the nurse can give is to
- ○ 1. rinse the latex gloves with running tap water before donning them.
- ○ 2. apply a petroleum ointment to both hands before donning latex gloves.
- ○ 3. eliminate wearing gloves, but wash both hands vigorously with alcohol afterward.
- ● 4. wear two pairs of vinyl gloves when there is a potential for contact with blood.

A person with prolonged exposure to cold consults a nurse about first-aid measures for treating frostbite.

109 Which measure is *best* for the nurse to recommend?
- ● 1. Soak affected body parts in a warm solution with a temperature of approximately 100°F.
- ○ 2. Begin the rewarming process by first applying cold skin compresses.
- ○ 3. Apply a heating pad on the highest setting to the affected body parts.
- ○ 4. Flood the surface of the affected skin with hot water at a temperature of approximately 140°F.

110 When a client develops pruritus, which nursing measure is *best* for relieving the client's discomfort?
- ○ 1. Use hypoallergenic or glycerin soap for bathing.
- ○ 2. Add extra wool blankets to the bedding for warmth.
- ● 3. Take showers rather than tub baths.
- ○ 4. Rub the skin dry after bathing.

Directions: Two numbers appear in parentheses following each rationale. The first number identifies the textbook listed in the references, page 512, and the second number identifies the page(s) in that textbook on which the correct answer can be verified. Occasionally two or more textbooks are given to verify the correct answer.

NURSING CARE OF CLIENTS WITH EYE DISORDERS

1 3. Irrigating the eyes is the most important first step in treating a chemical injury. Diluting and removing the chemical reduces the potential for corneal damage. Although identifying the chemical is important, immediate treatment is not compromised by taking time to determine what, if anything, will neutralize the chemical. Liability is affected if safety glasses are not worn, but the priority is treating the chemical splash if that has not already been done. It is too soon to evaluate the extent of sensory damage. (4:1068; 18:352; 21:620)

Nursing Process—Data collection
Client Need—Physiological integrity

2 1. Water is used in an emergency to flush the eye(s) and dilute the chemical. Tap water from a faucet or shower is generally available. The other chemical solutions may be appropriate depending on the specific chemical that caused the trauma, but they may need to be diluted to a specific strength to prevent additional damage to the eye. Valuable time is wasted by delaying first-aid measures. (18:352; 21:620)

Nursing Process—Planning
Client Need—Physiological integrity

3 2. The irrigating solution is directed so that it flows from the inner canthus toward the outer canthus. This is an especially important principle to follow so that substances in one eye do not come in contact with tissue of the other eye. It is best to instill the force of the water on the conjunctiva rather than onto the sensitive cornea, which may cause discomfort or reflex blinking. The anterior chamber is not an external eye structure. The nasolacrimal duct lies in the area of the inner canthus. (4:1070)

Nursing Process—Implementation
Client Need—Physiological integrity

4 2. An ophthalmologist is a physician who is licensed to diagnose and treat eye diseases and traumatic injuries. An optician fills prescriptions for corrective lenses. An optometrist tests vision and prescribes glasses or contact lenses to correct visual acuity. A podiatrist is trained in the care of feet. (18:1086)

Nursing Process—Implementation
Client Need—Safe, effective care environment

5 4. The eyes are patched loosely with the lids closed to reduce further injury by blinking and moving the eyes. Instilling antibiotic ointment interferes with the medical examination, although it may be prescribed after the object is removed. Attempts to remove an embedded object are left to others with medical training. (4:1069; 18:352)

Nursing Process—Implementation
Client Need—Physiological integrity

6 2. A Snellen chart is used to test far vision. Clients therefore stand 20 feet from the chart and are asked to read letters that progressively become smaller. A Jaeger chart is used to test near vision. Ishihara plates are used to test color vision. A tangent screen is used to assess the peripheral visual field. This test requires that the client indicate when he sees a stimulus in his peripheral vision. (4:1049; 25:178–179)

Nursing Process—Implementation
Client Need—Health promotion/maintenance

7 4. The term for nearsightedness is myopia. Presbyopia is a type of farsightedness associated with aging. It is caused by loss of elasticity in the lenses. Amblyopia is commonly referred to as "lazy eye." Untreated amblyopia results in the loss of vision in one eye from lack of use. Hyperopia is farsightedness. (4:1052; 18:1087; 21:615)

Nursing Process—Implementation
Client Need—Health promotion/maintenance

8 3. The Lions International organization has vision and hearing improvement as its major goal. Local or state chapters can provide information and assistance to those who need but cannot afford glasses, a guide dog, hearing aid, or surgery. The other organizations are both fraternal and philanthropic, but they have not named vision or hearing assistance as their projects. (18:1089)

Nursing Process—Implementation
Client Need—Health promotion/maintenance

9 2. Due to an irregularly shaped cornea or lens, a person with astigmatism has unequal refraction of images on the retina. Therefore, there is an area where objects appear blurred or distorted (wider or taller) than they actually are. People with hyperopia see far objects more clearly. People with myopia can see near objects more clearly. No visual acuity disorder causes objects to appear unusually small. (4:1052; 18:1087; 21:615)

> Nursing Process—Data collection
> Client Need—Physiological integrity

10 2. Glasses are washed first and wiped with a soft cloth to avoid scratching the surface with dirt and dust. Paper products are not used for drying because they are made from wood pulp, which could scratch the lenses, especially if they are made of plastic. Air drying is tedious and likely to leave the glasses streaked. (25:324)

> Nursing Process—Implementation
> Client Need—Safe, effective care environment

11 2. Anxiety occurs because a person feels threatened by an unexpected or unfamiliar situation. Having care explained before it is performed prepares a person for what is about to take place. A sightless client is always spoken to before being touched. Shutting the door increases a client's feeling of isolation and fear that help will be unavailable. Having adequate light helps the partially sighted but not someone who cannot see. (4:1050–1051; 21:616)

> Nursing Process—Planning
> Client Need—Psychosocial integrity

12 1. A blind person feels safer and more secure by following the lead of someone who is sighted. This is best accomplished by having the blind person stand slightly behind and to the side while taking the sighted person's arm. Safety is a higher priority in an unfamiliar environment than total independence. (4:1051; 25:617)

> Nursing Process—Evaluation
> Client Need—Safe, effective care environment

13 1. Using the imagery of a clock helps the sightless person locate food and feed himself or herself. Feeding a client does not promote self-reliance. Ordering liquid forms of nourishment without collaborating first with the client implies that he or she is not capable of eating like an adult and may lower self-esteem. Beverages in paper cups are more likely to spill during the client's attempts at eating independently and may reinforce a feeling of inadequacy. (4:1051; 21:617)

> Nursing Process—Planning
> Client Need—Psychosocial integrity

14 1. As senile cataracts form, they cause progressively diminished vision. The visual change is due to degeneration of the lenses of the eye due to aging. Fullness and ocular pain or discomfort are more likely due to trauma or an inflammatory process. Seeing flashes of light is a symptom described by someone with a detached retina. (4:1058; 21:628)

> Nursing Process—Data collection
> Client Need—Physiological integrity

15 3. When the eyes of someone with cataracts are examined, the usual black pupil appears white, gray, or yellow. This sign is due to an opacity of the lens, which lies behind the pupil, the opening in the center of the iris. Ruptured blood vessels on the eye are associated with conditions in which the blood pressure has been suddenly elevated, such as when performing Valsalva maneuver while vomiting or defecating. An irregularly shaped iris can be the result of surgery performed for the treatment of glaucoma. Abnormal tissue may appear as a growth on the cornea. (4:1058; 21:629)

> Nursing Process—Data collection
> Client Need—Physiological integrity

16 1. The time for cataract removal is left to the client. It largely depends on the person and when the impaired vision interferes with the quality of his or her life. Cataracts are painless. The opinions of others do not influence the timing of surgery. Postponing surgery until a cataract "ripens" is no longer considered a standard for care. (18:1091)

> Nursing Process—Evaluation
> Client Need—Health promotion/maintenance

17 2. The nurse clarifies any aspect of the medical orders that seem inaccurate. The nurse therefore consults with the physician who wrote the abbreviation *o.s.* for administering preoperative medication into the left eye, but plans to remove the cataract from the right eye. The client or the nurse scrubs the skin. It is not essential that the client do this himself. Usually, the nurse preparing the client for surgery is responsible for clipping the eyelashes on the operative eye. (25:697)

> Nursing Process—Implementation
> Client Need—Physiological integrity

18 4. Eye drops and ointments are placed in the exposed lower conjunctival sac. If they are placed on the cornea, they may cause discomfort and reflex blinking. Medication is systemically absorbed when instilled at the inner canthus. Placing eye drops and ointments at the outer canthus makes it difficult to distribute them in the eye. (18:724; 25:717)

Nursing Process—Implementation
Client Need—Physiological integrity

19 3. Coughing and other activities, like straining or squeezing the eyelids together, is avoided to prevent an increase in intraocular pressure. Raising intraocular pressure places strain on the delicate sutures and may dislodge an intraocular lens if one is implanted. The client can and should deep-breathe to prevent postoperative respiratory complications. All the other orders are appropriate for this patient. (4:1059; 26:799)

Nursing Process—Planning
Client Need—Physiological integrity

20 1. Severe pain is an indication that intraocular hemorrhage is occurring. It is essential to report these data to the nurse in charge, who may then contact the client's surgeon. Giving an analgesic masks the symptom and thereby decreases the perception of its significance. Assessing pupils does not reveal the cause of the symptom. The pupils will most likely be dilated and not respond to light. Postoperatively, cataract clients are not allowed to lie on their operative side. (4:1060; 21:632)

Nursing Process—Implementation
Client Need—Physiological integrity

21 2. A metal eye shield, called a Fox shield, is applied at night or before naps to prevent accidental injury to the operative eye. The shield is a mechanical barrier between the environment and the eye, but that is not the purpose for its use. Patching the eyes does not prevent the rapid eye movements that occur during sleep. If it is necessary to dilate the pupil, drugs are used that paralyze the ciliary muscle. (18:1084)

Nursing Process—Implementation
Client Need—Health promotion/maintenance

22 1. Bending over is contraindicated for approximately 2 weeks after eye surgery because it puts strain on the operative sutures. It is not necessary to keep both eyes patched at all times. Clients may sleep with or without a pillow, but they are to sleep on their unoperative side for about 1 week to prevent pressure on the operative eye and reduce tissue edema. External bleeding is not expected at any time postoperatively. Intraocular bleeding, indicated by sudden eye pain, is considered a complication that necessitates immediate examination. (18:1084)

Nursing Process—Planning
Client Need—Health promotion/maintenance

23 3. People with both chronic and acute glaucoma generally describe the appearance of rainbow halos or rings, particularly around lights. Itching and burning are likely an allergic response. Headaches may occur when a client who is in need of corrective lenses strains to read. The loss of central vision is a symptom of macular degeneration. (18:1090; 21:626)

Nursing Process—Data collection
Client Need—Safe, effective care environment

24 2. The symptoms of glaucoma occur as a result of increased intraocular pressure. This condition is diagnosed using an instrument called a tonometer. An ophthalmoscope is an instrument used for viewing the fundus or back portion of the eye. A retinoscope is used to measure visual acuity and determine refractory errors. A speculum is an instrument that widens a cavity. (4:1049; 21:626)

Nursing Process—Implementation
Client Need—Safe, effective care environment

25 1. The person with chronic glaucoma gradually loses peripheral vision. If untreated, the visual field is reduced to only the image that is focused directly on the macula. Clients describe this as looking through a tube or tunnel. Double vision is due to neurologic diseases or a weakness in eye muscles. Bulging eyes, also called exophthalmos, accompanies hyperthyroidism. Inflamed eyes can be due to various irritating substances. (4:1065; 18:1090–1091)

Nursing Process—Data collection
Client Need—Physiological integrity

26 3. Glaucoma is a chronic disease that requires lifelong treatment unless the client is treated surgically. Handwashing and replacing the cap are aseptic measures to prevent the transmission of organisms within the eye. Timolol maleate is a beta adrenergic blocking agent that decreases aqueous humor formation without constricting the pupil. (4:1065; 18:1091; 21:627, 643)

Nursing Process—Evaluation
Client Need—Health promotion/maintenance

27 1. Atropine sulfate and other anticholinergic drugs dilate the pupil. This blocks the drainage of aqueous humor. If administered, atropine sulfate may cause an acute attack by precipitating high intraocular pressure. If untreated, the client may become permanently blind. Morphine sulfate is a narcotic analgesic. Magnesium sulfate is known as Epsom salts. Ferrous sulfate is an iron preparation. None of these last three substances is contraindicated for clients with glaucoma. (4:1065; 21:627)

Nursing Process—Implementation
Client Need—Physiological integrity

28 2. When there is an acute increase in intraocular pressure, clients experience severe eye pain, nausea, vomiting, and loss of vision. Clients with retinal detachments or hypertension describe seeing "spots" in their fields of vision. During an acute attack of closed-angle glaucoma, the pupils are widely dilated; treatment involves administering drugs that both constrict the pupils and eliminate intraocular fluid. The eyes appear normal in size even during an acute attack of closed-angle glaucoma. (4:1065; 21:926)

Nursing Process—Data collection
Client Need—Physiological integrity

29 4. An iridectomy involves removing a piece of the iris to allow aqueous humor to flow from the posterior chamber into the anterior chamber and out Schlemm's canal. The iris no longer appears perfectly round postoperatively; the missing section appears black. (21:627)

Nursing Process—Data collection
Client Need—Physiological integrity

30 2. Retinal detachment has multiple etiologies. The more common etiologies include trauma, such as a blow to the head, myopia, and degenerative changes. Aging is a factor, but the most common period for retinal detachment is between the ages of 50 and 60. There is no causal relationship between a retinal detachment, infection, or allergies. (18:1092; 21:630)

Nursing Process—Data collection
Client Need—Physiological integrity

31 3. The purpose for patching the eyes of a client with a detached retina is to keep the eyes at rest; the patches therefore are applied to both eyes with the eyelids closed. Keeping the eyelids closed also protects them from contact with dust or fibers and prevents the eyes from becoming dry, because blinking is difficult once the eyes are patched. Light is not necessarily harmful; rather, it is the problem of looking about. Gravity rather than pressure has some therapeutic value when treating a detached retina. Patching the eyes, but facilitating vision is a contradiction in therapeutic principles. (21:631)

Nursing Process—Implementation
Client Need—Physiological integrity

32 2. Because the client whose eyes are patched has no visual cue as to whether the nurse is still in the room, it is important to indicate when the client is being left alone. It is frustrating and embarrassing to carry on a conversation when no one is there to respond. (4:1051)

Nursing Process—Implementation
Client Need—Psychosocial integrity

33 1. Giving an explanation of the purpose for bed rest helps the client to comply with the prescribed therapy. Bed rest and bilateral patching frequently are the initial conservative treatments for a detached retina before surgical alternatives are considered. Asking a client if he or she wants to be permanently blind may heighten a client's anxiety. Sedatives often are prescribed. In this case, however, the situation does not warrant the added risks from sedation. Responding in a superficial, belittling manner, as in the last example, implies that the client's question is frivolous. (9:138–139; 25:79–80)

Nursing Process—Implementation
Client Need—Psychosocial integrity

34 2. Vomiting raises intraocular pressure and requires immediate treatment. If an antiemetic is not ordered, the nurse notifies the charge nurse or the physician. Pain is expected following surgery for a detached retina. Although pain causes discomfort, its treatment, or lack thereof, does not affect the outcome of the surgical procedure. Anxiety and boredom are not physiologic problems and therefore do not rank as high on the list of priorities. (18:1084; 21:633; 26:800)

Nursing Process—Evaluation
Client Need—Physiological integrity

35 3. Radial keratotomy (RK) is performed to reshape the cornea so visual images converge directly on the retina. If successful, clients who undergo RK no longer need to wear corrective lenses. Radial keratotomy does *not* improve night vision, correct color blindness, or facilitate binocular vision. (4:1053; 21:616)

Nursing Process—Evaluation
Client Need—Physiological integrity

36 1. Clients with "pinkeye," which is a common name for conjunctivitis, have an obviously inflamed conjunctiva, sticky or crusty drainage that collects on the lid, itching or burning of the eyes, and possible edema of the eyelid. The disorder is not associated with any compromise in pupil response. The eyelid may be swollen, but the eye itself does not protrude. Tearing may be excessive. (4:1055; 21:622)

Nursing Process—Data collection
Client Need—Physiological integrity

37 3. Using individual bath linen and performing frequent handwashing are techniques for preventing the transmission of infectious microorganisms that are present in the inflammatory secretions. Eating a nutritious diet and using sunglasses to filter ultraviolet light are healthful behaviors, but they are unrelated to the client's disorder. The use of aspirin is not contraindicated; in fact, a mild analgesic may relieve some of the client's discomfort. (4:1055; 21:622)

> Nursing Process—Implementation
> Client Need—Health promotion/maintenance

38 4. Fluorescein is a tissue-staining substance that is applied topically to assess the condition of the cornea. Povidone iodine and gentian violet are used for their antimicrobial properties rather than for diagnostic purposes. Methylene blue is used to stain pathology slides and for the treatment of cyanide poisoning. (4:1056; 21:623)

> Nursing Process—Implementation
> Client Need—Safe, effective care environment

39 3. Having lost macular function, which is the point at which light rays converge to provide the clearest and most distinct visual information, clients are left with what appears to them as a "bull's-eye" visual defect. Peripheral vision remains, but it is not sufficient to read or perform any other activities that require acute vision. (4:1062; 21:625)

> Nursing Process—Data collection
> Client Need—Physiological integrity

40 2. Clients with diabetes mellitus are at risk for developing vascular pathology in the retina. Their retinal blood vessels tend to weaken and bleed. When treated early with photocoagulation using a laser, or by having a vitrectomy performed, loss of vision is delayed or prevented. Persons who take aspirin, have lactose intolerance, and use potassium supplements are not at any higher risk for ophthalmologic complications than others in the general population. (4:1062; 21:807)

> Nursing Process—Planning
> Client Need—Health promotion/maintenance

41 3. Following an enucleation, clients are taught how to remove, cleanse, and replace the shell-shaped prosthetic eye. The prosthetic eye is only cosmetic, not functional. A conformer, a round implant, is inserted during surgery to maintain the shape of the eye. The conformer remains permanently in place; the prosthetic eye is not inserted until healing takes place which, for most, is approximately 4 to 6 weeks postoperatively. (4:1071; 18:1092–1093; 25:325)

> Nursing Process—Evaluation
> Client Need—Health promotion/maintenance

42 2. Signs of corneal transplant rejection include redness, loss of vision, and sensitivity to light. If tearing, blinking, and itching occur, they deserve medical assessment. However, they are not the usual indications of tissue rejection. (4:1071)

> Nursing Process—Data collection
> Client Need—Physiological integrity

NURSING CARE OF CLIENTS WITH DISORDERS OF ACCESSORY EYE STRUCTURES

43 4. Incomplete closure of the eyelids leads to dry eyes. The tarsal muscles within the lids are generally atonic due to age; consequently, lid spasms are unlikely. Topical medications are used to treat the symptoms, but surgery provides a more permanent cosmetic and functional treatment. Neither double vision nor light sensitivity are common manifestations of structural disorders of the lids. (4:1057)

> Nursing Process—Data collection
> Client Need—Physiological integrity

44 1. Blepharitis is commonly associated with excessive oiliness of the skin, face, and scalp. Therefore, more frequent washing of the face and hair relieves the symptoms. In chronic or severe conditions, clients improve with the additional use of a topical antibiotic ointment. Modifying fluid and food intake and the amount of time spent watching television are not likely to prove therapeutic in managing the signs and symptoms of blepharitis. (21:623)

> Nursing Process—Implementation
> Client Need—Health promotion/maintenance

45 2. Warm moist heat improves circulation to the area that is inflamed and swollen. Vasodilation relieves the edema and promotes a reduction in exudate via absorption or phagocytosis. Incision and drainage may become necessary, but it is better performed by a physician than the client. Covering the lesion disguises the appearance of the stye, but it does not provide any therapeutic benefit. (18:1089; 21:623)

> Nursing Process—Implementation
> Client Need—Health promotion/maintenance

46 3. A chalazion, and other eyelid disorders, tend to be minor. If gentle massage does not relieve the obstruction, office surgery is performed to excise the cyst-like growth of tissue. A chalazion is more likely to produce a sensation of pressure than of pain. The eyelashes are lost from seborrheic blepharitis, not a chalazion. Blindness is not a common complication associated with a chalazion. (18:1089; 21:624)

> Nursing Process—Implementation
> Client Need—Health promotion/maintenance

NURSING CARE OF CLIENTS WITH EAR DISORDERS

47 3. Musicians, and others who are exposed to excessively loud sound without ear protection, acquire sensorineural hearing loss. There is no significant evidence that occupations involving computer programming, using the telephone, or accounting are associated with impaired hearing. (4:1074; 18:1093–1094)

> Nursing Process—Data collection
> Client Need—Physiological integrity

48 1. The accumulation of normal cerumen is best removed by washing the ears with soapy water and a soft cloth. Hard and sharp objects can injure the ear canal or tympanic membrane. A medical referral is appropriate only if the cerumen is excessively hard or impacted within the ear. (4:1045; 18:513)

> Nursing Process—Implementation
> Client Need—Health promotion/maintenance

49 2. A tuning fork is used to test for conductive and sensorineural hearing loss. Weber's test is performed by striking the tuning fork and placing it centrally on the forehead. The Rinne test is performed by striking the tuning fork and placing it on the mastoid bone and beside the ear. An otoscope is used to inspect the physical structures in the external ear. A reflex hammer is used to test deep tendon responses. A stethoscope is used to auscultate body sounds. (4:1073; 25:181–182)

> Nursing Process—Planning
> Client Need—Health promotion/maintenance

50 4. Tinnitus, ringing or buzzing in the ears, is a common symptom experienced by people who take repeated, high dosages of aspirin. Although tinnitus is associated with many ear disorders, the other questions in this item do not necessarily help to establish a cause-and-effect relationship with the client's symptom. (18:594; 20:124)

> Nursing Process—Data collection
> Client Need—Physiological integrity

51 1. Feedback, a loud shrill noise, occurs when a hearing aid is not positioned correctly within the ear. Cleaning, replacing the battery, and regulating the volume are important to the care of a client with a hearing aid, but they do not affect feedback. (25:326)

> Nursing Process—Implementation
> Client Need—Health promotion/maintenance

52 3. The aminoglycoside family of antibiotics, of which gentamicin is one example, is ototoxic and nephrotoxic. Beta adrenergic blocking agents cause vertigo but they do not affect hearing acuity. Neither nonsteroidal anti-inflammatory drugs nor histamine (H_2) antagonists are known to be ototoxic. (17:118; 20:73)

> Nursing Process—Evaluation
> Client Need—Physiological integrity

53 1. The correct technique for straightening the ear canal of an adult is to pull the ear upward and backward. For a child, the ear is pulled downward and backward. (4:137; 25:182)

> Nursing Process—Implementation
> Client Need—Physiological integrity

54 1. Maintaining a position, such as the head tilted to the side or a side-lying position, facilitates the movement of the medication to the lowest area of the ear canal. Cotton is loosely inserted within the ear to collect drainage and any excess volume of medication. The eustachian tube does connect the middle ear with the pharynx. However, if the tympanic membrane is intact, blowing the nose does not displace the medication. The temperature of beverages does not affect the instillation of ear drops. (4:414; 18:725)

> Nursing Process—Implementation
> Client Need—Physiological integrity

55 4. Swabbing the earlobes mechanically removes microorganisms from the area. The use of alcohol, which is an antimicrobial agent, inhibits the growth of pathogens that remain. Using quality metal, such as 14-kt gold, tends to reduce local inflammation due to hypersensitivity. Leaving the earrings in place temporarily and turning them facilitates the formation of a well-healed channel. (18:1096; 25:430–431)

> Nursing Process—Implementation
> Client Need—Health promotion/maintenance

56 1. The presence of drainage, called otorrhea, is most suggestive that an inflammatory process is the underlying problem. Because the drainage is foul smelling, the likelihood that the inflammation is due to a pathogen is highly probable. Hearing is diminished from swelling and drainage that blocks the transmission of sound on currents of air, but there are other preinfectious factors that can cause a loss of hearing. Trauma can rupture the eardrum, but the eardrum is intact according to the data. Injuring the head is most likely unrelated to an infection. Dandruff suggests a dry, flaky dermatitis of the scalp and not something that contributes to the acute symptoms with which the client presents. (4:1076)

> Nursing Process—Data collection
> Client Need—Physiological integrity

57 1. Organisms travel more easily through a pathway that is short and straight, which is the case in infants and children. With growth, the eustachian tube changes to a 45-degree angle. This natural curve provides a barrier against ascending pathogens. (16:729; 18:1098)

> Nursing Process—Implementation
> Client Need—Health promotion/maintenance

58 4. Antibiotic effectiveness is most evident when the client's ear discomfort is relieved. The inflamed area in the middle ear is beyond the reach of the fingers; therefore assessing the temperature of the tissue is impossible. Tinnitus, or disturbing sounds, is not generally a problem for a person during the acute phase of a middle ear infection. Watery or purulent drainage is an indication that the eardrum is perforated. (21:640)

> Nursing Process—Evaluation
> Client Need—Physiological integrity

59 4. Signs of labyrinthitis (inflammation of the labyrinth of the inner ear) include dizziness, nausea, vomiting, and nystagmus. Headaches indicate the infection has extended to the meningeal area of the brain. Sore throat and nasal congestion are more likely caused by the primary upper respiratory infection, which often precedes a middle ear infection. (4:1080)

> Nursing Process—Data collection
> Client Need—Physiological integrity

60 2. A myringotomy, which is the term for incising the tympanic membrane or eardrum, provides a pathway for drainage from the middle ear. As the exudate drains, the client's discomfort is reduced. A surgical incision is preferable to the spontaneous rupture of the eardrum since a surgical incision heals better. Although hearing may be permanently diminished, it is less affected with an incised tympanic membrane. Systemic drugs rather than topical drugs are more effective in treating a middle ear infection. Incising the eardrum is not done to preserve motion of the ossicles in the middle ear. (18:1097; 21:638)

> Nursing Process—Implementation
> Client Need—Health promotion/maintenance

61 2. Loosely packed cotton is more likely to absorb drainage than tightly packed cotton. The cotton pledget is replaced on a scheduled basis or as it becomes moist. It is incorrect to wait until the cotton is totally saturated. The ear canal is generally cleansed before inserting the dry cotton. (18:1097; 21:638)

> Nursing Process—Planning
> Client Need—Health promotion/maintenance

62 4. Although the cause of otosclerosis is unknown, most have a family history of this condition. The onset of this disorder usually becomes apparent when clients are in their twenties or thirties. Otosclerosis is caused by an ankylosing of the bones in the middle ear. Therefore having a high fever and having tonsils or adenoids has no relationship to the development of otosclerosis. (4:1082; 21:639)

> Nursing Process—Data collection
> Client Need—Physiological integrity

63 1. A conductive hearing loss occurs when there is a barrier in the transmission of vibrating sound waves from the external and middle ear to the inner ear. Common causes of conductive hearing loss include otosclerosis, otitis media, and a ruptured tympanic membrane. The other options in this item describe the causes of sensorineural hearing loss. (18:1093; 21:610)

> Nursing Process—Implementation
> Client Need—Health promotion/maintenance

64 1. Indicating an ability to understand staff is a measurable, client-centered goal. Accomplishing this goal indicates that the approaches used by staff to communicate with the hearing-impaired client are effective. The goal should not indicate what the nursing team hopes to accomplish. The client with normal speech but decreased hearing does not have difficulty verbally communicating to staff. (26:806; 25:22–23)

> Nursing Process—Planning
> Client Need—Safe, effective care environment

65 2. It is best to face the hearing-impaired client so that lip movements and facial expressions are seen because most have learned to adapt by lip reading or speech reading. Speaking into the client's ear distorts the words and masks the visual cues. Dropping the voice causes some of the words to be missed. Raising or lowering the pitch of the voice helps persons with a hearing loss in one or the other vocal registers. High tones are generally more difficult to hear. (4:1075; 26:806)

> Nursing Process—Planning
> Client Need—Physiological integrity

66 1. As long as the client is literate and is not visually impaired, reading a descriptive pamphlet is an appropriate alternative. Another stapedectomy client should not be the primary resource for explaining technical information. A client with otosclerosis is probably not so profoundly deaf that he or she uses sign language. Writing short sentences or words is appropriate, but writing lengthy technical information is too tedious and time-consuming. (4:1075; 26:805)

      Nursing Process—Planning
      Client Need—Safe, effective care environment

67 2. Encouraging a client to discuss his or her feelings is a therapeutic intervention. Endorsing or defending the expertise of the surgeon does not relieve the client's fears about the risks she is facing. Giving advice, offering a reassuring cliché, and changing the subject are nontherapeutic communication techniques. (9:140–141; 25:79–80)

      Nursing Process—Implementation
      Client Need—Psychosocial integrity

68 2. The facial nerve, which is cranial nerve VII, is assessed by having the client smile or raise the eyebrows. If there is facial asymmetry, it suggests there is damage to this nerve. The olfactory nerve is assessed by asking the client to identify familiar odors. The hypoglossal nerve is tested by having the client stick out his or her tongue. The optic nerve is tested by determining if the client can see. (4:1099; 18:591; 21:639)

      Nursing Process—Data collection
      Client Need—Physiological integrity

69 1. Keeping the client flat and the operative ear up helps to maintain the placement of the prosthetic stapes and reduce the occurrence of vertigo. None of the other positional choices accomplishes this goal. (4:1085; 21:639)

      Nursing Process—Planning
      Client Need—Physiological integrity

70 1. Both rebound swelling and packing within the ear contribute to a temporary decrease in hearing acuity after a stapedectomy. This setback is only temporary and eventually subsides in the absence of any complications. The success of the surgery is evident in a matter of weeks. If the surgery is successful, the client does not need a hearing aid. The prosthetic stapes is secured to the incus by a fine wire loop or hook. It moves immediately without any bone formation around it. (4:1085; 26:809)

      Nursing Process—Implementation
      Client Need—Health promotion/maintenance

71 3. To avoid displacing the device that replaces the stapes, it is best to keep the mouth widely open if and when a sneeze is unavoidable. Esthetically, chewing food with the mouth closed shows good table manners. To prevent transmitting infectious organisms, it is best to enclose the exudate from the nose in a paper tissue and dispose of it in a lined refuse container. Turning the head also reduces the potential for droplet transmission of pathogens. (26:809)

      Nursing Process—Implementation
      Client Need—Health promotion/maintenance

72 3. Vertigo is often experienced by stapedectomy clients due to a loss of perilymph, or labrynthitis. To avoid injury, the side rails are kept raised and the client is assisted with ambulation. The client undergoing stapedectomy is generally young or middleaged and is not likely to feel exceptionally tired. Diplopia is not associated with the effects of this surgery. There is some discomfort, but it is not a major postoperative problem predisposing the client to injury. (4:1085; 21:639)

      Nursing Process—Implementation
      Client Need—Safe, effective care environment

73 2. Flying in an airplane is temporarily contraindicated after a stapedectomy because of the potential damaging effects that may occur with sudden changes in air pressure. For the same reason, scuba diving also is avoided. None of the other activities are specifically contraindicated for a client who has had a stapedectomy. (21:642; 26:806)

      Nursing Process—Evaluation
      Client Need—Health promotion/maintenance

74 3. The major symptom of Ménière's disease is severe vertigo. This is not described as simply dizziness, but rather a sensation of seeing and feeling motion or rotation. The other symptoms are not associated with Ménèiere's disease. (18:1098; 21:640)

      Nursing Process—Data collection
      Client Need—Physiological integrity

75 1. A caloric test involves instilling cold and warm solution separately into each ear. An audiometric test requires headphones. Electrodes are used for electroencephalography and electronystagmography. A specimen of blood is not used in a caloric test. (18:1091; 21:611)

      Nursing Process—Planning
      Client Need—Health promotion/maintenance

76 1. A client with Ménière's disease develops a sudden onset of severe symptoms such as vertigo, nausea, vomiting, and tinnitus during a caloric test. If there is no response to the instillation of warm or cold solution within the ear, it indicates an auditory nerve tumor. Normal people experience slight dizziness and nystagmus during a caloric test. Aphasia and loss of consciousness are unrelated to the mechanics or physiology of a caloric test. (18:1081)

    Nursing Process—Data collection
    Client Need—Physiological integrity

77 1. Allowing the client to participate in the planning and implementation of nursing activities maintains an independent locus of control. The client, more so than anyone else, knows what movement will cause him the least discomfort. Discontinuing or restricting nursing activities does not reflect a high standard of care. Performing nursing activities quickly heightens the client's anxiety because unexpected movements can induce or aggravate his symptoms. (9:89; 10:91; 18:1098)

    Nursing Process—Planning
    Client Need—Psychosocial integrity

78 2. Ménière's disease seems to be related to an increase in endolymphatic fluid within the spaces of the labyrinth in the inner ear. Neither electrolyte or vitamin deficiency nor genetics is implicated as a cause of Ménière's disease. (18:1098; 21:639)

    Nursing Process—Implementation
    Client Need—Health promotion/maintenance

79 4. Sudden movement of the client's head or making sudden movements precipitate an attack that includes nausea and vomiting. Decreasing fluid intake is beneficial. Changing positions frequently is avoided. The intensity of room lights is not a factor in controlling the symptoms of Ménière's disease. (18:1098; 21:640)

    Nursing Process—Implementation
    Client Need—Physiological integrity

80 3. Hearing loss associated with Ménière's disease becomes progressively worse with each subsequent attack. Low-sodium diets are prescribed to control the volume of endolymph. The period of time that symptoms last is unpredictable. Surgery is performed in advanced cases to eliminate the vertigo, nausea, and vomiting. However, permanent deafness is a consequence of most surgical procedures. (4:1082; 21:639–640)

    Nursing Process—Evaluation
    Client Need—Health promotion/maintenance

NURSING CARE OF CLIENTS WITH NASAL DISORDERS

81 3. If not cared for, injuries to the nose, such as a fracture, bend the septum to one side or the other. Nasal polyps generally are due to chronic inflam-

mation. An enlarged, red, bulbous nose may be from a skin condition, such as acne rosacea. Serous drainage indicates concurrent irritation from an allergen or pathogen. (4:886)

    Nursing Process—Data collection
    Client Need—Physiological integrity

82 2. Nosebleeds occur when the arterial blood pressure becomes high. The hypertension causes capillaries in the nasal membrane to rupture and bleed. A pulse rate of 110 is the result, rather than the cause, of blood loss. Anxiety causes a transient elevation in both heart and respiratory rate. An oral temperature of 97.6°F (36.7°C) is slightly lower than normal. However, a low temperature is not likely to cause the nose to bleed. (21:280)

    Nursing Process—Data collection
    Client Need—Physiological integrity

83 3. Fear is an emotional response to a real or imagined danger. It occurs when a person feels helpless or powerless to control the situation in which he is involved. Eliminating or reducing the fear-provoking stimulus, in this case the bloody clothing, will probably diminish his fear. Having the client recline is not appropriate, because the first-aid treatment for a nosebleed involves having the client sit forward. A towel would not likely stay in place unless the client is reclining. An anxious or fearful person probably is not able to concentrate on reading. (21:106; 25:60)

    Nursing Process—Planning
    Client Need—Psychosocial integrity

84 3. The best first-aid measure for controlling a nosebleed is to apply direct pressure. Leaning forward allows blood to drain from the nose rather than down the nasopharynx into the throat. An upright position also tends to lower the blood pressure. Swallowing, mouth-breathing, and clenching the teeth do not control bleeding. (18:353; 21:281)

    Nursing Process—Implementation
    Client Need—Physiological integrity

85 4. Blowing the nose retraumatizes the ruptured nasal capillaries, causing bleeding to recur. There is no need to restrict fluid intake. Taking the carotid pulse is unnecessary. Keeping the client's head up helps lower the blood pressure, but it is not the most essential information that the client receives. (4:885)

    Nursing Process—Implementation
    Client Need—Health promotion/maintenance

86 2. Nasal polyps are associated with chronic inflammation of the nasopharynx, which is caused by inhalant allergies or upper respiratory infections. Nasal injuries are more correlated with a deviated septum. Previous nasal surgery or tonsillectomy are incidental to the development of nasal polyps. (4:886)

Nursing Process—Data collection
Client Need—Physiological integrity

87 1. Swallowing at frequent intervals is common when blood accumulates posteriorly in the pharynx. Impaired appetite, a hoarse voice, and diminished hearing are abnormal assessment findings, but they are not directly correlated with nasal bleeding. (4:885)

Nursing Process—Data collection
Client Need—Physiological integrity

88 4. Breathing through the mouth is very drying to the oral mucous membranes. A sore throat is relieved by offering cool or warm liquids or by using a medicated gargle. A bloody dressing indicates a need to change or reinforce the dressing. Many people are nauseated from swallowing blood; mouth care does not relieve this discomfort. (18:510)

Nursing Process—Data collection
Client Need—Physiological integrity

89 3. It is best for the nurse to remain objective and limit his or her response to describing the client's external appearance. Predicting that the client will look gorgeous is considered false reassurance because body image is a personal concept. The client most likely felt unattractive prior to the surgery; contradicting the client's opinion causes her to lose faith in future things the nurse says. Telling the client that personality is more important also is the nurse's subjective opinion. It borders on giving advice, which is a nontherapeutic communication technique. (10:70)

Nursing Process—Implementation
Client Need—Psychosocial integrity

NURSING CARE OF CLIENTS WITH DISORDERS OF THE SKIN AND RELATED STRUCTURES

90 4. The first response in helping a victim who is in flames is to smother the fire either by rolling the victim on the ground or smothering the flames with a blanket or other dense material. Nothing, other than cool water, is applied to the skin until the victim is examined by a physician. Clean cloth is used to cover the burn wound, but this is not the best action to take first. The use of ice is contraindicated since it causes hypothermia or causes further thermal injury to the burned tissue. (4:556; 18:349; 21:1045)

Nursing Process—Implementation
Client Need—Physiological integrity

91 2. Whenever a burn involves the head, neck, or chest, establishing and maintaining a patent airway is of vital importance. Many burn victims, regardless of the area that is burned, inhale smoke, which irritates the air passages and results in increased respiratory secretions and edema of the air passages. Taking the pulse and blood pressure are important, but this assessment can be delayed until determining that, for the time being, the airway is patent. Identifying the next of kin and determining the extent of burns are less important than making sure the victim is able to breathe. (4:556; 18:349; 21:1045)

Nursing Process—Implementation
Client Need—Physiological integrity

92 1. Full-thickness burns, which previously were identified as third- or fourth-degree burns, are generally white, cherry red, tan, dark brown, or black. The tissue is generally leathery and painless. Deep partial-thickness burns are pink to rosy red, dull white or tan, blistered, and painful. (4:1564–1565; 21:1045)

Nursing Process—Data collection
Client Need—Physiological integrity

93 3. The first major complication of a burn is hypovolemic shock. Therefore, urine output is monitored hourly to evaluate the effectiveness of fluid replacement therapy. Burn victims receive massive volumes of fluid initially to replace what is lost from the intracellular space and that which is transferred from the intravascular space to the interstitial space. Although it is difficult for burn victims to regulate body temperature, body temperature is monitored to detect the course of infection that more likely occurs in later phases of burn management. Clients with full-thickness burns do not experience as much pain as someone with a partial-thickness burn over a similar percent of body surface area. Range of motion is not a concern initially, but rather becomes a priority when contractures develop during the healing phases of burn care. (4:556–557; 18:969; 21:1050)

Nursing Process—Data collection
Client Need—Physiological integrity

94 1. Infection is a common complication when the burn wound is exposed to microorganisms in the environment and those that are present and reside in the burn victim's own tissues, secretions, and excretions. Hypothermia, rather than hyperthermia, occurs due to leaving the burn wound undressed.

Depression over the potential change in body image and malnutrition occur regardless of the method used to manage the burn wound. (4:558)
   Nursing Process—Data collection
   Client Need—Physiological integrity

95 2. Mafenide (Sulfamylon) is an excellent antimicrobial for preventing and treating post-burn wound infections. However, the pain it causes on application is an obvious disadvantage. Another topical antimicrobial, silver sulfadiazine (Silvadene), does not cause pain but can cause a skin rash. Silver nitrate, which is used for burn wound management, stains tissue and everything else it contacts. It also causes stinging on application and increases the potential for electrolyte imbalance. (4:560; 21:1048)
   Nursing Process—Implementation
   Client Need—Physiological integrity

96 3. Since debridement causes pain, it is essential that the burn victim receives an analgesic no earlier than 30 minutes before the procedure is performed. In the case of hydrotherapy when a whirlpool is used, it is not mandatory that the client refrain from food or fluids. In the case of surgical debridement under anesthesia, policies generally include that the client fast and that a separate consent form is obtained. (18:972; 21:1050)
   Nursing Process—Implementation
   Client Need—Physiological integrity

97 1. Minimal movement of the grafted area is best for approximately 48 hours to ensure that the graft is not displaced. Disturbance of the graft may result in problems, such as failure to adhere to underlying tissues, infection, and tissue necrosis. The graft dressing is only changed or reinforced by the physician. Wet soaks are not applied to the graft because this disturbs the contact between the graft and underlying tissues. (4:561; 18:972)
   Nursing Process—Planning
   Client Need—Physiological integrity

98 3. Pressure garments are worn for as long as 2 years to promote a smooth appearance to the burn scar and to help prevent or reduce wound contractures. Pressure garments are not used to prevent wound infection, exposure to sunlight, or social rejection, although the latter two are secondary benefits from their application. (21:1049)
   Nursing Process—Evaluation
   Client Need—Health promotion/maintenance

99 4. Repositioning the client every 2 hours is the best method of restoring or maintaining skin integrity. Application of a skin-toughening agent is not effec-

tive if the client's position is not changed at frequent intervals. Keeping the head of the bed elevated is of no value in preventing skin breakdown; a sitting position creates a shearing force that contributes to skin impairment. Massaging skin that does not blanch when pressure is relieved is contraindicated since it causes further skin disruption and damage. (25:568–569)
   Nursing Process—Implementation
   Client Need—Physiological integrity

100 1. At least two applications of a shampoo containing a pediculocide such as lindane (gamma benzene hydrochloride) are necessary. The first kills the adult lice, but a subsequent treatment is necessary to kill the lice that hatch from nits that adhere to the hair. As long as nits are seen, shampooing must be repeated. (18:966)
   Nursing Process—Evaluation
   Client Need—Health promotion/maintenance

101 1. Interventions to prevent pooling and congestion of blood are a priority when planning the nursing care of a client with a venous stasis ulcer. Therefore, elevating the legs is best among the choices for promoting venous circulation. Covering the legs with warm blankets promotes warmth and vasodilation, but the fibers may adhere to the ulcer and disrupt wound healing when removed. A bed cradle is used to keep the legs covered and warm, yet prevent contact between the skin and woven fabrics. Assessing arterial circulation does not promote venous circulation. Sitting contributes to venous congestion if the legs are not elevated. (4:776)
   Nursing Process—Planning
   Client Need—Physiological integrity

102 2. Male pattern baldness places fair-skinned individuals at risk for chronic exposure to ultraviolet radiation. Smoking cigarettes is a risk factor for other types of cancer. Dark green and yellow vegetables contain beta-carotene, which is considered an antioxidant that contributes to cellular integrity; their possible avoidance is not as strongly suggestive as a link to skin cancer as sun exposure. Although exposure to chemicals is a factor in causing cancer, deodorant soap is considered a safe product. (18:973)
   Nursing Process—Data collection
   Client Need—Physiological integrity

103 2. Since birth defects are associated with isotretinoin (Accutane), it is contraindicated during pregnancy. The literature does not indicate a relationship between breast cancer or increased vulnerability to

adverse effects at the time of ovulation. Acne vulgaris is not a sexually transmitted disease. (21:1030)
>Nursing Process—Implementation
>Client Need—Health promotion/maintenance

104 3. Wearing a different pair of shoes each day provides time for shoe moisture to evaporate. The growth of the fungus that causes tinea pedis is supported in an environment that is dark, moist, and warm. Eliminating one or more of these factors may reduce the frequency of tinea pedis. Avoiding bare feet, cutting the nails straight across, and wearing other than white socks does not promote nor eliminate tinea pedis. (21:1030–1031)
>Nursing Process—Implementation
>Client Need—Health promotion/maintenance

105 1. Shingles results from a reactivation of the varicella-zoster virus, which lies dormant in the sensory ganglia after a previous infection with chickenpox. The individual with shingles usually gives a history of chickenpox in childhood. Shingles also occurs in those who have not had chickenpox but come in contact with someone who has chickenpox or is immunocompromised. Shingles is not caused by the bite of an insect, a bacterial toxin, or antibody response. (21:1039)
>Nursing Process—Implementation
>Client Need—Health promotion/maintenance

106 2. Clients with herpes simplex virus type 1, also known as "cold sores" or "fever blisters," are cautioned to use good personal hygiene to prevent the spread of the infection to other areas, such as the eyes and genitals. The application of petroleum jelly delays healing and does not prevent the spread of the infection. Scabs, should they form, are allowed to dry and fall off. When cleaning the affected areas, care is taken to use tissues or gauze to gently clean and remove any fluid that has formed on the lesions. The tissues or gauze are used only once and then discarded. (4:535)
>Nursing Process—Implementation
>Client Need—Health promotion/maintenance

107 2. Psoriasis is characterized by areas of redness covered with silvery scales. Areas affected usually include the elbows, knees, and scalp, although other areas also are affected. (21:1031)
>Nursing Process—Data collection
>Client Need—Physiological integrity

108 4. Vinyl gloves are substituted for latex gloves, but since they are more permeable, two pairs are worn. Neither rinsing the gloves with tap water nor applying petroleum-based ointment eliminates an allergic reaction to latex. It is unsafe to work unprotected when there is a potential for contact with body fluids that may contain blood. (25:437)
>Nursing Process—Implementation
>Client Need—Safe, effective care environment

109 1. Soaking with a warm solution between 100° to 106°F (37.7° to 41.1°C) is recommended for the treatment of frostbite. Cold applications are contraindicated because this delays effective treatment. A heating pad or hot water are not used because they cause further tissue damage. (21:257)
>Nursing Process—Implementation
>Client Need—Physiological integrity

110 1. Hypoallergenic or glycerin soap decreases skin irritation and therefore lessens itching. Regular soap removes skin oils or adds to or causes itching. Rough fibers, like wool, irritate the skin and contribute to the itching sensation. Tepid water, rather than hot or cold water, is recommended for bathing. Patting the skin dry rather than rubbing reduces skin irritation and itching. (21:1033)
>Nursing Process—Implementation
>Client Need—Physiological integrity

Classification of Test Items

Unit I Review Test **10**

The Nursing Care of Clients with Disorders of Sensory Organs and the Integument

Directions: After each question the correct answer is given, as well as a classification of each test question. Compare the correct answer with your answer. If a question has been answered *incorrectly*, draw a line to the end of all the columns. When finished, add up the number of your correct answers in each column and place that number in the respective box at the end in the area identified as *Number Correct*.

To determine the percentage of questions you answered correctly and your performance in each of the test plan categories, divide the *Number Correct* in each column by the *Number Possible* in each column. Then multiply the decimal by 100. For example:

$$\frac{\text{Number Correct: 86}}{\text{Number Possible: 110}} = 0.781 \times 100 = 78\%$$

Any score that is less than 75% indicates an area where further review would be beneficial.

KEY TO ITEM CLASSIFICATION:

NURSING PROCESS

D = Data collection
P = Planning
I = Implementation
E = Evaluation

CLIENT NEEDS

S = Safe, effective care environment
P = Physiological integrity
M = Psychosocial integrity
H = Health promotion/maintenance

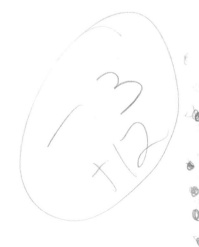

Question #	Answer #	Nursing Process				Client Needs			
		D	P	I	E	S	P	M	H
1	3	D					P		
2	1		P				P		
3	2			I			P		
4	2			I		S			
5	4			I			P		
6	2			I					H
7	4			I					H
8	3			I					H
9	2	D					P		
10	2			I		S			
11	2		P					M	
12	1				E	S			
13	1		P					M	
14	1	D					P		
15	3	D					P		

Question #	Answer #	Nursing Process				Client Needs			
		D	P	I	E	S	P	M	H
16	1				E				H
17	2			I			P		
18	4			I			P		
19	3		P				P		
20	1			I			P		
21	2			I					H
22	1		P						H
23	3	D				S			
24	2			I		S			
25	1	D					P		
26	3				E				H
27	1			I			P		
28	2	D					P		
29	4	D					P		
30	2	D					P		
31	3			I			P		
32	2			I				M	
33	1			I				M	
34	2				E		P		
35	3				E		P		
36	1	D					P		
37	3			I					H
38	4			I		S			
39	3	D					P		
40	2		P						H
41	3				E				H
42	2	D					P		
43	4	D					P		
44	1			I					H
45	2			I					H
46	3			I					H
47	3	D					P		

| | | Nursing Process | | | | Client Needs | | | |
Question #	Answer #	D	P	I	E	S	P	M	H
48	1			I					H
49	2		P						H
50	4	D					P		
51	1			I					H
52	3				E		P		
53	1			I			P		
54	1			I			P		
55	4			I					H
56	1	D					P		
57	1			I					H
58	4				E		P		
59	4	D					P		
60	2			I					H
61	2		P						H
62	4	D					P		
63	1			I					H
64	1		P			S			
65	2		P				P		
66	1		P			S			
67	2			I				M	
68	2	D					P		
69	1		P				P		
70	1			I					H
71	3			I					H
72	3			I		S			
73	2				E				H
74	3	D					P		
75	1		P						H
76	1	D					P		
77	1		P					M	
78	2			I					H

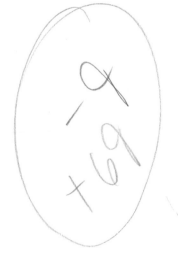

Question #	Answer #	Nursing Process				Client Needs			
		D	P	I	E	S	P	M	H
79	4			I			P		
80	3				E				H
81	3	D					P		
82	2	D					P		
83	3		P					M	
84	3			I			P		
85	4			I					H
86	2	D					P		
87	1	D					P		
88	4	D					P		
89	3			I				M	
90	4			I			P		
91	2			I			P		
92	1	D					P		
93	3	D					P		
94	1	D					P		
95	2			I			P		
96	3			I			P		
97	1		P				P		
98	3				E				H
99	4			I			P		
100	1				E				H
101	1		P				P		
102	2	D					P		
103	2			I					H
104	3			I					H
105	1			I					H
106	2			I					H
107	2	D					P		
108	4			I		S			
109	1			I			P		

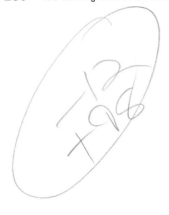

Question #	Answer #	Nursing Process				Client Needs			
		D	P	I	E	S	P	M	H
110	1			I			P		
Number Correct	98	27	14	45	12	7	53	7	32
Number Possible	110	31	17	50	12	10	59	7	34
Percentage Correct	89	87	82 90		100	70	90	100	94

4 35   3 6   2

Unit II

The Nursing Care of the Childbearing Family

Directions: With a pencil, blacken the circle in front of the option you have chosen for your correct answer.

ANATOMY AND PHYSIOLOGY OF THE MALE AND FEMALE REPRODUCTIVE SYSTEMS

A 25-year-old female attends a family planning class sponsored by one of the local hospitals. She is accompanied by her husband. They have no children but are seriously considering starting a family. They tell the nurse that they are attending this class to find out more about reproduction and the process of fertilization. The client and her husband ask the nurse where fertilization takes place.

1 The nurse would be *correct* to explain that fertilization usually takes place in the
- 1. fallopian tube.
- 2. ovary.
- 3. uterus.
- 4. vagina.

The client ask the nurse how long after ovulation the egg will remain viable.

2 The nurse would be *correct* to explain that, after ovulation, the ovum remains viable for
- 1. 12 hours.
- 2. 24 hours.
- 3. 48 hours.
- 4. 72 hours.

3 To prevent damage to the sperm, the nurse would instruct the client's husband to
- 1. avoid swimming in chlorinated water.
- 2. avoid taking hot baths.
- 3. avoid wearing boxer shorts.
- 4. avoid wearing colored underwear.

The client shares with the nurse that she really wants to have a baby but she is concerned that she will not be able to deliver the baby vaginally because of her small hips.

4 The nurse can *best* respond to the client's concern about being able to deliver vaginally by explaining that
- 1. the size of the baby's head is the only factor that will determine whether or not the infant can be delivered vaginally.
- 2. her hips should be measured in order to make an accurate determination of whether or not the infant can be delivered vaginally.
- 3. the size of her true pelvis, not the size of her hips, will determine whether or not she can deliver a baby vaginally.
- 4. it doesn't really matter whether she delivers vaginally or by cesarean section because the risk for both types of delivery is the same.

The client also tells the nurse that her breasts are small and asks the nurse if she will be able to breast feed.

5 The nurse can *best* respond to the client's concern about being able to breast-feed by telling her that
- 1. the size of her breasts will not affect her ability to breast-feed.
- 2. she can breast-feed and give the infant supplemental formula.
- 3. bottle-feeding an infant is just as nutritious as breast-feeding.
- 4. she can do exercises that will increase the size of her breasts.

The client's husband asks the nurse when the sex of the baby is determined.

6 The nurse would be *correct* to explain that the sex of the baby is determined
○ 1. during maturation of the ovum in the ovaries.
○ 2. during maturation of the sperm in the epididymis.
○ 3. when the fertilized ovum implants in the uterine lining.
● 4. when the sperm fertilizes the ovum in the fallopian tubes.

The client asks the nurse, "Where does the discharge come from when you have your monthly menstrual period?"

7 The nurse would be *correct* to explain that the menstrual discharge is mostly the result of the sloughing off of the
● 1. endometrium
○ 2. perimetrium
○ 3. myometrium
○ 4. epimetrium

SIGNS AND SYMPTOMS OF PREGNANCY

A 22-year-old female is visiting the prenatal clinic. She tells the nurse that she is not sure, but she thinks she is pregnant. During the initial visit with the client, the nurse obtains a history.

8 If the client reports the following signs and symptoms, which one represents a *probable* sign of pregnancy?
○ 1. Amenorrhea
● 2. Abdominal enlargement
○ 3. Nausea and vomiting
○ 4. Frequent urination

The physician orders a pregnancy test.

9 The nurse would be *correct* to send a requisition and specimen for which one of the following laboratory tests?
○ 1. Alpha-fetoprotein (AFP)
○ 2. Cortisol level
● 3. Human chorionic gonadotropin (HCG)
○ 4. Follicle stimulating hormone (FSH)

10 If the nurse collects the following data, which one represents a *positive* sign of pregnancy?
○ 1. Palpable fetal outline
○ 2. Blotchy tan facial skin
○ 3. Positive pregnancy test
● 4. Fetal heart tones

The client tells the nurse that if she is pregnant she couldn't be more than a couple of months. She also asks the nurse if an ultrasound would be capable of confirming whether or not she is pregnant.

11 The nurse would be *correct* to explain that
● 1. transvaginal ultrasound can be used to diagnose pregnancy as early as 2½ to 3 weeks.
○ 2. ultrasounds are not usually performed during the first trimester because of the possible risk to the baby.
○ 3. an x-ray would be just as reliable as an ultrasound and would pose less of a risk to the baby.
○ 4. ultrasounds cannot be used until the uterus ascends out of the pelvis into the abdomen.

The pregnancy test is positive. The physician informs the client of the results and tells her that during the pelvic examination she had a positive Chadwick's sign, which further supports the diagnosis of pregnancy. After the physician leaves, the client asks the nurse, "What is Chadwick's sign?"

12 The nurse would be *correct* to explain that Chadwick's sign is
○ 1. the spontaneous occurrence of intermittent painless contractions that begin early in pregnancy and continue throughout the entire period of gestation.
● 2. a bluish discoloration of the cervix, vagina, and vulva that occurs as a result of the presence of an increased number or blood vessels.
○ 3. a softening of the cervix that occurs because there is an increased amount of blood flowing to the reproductive organs.
○ 4. a dark brown line, extending from the umbilicus to the symphysis pubis, that appears as a result of hormonal changes.

When reviewing the client's medical record, the nurse notes that the physician documented the presence of ballottement.

13 Based on this finding, the nurse would be *correct* to inform the client that rather than being a couple of months pregnant, she is probably at least
● 1. 5 months pregnant.
○ 2. 6 months pregnant.
○ 3. 7 months pregnant.
○ 4. 8 months pregnant.

The client asks the nurse when she should be able to feel the baby move.

14 The nurse would be *correct* to tell the client that fetal movement is usually felt, for the first time, between
   ◉ 1. 10 and 14 weeks
   ○ 2. 16 and 20 weeks
   ○ 3. 22 and 26 weeks
   ○ 4. 28 and 32 weeks

ASSESSING THE PREGNANT CLIENT

A 32-year-old female is visiting the prenatal clinic for the first time. During the interview she informs the nurse that she has three children, a son and twin daughters. She states that she has not had any abortions or stillbirths.

15 When using the TPAL method, the nurse would be *correct* to record the client's obstetrical history as
   ○ 1. T-III, P-0, A-0, L-III
   ◉ 2. T-III, P-III, A-0, L-0
   ○ 3. T-III, P-II, A-0, L-II
   ○ 4. T-II, P-0, A-0, L-III

The client informs the nurse that her last menstrual period began on March 13. She asks when her baby will be due.

16 Using Nägele's rule, the nurse would be *correct* to tell the client that her expected delivery date will be approximately
   ○ 1. November 13.
   ◉ 2. November 23.
   ○ 3. December 3.
   ○ 4. December 20.

The client asks the nurse, "What is the normal weight gain during pregnancy?"

17 The nurse would be *correct* to explain that the recommended weight gain for a woman who has a normal prepregnancy weight is
   ○ 1. less than 15 pounds.
   ○ 2. 15 to 20 pounds.
   ◉ 3. 25 to 35 pounds.
   ○ 4. no more than 40 pounds.

The physician instructs the nurse to prepare the client for a pelvic examination.

18 The nurse would be *correct* to assist the client into which of the following positions?
   ◉ 1. Lithotomy
   ○ 2. Prone
   ○ 3. Sims
   ○ 4. Trendelenburg

19 Prior to the examination the nurse should
   ○ 1. give the client an enema.
   ◉ 2. have the client empty her bladder.

   ○ 3. shave and prep the client's perineum.
   ○ 4. give the client a mild sedative.

20 During the examination the nurse can *best* promote the client's comfort by
   ○ 1. instructing the client to rest her feet on the examining table.
   ○ 2. instructing the client to press her back into the examining table.
   ○ 3. instructing the client to tighten her buttocks.
   ◉ 4. instructing the client to let her knees fall outward.

The physician determines that the client is in her 12th week of pregnancy. The client asks if it is too early to hear the baby's heartbeat.

21 The nurse would be *correct* to explain that, with the use of a Doppler device, the fetal heartbeat can be heard as early as
   ○ 1. 4 to 6 weeks.
   ◉ 2. 8 to 10 weeks.
   ○ 3. 12 to 14 weeks.
   ○ 4. 16 to 18 weeks.

22 Which of the following actions by the nurse will *best* ensure that an accurate fetal heart rate is obtained?
   ○ 1. Assess the fetal heart rate when the client is lying on her right side.
   ○ 2. Assess the fetal heart rate when the client reports fetal movement.
   ○ 3. Assess the fetal heart rate between Braxton Hicks contractions.
   ◉ 4. Assess the maternal pulse and fetal heart rate and compare the two.

23 Which one of the following fetal heart rates should the nurse report *immediately* to the nurse in charge or to the physician?
   ◉ 1. 100
   ○ 2. 120
   ○ 3. 140
   ○ 4. 160

Prior to leaving the clinic, the client asks the nurse how often she should expect to have checkups.

24 The nurse can *best* respond by telling the client that the schedule for uncomplicated pregnancies is usually monthly for the first 28 weeks and then
   ○ 1. weekly for the remainder of the pregnancy.
   ○ 2. every 2 weeks for the remainder of the pregnancy.
   ◉ 3. every 2 weeks up to 36 weeks and weekly for the last month.
   ○ 4. weekly up to 36 months and twice weekly for the last month.

The client tells the nurse that she has a first cousin who had a baby with spina bifida. She asks the nurse if it is possible to detect the presence of this condition during pregnancy.

25 The nurse can *best* respond by explaining that the
○ 1. FTA-ABS test can detect this type of defect.
○ 2. HB$_s$Ag test can detect this type defect.
◉ 3. MSAFP test can detect this type defect.
○ 4. VDRL test can detect this type defect.

The client returns for follow-up visits on a regular basis.

26 At 20 weeks gestation, the nurse would expect to palpate the fundus
○ 1. just above the symphysis pubis.
○ 2. just below the xiphoid process.
◉ 3. near the level of the umbilicus.
○ 4. just below the symphysis pubis.

27 At 24 weeks gestation, the nurse would be *correct* to prepare the client for which one of the following routine tests?
○ 1. Coombs test
◉ 2. Glucose tolerance test
○ 3. Pap smear
○ 4. Rapid Plasma Reagin

The client is now in her last month of pregnancy. The physician orders a nonstress test.

28 When planning for this test, the nurse should have which one of the following available?
○ 1. Intravenous magnesium sulfate
○ 2. A cardiac monitor
○ 3. Intravenous oxytocin
◉ 4. A fetal monitor

COMMON DISCOMFORTS OF PREGNANCY

The nurse is conducting a class on common discomforts of pregnancy. One of the women attending the class asks the nurse what can be done to relieve constipation.

29 The nurse can *best* respond by telling the client that
○ 1. regular periods of rest will help to control constipation.
◉ 2. regular periods of exercise will help to control constipation.
○ 3. a low-fat diet will help to control constipation.
○ 4. prenatal vitamins will help to control constipation.

Several of the women attending the class ask the nurse to discuss what causes varicose veins and what treatments are available.

30 The nurse can *best* explain the cause of varicose veins by telling the participants that varicose veins occur during pregnancy because of the increased blood volume and
◉ 1. impaired venous return.
○ 2. decreased sodium level in the blood.
○ 3. changes in the body's center of gravity
○ 4. impaired kidney function.

31 The nurse would be *correct* to explain that the discomfort associated with varicose veins can be controlled by
○ 1. resting with the feet and legs in the dependent position.
◉ 2. sitting instead of standing when possible.
○ 3. wearing calf-length, elastic-top hose.
○ 4. moving around when standing for long periods of time.

The nurse teaches the class about correct application of elastic hose and complications associated with varicose veins.

32 Which one of the following statements would indicate that teaching has been effective?
○ 1. "The stockings should be put on before going to bed at night."
○ 2. "The stockings should be put on before getting out of bed in the morning."
◉ 3. "The stockings should be put on only if the veins become inflamed."
○ 4. "The stockings should be put on while in the standing position."

33 Which one of the following findings should the nurse instruct the participants to report *immediately*?
○ 1. The appearance of additional varicose veins.
○ 2. The presence of purple varicose veins.
○ 3. The legs begin to ache and feel heavy.
◉ 4. The legs become red, tender, and warm.

One of the participants tells the nurse, "My skin itches so much. What can I do about it?"

34 The *most* appropriate suggestion the nurse can make is that this discomfort may be relieved by
○ 1. increasing fluid intake.
○ 2. taking vitamin C.
◉ 3. taking alcohol baths.
○ 4. taking frequent rest periods.

One of the participants, who is in her third trimester, states that she has begun to experience shortness of breath. She asks the nurse if she should be concerned about this.

35 The nurse can *best* respond by explaining that shortness of breath
  ○ 1. is not a common discomfort and may be the result of a blood clot in the lungs.
  ○ 2. is probably the result of anxiety about the impending delivery of the baby.
  ● 3. is probably caused by the enlarged uterus pressing against the diaphragm.
  ○ 4. is probably caused by decreased oxygen secondary to slow venous circulation.

36 The nurse would be *correct* to instruct the woman to
  ○ 1. contact her health care provider immediately.
  ○ 2. decrease her activity level to conserve oxygen.
  ○ 3. ask her doctor for a mild sedative.
  ● 4. sleep with her upper body elevated on pillows.

Several of the participants complain of frequent urination.

37 The nurse would be *correct* to explain that frequent urination during early pregnancy usually subsides when the
  ○ 1. placenta is fully developed.
  ○ 2. fetal kidneys begin to function.
  ● 3. uterus rises into the abdominal cavity.
  ○ 4. hormone balance is re-established.

38 The nurse would be *correct* to explain that the *most probable* cause of frequent urination late in pregnancy is
  ○ 1. that the mother has alkaline urine.
  ○ 2. the presence of a urinary tract infection.
  ● 3. the enlarging uterus exerting pressure on the bladder.
  ○ 4. the growing fetus excreting increased amounts of waste.

39 Which one of the following statements by a participant indicates a need for additional teaching regarding management of urinary frequency.
  ● 1. "Limiting fluid intake will help to control this problem."
  ○ 2. "A burning sensation during urination should be reported."
  ○ 3. "Voiding before going to bed may help control this problem."
  ○ 4. "Avoiding fluids high in caffeine may help control this problem."

One of the participants, who is 5 months pregnant, complains of having annoying backaches.

40 To relieve this discomfort, the nurse can advise her to
  ○ 1. avoid taking tub baths.
  ○ 2. sleep on a soft mattress.
  ○ 3. avoid coffee and spicy food.
  ● 4. wear low-heeled shoes.

The nurse teaches the class ways to minimize the occurrence of heartburn and nausea.

41 Which one of the following statements by a participant about remedies for heartburn and nausea indicates that teaching was effective?
  ● 1. "I should eat frequent, small meals."
  ○ 2. "I should take an Alka-Seltzer after eating."
  ○ 3. "I should eat my largest meal of the day after 7 PM."
  ○ 4. "I should drink extra water with my meals."

One of the participants asks the nurse what she can do to relieve leg cramps. She also informs the nurse that she had problems with thrombophlebitis during her previous pregnancy.

42 The nurse would be *correct* to instruct her to
  ○ 1. increase her milk intake to 5 to 6 servings per day.
  ○ 2. place hot water bottles on the affected area.
  ● 3. stretch her legs by pointing her toes to the floor.
  ○ 4. massage her leg when she feels a cramp.

HIGH-RISK FACTORS AND PREGNANCY

The nurse is asked to discuss high-risk factors with a small group of women attending a prenatal clinic.

43 The nurse would be *correct* to identify which one of the following clients as having a high risk for developing complications of pregnancy?
  ○ 1. A 25-year-old gravida I client.
  ○ 2. A client with the placenta implanted on the fundus of the uterus.
  ○ 3. A client who has nausea and vomiting during the first trimester.
  ● 4. A 35-year-old gravida V client.

One of the participants asks the nurse if occasional consumption of alcohol will harm the unborn baby.

44 The nurse could *best* respond by explaining that
○ 1. any consumption of alcohol during pregnancy will cause the infant to have complications at birth.
○ 2. the minimal safe amount of alcohol consumption during pregnancy has not been determined.
○ 3. alcohol consumption has a harmful effect on the baby only if consumed during the first trimester of pregnancy.
○ 4. occasional intake of a small amount of alcohol during pregnancy will not adversely affect the unborn baby.

Another participant asks the nurse what effect smoking has on pregnancy.

45 The nurse would be *correct* to tell the participants that women who smoke during pregnancy have a greater risk of
○ 1. having a premature delivery.
○ 2. acquiring human immunodeficiency virus (HIV).
○ 3. developing hyperemesis gravidarum.
○ 4. developing prenatal infections.

A 38-year-old participant who is in her 10th week of pregnancy tells the nurse that she is concerned about how her age may affect the health of her baby. She asks the nurse what test can be done at this point in her pregnancy that will identify genetic disorders that the baby may have.

46 The nurse would be *correct* to tell the woman that at this point in her pregnancy the physician may order which one of the following tests to detect genetic disorders
○ 1. Amniocentesis
○ 2. Chorionic Villi Sampling
○ 3. Rapid Plasma Reagin
○ 4. Ultrasound

COMPLICATIONS OF PREGNANCY

A 25-year-old primigravida is being seen for the first time at the prenatal clinic. The physician determines that she is 4 months pregnant. She also is diagnosed as having trichomoniasis vaginitis.

47 If the nurse observes the following, which one is *most* indicative of trichomoniasis vaginitis?
○ 1. Painful blisters on the labia
○ 2. Generalized fine red rash
○ 3. Frothy vaginal discharge
○ 4. Clusters of tan lesions on vulva

48 Which of the following statements by the client indicates a need for additional teaching regarding trichomoniasis vaginitis?
○ 1. "My sex partner should be treated also."
○ 2. "I will have to have a cesarean delivery to protect my baby."
○ 3. "The physician will probably prescribe metronidazole (Flagyl)."
○ 4. "My Pap smear results may show atypical cells."

Before the client leaves the clinic, the nurse teaches her about danger signals that should be reported immediately to the physician.

49 The nurse would be *correct* to instruct the client to *immediately* contact the physician
○ 1. the first time fetal movement is noted.
○ 2. if her breasts become tender.
○ 3. if bleeding from the vagina occurs.
○ 4. if she experiences frequent urination.

The client returns to the clinic complaining of nausea. She tells the nurse she has been nauseous and vomiting frequently for the past 4 days. The physician determines that the client has hyperemesis gravidarum and is moderately dehydrated.

50 Which one of the following equipment should the nurse plan to have available for the treatment of this client?
○ 1. Intravenous start pack
○ 2. Warmed speculum
○ 3. Oxygen and face mask
○ 4. Cardiac monitor

A 31-year-old multipara client who is in her first trimester of pregnancy is being seen by the physician at the prenatal clinic. She tells the nurse that her last pregnancy ended in a spontaneous abortion because of an incompetent cervix. She asks the nurse to clarify what is meant by an incompetent cervix.

51 The nurse can *best* respond by explaining that incompetent cervix means that the cervix
○ 1. is not large enough for passage of the fetus.
○ 2. is not able to support the weight of the fetus.
○ 3. has an external opening but does not have an internal opening.
○ 4. has an internal opening but does not have an external opening.

At the end of the first trimester the physician puts a cerclage in the cervix. The client ask the nurse how long the cerclage will be in place.

52 The nurse would be *correct* to explain that the physician will probably leave the cerclage in place until
- ● 1. the client goes into labor.
- ○ 2. after the client delivers the baby.
- ○ 3. the end of the second trimester.
- ○ 4. the client is near term.

A 31-year-old primigravida client is in her 22nd week of pregnancy. The physician informs the client that she has pregnancy-induced hypertension (PIH), also called pre-eclampsia.

53 If the nurse observes the following, which is *most* indicative of mild PIH?
- ● 1. A 15 mm Hg rise in the baseline systolic blood pressure
- ○ 2. A weight gain of 1 lb per week in the second trimester
- ○ 3. A +1 protein reading on the urine reagent test strip
- ○ 4. The presence of ankle edema on a frequent basis

The physician decides that the client can be managed at home and requests that the nurse give the client instructions for home care.

54 The nurse would be *correct* to instruct the client to
- ○ 1. limit her fluid intake.
- ○ 2. return for bimonthly checkups.
- ○ 3. eat high-protein foods.
- ● 4. limit activity to light housework.

The client's condition worsens and she is admitted to the hospital. The physician orders magnesium (MgSO₄) for the client.

55 In addition to vital signs, the nurse should assess the client's
- ○ 1. urine for glucose.
- ● 2. deep tendon reflexes.
- ○ 3. stools for blood.
- ○ 4. skin for rashes.

56 The nurse would be *correct* to inform the nurse in charge or the physician of the presence of eclampsia if
- ● 1. the client develops convulsions.
- ○ 2. the client sleeps for long periods of time.
- ○ 3. the fetal heart tones are greater than 100.
- ○ 4. the client complains of being thirsty.

57 Which one of the following medications should the nurse have available when the client is receiving magnesium sulfate (MgSO₄)?

- ○ 1. Hydralazine (Apresoline)
- ○ 2. Oxytocin (Pitocin)
- ○ 3. Methyl ergonovine (Methergine)
- ● 4. Calcium gluconate

58 Which one of the following findings would indicate the presence of magnesium sulfate (MgSO₄) toxicity?
- ● 1. Brisk deep tendon reflexes
- ○ 2. Respiratory rate less than 14
- ○ 3. Presence of a skin rash
- ○ 4. Magnesium blood level of 5 mg/dL

A 28-year-old multipara is admitted to the hospital for observation during her 10th week of pregnancy. She has a history of spontaneous abortions and currently is experiencing spotting.

59 Which one of the following, if reported by the client, would be indicative of a spontaneous abortion?
- ○ 1. Ankle swelling
- ○ 2. Severe headache
- ○ 3. Persistent nausea
- ● 4. Abdominal cramping

The physician examines the client and determines that her cervix is dilated but the fetus and placenta are still in the uterus.

60 At this point, the nurse would be *correct* to
- ○ 1. prepare the client for dilation and curettage (D&C).
- ● 2. place the client in the Trendelenburg position.
- ○ 3. prepare the client for placement of a purse-string stitch.
- ○ 4. place the client in the side-lying position.

The client comments to the nurse, "This is like a recurring nightmare. I don't want to lose my baby."

61 Which one of the following responses by the nurse is *most* appropriate?
- ● 1. "I know this is painful for you. Would you like to talk about how you are feeling about this?"
- ○ 2. "Let's be positive. It is too early to know whether or not you will lose your baby."
- ○ 3. "I know you are scared, but you must try to stay calm. Stress will make the situation worse."
- ○ 4. "I know things seem really bad, but trust me, everything will work out for the best in the end."

A 22-year-old woman who has insulin-dependent diabetes mellitus (IDDM) is being seen by the obstetrician for the first time. She was diagnosed with diabetes when she was 6 years old. Her diabetes has been well controlled since her initial diagnosis. While waiting to see the doctor, she asks the nurse if the pregnancy will increase her need for insulin.

62 The nurse would be *correct* to explain that during pregnancy her need for insulin will
 ○ 1. increase.
 ○ 2. decrease.
 ◉ 3. fluctuate.
 ○ 4. not change.

The client also asks the nurse, "What kinds of complications might I have during my pregnancy?"

63 The nurse would be *correct* to tell the client that she is at risk to develop
 ○ 1. hyperemesis gravidarum.
 ◉ 2. pregnancy-induced hypertension.
 ○ 3. placenta previa.
 ○ 4. toxoplasmosis.

The client is now in her last trimester of pregnancy. Her diabetes has been well controlled throughout her pregnancy. She tells the nurse that she is excited but also scared that something might be wrong with her baby because of her diabetes.

64 The nurse can *best* respond to the client by explaining that she is most likely to
 ◉ 1. have a large but otherwise healthy baby.
 ○ 2. have a small but otherwise healthy baby.
 ○ 3. have a baby that will be diabetic.
 ○ 4. have a baby that will have a minor birth defect.

A 26-year-old multigravida who is 8 months pregnant is admitted to the obstetrical unit with a diagnosis of incomplete placenta previa.

65 On admission, the nurse would expect the client to report which one of the following?
 ○ 1. Sudden, sharp abdominal pain
 ◉ 2. Painless bleeding from the vagina
 ○ 3. Persistent headache
 ○ 4. Continuous, painless contractions

66 Which one of the following data should the nurse obtain *first*?
 ○ 1. Height and weight
 ◉ 2. Blood pressure and pulse
 ○ 3. History of previous pregnancies
 ○ 4. General health and drug history

The client's husband arrives at the hospital. He asks the nurse, "What is placenta previa and how do they treat it?"

67 The nurse would be *correct* to explain that placenta previa means that the placenta
 ◉ 1. is implanted over or close to the internal cervical opening.
 ○ 2. is not producing the hormones needed to maintain the pregnancy.
 ○ 3. is invaded by polyps that cause premature uterine contractions.
 ○ 4. is producing antibodies that are destroying the baby's red blood cells.

68 The nurse would be *correct* to explain the if the client's condition remains stable the physician probably will
 ○ 1. induce labor.
 ○ 2. perform an emergency cesarean section.
 ◉ 3. keep the client on bed rest until she is at full term.
 ○ 4. start the client on ritodrine (Yutopar)

A 30-year-old multigravida who is in her last trimester of pregnancy is diagnosed with abruptio placentae.

69 Which one of the following findings would the nurse be *correct* to identify as a predisposing factor for abruptio placentae?
 ○ 1. Gestational diabetes
 ○ 2. Hyperemesis gravidarum
 ◉ 3. Oligiohydraminous
 ○ 4. Pregnancy-induced hypertension

70 Which one of the following findings would be *most* indicative of abruptio placentae?
 ○ 1. Rigid, boardlike, tender abdomen
 ○ 2. Severe nausea and vomiting
 ◉ 3. Smaller uterus than expected for dates
 ○ 4. Painless vaginal bleeding

71 If the client develops a complete abruption, the nurse should plan to
 ◉ 1. obtain written consent for a cesarean section.
 ○ 2. give the client an enema and prep the abdomen.
 ○ 3. place the client in the Trendelenburg position.
 ○ 4. prepare the client for a contraction stress test.

NUTRITION DURING PREGNANCY

The physician determines that a client who is in her fourth month of pregnancy is not eating an appropriate diet. The nurse is asked to teach the client about nutritional needs during pregnancy.

72 Prior to teaching the client about the nutritional needs during pregnancy, the nurse should

○ 1. determine if the client needs to gain weight or lose weight.

● 2. assess the client's current eating pattern and preferences.

○ 3. determine if the client knows how to accurately count calories.

○ 4. develop a sample menu that includes the required nutrients.

After interviewing the client, the nurse determines that the client does not have an adequate intake of calcium.

73 The nurse would be *correct* to tell the client that in order to meet her calcium needs she should drink

○ 1. 1 to 2 cups of milk daily.

○ 2. 3 to 4 cups of milk daily.

○ 3. 5 to 6 cups of milk daily.

● 4. 7 to 8 cups of milk daily.

The client tells the nurse that it is hard for her to get the calcium she needs because she does not like milk.

74 The nurse would be *correct* to suggest which one of the following foods as an alternate source of calcium?

○ 1. Organ meats

○ 2. White bread

● 3. Leafy green vegetables

○ 4. Dark turkey meat

The physician also prescribes an iron supplement for the client.

75 The nurse would be *correct* to tell the client

○ 1. to take the supplement with meals.

○ 2. that the supplement may cause mild abdominal pain.

● 3. to drink plenty of fluids to alleviate constipation.

○ 4. that dietary sources of iron can be substituted for the medication.

TEACHING THE PREGNANT CLIENT

A 26-year-old primigravida visits her obstetrician for her first prenatal visit. She is in the ninth week of her pregnancy. The nurse is assigned to discuss general health needs during pregnancy with the client.

76 Which one of the following statements made by the client about bathing indicates a need for additional teaching?

○ 1. "Tub baths should be discontinued if my membranes rupture."

● 2. "Tub baths should not be taken at any time during pregnancy."

○ 3. "Hot tub baths should be avoided because of possible harmful fetal effects."

○ 4. "Safety mats and hand rails should be used to prevent falls from occurring."

The client asks the nurse if it is okay to have sex while she is pregnant.

77 The nurse would be *correct* to explain that sexual intercourse should be avoided

○ 1. throughout pregnancy.

○ 2. until the baby is fully developed.

○ 3. once the abdomen starts to enlarge.

● 4. once the membranes rupture.

The client informs the nurse that she and her husband are planning to take their vacation in the near future and asks if there are any special instructions she should follow.

78 The nurse would be *correct* to recommend that the client

○ 1. carry a copy of her medical record with her when traveling.

○ 2. refrain from traveling after the first trimester of pregnancy.

○ 3. travel no farther than 100 miles from her home.

● 4. refrain from using a seatbelt for extended periods of time.

The client asks the nurse why some women have identical twins and other women have twins that do not look anything alike.

79 The nurse would be *correct* to explain that identical twins occur when

○ 1. two eggs are fertilized by identical sperm.

○ 2. the mother releases two identical eggs.

● 3. one fertilized egg divides into two identical halves.

○ 4. two identical eggs are fertilized by two identical sperm.

The client ask the nurse if she should tell the doctor about the spotting she had about 8 weeks ago, when she was at about 1 week gestation.

80 The nurse would be *correct* to explain that the spotting she experienced probably is normal and the result of

● 1. the baby implanting in the lining of the uterus.

○ 2. increased circulation of blood to the vaginal area.

○ 3. hormonal changes that occur during pregnancy.

○ 4. the cervical opening enlarging and thinning out.

The client asks the nurse, "What does my baby look like now?"

81 The nurse would be *correct* to explain that between 8 and 12 weeks, the baby is called
  ○ 1. a zygote and looks like a bumpy ball.
  ◉ 2. an embryo and has a well-defined head.
  ○ 3. an embryo and the sex is distinguishable.
  ○ 4. a fetus, and has fully developed arms and legs.

The client asks the nurse the purpose of the amniotic fluid.

82 The nurse can *best* respond by explaining that the amniotic fluid
  ○ 1. provides the embryo or fetus with antibodies from the mother.
  ◉ 2. helps protect the embryo or fetus from external injury.
  ○ 3. provides oxygen for the embryo or fetus.
  ○ 4. helps lower the body temperature of the mother.

ELECTIVE ABORTION

An 18-year-old primigravida is considering terminating her pregnancy. She tells the nurse that she needs more information before making her decision. She asks the nurse, "At what point during pregnancy can a baby live outside of the mother?"

83 The nurse can *best* respond by explaining that the legal threshold of viability is usually estimated to be
  ○ 1. 36 to 40 weeks.
  ◉ 2. 30 to 35 weeks.
  ○ 3. 20 to 24 weeks.
  ○ 4. 10 to 15 weeks.

The client is approximately 9 weeks gestation. She informs the nurse that she has decided to have the abortion. She asks the nurse how the abortion will be performed.

84 The nurse can *best* respond by explaining that the preferred techniques for terminating a pregnancy of less than 3 months are aspiration and
  ○ 1. abdominal hysterotomy.
  ◉ 2. dilation and curettage.
  ○ 3. hypertonic saline instillation.
  ○ 4. prostaglandin administration.

INDIVIDUAL TEST ITEMS

85 A client visiting the prenatal clinic for the first time informs the nurse that this is her first pregnancy. The nurse would be *correct* to record which one of the following terms on the client's prenatal records?
  ○ 1. Multipara
  ○ 2. Primipara
  ◉ 3. Primigravida
  ○ 4. Multigravida

86 When assessing a client with a history of PIH, the nurse should observe for
  ○ 1. a decrease in urine proteins.
  ○ 2. an increase in urine output.
  ○ 3. a decrease in the pulse rate.
  ◉ 4. any sudden gain in weight.

87 A client who is 3 months pregnant tells the nurse that she had rubella (German measles) 2 months ago. The nurse would be *correct* to discuss which one of the following possible complications with the client?
  ○ 1. Premature labor
  ◉ 2. Fetal deformities
  ○ 3. Severe preeclampsia
  ○ 4. Hydatidiform mole formation

88 Which one of the following should alert the nurse that the client may be in a high-risk group for the development of complications during pregnancy?
  ○ 1. The client is pregnant for the third time.
  ○ 2. The client's husband is overweight.
  ○ 3. The client has a history of twins in the family.
  ◉ 4. The client has primary hypertensive disease.

89 Which one of the following is *most* indicative of the presence of hydatidiform mole?
  ○ 1. A blotchy brown discoloration on the face
  ○ 2. A positive Chadwick's sign
  ○ 3. The presence of ballottement
  ◉ 4. A uterus that is larger than expected for dates

90 A client who has an active case of herpes simplex type 2 (genital herpes) is admitted in active labor. The nurse would be correct to prepare the client for a
  ◉ 1. cesarean delivery.
  ○ 2. forceps delivery.
  ○ 3. precipitate delivery.
  ○ 4. vaginal delivery.

91 Which one of the following individuals should the nurse encourage to be tested for hepatitis B?
  ○ 1. The client with a history of cigarette smoking
  ○ 2. The client who is single and pregnant for the first time
  ◉ 3. The client who is an immigrant from Haiti
  ○ 4. The client who had a recent exposure to H. Influenza

Directions: Two numbers appear in parentheses following each rationale. The first number identifies the textbook listed in the references, page 512, and the second number identifies the page(s) in that textbook on which the correct answer can be verified. Occasionally two textbooks are given for verifying the correct answer.

ANATOMY AND PHYSIOLOGY OF THE MALE AND FEMALE REPRODUCTIVE SYSTEMS

1 1. The ovum is released from the ovaries and enters into the outer third of the fallopian tube, where it is fertilized by the sperm. After fertilization, the fertilized ovum will travel through the remainder of the fallopian tube and enter the uterus, where it will implant and remain throughout pregnancy. (14:79)
> Nursing Process—Implementation
> Client Need—Health promotion/maintenance

2 2. The ovum remains viable for 24 hours after being released from the ovary. If fertilization does not occur within this time conception cannot take place. (14:47)
> Nursing Process—Implementation
> Client Need—Health promotion/maintenance

3 2. Hot baths should be avoided because they may cause damage or death to the sperm. Tight clothing, such as briefs, also may have the same effect by trapping body heat and thus elevating the temperature of the testicular area. (14:54)
> Nursing Process—Implementation
> Client Need—Health promotion/maintenance

4 3. The false pelvis is formed by the iliac portion of the innominate bone and is what accounts for hip measurements. The true pelvis is the part of the pelvis that influences the ability of the woman to deliver vaginally. Furthermore, the fetus must be in an appropriate position and small enough to pass through the true pelvis for a successful vaginal delivery to occur. (14:154; 16:45)
> Nursing Process—Implementation
> Client Need—Health promotion/maintenance

5 1. Each breast consist of lobules that contain alveoli, which house the milk-secreting cells. The size of the breast is determined by the adipose tissue, not the milk-secreting cell. Thus the size of the breast

has nothing to do with the woman's ability to breast-feed. (14:46)
> Nursing Process—Implementation
> Client Need—Health promotion/maintenance

6 4. The sex of the baby is determined at fertilization. Each parent contributes one sex chromosome. The mother will always contribute an X chromosome. The father may contribute an X or a Y chromosome. If the ovum is fertilized by a sperm containing an X chromosome, the offspring will be a female. If the ovum is fertilized by a sperm containing a Y chromosome, the offspring will be a male. (16:84)
> Nursing Process—Implementation
> Client Need—Health promotion/maintenance

7 1. The menstrual discharge consist of endometrial cells sloughed from the uterine lining, mucus, and blood. The myometrium is the muscle layer of the uterus. The perimetrium is the thin outer layer of the uterus. (14:49)
> Nursing Process—Implementation
> Client Need—Health promotion/maintenance

SIGNS AND SYMPTOMS OF PREGNANCY

8 2. Abdominal enlargement is a probable sign of pregnancy. Amenorrhea, nausea, vomiting, and frequent urination all are considered to be presumptive signs of pregnancy because they also can be indications of conditions other than pregnancy. (16:103)
> Nursing Process—Data collection
> Client Need—Health promotion/maintenance

9 3. Levels of HCG rise significantly shortly after implantation of the ovum. Blood and urine pregnancy testing for HCG is the basis for most pregnancy tests. The alpha-fetoprotein (AFP) test may be performed during pregnancy to determine the presence of neural tube defects. The primary purpose of cortisol laboratory studies is to evaluate adrenal hormone function. (16:104; 14:94)
> Nursing Process—Implementation
> Client Need—Safe, effective care environment

10 4. Detection of the fetal heartbeat by the health care provider confirms pregnancy. A palpable fetal outline and positive pregnancy test are probable signs of pregnancy but are not conclusive evidence of pregnancy. A blotchy tan discoloration of the face is known as chloasma and is a presumptive sign of pregnancy. (14:95)
    Nursing Process—Data collection
    Client Need—Health promotion/maintenance

11 1. Transvaginal ultrasounds can detect pregnancy as early as 2Z\x to 3 weeks. Abdominal ultrasounds can detect pregnancy as early as 5 to 6 weeks. Ultrasounds have replaced x-rays as a diagnostic tool for pregnancy and have eliminated the danger of radiation exposure of the fetus associated with x-rays. (14:96)
    Nursing Process—Implementation
    Client Need—Health promotion/maintenance

12 2. Chadwick's sign is a bluish discoloration of the cervix, vagina, and vulva caused by increased vascularization of the reproductive organs. Spontaneous intermittent contractions are referred to as Braxton Hicks contractions. Goodell's sign is the softening of the cervix, and linea nigra is the dark brown line that extends from the umbilicus to the symphysis pubis. (14:94)
    Nursing Process—Implementation
    Client Need—Health promotion/maintenance

13 1. Ballottement is observed when the fetus floats away and then rebounds after a gentle push of the uterus. Ballottement usually is first observed during the fourth or fifth month of pregnancy. (14:95)
    Nursing Process—Implementation
    Client Need—Health promotion/maintenance

14 2. The first fetal movement felt by the mother is referred to as quickening. Quickening usually is experienced between 16 and 20 weeks gestation. (14:93; 16:104)
    Nursing Process—Implementation
    Client Need—Health promotion/maintenance

ASSESSING THE PREGNANT CLIENT

15 4. TPAL is an acronym used when documenting the client's obstetrical history. T represents the number of term pregnancies; P represents the number of premature infants delivered; A represents the number of abortions or miscarriages; and L represents the number of living children. The client in this situation has had 3 term pregnancies, no premature

deliveries, no abortions, and has three living children. (14:92; 16:115)
    Nursing Process—Implementation
    Client Need—Health promotion/maintenance

16 4. Nägele's rule is one method of determining the estimated date of delivery (EDD). When using Nägele's rule you add 7 days to the first day of the last menstrual period, and count back 3 months. In this situation, the estimated delivery date would be December 20. (14:92)
    Nursing Process—Implementation
    Client Need—Health promotion/maintenance

17 3. The weight gain recommended during pregnancy must be individualized and the client's prepregnancy weight must be taken into consideration. The guidelines for weight gain for the client with normal prepregnant weight is 25 to 30 pounds. A weight gain between 28 and 40 pounds is recommended for the client who is underweight. Clients who are moderately overweight should gain between 15 and 25 pounds. Clients who are very overweight should gain approximately 15 pounds. (16:124)
    Nursing Process—Implementation
    Client Need—Health promotion/maintenance

18 1. When preparing the client for a pelvic examination, the nurse should assist the client to the lithotomy position. All of the other positions (prone, Sims, and Trendelenburg) do not accommodate this type of examination. (22:86)
    Nursing Process—Implementation
    Client Need—Safe, effective care environment

19 2. Prior to the pelvic examination, the client should be encouraged to empty her bladder. This action will increase the client's comfort during the examination and will facilitate a more accurate assessment of the pelvic structures. It is not necessary nor is it routine for the client to receive an enema, sedative, or shave and prep prior to having a pelvic examination. (14:107; 16:116)
    Nursing Process—Implementation
    Client Need—Safe, effective care environment

20 4. The nurse should instruct the client to let her knees fall outward and to relax during the examination. This will increase the client's comfort level during the examination. The examination cannot be performed with the client's feet on the examination table. Pressing her back into the examining table and tightening her buttocks will not promote relaxation because these actions cause increased tension in the muscles of the perineum.(16:116)

Nursing Process—Implementation
Client Need—**Safe, effective care environment**

21 2. With the use of a Doppler device, the examiner can detect fetal heart tones as early as 8 to 10 weeks gestation. The fetal heartbeat can be heard between 18 and 20 weeks gestation with a standard fetoscope. (14:96)

Nursing Process—Implementation
Client Need—Health promotion/maintenance

22 4. When auscultating for the fetal heart rate, the nurse may also hear the uterine souffle (a soft whirling sound produced by the maternal blood moving through the uterine vessels). To differentiate between fetal heart tones and the uterine souffle, the nurse should count the maternal pulse rate and compare it to the rate obtained when listening for the fetal heart tones. (14:96)

Nursing Process—Data collection
Client Need—Health promotion/maintenance

23 1. The fetal heart rate should be between 120 and 160 beats per minute. A fetal heart rate less than 120 or greater than 160 beats per minute may indicate fetal distress. (14:95; 22:209)

Nursing Process—Data collection
Client Need—Health promotion/maintenance

24 3. The pregnant woman who is not experiencing complications usually visits the health care provider every 4 weeks for the first 28 weeks of pregnancy, every 2 weeks from 28 weeks to 36 weeks gestation, and weekly from the 37th week to delivery. (14:109; 16:118)

Nursing Process—Implementation
Client Need—Health promotion/maintenance

25 3. The maternal serum alpha-fetoprotein test is used to screen for neural tube defects such as spina bifida. This test should be performed between 14 and 16 weeks gestation. The HB_xAg test is used to detect hepatitis B. The VDRL and FTA-ABS test are used to screen for syphilis. (16:118)

Nursing Process—Implementation
Client Need—Health promotion/maintenance

26 3. At 20 weeks gestation, the fundus of the uterus can be palpated near the level of the umbilicus. At 16-weeks gestation, the fundus is located halfway between the top of the symphysis pubis and the umbilicus. (16:103)

Nursing Process—Planning
Client Need—Health promotion/maintenance

27 2. The glucose tolerance test is a routine test performed between 24 and 28 weeks gestation as a screening tool for gestational diabetes. A Pap smear and RPR usually are performed at the first prenatal visit. The Coombs test is not a routine test performed during pregnancy. This test is performed when there is a possibility of Rh incompatibility between the mother and fetus or neonate. (14:108; 16:119)

Nursing Process—Implementation
Client Need—**Safe, effective care environment**

28 4. To perform the nonstress test, the nurse will attach a fetal monitor to the client's abdomen in order to monitor the response of the fetal heart rate to fetal movement. Intravenous magnesium sulfate is given to the client experiencing severe preeclampsia. Intravenous oxytocin can be given for several reasons, including augmentation of labor and control of postpartum hemorrhage. A cardiac monitor is not utilized during a nonstress test. (14:109; 16:100)

Nursing Process—Planning
Client Need—**Safe, effective care environment**

COMMON DISCOMFORTS OF PREGNANCY

29 2. Constipation may occur during pregnancy because of hormonal changes, increased uterine size, and the use of iron supplements. A diet containing fresh fruit and vegetables, whole grains, and increased intake of fluids will assist with controlling or relieving constipation. Also, exercise may assist with the control or relief of this discomfort. (14:104; 16:132)

Nursing Process—Implementation
Client Need—Health promotion/maintenance

30 1. During pregnancy, the client may develop varicose veins, especially in the lower extremities and rectal area (hemorrhoids). Varicose veins occur during pregnancy primarily because of impaired venous return, which is caused by the pressure of the enlarged uterus on venous circulation and the increased blood volume normally associated with pregnancy. Decreased sodium levels in the blood and changes in the body's center of gravity are not associated with the occurrence of varicose veins. Kidney function is not normally impaired during pregnancy. (16:132; 22:118)

Nursing Process—Implementation
Client Need—Health promotion/maintenance

31 4. It is recommended that the pregnant woman with varicose veins move around when standing for extended periods of time in order to prevent the stasis of blood in the lower extremities. The client should rest with her feet elevated and should not wear

round garters, knee- or calf-length elastic-top hose. (16:132; 22:118)
>Nursing Process—Implementation
>Client Need—Health promotion/maintenance

32 2. If elastic hose are used, they should be applied after the legs have been elevated for a period of time. It is recommended that the hose be applied before the client gets out of bed in the morning because at that time the veins are less likely to be distended by blood that has pooled in the extremities. (14:105; 16:132)
>Nursing Process—Evaluation
>Client Need—Health promotion/maintenance

33 4. Varicose veins normally are purple in color. The client with varicose veins may complain of her legs aching and feeling tired and heavy. If the client complains of the legs becoming red, tender, or warm to the touch, then the health care provider should be notified immediately, because the client may have developed thrombophlebitis, a more serious problem. (14:105; 16:132)
>Nursing Process—Implementation
>Client Need—Health promotion/maintenance

34 1. Itching of the skin is not uncommon and is an annoying discomfort of pregnancy. It may occur during pregnancy because the enlarging uterus causes the abdominal skin to stretch. Drying agents such as soaps and alcohol also might cause itching and should be avoided. Increased fluid intake may improve elasticity of the skin and decrease the occurrence of itching. (22:124)
>Nursing Process—Implementation
>Client Need—Health promotion/maintenance

35 3. As the uterus rises in the abdomen, pressure is exerted on the diaphragm, thus decreasing lung capacity. This decrease in lung capacity results in shortness of breath. This problem usually is seen in the third trimester of pregnancy and usually is not abnormal. Shortness of breath during the third trimester of pregnancy is not the result of anxiety about the impending delivery, nor is it associated with a decreased oxygen supply secondary to slow venous circulation. (14:105)
>Nursing Process—Implementation
>Client Need—Health promotion/maintenance

36 4. Elevating the upper body on pillows while resting may help to relieve the shortness of breath. Maintaining an erect posture when sitting or standing also may help to relieve this problem by increasing oxygen intake. It is not necessary for the client to notify the physician immediately, but the physician should be made aware of any difficulty in breathing

in order to rule out the presence of a serious problem. (14:105)
>Nursing Process—Implementation
>Client Need—Health promotion/maintenance

37 3. Frequent urination is common early in pregnancy because the enlarging uterus causes pressure on the urinary bladder. When the uterus rises into the abdominal cavity, urinary frequency may subside. Placental maturity, fetal kidney function, and hormonal balance are not usually causes of urinary frequency during early pregnancy. (14:104)
>Nursing Process—Implementation
>Client Need—Health promotion/maintenance

38 3. Frequent urination is common in late pregnancy because the enlarged uterus drops into the pelvis, causing pressure on the urinary bladder. Frequency is unrelated to having alkaline urine or increasing waste from the fetus. A urinary tract infection could cause frequency, but this is not the most probable cause late in pregnancy, and it would be likely to cause additional symptoms, such as burning and painful urination. (22:125; 14:104)
>Nursing Process—Implementation
>Client Need—Health promotion/maintenance

39 1. Limiting fluid intake prior to going to bed at night may be advised, but the patient should be advised to maintain adequate intake during the day. If the client does not consume an adequate amount of fluid, dehydration may occur. Reducing the intake of high-caffeine fluids and voiding before going to bed are acceptable means of controlling urinary frequency. The client also should be taught to recognize and report signs of a urinary tract infection. (16:130)
>Nursing Process—Evaluation
>Client Need—Health promotion/maintenance

40 4. Low-heeled shoes place the back in a more proper alignment and therefore may relieve backaches associated with pregnancy. A firm mattress also may help to relieve the backache by providing increased support to the lower back. The remaining suggestions are not likely to relieve the client's backache. (14:105; 22:120)
>Nursing Process—Implementation
>Client Need—Health promotion/maintenance

41 1. Nausea and heartburn are common discomforts during pregnancy that are believed to occur because of hormonal changes, decreased gastric motility, and displacement of the stomach and duodenum by the enlarging uterus. Eating small frequent meals, avoiding liquids during meals, and avoiding lying down after meals may prevent or limit nausea and heartburn. Antacid preparations may relieve these discomforts but should be taken only under the direction of a physician. Sodium bicarbonate and baking soda should be avoided because of the danger of fluid and electrolyte imbalances. (14:104; 22:114)

> Nursing Process—Evaluation
> Client Need—Health promotion/maintenance

42 2. Placing a hot water bottle on the affected area may help to prevent or relieve the client's leg cramps. Pointing the toes to the knee instead of to the floor also may help to relieve leg cramps. Because the client has a history of thrombophlebitis, she also should be instructed not to massage her legs because of the danger of clot formation. (22:118)

> Nursing Process—Implementation
> Client Need—Health promotion/maintenance

HIGH-RISK FACTORS AND PREGNANCY

43 4. A client who is younger than 18 or older than 35 years of age is considered to be at risk for complications during pregnancy. A client who has had more than four pregnancies also is considered to be at risk for complications. The other factors listed in this question are not identified as high-risk factors. (16:242)

> Nursing Process—Data collection
> Client Need—Physiological integrity

44 2. There is no known safe amount of alcohol that can be consumed by the mother during pregnancy. Pregnant women should be encouraged to stop drinking all alcoholic beverages throughout their pregnancies. Women with alcohol abuse problems should be referred to a rehabilitation program. (16:97; 14:113)

> Nursing Process—Implementation
> Client Need—Health promotion/maintenance

45 1. A woman who smokes during pregnancy increases the risk of complications for herself and her unborn child. Smoking during pregnancy has been linked to premature births, low-birth-weight infants, spontaneous abortions, and delayed mental and physical development of the child. There is no known association between cigarette smoking, hyperemesis gravidarum, or acquiring HIV.
(14:114; 16:97)

> Nursing Process—Implementation
> Client Need—Health promotion/maintenance

46 2. Chorionic villi sampling (CVS) would be the preferred procedure for the client because CVS can be done as early as 8 to 11 weeks gestation. An additional advantage of CVS is that the results can

be obtained within 1 to 7 days of the procedure. The amniocentesis cannot be performed until the client is between 14 and 20 weeks gestation and the results are not usually available for 10 days to 4 weeks. Ultrasound can detect some congenital anomalies but is more useful as an adjunct to other tests such as the amniocentesis. The rapid plasma reagin test is designed to screen for syphilis and does not detect genetic defects in the fetus. (16:100)

> Nursing Process—Implementation
> Client Need—Safe, effective care environment

COMPLICATIONS OF PREGNANCY

47 3. Trichomoniasis is a sexually transmitted disease. The female client with this infection usually will present with a frothy vaginal discharge, swelling of the vulva, and a complaint of intense itching. The other signs and symptoms presented in this question are not usual manifestations of trichomoniasis. (14:142)

> Nursing Process—Data collection
> Client Need—Physiological integrity

48 2. Clients diagnosed with trichomoniasis usually are treated with metronidazole (Flagyl). In the past, the use of metronidazole was contraindicated during the first trimester of pregnancy, but recent research findings have indicated that there is no increased risk of birth defects with the use of metronidazole (Flagyl) during the first trimester. Sexual partners of the client with trichomoniasis should be treated since this is a sexually transmitted disease. Atypical cells may show up on the Pap smear results because of the irritation of vaginal tissue. The pregnant woman with trichomoniasis is not required to deliver by cesarean section. (14:143; 16:133)

> Nursing Process—Evaluation
> Client Need—Health promotion/maintenance

49 3. Bleeding from the vagina may indicate a complication of pregnancy, such as abruptio placentae, spontaneous abortion, or placenta previa. This problem must be brought to the attention of the physician immediately. Breast tenderness, fetal movement, and frequent urination usually are normal occurrences during pregnancy and can be discussed with the physician during a routine visit. (22:89)

> Nursing Process—Implementation
> Client Need—Health promotion/maintenance

50 1. Hyperemesis gravidarum is persistent vomiting, is serious, and can result in dehydration and electrolyte imbalances. Severe cases of hyperemesis gravidarum require hospitalization of the client for intravenous therapy to correct the dehydration and electrolyte imbalances. The other equipment identified in this question may be ordered for various other reasons, but are not routinely used in the care of the client hospitalized for hyperemesis gravidarum. (14:134; 22:143)

Nursing Process—Planning
Client Need—Physiological integrity

51 2. An incompetent cervix dilates prematurely because it is unable to support the weight of the growing fetus. This complication usually occurs during the second trimester of pregnancy. If untreated, an incompetent cervix may result in a spontaneous abortion. Incompetent cervix is not described as a condition in which the cervix is not large enough for the passage of the fetus, nor does it have any relationship to the patency of the internal and external os. (14:126)

Nursing Process—Implementation
Client Need—Health promotion/maintenance

52 4. The treatment of choice for the client with an incompetent cervix who is not experiencing labor contractions is the placement of a purse-string suture (cerclage) in the cervix to pull closed the cervical os. The suture is left in place until the client is near term, when the client may go into labor spontaneously or be a candidate for a cesarean delivery. (14:126)

Nursing Process—Implementation
Client Need—Health promotion/maintenance

53 3. Clients experiencing mild preeclampsia will have a 30 mm Hg rise in the baseline systolic blood pressure or a 15 mm Hg rise in the baseline diastolic blood pressure; proteinuria with a +1 or +2 reading on the urine reagent test strip; and a weight gain of 2 or more pounds per week during the second trimester. Edema may be present but usually is observed in the face, hands, and ankles. Ankle edema may be present during pregnancy for reasons other than preeclampsia. (14:130; 16:261)

Nursing Process—Data collection
Client Need—Physiological integrity

54 3. The care of the client with mild preeclampsia usually can be managed at home. It is important that the client be monitored on a weekly basis, eat a diet high in protein and with an adequate fluid intake because of the protein lost during urination, and remain on bed rest. The client also should be taught danger signs that should be reported to the physician immediately. (14:131)

Nursing Process—Implementation
Client Need—Physiological integrity

55 2. In addition to assessing the vital signs, the nurse should assess the client's deep tendon reflexes, urine output, fetal heart tones, and monitor magnesium serum blood levels. These parameters are monitored because they will indicate the presence of or potential for magnesium toxicity. The presence of glucose in the urine, blood in the stool, and a skin rash are not significant to magnesium toxicity. (14:133; 16:265)

Nursing Process—Implementation
Client Need—Physiological integrity

56 1. The client with PIH is said to have developed eclampsia if she begins to have convulsions. Severe headache, abdominal pain, hyperirritability of the muscles, apprehension, and twitching often precede convulsions that are associated with eclampsia. The other signs and symptoms are not manifestations of eclampsia. (14:132; 16:262)

Nursing Process—Implementation
Client Need—Physiological integrity

57 4. The antidote for magnesium toxicity is a 10% solution of calcium gluconate. The medication usually is given intravenously and is injected over 3 or more minutes to prevent the occurrence of ventricular fibrillation. Hydralazine (Apresoline) is an antihypertensive; methyl ergonovine (Methergine) usually is given to control postpartum bleeding; and oxytocin (Pitocin) is used to augment labor and control postpartum bleeding. 14:132; 16:265)

Nursing Process—Implementation
Client Need—Physiological integrity

58 2. A respiratory rate of less than 14 is associated with magnesium toxicity. In addition, if the deep tendon reflexes are diminished, the urine output is less than 100 mL in 4 hours, there are signs of fetal distress, or the magnesium serum level is above 10 mg/dL, the magnesium sulfate should be discontinued and the physician should be notified because these are also signs of magnesium toxicity. (16:265)

Nursing Process—Data collection
Client Need—Physiological integrity

59 4. Vaginal bleeding and abdominal cramping or backaches are typical symptoms clients report with the occurrence of a spontaneous abortion. Ankle swelling is a common discomfort of pregnancy. Severe headaches and persistent nausea are not normal discomforts and should be reported to the health care provider, but are not usual manifestations reported by the client experiencing a spontaneous abortion. (14:126)

Nursing Process—Data collection
Client Need—Physiological integrity

60 1. When the cervix is dilated but the fetus and placenta remain in the uterus, spontaneous abortion is inevitable and the client will more than likely have to have a dilation and curettage to remove the remaining products of conception. The client should be prepared for the procedure both physically and emotionally. The other options are not usually included in the care of the client experiencing an inevitable spontaneous abortion. (14:126)

   Nursing Process—Implementation
   Client Need—Safe, effective care environment

61 1. An inevitable spontaneous abortion means that there is no hope of saving the baby. The nurse must be honest with the client and provide much-needed emotional support. The client and family members should be encouraged to verbalize their feelings to facilitate the client's and family's ability to cope with the situation. Telling the client that the outcome is not certain at this point is untrue. Suggesting that the client remain calm does not facilitate expression of her feelings and thus hinders her ability to cope with the situation. Telling the client that things will work out for the best does not acknowledge the justifiable sorrow that the client is experiencing. It also does not show emotional support that is much needed. (14:131)

   Nursing Process—Implementation
   Client Need—Psychosocial integrity

62 3. The insulin requirement for the pregnant client who is diabetic will fluctuate during pregnancy. During the first 18 weeks of pregnancy, the need for insulin decreases because increased amounts of glucose are being transported to the growing fetus by the mother. Later in pregnancy, the need for insulin usually increases because of the increasing amounts of hormones that cause insulin resistance in the client. During the postpartum period, the hormone levels drop and therefore decrease the need for insulin. (14:138; 16:244)

   Nursing Process—Implementation
   Client Need—Health promotion/maintenance

63 2. The pregnant diabetic client has an increased risk for developing pregnancy-induced hypertension. Some of the other complications that may occur secondary to diabetes during pregnancy are infection, hydramnios, possible birth trauma secondary to fetal size, and postpartum hemorrhage. (14:137; 16:245)

   Nursing Process—Implementation
   Client Need—Health promotion/maintenance

64 1. The pregnant diabetic client is at greatest risk for having a baby that is larger than average. Other fetal effects of diabetes include hypoglycemia, con-genital anomalies, prematurity, and respiratory distress syndrome. However, women who are well controlled during pregnancy rarely experience the other fetal effects listed here. (14:138)

   Nursing Process—Implementation
   Client Need—Health promotion/maintenance

65 2. The most characteristic sign of placenta previa is painless bleeding from the vagina. It occurs late in pregnancy, and is the most common cause of bleeding during the second and third trimesters of pregnancy. Sharp abdominal pain, elevated blood pressure, and continuous, painless contractions are not associated with placenta previa. (14:128; 16:256)

   Nursing Process—Data collection
   Client Need—Physiological integrity

66 2. The client with placenta previa is at risk for hemorrhaging. Therefore, a baseline blood pressure and pulse rate should be obtained so that further changes can be evaluated by those involved in the care of the client and significant findings can be reported to the physician in a timely manner. When a client is admitted to the hospital, height, weight, obstetrical history, and general health and drug history are obtained but do not take priority, in this situation, over obtaining the client's blood pressure and pulse. (14:129; 16:256)

   Nursing Process—Data collection
   Client Need—Physiological integrity

67 1. Placenta previa is a condition in which the placenta totally (complete or total placenta previa) or partially (partial placenta previa) covers the cervical os (opening), or the placenta may be implanted low in the uterus (marginal placenta previa) without covering any part of the os. The painless bleeding associated with placenta previa is due to a separation of the placenta from the uterus in the area that is near or covers the cervical os. The separation is caused by normal changes in the cervix that are occurring in preparation for labor. Placenta previa is unrelated to the development of polyps, hormonal deficiencies, or antibody production. (14:32; 16:256)

   Nursing Process—Implementation
   Client Need—Physiological integrity

68 3. The preferred course of treatment is to maintain the pregnancy as close to term as is possible. If the client is stable, the physician usually will order bed rest and continuous observation of the client. With marginal or partial placenta previa, vaginal delivery is possible. Uncontrolled hemorrhaging, fetal distress, or complete placenta previa will require immediate delivery of the baby, usually by cesarean section. Ritodrine may be indicated if the client goes into premature labor; however, this medication is not routinely used for clients with placenta previa. (14:128; 16:256)

> Nursing Process—Implementation
> Client Need—Physiological integrity

69 4. The client with pregnancy-induced hypertension is at risk for developing abruptio placentae. Other factors associated with the occurrence of abruptio placentae include essential hypertension, previous history of placenta previa, dietary deficiencies, trauma to the abdomen, multiparity, and a history of alcohol or drug abuse. Gestational diabetes, hyperemesis gravidarum, and oligiohydraminous are not associated with the occurrence of abruptio placentae. (14:129; 16:257)

> Nursing Process—Data collection
> Client Need—Physiological integrity

70 1. A rigid, boardlike abdomen is often observed in the client with abruptio placentae who has concealed hemorrhaging. Other signs and symptoms of abruptio placentae include severe pain, dark red vaginal bleeding, maternal shock, and fetal distress. Severe nausea and vomiting, smaller uterus than expected for dates, and painless vaginal bleeding are not manifestations of abruptio placentae. (14:129; 16:257)

> Nursing Process—Data collection
> Client Need—Physiological integrity

71 1. A complete abruption requires emergency cesarean delivery. Written consent should be obtained immediately from the client or a family member. Clients with vaginal bleeding should not be given enemas. The client with a complete abruption is not usually placed in the Trendelenburg position. A contraction stress test would be inappropriate for the client with any type of abruptio placentae. (14:129; 16:259)

> Nursing Process—Planning
> Client Need—Safe, effective care environment

NUTRITION DURING PREGNANCY

72 2. The client's current eating pattern and preferences must be known before a teaching plan can be formulated and implemented. Once this information is obtained, the nurse can show the client what foods must be added to or deleted from the diet. Also, the nurse can, with the assistance of the client, develop a plan that is more likely to be followed by the client. Calorie recommendations may be made; however, the client needs to be provided with information that will assist her in the selection of items that will supply the nutrients she needs (a cup of milk instead of 10 g of calcium). Once teaching is

initiated, it might be useful to develop sample menus with the client. (14:115; 16:123)

> Nursing Process—Planning
> Client Need—Health promotion/maintenance

73 2. During pregnancy, the recommended intake of milk is 3 to 4 servings (3 to 4 cups) daily. Milk is an excellent source of calcium and protein, both of which are essential for the proper development of strong bones, healthy teeth, healthy nerves and muscles, and normal blood clotting. (14:115; 16:125)

> Nursing Process—Implementation
> Client Need—Health promotion/maintenance

74 3. Of the foods listed in this question, leafy green vegetables, would contain the highest amount of calcium. (16:123)

> Nursing Process—Implementation
> Client Need—Health promotion/maintenance

75 3. Women who are receiving iron supplements sometimes complain of constipation. The nurse should encourage the client to increase her fiber intake and fluid intake to help prevent or control this problem. The RDA of iron doubles during pregnancy. The demand for iron usually exceeds the amount that can be provided from dietary sources; if the physician orders an iron supplement, the client should not attempt to substitute dietary sources of iron for the prescribed iron supplement. Iron supplements are best absorbed when taken between meals. (14:117; 16:122)

> Nursing Process—Implementation
> Client Need—Health promotion/maintenance

TEACHING THE PREGNANT CLIENT

76 2. Daily tub baths or showers are recommended for the client during pregnancy because women usually perspire more heavily and have a heavier vaginal discharge during pregnancy. Tub baths may increase the risk for fall during the latter part of pregnancy because of the shift in the center of gravity produced by the protruding abdomen. It is recommended that safety mats, hand grips, and other safety precautions be used to prevent falls. Hot tub baths should be avoided because of the danger of harmful fetal effects from elevated maternal core body temperature. Also, tub baths should be avoided once the membranes rupture because of the increased risk of the development of infection. (14:109; 16:128)

> Nursing Process—Evaluation
> Client Need—Health promotion/maintenance

77 4. During healthy pregnancies no restrictions are placed on sexual intercourse. However, sexual intercourse is contraindicated if the client experiences vaginal bleeding or if the membranes have ruptured. Also, clients with a history of premature labor should be cautioned about the danger of premature labor reoccurring with orgasms after 32 weeks gestation. (16:129)
> **Nursing Process—Implementation**
> **Client Need—Health Promotion/maintenance**

78 1. Restriction of travel during pregnancy is indicated only when the client is unhealthy or experiencing complications. The optimal time for travel is during the second trimester of pregnancy, when the client is most comfortable. The client should be encouraged to carry a copy of her medical records with her whenever she is traveling. (14:110; 16:129)
> **Nursing Process—Implementation**
> **Client Need—Health promotion/maintenance**

79 3. Identical twins result when one fertilized ovum divides into two identical halves that develop into two individuals with the same appearance and same sex. Fraternal twins are the result of two separate ovum being fertilized by two different sperm but at the same time. They may or may not resemble each other and may or may not be of the same sex. (16:96)
> **Nursing Process—Implementation**
> **Client Need—Health promotion/maintenance**

80 1. Once the ovum is fertilized it will travel through the fallopian tube to the uterus, where it will implant. The time required for the ovum to travel to the uterus and implant is approximately 7 days. At the time of implantation there may be a small amount of bleeding, similar to menstrual spotting. (16:84)
> **Nursing Process—Implementation**
> **Client Need—Health promotion/maintenance**

81 4. By the eighth week of gestation, the embryo has developed enough to be called a fetus. The fetal stage of development mostly involves growth and maturation of structures begun during the embryonic stage. At 8 weeks, the extremities are developed, and by the 12th week, the fetus not only has arms and legs but has fingers and toes. (14:81; 16:88)
> **Nursing Process—Implementation**
> **Client Need—Health promotion/maintenance**

82 2. The amniotic fluid protects the fetus, allows the fetus to move, keeps the environment for the fetus at a constant temperature, provides some nourishment for the fetus, and prevents the amnion from adhering to the fetus. Providing the fetus with antibodies, providing oxygen for the fetus, and lowering the body temperature of the mother are not functions of amniotic fluid. (14:82)
> **Nursing Process—Implementation**
> **Client Need—Health promotion/maintenance**

ELECTIVE ABORTION

83 3. During the first trimester of pregnancy, a woman has the legal right to have an abortion without legal restraints. During the second trimester, states can regulate the conditions under which an abortion is performed but cannot prohibit abortion. After viability, which according to legal guidelines is considered to be after 20 to 24 weeks gestation, the state may, and usually does, prohibit abortion except in a situation in which there is a threat to the life or health of the pregnant woman. (16:74)
> **Nursing Process—Implementation**
> **Client Need—Health promotion/maintenance**

84 2. Aspiration (or vacuum) and dilation and curettage are methods of abortion that are used during the first trimester of pregnancy. Hypertonic saline instillation, abdominal hysterotomy, and prostaglandin administration are methods used for second-trimester abortions. (16:75)
> **Nursing Process—Implementation**
> **Client Need—Health promotion/maintenance**

INDIVIDUAL TEST ITEMS

85 3. Primigravida describes a woman pregnant for the first time. A primipara describes a woman who has delivered her first viable infant. Multipara describes a woman who has delivered more than one viable infant. Multigravida describes a woman who has been pregnant more than once. (14:92; 16:110)
> **Nursing Process—Data collection**
> **Client Need—Health promotion/maintenance.**

86 4. Any sudden weight gain brings suspicion of PIH. Other signs include proteinuria, a decrease in urine output, and a rise in blood pressure (over 140/90). (16:262)
> **Nursing Process—Data collection**
> **Client Need—Physiological integrity**

87 2. Exposure to rubella (German measles) during the first trimester of pregnancy increases the risk of the fetus developing congenital rubella syndrome. Major manifestations of congenital rubella syndrome include blindness, deafness, heart defects, mental retardation, cleft lip, and cleft palate. (14:140)

> Nursing Process—Implementation
> Client Need—Health promotion/maintenance

88 4. Pregnant clients who have a preexisting disease, such as hypertensive disease, have an increased risk of developing complications during pregnancy. Pregnant clients who have more than 4 pregnancies also are considered to have an increased risk for complications. The husband's weight and a family history of twins does not increase the client's risk for the development of complications during pregnancy. (16:243)

> Nursing Process—Data collection
> Client Need—Health promotion/maintenance

89 4. Hydatidiform mole is suspected when there is abnormally rapid uterine growth. This condition also is suspected when fetal heart tones and fetal movement cannot be detected, when there is excessive or persistent nausea and vomiting, and when pregnancy-induced hypertension develops prior to 20 to 24 weeks gestation. Vaginal bleeding may be continuous or intermittent and the HCG level is greatly elevated. (16:255; 14:127)

> Nursing Process—Data collection
> Client Need—Physiological integrity

90 1. When a pregnant woman has herpes simplex virus type 2 (genital herpes), a cesarean delivery is most often performed to prevent infecting the infant during vaginal delivery. The infant mortality rate for infants who contract neonatal infections during vaginal delivery is high. Newborns who survive often have serious neurological damage. (16:251; 14:143)

> Nursing Process—Implementation
> Client Need—Safe, effective care environment

91 3. The Centers for Disease Control recommends that pregnant women who are at risk for having the hepatitis B virus be tested during pregnancy. Risk groups include: women of Asian, Pacific Island, Alaskan Eskimo, and Haitian descent; recipients of repeated blood transfusions; intravenous (IV) drug users or partners of IV drug users; women who have been exposed to hepatitis B; and women who have multiple sex partners. (14:108)

> Nursing Process—Implementation
> Client Need—Health promotion/maintenance

Classification of Test Items

Unit **II** Review Test **11**

The Nursing Care of Clients During the Antepartum Period

Directions: After each question the correct answer is given, as well as a classification of each test question. Compare the correct answer with your answer. If a question has been answered *incorrectly*, draw a line to the end of all the columns. When finished, add up the number of your correct answers in each column and place that number in the respective box at the end in the area identified as *Number Correct*.

To determine the percentage of questions you answered correctly and your performance in each of the test plan categories, divide the *Number Correct* in each column by the *Number Possible* in each column. Then multiply the decimal by 100. For example:

$$\frac{\text{Number Correct: 78}}{\text{Number Possible: 91}} = 0.857 \times 100 = 86\%$$

Any score that is less than 75% indicates an area where further review would be beneficial.

KEY TO ITEM CLASSIFICATION:

NURSING PROCESS

D = Data collection
P = Planning
I = Implementation
E = Evaluation

CLIENT NEEDS

S = Safe, effective care environment
P = Physiological integrity
M = Psychosocial integrity
H = Health promotion/maintenance

Question #	Answer #	D	P	I	E	S	P	M	H
1	1			I					H
2	2			I					H
3	2			I					H
4	3			I					H
5	1			I					H
6	4			I					H
7	1			I					H
8	2	D							H
9	3			I		S			
10	4	D							H
11	1			I					H
12	2			I					H
13	1			I					H
14	2			I					H
15	1			I					H

Question #	Answer #	Nursing Process				Client Needs			
		D	P	I	E	S	P	M	H
16	4			I					H
17	3			I					H
18	1			I		S			
19	2			I		S			
20	4			I		S			
21	2			I					H
22	4	D							H
23	1	D							H
24	3			I					H
25	3			I					H
26	3		P						H
27	2			I		S			
28	4		P			S			
29	2			I					H
30	1			I					H
31	4			I					H
32	2				E				H
33	4			I					H
34	1			I					H
35	3			I					H
36	4			I					H
37	3			I					H
38	3			I					H
39	1				E				H
40	4			I					H
41	1				E				H
42	2			I					H
43	4	D					P		
44	2			I					H
45	1			I					H
46	2			I		S			
47	3	D					P		

Question #	Answer #	Nursing Process				Client Needs			
		D	P	I	E	S	P	M	H
48	2				E				H
49	3			I					H
50	1		P				P		
51	2			I					H
52	4			I					H
53	3	D					P		
54	3			I			P		
55	2			I			P		
56	1			I			P		
57	4			I			P		
58	2	D					P		
59	4	D					P		
60	1			I		S			
61	1			I				M	
62	3			I					H
63	2			I					H
64	1			I					H
65	2	D					P		
66	2	D					P		
67	1			I			P		
68	3			I			P		
69	4	D					P		
70	1	D					P		
71	1		P			S			
72	2		P						H
73	2			I					H
74	3			I					H
75	3			I					H
76	2				E				H
77	4			I					H
78	1			I					H
79	3			I					H

Question #	Answer #	Nursing Process				Client Needs			
		D	P	I	E	S	P	M	H
80	1			I					H
81	4			I					H
82	2			I					H
83	3			I					H
84	2			I					H
85	3	D							H
86	4	D					P		
87	2			I					H
88	4	D							H
89	4	D					P		
90	1			I		S			
91	3			I					H
Number Correct	69	13	5	49	4	8	13	1	58
Number Possible	91	17	5	64	5	10	18	1	62
Percentage Correct	76	76	100	77	80	80	72	100	81

Directions: With a pencil, blacken the circle in front of the option you have chosen for your correct answer.

ADMISSION OF THE CLIENT TO A LABOR AND DELIVERY FACILITY

A 25-year-old primigravida, who is in her last trimester of pregnancy, calls her physician's office and tells the nurse that she thinks she is in labor.

1 The nurse would be *correct* to instruct the client to report *immediately* to the hospital's labor and delivery unit if the client states that
- ○ 1. she is having contractions every 10 minutes.
- ○ 2. she experienced a sudden burst of energy last night.
- ● 3. she experienced a sudden gush of fluid from her vagina.
- ○ 4. she has begun to experience urinary frequency.

The client arrives at the hospital and is admitted to the labor, delivery, recovery, postpartum (LDRP) unit. The nurse obtains a history on the client.

2 Which one of the following questions is *least* pertinent for the nurse the ask during the admission interview?
- ○ 1. "When did you last eat?"
- ● 2. "Have you ever had an enema?"
- ○ 3. "When did your contractions start?"
- ○ 4. "When is your baby due?"

3 The nurse can *best* obtain an accurate blood pressure reading by assessing the blood pressure
- ○ 1. at the peak of a contraction with the client positioned on her left side.
- ○ 2. at the peak of a contraction with the client positioned on her right side.
- ● 3. between contractions with the client positioned on her right side.
- ○ 4. between contractions with the client positioned on her left side.

NURSING CARE OF CLIENTS DURING THE FIRST STAGE OF LABOR

A 30-year-old primigravida is admitted to the labor, delivery, recovery, postpartum unit of a local hospital. On the client's admission record the physician writes that the client is in the latent phase of the first stage of labor.

4 Which one of the following would the nurse expect to observe when assessing the client?
- ● 1. Contractions occurring every 3 to 5 minutes
- ○ 2. Fetal heart rate of 120 to 160 beats per minute
- ○ 3. Bulging perineum
- ○ 4. Early decelerations

5 The nurse would be *correct* to encourage the client to
- ○ 1. remain in bed on her left side.
- ○ 2. continue oral intake of clear liquids.
- ○ 3. pant when she experiences a contraction.
- ● 4. avoid bathing until after delivery.

6 During the latent phase of the first stage of labor, the nurse should plan to assess the fetal heart rate every
- ○ 1. 5 minutes.
- ● 2. 15 minutes.
- ○ 3. 30 minutes.
- ○ 4. 60 minutes.

The client tells the nurse that she plans to have an epidural. She ask the nurse when she should expect to receive the epidural.

7 The nurse can *best* respond by explaining that the physician will probably perform the epidural when the client is
   ○ 1. 3 to 4 cm dilated.
   ● 2. 5 to 6 cm dilated.
   ○ 3. 7 to 8 cm dilated.
   ○ 4. 9 to 10 cm dilated.

The registered nurse performs a vaginal examination on the client and determines that the cervix is dilated 6 cm.

8 When assessing the frequency and duration of the client's contractions, the nurse would expect to find that the contractions are occurring every 3 to 5 minutes and lasting up to
   ○ 1. 30 seconds.
   ○ 2. 40 seconds.
   ● 3. 60 seconds.
   ○ 4. 90 seconds.

The client states that she thinks her membranes have ruptured. The nurse performs a nitrazine test.

9 Which one of the following test results would *indicate* that the membranes have ruptured?
   ● 1. The test strip turns blue.
   ○ 2. The test strip turns yellow.
   ○ 3. The test strip turns red.
   ○ 4. The test strip turns green.

The test results indicate that the membranes have ruptured. The physician orders internal electronic fetal monitoring. The client ask the nurse, "Is there any danger of this procedure causing harm to my baby?"

10 The nurse can *best* respond by explaining that the procedure requires
   ● 1. attachment of a small spiral electrode to the fetal scalp and poses a slight risk for soft tissue injury and infection.
   ○ 2. insertion of a soft, water-filled catheter into the uterus and poses no risk for injury to the fetus or the client.
   ○ 3. application of an ultrasound transducer over the maternal abdomen and poses no risk to the fetus or the client.
   ○ 4. application of a suction cup to the fetal scalp and poses a slight risk for the development of a hematoma.

The client has entered the transition phase of the first stage of labor.

11 Which one of the following findings would the nurse expect to observe during this phase?
   ● 1. Cervix dilated to 10 cm
   ○ 2. Crowning of the presenting part
   ○ 3. Increased bloody show
   ○ 4. Contractions lasting up to 60 seconds

12 Which one of the following actions would *best* meet the client's needs during the transition phase?
   ○ 1. Encourage the client to ambulate
   ● 2. Praise the client on a frequent basis
   ○ 3. Instruct the client to push with each contraction
   ○ 4. Massage the clients back between contractions

A 29-year-old multipara who has had an uneventful healthy pregnancy is admitted to the LDRP. The physician informs the client that she is in the active phase of the first stage of labor. The records also show that the baby is in the left occiput posterior (LOP) position.

13 Which one of the following would the nurse include when the fetus is in the LOP position?
   ● 1. Assist the client to the knee-chest position to relieve her back pain.
   ○ 2. Place the client in the Trendelenburg position to prevent cord prolapse.
   ○ 3. Assist with preparation of equipment for a precipitous delivery.
   ○ 4. Have the client void frequently to minimize displacement of the uterus.

14 Which one of the following interventions is *most* appropriate for preventing distention of the client's bladder?
   ○ 1. Instruct the client to limit her fluid intake.
   ○ 2. Decrease the rate of the intravenous infusion.
   ○ 3. Offer solid foods instead of liquids.
   ● 4. Encourage the client to void every 2 hours.

15 When assessing the duration of a contraction, the nurse would be *correct* to count the time interval between the
   ● 1. beginning of one contraction and the end of the same contraction.
   ○ 2. end of one contraction and the beginning of the next contraction.
   ○ 3. beginning of one contraction and the end of the next contraction.
   ○ 4. beginning of one contraction and the beginning of the next contraction.

16 When assessing the client's contractions, the nurse would be *correct* to place her hand
   ○ 1. over the fundus of the uterus, which is located just above the umbilicus in the full-term client.
   ○ 2. over the corpus of the uterus, which is located just above the umbilicus in the full-term client.
   ○ 3. over the fundus of the uterus, which is located midway between the umbilicus and the symphysis pubis in the full-term client.
   ◉ 4. over the corpus of the uterus, which is located midway between the umbilicus and the symphysis pubis in the full-term client.

17 During the active phase of the first stage of labor, the nurse would be *correct* to assess the fetal heart rate (FHR)
   ○ 1. every 5 minutes.
   ○ 2. every 10 minutes.
   ◉ 3. every 15 minutes.
   ○ 4. every 30 minutes.

The client tells the nurse that she thinks her membranes have ruptured. The nurse performs a nitrazine test and confirms that the membranes are ruptured.

18 Which of the following actions should the nurse perform *immediately* after the membranes are ruptured?
   ○ 1. Check the client's pulse
   ○ 2. Insert an indwelling catheter
   ○ 3. Perform a vaginal exam
   ◉ 4. Check the fetal heart tones

19 The nurse would be *correct* to assess the client's temperature
   ◉ 1. every hour.
   ○ 2. every 2 hours.
   ○ 3. every 4 hours.
   ○ 4. every 8 hours.

20 Which one of the following findings is *most* indicative of the presence of fetal distress?
   ○ 1. FHR of 140 beats per minute
   ○ 2. Presence of FHR accelerations
   ◉ 3. Presence of green amniotic fluid
   ○ 4. Increase in amount of bloody show

A 21-year-old primigravida client is admitted to the LDRP unit to evaluate whether or not the client is in true labor. The physician decides to perform a vaginal examination on the client.

21 The nurse can *best* prepare to assist with the vaginal examination by
   ◉ 1. having sterile gloves available for the examiner.

   ○ 2. placing the client in the left side-lying position.
   ○ 2. instructing the client to hold her breath during the examination.
   ○ 4. giving the client an enema before the examination is performed.

After performing the vaginal examination, the physician decides that the client is in the latent phase of the first stage of labor. A progress note is written in the client's admission records.

22 The nurse reviews the client's admission records. Which one of the following findings, in the records, is the *most reliable* indicator that the client is in true labor?
   ○ 1. Contractions are regular and increasing in duration and intensity.
   ○ 2. Contractions radiate from the lower back to the lower abdomen.
   ○ 3. Bloody show is present.
   ◉ 4. The cervix is dilating.

The client tells the nurse that she has not had anything to eat in the past 24 hours and asks the nurse if she can bring her some food because she is hungry.

23 The nurse would be *correct* to explain that solid foods cannot be given because they may
   ○ 1. alter the absorption of regional anesthetics.
   ○ 2. alter the duration and frequency of contractions.
   ○ 3. cause fetal distress to occur.
   ◉ 4. cause nausea and vomiting.

The client tells the nurse she heard the physician say that her baby was in the vertex position. She asks the nurse what the vertex position is.

24 The nurse would be *correct* in explaining that vertex position means the baby's
   ◉ 1. head is entering the birth canal first.
   ○ 2. feet are entering the birth canal first.
   ○ 3. buttocks are entering the birth canal first.
   ○ 4. shoulder is entering the birth canal first.

25 When evaluating the client's contractions during the active phase of the first stage of labor, the nurse should notify the physician or the nurse in charge *immediately* if the
   ○ 1. contractions occur every 3 to 5 minutes.
   ○ 2. contractions last longer than 45 seconds.
   ○ 3. uterus relaxes between contractions.
   ◉ 4. FHR drops after the acme of a contraction.

The physician visits the client and explains that she may have to have an episiotomy. The client begins to cry and asks the nurse, "Why do I have to have an episiotomy?"

26 The nurse would be *correct* to explain that an episiotomy may be necessary in order to prevent
  ○ 1. uterine rupture.
  ○ 2. postpartum infection.
  ◉ 3. perineal laceration.
  ○ 4. bowel trauma.

NURSING CARE OF CLIENTS DURING THE SECOND STAGE OF LABOR

The nurse is caring for a 30-year-old multipara client who is in the transition phase of the first stage of labor.

27 Which one of the following findings *best* indicates to the nurse that the client has entered the second stage of labor?
  ◉ 1. The perineum is bulging.
  ○ 2. Contractions are lasting 30 to 60 seconds.
  ○ 3. The cervix is dilated to 8 cm.
  ○ 4. The uterus is at the level of the umbilicus.

28 The nurse would be *correct* to plan to begin preparation for delivery of the baby when
  ○ 1. the client is about 7 cm dilated.
  ○ 2. the fetal head begins to crown.
  ○ 3. the physician or midwife arrives.
  ◉ 4. the client is completely dilated.

The client tells the nurse that she feels the urge to push down.

29 Which of the following actions should the nurse take *initially?*
  ○ 1. Instruct the client to push when she feels the next contraction.
  ○ 2. Ensure that the client is in the semi-Fowler's position.
  ◉ 3. Ensure that client's cervix is fully dilated.
  ○ 4. Instruct the client to take a cleansing breath before pushing.

The client complains of pain and asks the nurse, "Can I have some more Demerol?"

30 The nurse can respond *best* by explaining that Demerol should not be given at this time, because administering narcotic analgesics during the second stage of labor may
  ○ 1. decrease the effectiveness of the contractions.
  ○ 2. cause the uterus to rupture.
  ◉ 3. result in respiratory depression in the newborn.
  ○ 4. cause increased fetal activity.

The physician visits and request that the client be prepared for a saddle block (subarachnoid block).

31 When preparing the client for the saddle block (subarachnoid block), the nurse would be *correct* to explain that the anesthetic will take effect
  ○ 1. immediately.
  ◉ 2. in 10 to 20 minutes.
  ○ 3. 30 to 40 minutes.
  ○ 4. in approximately 1 hour.

The saddle block is performed successfully by the physician.

32 Which one of the following is it *most* important for the nurse to watch for during the *immediate* postprocedural period?
  ○ 1. Maternal hypotension
  ○ 2. Fetal tachycardia
  ○ 3. Spinal headache
  ◉ 4. Lower extremity paralysis

33 Which one of the following modifications in the plan of care is required after the client has undergone the saddle block (subarachnoid block)?
  ○ 1. Oxygen must be administered.
  ◉ 2. The nurse must instruct the client when to push.
  ○ 3. Oxytocin (Pitocin) must be given to augment labor.
  ○ 4. The client must be catheterized.

The client progresses and the physician request that the client be prepared for delivery.

34 The nurse would be *correct* to use which one of the following sequences when cleansing the perineum in preparation for delivery of the baby?
  ◉ 1. Pubic bone to lower abdomen, both inner thighs, right and left labia, vagina to anus.
  ○ 2. Vagina to anus, right and left labia, both inner thighs, pubic bone to lower abdomen.
  ○ 3. Both inner thighs, right and left labia, vagina to anus, pubic bone to lower abdomen
  ○ 4. Left and right labia, vagina to anus, both inner thighs, pubic bone to lower abdomen

NURSING CARE OF CLIENTS DURING THE THIRD STAGE OF LABOR

A 31-year-old client delivers a baby girl who appears to be in no apparent distress.

35 Which one of the following should the nurse plan to have available so that the physician can meet the *priority* need of the newborn immediately after delivery?

○ 1. Cord clamp
○ 2. Identification bracelet
◉ 3. Bulb syringe
○ 4. Oxygen supply

36 To *best* facilitate mother-infant attachment and prevent the infant from developing distress, the nurse should
   ○ 1. give the infant to the mother immediately after initial care is given in the delivery room.
   ◉ 2. immediately dry the infant, then place it skin-to-skin on the mother's abdomen.
   ○ 3. place the infant on a radiant warmer for 5 minutes, then wrap and give the infant to the mother.
   ○ 4. place the infant on a radiant warmer and position the warmer so that the mother can see the infant.

The newborn is given an Apgar score of 7 at 5 minutes.

37 The nurse would be *correct* to prepare to provide care to a newborn that is
   ◉ 1. experiencing severe distress.
   ○ 2. experiencing moderate distress.
   ○ 3. stable but needs to monitored closely.
   ○ 4. is vigorous and has no signs of distress.

38 Which one of the following actions is *most* important for the nurse to implement before transporting the infant from the delivery area to the nursery?
   ◉ 1. Application of matching identification bracelets
   ○ 2. Administration of prophylactic eye medication
   ○ 3. Administration of intramuscular vitamin K
   ○ 4. Performance of phenylketonuria (PKU) testing

The nurse is instructed by the physician to observe the client for signs of impending delivery of the placenta.

39 Which one of the following observations should the nurse report to the physician as a sign of impending delivery of the placenta?
   ◉ 1. Bulging perineum
   ○ 2. Shortening of the umbilical cord
   ○ 3. Rise of the fundus in the abdomen
   ○ 4. Decreased vaginal discharge

40 The nurse would be *correct* to encourage the client to do which of the following to facilitate delivery of the placenta?
   ○ 1. Turn on her right or left side.
   ○ 2. Breathe slowly and deeply.
   ○ 3. Tighten and relax the perineum intermittently.
   ◉ 4. Push when she feels a contraction occurring.

The placenta is delivered and the episiotomy is sutured by the physician. The physician instructs the nurse to add oxytocin (Pitocin) to the client's current bag of intravenous fluids. The client asks the nurse why she has to have oxytocin.

41 The nurse would be *correct* to explain that oxytocin is given after delivery of the baby and placenta in order to
   ○ 1. decrease the blood pressure.
   ○ 2. prevent the uterus from inverting.
   ◉ 3. decrease likelihood of hemorrhage.
   ○ 4. prevent rupture of the uterus.

NURSING CARE OF CLIENTS DURING THE FOURTH STAGE OF LABOR

A midline episiotomy is performed and the client delivers a healthy baby boy without complications. Thirty minutes after delivery of the infant, the placenta is delivered intact. The client complains of uncontrollable shaking and of being cold.

42 The nurse can *best* respond to the client's complaint by
   ○ 1. explaining that the shaking is normal and will go away.
   ○ 2. placing a warmed blanket over the client.
   ○ 3. suggesting that the client try not to think about the shaking.
   ◉ 4. notifying the physician or nurse in charge.

The nurse is assigned to provide care to the client during the fourth stage of labor.

43 During the fourth stage of labor, the nurse would expect to palpate the fundus of the uterus
   ○ 1. at or just below the level of the umbilicus.
   ◉ 2. just above the level of the umbilicus.
   ○ 3. just above the level of the symphysis pubis
   ○ 4. midway between the umbilicus and symphysis pubis.

44 Which one of the following findings should be reported *immediately* to the nurse in charge or the physician?
   ○ 1. A pulse rate between 70 and 80 beats per minute.
   ○ 2. Presence of dark red, fleshy-smelling lochia.
   ○ 3. Saturation of one perineal pad per hour.
   ◉ 4. A systolic blood pressure between 60 and 90 mm Hg.

45 Which one of the following would be *most* appropriate for relieving discomfort associated with episiotomy repair during this period?
   ○ 1. Sitz bath
   ◉ 2. Ice pack
   ○ 3. Heat lamp
   ○ 4. Topical cortisone

46 The nurse would be *correct* to massage the fundus if the
   ○ 1. fundus is firm and hard.
   ○ 2. fundus is at the level of the umbilicus.
   ○ 3. amount of lochia flow decreases.
   ● 4. fundus is soft and boggy.

47 The nurse would be *correct* to massage the fundus by placing one hand on the fundus and the other hand
   ● 1. just above the symphysis pubis.
   ○ 2. to the right side of the abdomen.
   ○ 3. just below the xiphoid process.
   ○ 4. to the left side of the abdomen.

NURSING CARE OF CLIENTS DURING THE POSTPARTUM PERIOD

A 33-year-old primigravida client delivered a healthy baby girl 6 hours ago. A mediolateral episiotomy was performed by the physician during the delivery. The client's condition is stable and she complains of no discomfort at present. During the initial assessment, the nurse notes that the client's fundus is one finger's breadth above the umbilicus and displaced to the right of the abdominal midline.

48 Which one of the following actions would be *most* appropriate for the nurse to take in response to this finding?
   ○ 1. Assist with repositioning the client onto her left side.
   ● 2. Have the client void and recheck the uterus afterward.
   ○ 3. Massage the fundus until it becomes firm and returns to its normal position.
   ○ 4. Document the findings and continue to check the fundus at least every 8 hours.

49 In which one of the following positions would it be *most* appropriate to place the client when assessing the perineum?
   ○ 1. Prone
   ○ 2. Supine
   ○ 3. Sims
   ● 4. Lithotomy

50 Which one of the following findings would be *most* indicative of the presence of a perineal hematoma?
   ○ 1. The client complains of a feeling of fullness in the vagina.
   ○ 2. The presence of heavy and foul-smelling lochia rubra.
   ○ 3. Separation and purulent drainage from the episiotomy.
   ● 4. The client complains of severe pain in the perineal area.

The patient care technician is assisting the client with perineal hygiene.

51 Which one of the following observations by the nurse would indicate that the patient care technician needs additional teaching regarding perineal hygiene?
   ● 1. Peri pad is applied from back to front.
   ○ 2. Gloves are worn while providing perineal care.
   ○ 3. Peri bottle is filled with warm tap water.
   ○ 4. Washes hands before and after giving perineal care.

The client tells the nurse that she has gone to the bathroom several times to void but has been unsuccessful. She states that she feels the urge to void but nothing will come out.

52 Which one of the following actions would be *most* appropriate to implement *initially*?
   ○ 1. Catheterize the client with a straight catheter.
   ○ 2. Catheterize the client with an indwelling catheter.
   ○ 3. Have the client drink more fluids .
   ● 4. Assist the client with a warm sitz bath.

When reviewing the client's medical records, the nurse notes that the client's rubella titer is low (less than 1:10) and that the client is to receive the rubella vaccine prior to discharge.

53 Before giving the vaccine, the nurse should determine if the client is allergic to
   ○ 1. neomycin sulfate (Mycifradin).
   ● 2. erythromycin estolate (Ilosone).
   ○ 3. tetracycline (Panmycin).
   ○ 4. doxycycline (Vibramycin).

One day after delivery, the client's condition is stable. The physician visits and leaves discharge orders. The nurse reviews home care instructions with the client in anticipation of her discharge.

54 Which of the following statements by the client indicates a need for additional teaching about ways to avoid constipation after being sent home? The client states that she will
   ○ 1. drink at least 2 to 3 quarts of fluid daily.
   ● 2. take a stool softener every other day.
   ○ 3. include raw fruits and vegetables in her diet.
   ○ 4. continue to ambulate on a regular basis.

55 The nurse would be *correct* to instruct the client to notify her health care provider if
- 1. she experiences any difficulty urinating.
- ○ 2. her lochia becomes creamy yellow after the first postpartum week.
- ○ 3. she experiences unexplainable feelings of tearfulness and sadness.
- ○ 4. her breasts become slightly firm after 48 hours.

The client tells the nurse that she is breast-feeding and plans to continue when she is discharged home. She asks the nurse what she should do if her breasts become engorged after she gets home.

56 The nurse can respond *best* by instructing the client to
- ○ 1. pump her breast between breast-feedings of the infant.
- ○ 2. limit her fluid intake for 24 hours.
- ● 3. feed the infant every 2 to 3 hours.
- ○ 4. wear a support bra and apply ice packs to the breast.

The client asks the nurse how long she should wait before having sexual intercourse?

57 The nurse can respond *best* by explaining that sexual intercourse
- ● 1. may be resumed as soon as the lochia has ceased and the perineum is healed.
- ○ 2. may be resumed as soon as an acceptable birth control method has been selected.
- ○ 3. may be resumed after the postpartum checkup in 4 to 6 weeks.
- ○ 4. may be resumed after the uterus has returned to its normal position.

The client tells the nurse that she is nervous about going home with a new baby.

58 Which one of the following actions by the nurse would be *most* appropriate?
- ○ 1. Suggest that the client ask the physician to postpone her discharge.
- ○ 2. Tell the client that this is a normal feeling that will go away in time.
- ● 3. Make sure the client has written instructions on infant care before being discharged.
- ○ 4. Give the client the facility's telephone number and encourage her to call as needed.

NURSING CARE OF CLIENTS HAVING A CESAREAN DELIVERY

A 26-year-old gravida I client is admitted to the hospital in active labor. The physician examines the client and determines that she has cephalopelvic disproportion. A cesarean delivery is scheduled to be performed using epidural anesthesia. The physician orders an indwelling catheter to be inserted before surgery. The client asks the nurse why it is necessary for her to have an indwelling catheter?

59 The nurse can respond *best* by explaining that an indwelling or retention catheter is usually inserted to
- ○ 1. prevent the development of postpartum hemorrhaging.
- ● 2. keep the bladder empty during the surgical procedure.
- ○ 3. prevent the development of a urinary tract infection.
- ○ 4. provide a safe way of collecting urine specimens.

The client asks the nurse if she will feel any pain while the surgery is being performed?

60 The nurse can respond *best* by telling the client that
- ● 1. she may experience pressure but will not feel any pain during the procedure.
- ○ 2. she may experience a brief sting when the first incision is made.
- ○ 3. she will not remember anything about the procedure because she will be asleep.
- ○ 4. she will not feel anything once the anesthesia takes effect.

The client's husband asks the nurse if he can remain with his wife during the procedure.

61 The nurse would be *correct* to tell the client's husband that
- ○ 1. only the client and surgical personnel are allowed in the operating room because of the need to maintain a sterile environment.
- ○ 2. he will be allowed to join his wife in the operating room after the baby has been delivered and his wife and baby are stable.
- ● 3. he will be allowed to join his wife in the operating room once he changes into the appropriate attire and the procedure is about to begin.
- ○ 4. he will be allowed to join his wife when she is transferred to the recovery area and she no longer is under the influence of the anesthesia.

The client is transferred to the operating room. The physician plans to perform a lower segment transverse incision and requests that a surgical skin prep be performed.

62 The nurse would be *correct* to cleanse the entire abdomen beginning
  ○ 1. at the level of the nipple line.
  ○ 2. at the top of the uterine fundus.
  ○ 3. at the level of the umbilicus.
  ● 4. Six inches above the mons pubis.

The cesarean is performed as planned and is without complications during the procedure. One and one-half hours after surgery the client is transferred in stable condition to the postpartum unit from the postanesthesia care unit. The abdominal dressing is dry and intact, the Foley catheter is patent and draining clear yellow urine, and intravenous fluids are infusing at the prescribed rate without signs of infiltration at the insertion site. The client also has a continuous infusion of epidural morphine sulfate in progress.

63 The nurse would be *correct* to monitor the client closely for which one of the following adverse reactions while the client is receiving epidural morphine sulfate?
  ○ 1. Urinary incontinence
  ○ 2. Pupil dilation
  ● 3. Respiratory depression
  ○ 4. Elevated blood pressure

64 Which one of the following medications should the nurse plan to have readily available while the client is receiving epidural morphine sulfate?
  ○ 1. Buprenorphine hydrochloride (Buprenex)
  ○ 2. Calcium gluconate
  ○ 3. Atropine sulfate
  ● 4. Naloxone hydrochloride (Narcan)

Twenty-four hours after surgery, the physician leaves orders for the morphine epidural, intravenous therapy, and Foley catheter to be discontinued. An order is written for Demerol 50 mg p.o. every 3 to 4 hours p.r.n. pain. The physician also removes the abdominal dressing and tells the client that she may shower and can be out of bed.

65 Which one of the following findings is most indicative of the presence of infection of the abdominal incision line?
  ○ 1. The client states that the incision line feels numb.
  ○ 2. The client's oral temperature is 99°F.
  ○ 3. The incision line is approximated.
  ● 4. The incision line is red and swollen.

The client complains of abdominal pain and the nurse notes that the client's abdomen is distended.

66 Which one of the following interventions would be *most* appropriate for relieving the client's discomfort?
  ● 1. Assist the client to ambulate in the hall.
  ○ 2. Instruct the client to lie on her abdomen periodically.
  ○ 3. Administer the prescribed pain medication.
  ○ 4. Instruct the client to use a straw when drinking fluids.

The client tells the nurse that she is disappointed that she had to deliver by cesarean. She asks the nurse, "If I have another baby, will I have to have another cesarean?"

67 The nurse can respond *best* by explaining that vaginal delivery
  ○ 1. after cesarean delivery may be possible if the previous cesarean incision was a classical incision.
  ○ 2. is contraindicated after cesarean delivery because of the danger of uterine rupture.
  ○ 3. is just as painful as a cesarean delivery because an episiotomy has to be performed.
  ● 4. after cesarean delivery may be possible if there is no history of medical conditions that prohibit VBAC.

NURSING CARE OF CLIENTS HAVING AN EMERGENCY DELIVERY

A 25-year-old primigravida client is in the active phase of the first stage of delivery when her membranes rupture. The nurse notes a decrease in the fetal heart tones on the electronic monitor and immediately checks the client's perineum. Upon inspection of the perineum, the nurse observes that the umbilical cord is protruding through the vagina.

68 Which one of the following actions would be *most* appropriate for the nurse to take *initially?*
  ○ 1. Turn the client on her left side and administer oxygen.
  ○ 2. Notify the physician or nurse in charge of the findings.
  ● 3. Place the client in the Trendelenburg position.
  ○ 4. Prepare a sterile field for delivery of the baby.

A 32-year-old client with a history of precipitous labor is admitted to the labor and delivery department. She states that her contractions are occurring every 2 to 3 minutes. When the nurse observes the client's perineum, she notes that the baby's head is crowning. The nurse is alone with the client and unable to obtain assistance.

69 At this point it would be *most* appropriate for the nurse to put on gloves, and then
- ○ 1. gently place one hand on the crowning head and allow the head to emerge slowly between contractions.
- ○ 2. push back firmly on the head and place pressure on the vaginal meatus until the physician arrives.
- ○ 3. place a sterile towel over the perineal area and have the client bring her legs close together.
- ● 4. slide a finger into the vagina and enlarge its exit while delivering the head during a contraction.

NURSING CARE OF CLIENTS HAVING A STILLBORN OR A NEWBORN WITH COMPLICATIONS

A 25-year-old, 40-week gestation primigravida is admitted to the labor and delivery department with a possible fetal demise. The client states that she has not felt the fetus move all day long. The nurse is unable to detect a fetal heartbeat using the external fetal monitor. The physician visits, examines the client, and determines that the fetus is dead. An infusion of oxytocin (Pitocin) is ordered for induction of labor. The client is crying and tells the nurse, "This can't be true. You must have made a mistake."

70 The nurse can respond *best* by
- ○ 1. rechecking the fetal heart tones with the electronic external fetal monitor so that the client can listen.
- ● 2. expressing sorrow about the client's loss and encouraging the client to express her feelings.
- ○ 3. redirecting the client's attention to the laboring process and correct use of breathing techniques.
- ○ 4. explaining that the baby probably would have been born with severe long-term health problems.

The baby is delivered stillborn. The client's condition is stabilized and she is transferred to a private room on a wing adjacent to the labor, delivery, recovery, postpartum (LDRP) unit. The client's husband is present. The client asks the nurse if she can see her baby.

71 Which one of the following actions would be *most* appropriate for the nurse to take at this point?
- ○ 1. Prepare a memory packet, including items such as a picture of the baby and footprints, and give it to the client.
- ● 2. Bring the infant to the client and her husband and allow them to visit with the baby privately.
- ○ 3. Encourage the client to postpone viewing the baby until she and her husband have had an opportunity to receive counseling.
- ○ 4. Bring the infant to the client and her husband but do not allow the parents to hold or touch the infant.

A 38-year-old multipara client gave birth 1 day ago to a full-term infant with myelomeningocele.

72 Which one of the following *best* indicates that the client is experiencing anticipatory grieving?
- ○ 1. The client states that she has not selected a name for the baby.
- ● 2. The client visits the nursery frequently and stays for long periods.
- ○ 3. The client asks her doctor to postpone her discharge from the hospital.
- ○ 4. The client leaves the nursery when the infant is receiving treatments.

73 Which one of the following actions by the nurse will *best* facilitate the client's acceptance and care of the infant?
- ○ 1. Show the client before and after pictures of other infants born with myelomeningocele.
- ● 2. Serve as a role model for the client by feeding, holding, and changing the infant in the client's presence.
- ○ 3. Explain to the client that surgery will most probably eliminate the defect and its consequences.
- ○ 4. Assure the client that social agencies will most likely assume full care of the newborn.

NURSING CARE OF FAMILIES CONSIDERING FAMILY PLANNING

The nurse is assigned to discuss family planning and various methods of contraception with a group of women who have expressed an interest in this topic. One of the participants asks the nurse, "How do oral contraceptives prevent pregnancy?"

74 The nurse would be *correct* to explain that the combination oral contraceptive prevents pregnancy by interfering with the sperm reaching the ovum, and by
- ● 1. preventing ovulation.
- ○ 2. depressing progesterone secretion.
- ○ 3. depressing corpus luteum formation.
- ○ 4. thickening the uterine lining.

Another participant asks the nurse to explain the difference between oral contraceptive packages that have 21 pills and those that have 28 pills.

75 The nurse would be *correct* to explain that packages that contain 28 pills
○ 1. are biphasic and release a constant amount of estrogen and an increasing amount of progesterone throughout the cycle.
◉ 2. have 7 placebo pills and allow a woman to maintain a routine of taking a pill a day without missing a dose.
○ 3. have 21 pills that contain estrogen and 7 pills that contain progesterone and are called combination oral contraceptives.
○ 4. are prescribed for women who have a 28-day menstrual cycle instead of a 21-day menstrual cycle.

76 Which one of the following statements by a participant indicates a need for additional teaching regarding safe and effective use of oral contraceptives?
○ 1. An alternate form of contraceptive should be used if more than one dose of the oral contraceptive has been missed.
○ 2. Oral contraceptives should not be taken by women who have a history of primary dysmenorrhea.
◉ 3. Oral contraceptives should be discontinued 3 to 4 months before a planned pregnancy.
○ 4. Oral contraceptives may cause breakthrough bleeding when used concurrently with some antibiotics and antihistamines.

A participant asks the nurse how long is the Norplant form of contraception effective?

77 The nurse would be *correct* to inform the client that the Norplant contraceptive device
○ 1. must be discarded after each use.
○ 2. must be replaced every 3 to 6 months.
◉ 3. is effective for up to 5 years.
○ 4. is effective as long as it remains in place.

The nurse describes to the participants the various barrier methods of contraception.

78 Which one of the following statements by the participants indicates a need for additional teaching about the barrier methods of contraception?
○ 1. A diaphragm may have to be refitted or replaced if there is a weight gain or loss of 10 lb or more.
◉ 2. Use of the intrauterine device is not recommended for clients who have never been pregnant.

○ 3. Toxic shock syndrome is a potential side effect associated with the use of the cervical cap.
○ 4. Use of the female condom is not recommended for women who are allergic to latex.

One of the participants states that she is considering using the basal body temperature method of natural family planning and asks the nurse the correct way to use this method.

79 The nurse would be correct to explain that to this method requires the woman to
○ 1. record the pattern of her menstrual cycle for 6 to 8 months before actually using the method.
○ 2. regularly monitor the consistency of vaginal secretions along with the body temperature.
◉ 3. take her temperature every morning before arising for 6 months before using the method.
○ 4. have her sex partner withdraw his penis from the vagina just before ejaculation occurs.

NURSING CARE OF THE NEWBORN CLIENT

A full-term newborn baby girl is transferred to the well baby nursery in stable condition after an uneventful vaginal delivery. The infant is accompanied to the nursery by her father. The nurse tells the father that the infant will receive an injection of vitamin K (Aquamephyton) and erythromycin (Ilotycine) eye ointment. The father asks the nurse why the infant has to receive these medications.

80 The nurse would be *correct* to explain that vitamin K (Aquamephyton) is given to help
○ 1. stimulate respiration.
○ 2. start peristaltic movements.
◉ 3. decrease risk for hemorrhage.
○ 4. increase calcium absorption.

81 When preparing to give vitamin K (Aquamephyton), the nurse would be *correct* to choose which one of the following sites for injection of the medication?
○ 1. The ventrogluteal muscle.
○ 2. The deltoid muscle.
◉ 3. The vastus lateralis muscle.
○ 4. The gluteus maximus muscle.

82 The nurse would be *correct* to explain that erythromycin (Ilotycine) is given to protect the infant from neonatal blindness, which can occur if the infant develops an eye infection cause by the gonococcal or
◉ 1. chlamydia organisms.
○ 2. streptococcal organisms.
○ 3. *Candida albicans* organisms.
○ 4. *Pneumocystis carinii* organisms.

83 The nurse would be *correct* to explain that the new-born may experience which one of the following after instillation of the eye ointment?
○ 1. Swelling of the eyes
○ 2. Temporary blurred vision
● 3. A purulent eye drainage
○ 4. A conjunctival hemorrhage

The patient care technician is assigned to weigh the infant.

84 Which one of the following actions by the patient care technician indicates a need for additional teaching regarding accurate and safe assessment of the new-born's weight?
○ 1. The infant is undressed before the weight is obtained.
○ 2. A diaper or paper barrier is placed on the scale before it is balanced.
● 3. One hand remains on the infant while the weight is being obtained.
○ 4. The scale is cleansed with an antiseptic before it is used.

Two hours have elapsed since the infant was admitted to the nursery. The infant's temperature has stabilized and the nurse is giving the infant a bath.

85 If the nurse observes all of the following during the bath, which one of the findings should be reported *immediately* to the nurse in charge or the physician?
○ 1. The hands and feet are bluish in color.
○ 2. The pulse rate is 140 beats per minute.
● 3. The skin has a yellowish discoloration.
○ 4. The labia appear to be slightly swollen.

After the bath is completed, the nurse rechecks the infant's temperature and finds that it is 97°F axillary.

86 Which one of the following nursing interventions would be *most* appropriate?
○ 1. Dress the infant, wrap in a blanket, place in an open crib, and recheck the temperature every 4 to 8 hours.
● 2. Place the infant on a preheated radiant warmer and gradually rewarm the infant over a period of 2 or more hours.
○ 3. Dress the infant, wrap in double blankets, place in an open crib, and recheck the temperature in 30 to 60 minutes.
○ 4. Place the infant on a preheated radiant warmer and rewarm the infant over a period of 15 to 30 minutes.

Fours hours after admission to the nursery, the infant's condition is stable and there are no signs of distress. The infant is taken to the mother for a visit and the first

feeding. The father is also present. Before leaving the infant with the parents, the nurse gives the mother the infant's bulb syringe and instructs the mother on proper use of the bulb syringe.

87 Which one of the following statements, by the mother, indicates a need for additional teaching regarding proper use of the bulb syringe?
○ 1. The mother states that the infant's mouth should be suctioned before the nose is suctioned.
○ 2. The mother states that the bulb syringe should be compressed before it is placed in the infant's mouth or nose.
○ 3. The mother states that when suctioning the mouth, the bulb syringe should not touch the back of the throat.
● 4. The mother states that the bulb syringe should remain compressed until it is removed from the nose or mouth.

The infant's mother tells the nurse that she would like to breast-feed the infant but wants to give the infant formula until her milk comes in. She tells the nurse that she has one other child. She also tells the nurse that she started out breast-feeding her first child but changed over to bottle feeding because the baby experienced a 5% weight loss before being discharged from the hospital.

88 The nurse can respond *best* by explaining that
● 1. it is normal for both bottle-fed and breast-fed infants to lose up to 10% of their birth weight during the first few days after birth.
○ 2. if she begins bottle-feeding the infant, she will not be successful with breast-feeding because the infant will prefer the bottle nipple.
○ 3. the infant is more prone to lose weight with bottle-feeding than breast-feeding because formula is more difficult to digest.
○ 4. she should pump her breast until she is ready to begin breast-feeding in order to facilitate the milk letdown reflex.

89 The nurse also would be *correct* to explain that, during the first few days after the birth of her baby, her breast will secrete colostrum, which is beneficial to the baby because it contains
○ 1. estrogen, which will prevent the infant from developing breakthrough bleeding.
● 2. antibodies, which provide protection against certain types of infections.
○ 3. predigested fats, which increase the infant's ability to absorb fat-soluble vitamins.
○ 4. digestive enzymes, which increases the newborn's ability to absorb nutrients.

The infant's mother tells the nurse that she was not aware of all of these things and states that she would like to begin breast-feeding the infant right away. The nurse gives the mother verbal instructions on how to breast-feed the infant correctly, and remains present to assist the mother with starting the breast-feeding.

90 Which one of the following actions by the infant's mother indicates a need for additional teaching regarding proper breast-feeding technique?
- ○ 1. The mother uses the thumb of her free hand to gently press the breast away from the infant's nose.
- ○ 2. The mother gently strokes the infant's lips with her nipple when she is ready to breast-feed.
- ○ 3. The mother places a breast shield over her nipple before placing the nipple in the infant's mouth.
- ● 4. The mother gently pulls down on the infant's chin before removing the nipple from the infant's mouth.

The infant's father asks the nurse how he should position the infant when placing it in the crib after his wife finishes breast-feeding.

91 The nurse would be *correct* to explain that the *most* appropriate position in which to place the infant after the feeding would be the
- ● 1. right side-lying position.
- ○ 2. left side-lying position.
- ○ 3. prone position.
- ○ 4. supine position

The pediatrician visits when the infant is 1 day old and discharges the infant. The mother also has been discharged by her physician. Prior to discharge, the mother asks the nurse, "How will I know that my baby is getting enough to eat?"

92 The nurse can respond *best* by explaining that the infant whose nutritional needs are *not* being adequately met
- ○ 1. will awaken during the night for a feeding.
- ● 2. will have fewer than 6 wet diapers per day.
- ○ 3. will have loose, pale-yellow stools.
- ○ 4. will breast-feed every 2 to 3 hours.

The infant's mother tells the nurse that she plans to continue to breast-feed after she returns to work. She also states that she plans to pump her breast when she cannot breast-feed and asks the nurse how long she can store the breast milk that she pumps.

93 The nurse would be *correct* to explain that breast milk can be stored at room temperature for up to 40 minutes and can be stored in the refrigerator for up to

- ○ 1. 48 hours.
- ● 2. 1 week.
- ○ 3. 3 months.
- ○ 4. 1 year.

A full-term newborn baby boy is admitted to the nursery, in no apparent distress, after an uneventful planned cesarean delivery that was performed because the mother had a previous cesarean section.

94 Which one of the following assessment findings would the nurse consider *abnormal* for the full-term newborn?
- ○ 1. A scrotal sac that has numerous rugae
- ● 2. An umbilical cord that has one vein and one artery
- ○ 3. Vernix caseosa in the creases of the groin area
- ○ 4. Bluish discoloration of the hands and feet

95 Which one of the following assessment findings would the nurse consider *abnormal* when performing the gestational age assessment?
- ● 1. Lanugo over the shoulders, back, and forehead
- ○ 2. A strong Moro reflex
- ○ 3. Anterior transverse crease on the soles of the feet
- ○ 4. Fully flexed posture

Six hours after admission to the nursery, the infant is taken to the mother for the first feeding. The mother states that she has decided to bottle-feed the infant. The nurse reviews basic principles of bottle-feeding with the mother before the infant is fed.

96 Which one of the following observations by the nurse indicates that the client has a *incorrect* understanding of basic principles of bottle-feeding?
- ○ 1. The mother places the nipple of the bottle on top of the infant's tongue.
- ● 2. The mother places the infant in the supine position when feeding the infant.
- ○ 3. The mother burps the infant after each ounce of formula that is taken.
- ○ 4. The mother places the infant in the right side-lying position after the feeding.

The infant's mother ask the nurse why it is important to keep the bottle nipple full of formula?

97 The nurse would be *correct* to explain that the bottle should be held so that the nipple is always full of formula because this will prevent the baby from
- ○ 1. getting too much formula at once.
- ○ 2. getting tired while feeding.
- ○ 3. regurgitating the formula.
- ● 4. swallowing air when sucking.

The infant's mother tells the nurse that she plans to use concentrated liquid formula at home. The nurse reviews general principles of formula preparation with the infant's mother.

98 Which one of the following statements by the infant's mother indicates a need for additional teaching?
   ○ 1. The mother states that the formula bottles can be washed in a dishwasher.
   ● 2. The mother states that warm tap water can be used to dilute the concentrate.
   ○ 3. The mother states that the formula should be used immediately after it is prepared.
   ○ 4. The mother states that the lid of the formula can must be wiped before opening it.

When the infant is 3 days old the nurse observes that the skin is slightly yellow in appearance.

99 A routine assessment checklist is used for documentation in the nursery. If all of the following terms appear on the checklist, which one should the nurse check to *correctly* document the infant's skin appearance?
   ○ 1. Mottle
   ● 2. Jaundice
   ○ 3. Acrocyanosis
   ○ 4. Erythematous

The infant's total bilirubin level is 11 mg/dL. The physician orders phototherapy treatment.

100 When providing care to the infant who is receiving phototherapy treatment, the nurse would be *correct* to
   ● 1. remove all clothing when the infant is receiving the treatment.
   ○ 2. feed the infant by the nasogastric route.
   ○ 3. maintain the infant in the supine position.
   ○ 4. monitor the intravenous infusion site at least every 2 hours.

After 2 days of therapy, the infant's total bilirubin level decreases to 9 mg/dL. Phototherapy treatment is discontinued as ordered by the physician. A circumcision using the plastibell technique is performed by the physician.

101 Following the circumcision, the nurse should
   ○ 1. maintain a Vaseline gauze dressing over the glans penis.
   ○ 2. monitor the vital signs every 15 minutes for the first hour.
   ● 3. frequently monitor the penis for bleeding and swelling.
   ○ 4. apply alcohol to any area that appears to be infected.

The physician leaves orders for the infant to be discharged home with the parents if no complications occur within 4 hours of the circumcision. The nurse visits with the parents and goes over home care of the circumcision.

102 Which one of the following statements by the parents indicates that teaching has been effective?
   ○ 1. The parents state that the physician should be notified of any drainage from the penis.
   ● 2. The parents state that the penis should be cleansed 3 times a day with alcohol.
   ○ 3. The parents state that the plastibell should be removed if it has not fallen off in 1 week.
   ○ 4. The parents state that Vaseline should be applied to the penis after each diaper change.

Prior to discharge, the nurse prepares to perform the phenylketonuria (PKU) test.

103 Which one of the following is *most* important for the nurse to determine prior to performing the PKU test?
   ● 1. Whether or not the infant has been drinking formula for at least 2 to 3 days.
   ○ 2. Whether or not the infant was large for gestational age at birth.
   ○ 3. Whether or not the mother had gestational diabetes during her pregnancy.
   ○ 4. Whether or not there is a family history of mental retardation.

104 When obtaining the blood specimen for the PKU, the nurse should perform all of the following actions *except*
   ○ 1. Warm the heel for 5 to 10 minutes prior to obtaining the specimen.
   ● 2. Puncture the lateral aspect of the heel.
   ○ 3. Discard the first drop of blood obtained.
   ○ 4. Apply pressure with an alcohol wipe after the specimen is obtained.

INDIVIDUAL TEST ITEMS

105 The physician leaves orders for a client who is in preterm labor to receive terbutaline sulfate. The nurse should withhold the medication and notify the nurse in charge or the physician if
   ○ 1. the electronic monitor reveals that the client is having mild contractions.
   ● 2. the cervix is dilated 4 cm or more and/or effaced 50% or more.
   ○ 3. the electronic monitor reveals the presence of fetal heart rate variability.
   ○ 4. the client states that the contractions are milder and occurring less frequently.

106 When administering rho(d) immune globulin (Rho-GAM) to an Rh negative mother who has delivered an Rh positive infant, the nurse would be *correct* to give the medication
- ○ 1. no sooner than 48 hours after delivery.
- ○ 2. no later than 72 hours after delivery.
- ○ 3. at the 6-week postpartum checkup.
- ● 4. no later than 24 hours after delivery.

107 Which one of the following observations would the nurse consider *most* indicative of cystitis in the postpartum client?
- ○ 1. Boggy uterus displaced to right of the abdominal midline
- ○ 2. Complaint of increased thirst and voiding large amounts of urine
- ○ 3. Urinary retention and swelling of the lower extremities
- ● 4. Complaint of painful urination and presence of blood in the urine

108 Which one of the following instructions should the nurse plan to include in the discharge teaching plan for the client who at risk for developing mastitis?
- ○ 1. Wear a breast binder between breast-feedings.
- ○ 2. Apply petroleum jelly to the nipples before breast-feeding.
- ● 3. Clean nipples with soap and water after breast-feeding.
- ○ 4. Wash both hands before handling the breast.

109 Which one of the following findings would the nurse consider most indicative of congenital hip dislocation in the newborn?
- ● 1. Asymmetry of the gluteal skin folds
- ○ 2. Limited adduction of the affected hip
- ○ 3. No spontaneous movement of the affected leg
- ○ 4. Exaggerated curvature of the lumbar spine

110 Which one of the following findings would the nurse consider *abnormal* for the postpartum client who delivered within the past 24 hours?
- ○ 1. The client states that she passed a couple of nickel-sized clots.
- ● 2. The client complains of calf pain when the foot is dorsiflexed.
- ○ 3. The client complains of abdominal cramping while breast-feeding.
- ○ 4. The client states that her vaginal discharge is dark red in color.

111 A client is readmitted to the hospital on her fifth postpartum day with a tentative diagnosis of puerperal infection. Which one of the following manifestation would the nurse consider *most* indicative of the presence of a puerperal infection?
- ○ 1. Slower than normal pulse rate
- ● 2. Complaint of abdominal tenderness
- ○ 3. A decrease in the size of the uterus
- ○ 4. Presence of lochia serosa

Directions: Two numbers appear in parentheses following each rationale. The first number identifies the textbook listed in the references, page 512, and the second number identifies the page(s) in that textbook on which the correct answer can be verified. Occasionally two textbooks are given for verifying the correct answer.

ADMISSION OF THE CLIENT TO A LABOR AND DELIVERY FACILITY

1 3. A sudden gush of fluid from the vagina may indicate that the bag of water has ruptured, in which case the client should report to the hospital or designated health care facility because, once the membranes are ruptured, there is an increased risk for intrauterine infection and also for prolapse of the umbilical cord if the fetus head has not engaged. A sudden burst of energy, also referred to as the nesting instinct, is a preliminary sign of approaching labor that may occur a few days prior to the beginning of labor and does not require that the client report to the health care facility. Urinary frequency may occur as the fetus settles into the pelvic brim. The client may experience urinary frequency as early as 2 to 3 weeks prior to the beginning of labor for the primigravida. The client generally is told to report to the hospital or health care facility when contractions are 5 minutes apart. (14:178)
Nursing Process—Implementation
Client Need—Health promotion/maintenance

2 2. Pertinent questions to ask a woman having uterine contractions when she is being admitted to the hospital include questions related to whether membranes have ruptured, when contractions started, and when the client last ate. The anesthesiologist is especially interested in knowing when the client last ate. Least pertinent of the questions given in this item deals with the administration of an enema. Not all clients have enemas. The appropriate time to ask a client if she has ever had an enema is shortly before administration of the enema. (14:179; 16:160)
Nursing Process—Data collection
Client Need—Health promotion/maintenance

NURSING CARE OF CLIENTS DURING THE FIRST STAGE OF LABOR

3 4. To obtain the most accurate blood pressure reading, the blood pressure should be assessed between contractions with the client in the left side-lying position. This method of assessing the blood pressure minimizes the possibility of obtaining an inaccurate blood pressure reading because of a decrease in circulating blood volume that may occur with contractions and if the inferior vena cava is compressed by the enlarged uterus. (14:153)
Nursing Process—Data collection
Client Need—Health promotion/maintenance

4 2. The normal fetal heart rate ranges from 120 to 160 beats per minute. During the latent phase of the first stage of labor, the contractions occur every 5 to 30 minutes. The perineum does not begin to bulge until the transition phase of the first stage of labor, and early decelerations usually occur late in labor and are a response to head compression. (22:201)
Nursing Process—Data collection
Client Need—Health promotion/maintenance

5 2. During the latent phase of the first stage of labor, the client is encouraged to drink clear liquids in order to prevent the occurrence of dehydration. If the client's membranes are intact and her contractions are not very frequent or intense, she may be allowed to ambulate and take a warm shower or Jacuzzi bath. The client does not use a panting breathing pattern until the transition phase of the first stage of labor. (14:184; 16:161)
Nursing Process—Implementation
Client Need—Health promotion/maintenance

6 3. The fetal heart rate should be assessed every 30 minutes during the latent phase of the first stage of labor, every 15 minutes during the active phase of the first stage of labor, and every 5 minutes during the second stage of labor. (14:179)
Nursing Process—Planning
Client Need—Health promotion/maintenance

7 2. Epidural anesthesia can be administered at any time but is usually administered to the primigravida cli-

ent when she is 5 to 6 cm dilated, and to the multigravida client when she is 3 to 4 cm dilated. (14:172)
Nursing Process—Implementation
Client Need—Safe, effective care environment

8 3. Contractions usually occur every 3 to 5 minutes and last between 45 and 60 seconds during the active phase of the first stage of labor. Contractions last up to 30 seconds during the latent phase of the first stage of labor, and up to 90 seconds during the transition phase of the first stage of labor and during the second stage of labor. (14:184)
Nursing Process—Data collection
Client Need—Health promotion/maintenance

9 1. When there is a question concerning whether or not the membranes have ruptured, a nitrazine test may be performed. Amniotic fluid turns the nitrazine test strip blue because amniotic fluid is alkaline. The nitrazine test will remain yellow when exposed to vaginal secretions and urine because they are usually acidic. (14:153; 16:161)
Nursing Process—Evaluation
Client Need—Health promotion/maintenance

10 1. Internal electronic fetal monitoring requires the application of a scalp electrode to the fetal scalp. Infection and soft tissue injury can occur with the use of internal electronic fetal monitoring, but both are rare. A soft, water-filled catheter is inserted into the uterus for internal electronic monitoring of uterine contractions. A transducer is applied to the mother's abdomen when external electronic monitoring is being utilized. A suction cap is applied to the fetal scalp when a vacuum extraction is being performed to assist with delivery of the fetal head. (16:168)
Nursing Process—Implementation
Client Need—Safe, effective care environment

11 3. During the transition phase of the first stage of labor, the client usually will have an increase in bloody show and the contractions will last up to 90 seconds. Crowning of the presenting part does not occur until the cervix is completely dilated, which occurs during the second stage of labor. (14:185)
Nursing Process—Data collection
Client Need—Health promotion/maintenance

12 2. During the transition phase of the first stage of labor, the client is at risk for losing control because of the intense discomfort, fatigue, frequency, and length of contraction. Praising the client on a frequent basis will help her maintain control of the situation. During the transition phase of labor the membranes usually rupture, if they are not already

ruptured, and the client may be receiving a narcotic analgesic or regional anesthetic; therefore it is not usually recommended that the client be ambulatory. The client should not push until the cervix is completely dilated, which occurs during the second stage of labor. Application of sacral pressure can relieve back discomfort. Some women have a low tolerance to touch during this phase of labor, however; therefore each client should be assessed individually to determine her preference. (14:186; 16:179)
Nursing Process—Implementation
Client Need—Psychosocial integrity

13 1. When the fetus presents in the posterior instead of the anterior position, the client experiences back discomfort and there is a danger of maternal laceration if the fetus does not rotate before delivery. The client should be assisted to a position that increases her comfort. The knee-chest position is a position often recommended because it not only relieves the discomfort associated with the posterior presentation of the head, but it also facilitates rotation of the head. The Trendelenburg position will not assist with rotation of the head to the anterior position. During this phase it also is recommended that the client not be placed on her back to avoid vena cava compression by the uterus. The uterus is not usually displaced with a posterior presentation. Also, the posterior position usually prolongs labor. (14:195)
Nursing Process—Implementation
Client Need—Psychosocial integrity

14 4. The client should be encouraged to void every 2 hours in order to minimize the occurrence of bladder distention, which may prolong labor. The client should be encourage to drink clear liquids at frequent intervals to prevent dehydration. The intravenous infusion rate should not be decreased unless the physician orders the rate to be decreased. Maintaining the prescribed intravenous infusion rate also will prevent dehydration. No solid foods are given during labor because peristalsis is slowed during labor. (14:184; 16:180)
Nursing Process—Implementation
Client Need—Health promotion/maintenance

15 1. The duration of a contraction is defined as the time interval between the beginning of a contraction and the end of the same contraction. The time interval between the end of one contraction and the beginning of the next contraction is called the relaxation period. The time interval between the beginning of one contraction and the end of the next contraction is not significant when assessing the client's labor pattern. The time interval between the begin-

ning of one contraction and the beginning of the next contraction is defined as the frequency of the contractions. (14:157; 16:164)
Nursing Process—Data collection
Client Need—Health promotion/maintenance

16 1. The nurse should palpate the fundus of the uterus, which usually is located just above the umbilicus in the full-term client. The fundus is palpated because muscular contractions are strongest at this location; contractions therefore are easier to assess at this location. (18:773)
Nursing Process—Data collection
Client Need—Health promotion/maintenance

17 3. The fetal heart rate should be assessed every 30 minutes during the latent phase of the first stage of labor, every 15 minutes during the active phase of the first stage of labor, and every 5 minutes during the second stage of labor. (14:179)
Nursing Process—Planning
Client Need—Health promotion/maintenance

18 4. The fetal heart tones should be checked immediately after the membranes rupture. A drop in the fetal heart rate may indicate prolapse of the umbilical cord. Prolapse of the umbilical may occur because of the sudden gush of fluid from the vagina, especially if the presenting part is not engaged. The client's pulse is not affected by the rupturing of the membranes. The registered nurse usually performs vaginal exams, and an indwelling catheter is not usually indicated when the membranes rupture. (14:184; 16:181)
Nursing Process—Implementation
Client Need—Physiological integrity

19 1. The client's temperature should be assessed every hour once the membranes rupture because of the increased risk for infection. The temperature is assessed every 4 hours if the membranes are intact. (14:184)
Nursing Process—Data collection
Client Need—Physiological integrity

20 3. The presence of green amniotic fluid indicates that the fetus has passed a meconium stool in utero. Passage of meconium in utero when the fetus is presenting in the vertex position is an indication of fetal distress and should be reported immediately. The normal range for the fetal heart rate is 120 to 140 beats per minute. It is normal for the fetal heart to accelerate. An increase in bloody show usually indicates that the second stage of labor is imminent. (16:161)
Nursing Process—Evaluation
Client Need—Physiological integrity

21 1. When a vaginal examination is performed, the examiner should be provided with a pair of sterile gloves in order to decrease the risk of the client developing an infection. The client should be assisted to the supine position and assisted to use breathing techniques (breathing slowly through an open mouth) to help her relax. An enema usually is not a part of the preparation of the client for a vaginal examination. (16:181)
Nursing Process—Planning
Client Need—Safe, effective care environment

22 4. Although regular contractions of increasing frequency and duration radiating from the lower back to the lower abdomen, as well as the presence of bloody show, also suggest that the client is in true labor, dilation and effacement of the cervix is the only definite indicator of true labor. (14:154)
Nursing Process—Data collection
Client Need—Health promotion/maintenance

23 4. Solid foods usually are not given when the client is in labor because they may cause nausea and vomiting. This may occur because peristalsis is slow during labor. Solid foods are not known to alter the absorption of regional anesthetics, alter the duration and frequency of contraction, or cause fetal distress. (14:184; 18:775)
Nursing Process—Implementation
Client Need—Health promotion/maintenance

24 1. When the fetus is presenting in the vertex position, the head is descending into the birth canal first. If the feet or buttocks enter the birth canal first, the presentation is defined as breech. Both breech and shoulder presentations are considered malpresentations and make delivery more difficult. (14:155)
Nursing Process—Implementation
Client Need—Health promotion/maintenance

25 4. A drop in the fetal heart rate after the contraction acme is defined as a late decelerations. Late decelerations are usually a sign of fetal distress and should be reported immediately. The other options describe processes that normally occur during the active phase of the first stage of labor. (14:182; 16:173)
Nursing Process—Data collection
Client Need—Physiological integrity

26 3. An episiotomy is an incision made into the perineum tissue that enlarges the vaginal opening. It is usually performed to prevent lacerations or damage of the perineum. An episiotomy also diminishes the possibility of prolonged pressure on the fetal head and speeds up the delivery process. (16:189)
Nursing Process—Implementation
Client Need—Psychosocial integrity

NURSING CARE OF CLIENTS DURING THE SECOND STAGE OF LABOR

27 1. The perineum usually begins to bulge and the presenting part begins to crown during the second stage of labor. The contractions usually last for 60 to 90 seconds and the cervix is completely dilated (10 cm). The level of the uterus is not an indicator of the stage of labor. (14:186)

   Nursing Process—Data collection
   Client Need—Health promotion/maintenance

28 1. Preparation for delivery for the multipara client should begin when the client is 6 to 7 cm dilated. Preparation for the primipara client can be delayed until the client is completely dilated (10 cm) because the time between complete dilation for the multipara client is shorter than it is for the primigravida client. The time of arrival of the physician or midwife varies and should not be used as an indicator of when to begin to prepare for delivery. (16:182)

   Nursing Process—Planning
   Client Need—Health promotion/maintenance

29 3. The client's cervix should be completely dilated before she begins to push in order to prevent edema of the cervix, which will prolong labor and possibly require delivery by cesarean section. (14:188)

   Nursing Process—Implementation
   Client Need—Physiological integrity

30 3. If a narcotic analgesic is given to late in labor it may cause respiratory depression. The medication can cross the placental barrier and may continue to be present after the infant is delivered, thus resulting in respiratory depression. Giving a narcotic analgesic too early in labor may interfere with the progression of labor. Administration of a narcotic analgesic is not associated with uterine rupture or increased fetal activity. (14:160; 16:205)

   Nursing Process—Implementation
   Client Need—Psychosocial integrity

31 1. A saddle block, also called a subarachnoid block, usually takes effect immediately and reaches its maximum potency within 3 to 5 minutes of administration. (16:208)

   Nursing Process—Implementation
   Client Need—Safe, effective care environment

32 1. During the immediate postprocedural period the client's blood pressure should be assessed and evaluated for the presence of hypotension; a drop in blood pressure occasionally occurs secondary to sympathetic blockade and may decrease the oxygen supply to the infant, which would be mani-

fested by fetal bradycardia. Paralysis of the lower extremities is an expected result of the saddle block (subarachnoid block). The client may experience a spinal headache within 24 to 72 hours after the procedure, but not immediately. Both maternal hypotension and spinal headache usually can be minimized by ensuring that the client is well hydrated (usually by method of intravenous infusion) before, during, and after the procedure. (14:171; 16:209)

   Nursing Process—Data collection
   Client Need—Safe, effective care environment

33 2. The client who has had saddle block (subarachnoid block) anesthesia has to be instructed when to push because she is unable to feel contractions occurring. Oxygen is not routinely required unless complications arise. The client is not usually catheterized following this type of anesthesia, and the anesthesia is usually given late in labor (second stage) or for cesarean delivery; thus it usually does not slow the progress of labor. (16:209)

   Nursing Process—Planning
   Client Need—Health promotion/maintenance

34 1. When cleansing the perineum in preparation for delivery, the nurse should use the technique that decreases the possibility of infection and increases visibility of the area. The usual procedure of cleaning the area is pubic bone to lower abdomen, both inner thighs, the right and left labia, and the vagina to the anus. The vagina should always be the last area cleaned. (16:187)

   Nursing Process—Implementation
   Client Need—Safe, effective care environment

NURSING CARE OF CLIENTS DURING THE THIRD STAGE OF LABOR

35 3. The priority need of the newborn immediately after delivery is establishment of a patent airway. This can best be accomplished by bulb suctioning the infant before complete delivery of the body. Oxygen should not be given before the airway is cleared and only given if needed. Application of the cord clamp and the identification bracelet do not take priority over establishment and maintenance of respirations. (16:191)

   Nursing Process—Implementation
   Client Need—Health promotion/maintenance

36 2. The infant should be dried first, to prevent heat loss secondary to evaporation, and then placed on the mother's abdomen in skin-to-skin contact and covered with a warmed blanket. The mother's abdomen is usually warm; thus there is not a danger of heat loss because of the contact with the mother's warm body. The other options either interfere with maintaining warmth of the infant or promoting mother-infant attachment. (16:192)

> Nursing process—Implementation
> Client Need—Health promotion/maintenance

37 4. An Apgar score of 7 to 10 is considered to be good and does not require any intervention. A score of between 4 and 6 indicates moderate distress, in which case the infant should be monitored closely and may require intervention. A score between 0 and 3 is considered to be poor and indicates a definite need for intervention. (16:192; 22:260)

> Nursing Process—Planning
> Client Need—Health promotion/maintenance

38 1. Matching identification bracelets should be applied to the infant and mother prior to the infant leaving the delivery area to prevent the risk of a mother receiving the wrong baby. Eye prophylaxis and administration of the vitamin K (Aquamephyton) are usually delayed to facilitate early bonding between the mother and the infant. The phenylketonuria (PKU) testing should be performed once the client has begun to take formula. (16:192)

> Nursing Process—Implementation
> Client Need—Health promotion/maintenance

39 3. A rise of the fundus in the abdomen, lengthening of the umbilical cord, and a sudden gush of blood from the vagina are all signs of impending delivery of the placenta. The perineum does not bulge with delivery of the placenta. (14:189)

> Nursing Process—Evaluation
> Client Need—Health promotion/maintenance

40 4. Once the placenta has separated from the wall of the uterus, it may be delivered by having the client to bear down, or it may be manually expressed by the attending health care provider. Breathing slowly and deeply, assuming the side-lying position, and tightening and relaxing the perineum will not facilitate delivery of the placenta. (16:193)

> Nursing Process—Implementation
> Client Need—Health promotion/maintenance

41 3. Oxytocin (Pitocin) decreases the risk for hemorrhage after delivery because the medication causes the uterus to continue to contract. The client's blood pressure should be monitored closely because hypertension is a side effect of this medication. Also, uterine rupture may occur with the administration of oxytocin if hyperstimulation of the uterus occurs secondary to a toxic dose of the medication. Administering oxytocin does not prevent the uterus from inverting; instead, supporting the uterus just above the symphysis pubis when palpating the uterus is

most commonly used to prevent the uterus from inverting. (14:189)

> Nursing Process—Implementation
> Client Need—Health promotion/maintenance

NURSING CARE OF CLIENTS DURING THE FOURTH STAGE OF LABOR

42 2. The client's needs can best be met by applying a warm blanket. In addition to applying the warm blanket, the nurse can explain that the shaking that she is experiencing is a normal response. It is believed that this response occurs because of the sudden physiological changes occurring as result of childbirth. Suggesting that the client try not to think about the shaking will not resolve the shaking because of the underlying cause; therefore this will not adequately address the client's complaint. It is not necessary to notify the physician since this is a normal physiological process. (14:212; 16:193)

> Nursing Process—Implementation
> Client Need—Health promotion/maintenance

43 1. Following delivery of the placenta, the fundus of the uterus should be firmly contracted and located at or just below the level of the umbilicus. (16:216; 22:291)

> Nursing Process—Data collection
> Client Need—Health promotion/maintenance

44 4. A systolic blood pressure of 100 mm Hg or less should be reported. The normal pulse rate is slightly lower during the fourth stage of labor than during previous stages of labor because of decreased cardiac strain. The pulse can range between 40 and 80 beats per minute and still be considered normal. During the fourth stage of labor the lochia is usually dark red with a fleshy but not foul odor, and the client may saturate one perineal pad within one hour. (16:216)

> Nursing Process—Evaluation
> Client Need—Physiological integrity

45 2. If the client has an episiotomy, ice is applied to the perineum to reduce the swelling and subsequently decrease the discomfort that may occur as a result of the swelling. Sitz baths, heat lamp treatments, and topical cortisone are usually ordered for use after the fourth stage of labor. (16:193; 22:293)

> Nursing Process—Implementation
> Client Need—Physiological integrity

46 4. A soft and boggy fundus can lead to uterine bleeding. Normally the fundus is firm, hard, and located at or just below the level of the umbilicus. The uterus should be massaged if there is an increase in the lochia flow. (22:262)

> Nursing Process—Evaluation
> Client Need—Physiological integrity

47 1. Placing one hand on the fundus of the uterus and the other hand just above the symphysis pubis prevents the uterus from becoming inverted. The hand placement in the other options will not prevent the uterus from inverting. (14:209)
Nursing Process—Implementation
Client Need—Health promotion/maintenance

NURSING CARE OF CLIENTS DURING THE POSTPARTUM PERIOD

48 4. A high fundus that is displaced from the midline is consistent with urinary retention. Therefore, the client should be encouraged to void and the fundus rechecked afterwards. The client may need to be catheterized if she is unable to void voluntarily. Repositioning the client and massaging the uterus will not resolve the urinary retention. (16:216)
Nursing Process—Implementation
Client Need—Health promotion/maintenance

49 3. When assessing the perineum of the client who delivered vaginally, the client should be assisted to the left side-lying position with the right leg flexed at the knee (Sims position). The upper buttock is lifted to expose the anus and perineum. This technique allows for the best visualization of the perineum area. The positions identified in the other options do not allow for maximal visualization of the perineum. (14:214; 16:225)
Nursing Process—Implementation
Client Need—Health promotion/maintenance

50 4. A client who develops a perineal hematoma usually complains of a great deal of pain in the perineal area, especially when there are sutures following an episiotomy. The condition should be reported promptly. A hematoma is not associated with a feeling of fullness in the vagina, the presence of heavy and foul-smelling lochia rubra, or separation and purulent drainage from the episiotomy. (16:217)
Nursing Process—Data collection
Client Need—Physiological integrity

51 1. The peri pad should always be applied and removed from front to back to avoid contamination of the perineum. The hands should be washed before and after assisting with peri care, gloves should be worn, and if a peri bottle is used it should be filled with warm water. (14:214; 16:227)
Nursing Process—Evaluation
Client Need—Safe, effective care environment

52 4. A warm sitz bath or warm shower may assist the ambulatory client to void. If these techniques are not successful, the client will have to be catheterized with a straight catheter. If the client has to be catheterized more than once, the health care provider may order an indwelling catheter be inserted. Having the client drink more fluid usually makes the situation worse instead of better because it increases the bladder distention. (16:218)
Nursing Process—Implementation
Client Need—Physiological integrity

53 1. The client should be asked if she is allergic to neomycin sulfate (Mycifradin) because the rubella vaccine contains neomycin. It would not be necessary to ask if the client is allergic to any of the medications listed in the other options because the rubella vaccine does not contain any of those medications. (16:229)
Nursing Process—Implementation
Client Need—Physiological integrity

54 2. Stool softeners are used only when the client has difficulty passing stools. Drinking at least 2 to 3 quarts of fluids daily, including raw fruits and vegetables in the diet, and ambulating are ways to *prevent* the occurrence of constipation. (16:229)
Nursing Process—Evaluation
Client Need—Health promotion/maintenance

55 1. Normal bladder function usually returns within a few days of delivery. The client should notify the health care provider of difficult or burning urination. The health care provider should be notified if the client is unable to void. These are considered danger signs and may indicate infection or some other complication. The other options identify normal findings during the postpartum period. (14:221)
Nursing Process—Implementation
Client Need—Health promotion/maintenance

56 3. The best method for alleviating breast engorgement is to breast-feed the infant frequently. Pumping the breast will usually increase the supply of milk and further aggravate the engorgement. Limiting the fluid intake may interfere with the production of an adequate amount of milk for feeding the infant. Wearing a support bra will also assist with controlling breast engorgement; warmth instead of cold should be applied to the breast, however. The application of cold will suppress lactation and thus may interfere with the production of an adequate supply of milk for feeding the infant. (16:223)
Nursing Process—Implementation
Client Need—Health promotion/maintenance

57 1. The client may resume sexual intercourse once the perineum is healed and the lochia has ceased. The generally occurs by the third postpartum week. The client may be able to resume sexual intercourse before the postpartum checkup because the perineum may be healed and lochia flow may have ceased by that time. It is not necessary to wait for complete involution of the uterus before having sexual intercourse. Also, the client makes the decision regarding use or lack of use of a birth control method. If the client chooses to use a birth control method, selection of the method may occur before or after the perineum has healed and lochia flow has ceased; thus this is not the most significant factor that should be considered when deciding whether or not to have sexual intercourse. (14:220; 16:233)

Nursing Process—Implementation
Client Need—Health promotion/maintenance

58 4. The client who feels nervous about going home with a new baby will benefit most from knowing that she can make contact with the health care facility after her discharge if she has questions. Some facilities also make follow-up phone calls to check on the new mother. The client probably will have the same nervous feeling at the time of the rescheduled discharge if the discharge is postponed, so this action will only relieve the nervousness temporarily. Also, nervousness is not usually an acceptable reason for postponing the client's discharge. The nurse should acknowledge that the client's feelings are normal and should provide the client with written instructions on infant care, but these actions alone will not decrease the client's nervousness. (14:221)

Nursing Process—Implementation
Client Need—Psychosocial integrity

NURSING CARE OF CLIENTS HAVING A CESAREAN DELIVERY

59 2. The client is catheterized prior to abdominal surgery in order to prevent trauma to the bladder that may occur if the bladder becomes distended during surgery. Catheterization prior to abdominal surgery is not performed to reduce postpartum hemorrhage, prevent urinary tract infection, or provide a safe way of collecting urine specimens. (21:230)

Nursing Process—Implementation
Client Need—Safe, effective care environment

60 1. When a cesarean delivery is performed using epidural anesthesia, the client may feel pressure but does not experience pain because the nerve roots (source of pain) are blocked. (14:202)

Nursing Process—Implementation
Client Need—Safe, effective care environment

61 3. The client's husband or coach is usually allowed to be present during the cesarean delivery. The husband or coach is directed to scrub and change into the appropriate attire. Once this process is completed and the procedure is ready to begin, the husband or coach is brought into the surgical area and placed near the client's head. (14:202)

Nursing Process—Implementation
Client Need—Psychosocial integrity

62 1. Prior to a cesarean section delivery, the nurse performs an abdominal-perineal preparation. The area prepared begins at the nipple line and extends vertically to perineal area that is visible when the legs are parallel, and extends horizontally from one side of the abdomen to the other side of the abdomen. (14:203; 16:199)

Nursing Process—Implementation
Client Need—Safe, effective care environment

63 3. The client should be monitored for respiratory depression when receiving a narcotic by the epidural route; respiratory depression is the most serious adverse effect associated with administration of narcotics by this route. The client may also experience urinary retention, pinpoint pupils, and circulatory collapse. (20:137)

Nursing Process—Data collection
Client Need—Physiological integrity

64 4. A narcotic antagonist such as naloxone hydrochloride (Narcan) should be readily available in case respiratory depression occurs. The medications identified in the other options are not required when the client is receiving epidural morphine sulfate. (20:137)

Nursing Process—Planning
Client Need—Physiological integrity

65 4. Redness and swelling around the incision is usually an indication of the presence of an infection. Other signs of infection include an elevated temperature (100.4°F or greater orally) 2 to 3 days after delivery, severe pain, or incisional drainage. It is normal for the incision line to feel numb for several months. (16:231; 18:636)

Nursing Process—Evaluation
Client Need—Physiological integrity

66 1. Ambulation, a diet low in gas-forming foods, small enemas, and antiflatulence medications are some of the methods utilized to reduce abdominal discomfort that may be experienced by the client who has had a cesarean delivery. Pain medications such as meperidine hydrochloride (Demerol) and morphine sulfate can contribute to the abdominal discomfort instead of relieving it because they slow peristalsis. Also, drinking from a straw should be discouraged because it causes the client to swallow more air, which further aggravates the problem. (16:230)

> Nursing Process—Implementation
> Client Need—Physiological integrity

67 1. Vaginal birth after a previous cesarean delivery (VBAC) may be possible if the client has had a low transverse incision, the woman wishes to attempt to have a vaginal delivery, and there is no history of medical conditions that prohibit a vaginal birth. (14:203)

> Nursing Process—Implementation
> Client Need—Psychosocial integrity

NURSING CARE OF CLIENTS HAVING AN EMERGENCY DELIVERY

68 3. If the nurse observes prolapse of the umbilical cord, the client should be placed in the Trendelenburg or knee-chest position. Both of these positions assist to relieve the pressure of the presenting part on the umbilical cord. The nurse also may attempt to lift the presenting part off the cord with a gloved finger until the health care provider arrives. Oxygen usually is administered but the client is not positioned on the left side. The client is usually delivered by cesarean delivery. Preparation of the delivery area and notification of the nurse in charge nurse do not take priority over relieving cord compression. (16:181)

> Nursing Process—Implementation
> Client Need—Physiological integrity

69 1. When birth is imminent and no help is available, the nurse should gently control the delivery of the head, allow it to emerge, and deliver it between contractions. The nurse should not hold back the baby's head to prevent birth, nor should the nurse attempt to enter or enlarge the vaginal opening. (16:196)

> Nursing Process—Implementation
> Client Need—Physiological integrity

NURSING CARE OF CLIENTS HAVING A STILLBORN OR A NEWBORN WITH COMPLICATIONS

70 2. The nurse should encourage the client to express her feelings and should express sorrow over the client's loss. These actions allow the client to sort through her feelings and facilitate the establishment of a trusting relationship between the client and nurse. The fetal heart tones should be checked by an experienced nurse and, once checked, should not be rechecked; the client should not be given

any false hope, only to be disappointed and discouraged when the inevitable happens. Redirecting the client's attention to the laboring process does not allow the client the opportunity to sort through her feelings. Explaining that the baby probably would have been born with severe long-term health problems is not necessarily an accurate statement and also does not ease the sorrow experienced by the client. (14:233)

> Nursing Process—Implementation
> Client Need—Psychosocial integrity

71 2. Allowing the parents to visit with the infant will allow them to say their last goodbyes to the infant and may help them to accept that the infant is actually dead. The infant should be clean and the parents should be allowed to hold and touch the infant. A memory packet may also be given to the parent, but it should not substitute for an actual visit with the infant if the parents so desire. Postponing the visit may interfere with the grieving process. (14:234)

> Nursing Process—Implementation
> Client Need—Psychosocial integrity

72 1. The client who is experiencing anticipatory grieving may delay naming the infant, may be reluctant to visit the infant in the nursery, and may focus on equipment and treatments when visiting the child. Asking the physician to postpone her discharge from the hospital is not a sign of anticipatory guidance; instead, this request is often made because the client does not want to leave the infant. (14:258)

> Nursing Process—Evaluation
> Client Need—Psychosocial integrity

73 2. The nurse can act as a role model and encourage the parents to interact with the newborn. This establishes an early bond between the newborn and the parents. Surgery will result in closure of the defect but may not correct the neurologic deficit that accompanies this condition. Showing the parents before and after surgery picture is usually most effective when the surgical intervention results in correction of the deformity or disorder; this is not the case with myelomeningocele. (14:234)

> Nursing Process—Implementation
> Client Need—Psychosocial integrity

NURSING CARE OF CLIENTS CONSIDERING FAMILY PLANNING

74 1. Combination oral contraceptives contain estrogen and progesterone. The estrogen is thought to prevent maturation of the follicle and thus prevent ovulation. The progesterone is thought to inhibit thickening of the uterine lining. The other two op-

tions do not reflect correct functions of the combination oral contraceptive. (14:58; 16:72)
> Nursing Process—Implementation
> Client Need—Health promotion/maintenance

75 2. The 28-pill package has 7 placebo pills that serve the purpose of allowing the woman to maintain a routine of taking the pills daily. This cuts down the possibility of the client forgetting to take a pill. The length of the menstrual cycle has nothing to do with the number of pills that are dispensed in the package. Monophasic, biphasic, and triphasic are categories of combination pills that have to do with how the estrogen and progesterone are released over the course of the menstrual cycle. All combination oral contraceptives have estrogen and progesterone in each pill. (14:58)
> Nursing Process—Implementation
> Client Need—Health promotion/maintenance

76 2. Oral contraceptives are sometimes prescribed for women who have primary dysmenorrhea because the oral contraceptive is thought to create a better hormonal balance and possibly decrease the discomfort experienced by the client. All of the other statements are accurate statements about oral contraceptives. (14:61)
> Nursing Process—Evaluation
> Client Need—Health promotion/maintenance

77 3. The Norplant system of contraception delivers a constant low dose of progesterone over 5 years and does not require any type replacement or maintenance during the 5-year period of time. (14:60)
> Nursing Process—Implementation
> Client Need—Health promotion/maintenance

78 4. The female condom is made of polyurethane, not latex; thus the client who has an allergy to latex can use a female condom without experiencing an allergic reaction. All of the other statements relate accurate information about the barrier form of contraception. (14:63; 16:69)
> Nursing Process—Evaluation
> Client Need—Health promotion/maintenance

79 3. The client who wishes to use the basal body temperature method of natural family planning should take her temperature every morning before arising for 6 months with a special thermometer. Recording the pattern of the menstrual cycle for 6 to 8 months is utilized when using the rhythm or calendar method of natural family planning. Monitoring the consistency of the vaginal secretions is used with Billings or ovulation method of natural family planning. Having the male sex partner to withdraw the penis from the vagina before ejaculation is called coitus interruptus. (14:65)
> Nursing Process—Implementation
> Client Need—Health promotion/maintenance

NURSING CARE OF THE NEWBORN CLIENT

80 3. Vitamin K is synthesized by bacteria normally found in the intestines. The newborn infant is given vitamin K because at birth the intestines are sterile and therefore vitamin K cannot be synthesized. Vitamin K is needed for the formation of prothrombin and other clotting factors that help to prevent bleeding. Vitamin K does not stimulate respirations, start peristalsis, or increase calcium absorption. (22:339)
> Nursing Process—Implementation
> Client Need—Health promotion/maintenance

81 3. The preferred site for intramuscular injections in the infant is the vastus lateralis. The rectus femoris may also be used. The ventrogluteal muscle and the gluteus maximus muscles are not used in the infant because of the risk for sciatic nerve damage. The deltoid muscle should not be used before the child is 3 years of age. (14:430)
> Nursing Process—Implementation
> Client Need—Health promotion/maintenance

82 1. Neonatal blindness can occur as a result of eye infections caused by the gonococcus and chlamydia organisms. Erythromycin (Ilotycine) ophthalmic ointment is used prophylactically in the newborn to prevent blindness that may result from exposure to these organisms during passage through the mother's birth canal. (16:317; 22:339)
> Nursing Process—Implementation
> Client Need—Health promotion/maintenance

83 2. The infant may experience temporary blurring of the vision following administration of erythromycin (Ilotycine) ophthalmic ointment. The infant's eyes may be swollen, but this is more likely the result of pressure exerted on the soft tissue of the lids during passage through the birth canal. Purulent eye drainage and conjunctival hemorrhage are not associated with the use of erthromycin (Ilotycine). (16:317; 22:339)
> Nursing Process—Implementation
> Client Need—Health promotion/maintenance

84 3. The nurse should have a hand *over* the baby but the hand should not be placed on the infant because this action may affect the accuracy of the weight obtained. Undressing the infant before the weight is obtained, placing a diaper or paper barrier on the scale before it is balanced, and cleansing the scale with an antiseptic before it is used are all correct techniques to implement when weighing the infant. (11:42; 18:796)

Nursing Process—Evaluation
Client Need—Safe, effective care environment

85 3. Yellow discoloration of the skin occurring within 24 hours of birth of the infant indicates a condition known as pathologic jaundice. This finding should be reported immediately so that the health care provider can order the appropriate treatment. Bluish discoloration of the hands and feet, a pulse rate of 140, and slightly swollen labia are all normal finding in the newborn. 14:244; 16:291)

Nursing Process—Evaluation
Client Need—Physiological integrity

86 2. The axillary temperature for the normal newborn should range between 97.7°F and 98.6°F. A temperature lower than this range is associated with hypothermia. The newborn who is hypothermic should be placed on a prewarmed radiant warmer and rewarmed gradually over a period of approximately 2 hours. Warming the infant too rapidly can result in apnea and acidosis. When the temperature falls within the acceptable range, the infant can be dressed, wrapped in a blanket, and placed in an opened crib; the temperature should be rechecked in 4 to 8 hours. Dressing the infant, wrapping the infant in double blankets, placing the infant in an opened crib, and rechecking the temperature in 30 to 60 minutes is not an appropriate method of rewarming an infant whose temperature is as low as 97°F. (16:311)

Nursing Process—Implementation
Client Need—Physiological integrity

87 4. When suctioning the infant with a bulb syringe, the bulb should be compressed before it is placed in the infant's nose or mouth. The mouth should be suctioned before the nose to prevent aspiration that may occur during the gasp response. Also, the back of the throat should not be touched when suctioning the mouth because the gag reflex may be stimulated. Once the bulb syringe has been inserted into the mouth or nose, the bulb should be decompressed so that the mucus can be aspirated. (16:310; 22:510)

Nursing Process—Evaluation
Client Need—Health promotion/maintenance

88 1. During the first few days after delivery, all newborns normally lose up to 10% of their birth weight. It is not necessarily true that the infant who bottle-feeds first will not successfully breast-feed because of a preference for the bottle nipple. It is preferable for the client to breast-feed instead of pumping the breast because the infant's sucking will stimulate

the production of an adequate amount of milk to meet his or her needs. Also, the infant benefits from the colostrum initially present in the breast. (14:240; 16:324)

Nursing Process—Implementation
Client Need—Health promotion/maintenance

89 2. Colostrum is a thin, yellowish fluid that contains maternal antibodies, salt, protein, and fat. The maternal antibodies found in the colostrum provides the infant with limited immunity to certain disorders. Also, the colostrum has a laxative effect and helps the newborn to expel the thick meconium normally present in the intestinal tract at birth. Colostrum does not contain estrogen, predigested fats, or digestive enzymes. (22:350)

Nursing Process—Implementation
Client Need—Health promotion/maintenance

90 3. A breast shield is not routinely used for breast-feeding. A breast shield may be worn when the nipples are flat or inverted, and occasionally when the nipples are sore and cracked. The other options identify correct techniques for breast-feeding. (16:320; 22:351)

Nursing Process—Evaluation
Client Need—Health promotion/maintenance

91 1. The infant should be placed in the right side-lying position. This position facilitates gastric emptying and also prevents aspiration if the infant should regurgitate the formula. The infant is not placed in the prone position because of its association with sudden infant death syndrome (SIDS). The infant is not placed in the supine position because there is a risk that the infant may aspirate regurgitated formula. The left-side lying position may prevent aspiration but does not facilitate gastric emptying. (14:253)

Nursing Process—Implementation
Client Need—Health promotion/maintenance

92 2. The infant whose nutritional needs are not being met is at risk to develop dehydration. One indication of dehydration is that the infant will have fewer than 6 wet diapers per day. It is normal for the breast-fed infant to have loose, pale-yellow stools; to awaken during the night for a feeding; and to feed every 2 to 3 hours. (14:240)

Nursing Process—Implementation
Client Need—Health promotion/maintenance

93 1. Breast milk can be stored in the refrigerator for up to 48 hours. It can be stored in a freezer (separate refrigerator and freezer doors) for up to 3 months, and can be stored in a deep freezer for up to 12 months. (16:320)

Nursing Process—Implementation

Client Need—Health promotion/maintenance

94 2. The umbilical cord should have two arteries and one vein. Variations in this configuration may be associated with congenital anomalies, particularly kidney anomalies. The scrotum normally is pendulous with numerous rugae, vernix caseosa is normally present (particularly in the body creases), and bluish discoloration of the hands and feet (acrocyanosis) is a normal finding. (16:299)

Nursing Process—Data collection

Client Need—Health promotion/maintenance

95 3. The full-term infant usually has plantar creases over the entire surface of the soles of the feet. The presence of anterior transverse creases is associated with prematurity. Lanugo over the shoulders, back, and forehead is a normal finding in the full-term newborn. A strong Moro reflex and a fully flexed posture are also characteristic of the full-term newborn. (16:301)

Nursing Process—Data collection

Client Need—Health promotion/maintenance

96 2. The infant should not be placed in the supine position because of the danger of aspiration. Infants seem to bottle-feed best when the client is held close and at a 45-degree angle. The techniques stated in the other options are correct techniques for bottle-feeding the infant. (16:323)

Nursing Process—Evaluation

Client Need—Health promotion/maintenance

97 4. Positioning the bottle so that the nipple remains full of formula throughout the feeding will help to prevent the baby from swallowing air. Keeping the nipple full of formula will not prevent the infant from getting formula, nor will it prevent regurgitation. Also, this technique is not known to prevent the infant from getting tired while feeding. (14:220)

Nursing Process—Implementation

Client Need—Health promotion/maintenance

98 3. Prepared formula can be refrigerated for up to 48 hours. Formula remaining in the bottle once the infant has finished feeding should be discarded. Bottles can be washed in a dishwasher. Warm tap water usually can be used. If the water source is questionable, the tap water should be boiled first. Also, the lid of the can of the formula concentrate should be wiped off before it is opened. (16:323)

Nursing Process—Evaluation

Client Need—Health promotion/maintenance

99 2. A yellowish discoloration of the skin is known as jaundice. Acrocyanosis indicates a bluish discoloration of the hands and feet. Erythematous means that the skin is red in color. Mottling is an irregular discoloration of the skin. (22:370)

Nursing Process—Data collection

Client Need—Physiological integrity

100 1. The infant who is receiving phototherapy treatment should have all clothes removed. Protective eye pads are applied to protect the retina of the eye from damage from the ultraviolet lights used for this type of treatment. The infant does not routinely have an intravenous infusion. It is not necessary to feed the infant by the nasogastric route solely on the basis of phototherapy treatment being in progress. The infant's position should be changed frequently to ensure exposure of all body surface areas to the ultraviolet light. (22:371)

Nursing Process—Implementation

Client Need—Physiological integrity

101 3. The penis should be monitored frequently for swelling and bleeding, which are the most common complications associated with the circumcision procedure. Vaseline gauze dressings are not required when a plastibell is in place. It usually is not necessary to check the vital signs more frequently unless there are complications such as hemorrhage. Alcohol should not be applied to the penis. Bacteriostatic ointments may be used if a Gomco circumcision is performed; otherwise the health care provider should be consulted for further instructions when an infection is suspected. (16:326)

Nursing Process—Implementation

Client Need—Physiological integrity

102 1. The physician should be notified if there is any drainage from the penis, if there are any blood spots larger than a quarter, if the infant is not voiding, and if the plastibell has not fallen off in 7 days; the plastibell should not be manually removed. The penis should be gently cleaned with soap and water. It is not necessary to apply petroleum jelly (Vaseline) to the penis if a plastibell is in place. (16:328)

Nursing Process—Evaluation

Client Need—Health promotion/maintenance

103 1. The newborn infant should be drinking breast milk or formula for at least 2 to 3 days before the phenylketonuria test (PKU) is performed. If the infant has not been receiving formula for the prescribed times, the result may be inaccurate. Babies who are discharged prior to this time should have the test performed within the prescribed amount of time in an outpatient setting such as the physician's office or a clinic. The data identified in the remaining options are not pertinent to have before performing the PKU test. (14:249)

> Nursing Process—Data collection
> Client Need—Health promotion/maintenance

104 4. After the heel stick, pressure should be applied to the heel with a dry gauze to prevent further bleeding. The nurse would be correct to warm the heel, puncture the lateral aspect of the heel, and discard the first drop of blood when performing the phenylketonuria (PKU) test. (16:311)

> Nursing Process—Implementation
> Client Need—Safe, effective care environment

INDIVIDUAL TEST ITEMS

105 2. Tocolytic agents should not be given if the client's cervix is dilated 4 cm or more and/or effaced 50% or more. Also, they should not be given if the client is hemorrhaging, has severe pregnancy-induced hypertension, or if fetal distress is indicated. The contractions indicate that the client continues to be in premature labor and thus it would be appropriate to give the client the tocolytic medication. Fetal heart variability is a normal finding and indicates fetal well-being. A statement of the client's perception of the contraction is not substantial enough to withhold this medication. (14:199)

> Nursing Process—Implementation
> Client Need—Physiological integrity

106 2. During the postpartum period, rho(d) immune globulin (RhoGAM) should be administered within 72 hours of delivery of the infant. If it is not administered within this time frame, there is an increased risk for the mother to develop antibodies that may cause hemolytic disease if she has an Rh positive infant in the future. (14:221; 16:229)

> Nursing Process—Implementation
> Client Need—Physiological integrity

107 4. Dysuria and hematuria are clinical manifestations that occur when the client has cystitis. A boggy displaced uterus is usually associated with bladder distention. Urinary retention and swelling of the lower extremities may be associated with kidney or circulation problems. Increased thirst and voiding large amounts of urine (polydipsia and polyuria) are two manifestations associated with diabetes mellitus. (22:298)

> Nursing Process—Data collection
> Client Need—Physiological integrity

108 4. It is important for the client to wash her hands thoroughly before handling the breast. This action will prevent contamination. The client who is breast-feeding should not wear a breast binder because this may suppress milk production. The nipples should not be cleansed with soap because soap will contribute to drying and cracking of the nipples. Petroleum jelly should not be applied to the nipples. (14:230)

> Nursing Process—Implementation
> Client Need—Health promotion

109 1. Asymmetry of the gluteal skin folds, limitation of abduction of the affected hip, and apparent shortening of the femur are signs of congenital hip dysplasia. Absence of spontaneous movement of the leg may be associated with other musculoskeletal disorders and is not usually seen in the infant with congenital hip dysplasia. An exaggerated curvature of the lumbar spine is called lordosis. (11:156; 16:357)

> Nursing Process—Data collection
> Client Need—Physiological integrity

110 2. Calf pain when the foot is dorsiflexed is a manifestation of thrombophlebitis. This response is also called a positive Homans sign. It is normal for the client to pass a couple of nickel-sized clots during the first 24 hours after delivery. The client may experience abdominal cramping similar to contraction pains during labor; these are caused by the release of oxytocin that occurs when the client is breast-feeding. They are more common among multiparas. The vaginal discharge is normally dark red in color during this time period. (14:227)

> Nursing Process—Data collection
> Client Need—Physiological integrity

111 2. Puerperal infection may be manifested by an elevated temperature, abdominal tenderness, foul-smelling lochia, abnormally large uterus, and chills. When infection is present, the pulse usually increases. Also the presence of lochia serosa on the fifth postpartum day is considered to be within the normal limits. (16:271)

> Nursing Process—Data collection
> Client Need—Physiological integrity

Classification of Test Items

Unit **II**   Review Test **12**

The Nursing Care of Clients During the Intrapartum and Postpartum Periods

Directions: After each question the correct answer is given, as well as a classification of each test question. Compare the correct answer with your answer. If a question has been answered *incorrectly*, draw a line to the end of all the columns. When finished, add up the number of your correct answers in each column and place that number in the respective box at the end in the area identified as *Number Correct*.

To determine the percentage of questions you answered correctly and your performance in each of the test plan categories, divide the *Number Correct* in each column by the *Number Possible* in each column. Then multiply the decimal by 100. For example:

$$\frac{\text{Number Correct: } 78}{\text{Number Possible: } 94} = 0.83 \times 100 = 83\%$$

Any score that is less than 75% indicates an area where further review would be beneficial.

KEY TO ITEM CLASSIFICATION:

NURSING PROCESS

D = Data collection
P = Planning
I = Implementation
E = Evaluation

CLIENT NEEDS

S = Safe, effective care environment
P = Physiological integrity
M = Psychosocial integrity
H = Health promotion/maintenance

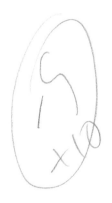

Question #	Answer #	Nursing Process				Client Needs			
		D	P	I	E	S	P	M	H
1	3			I					H
2	2	D							H
3	4	D							H
4	2	D							H
5	2			I					H
6	3		P			S			
7	2			I					H
8	3	D							H
9	1				E				H
10	1			I		S			
11	3	D							H
12	2			I				M	
13	1			I				M	
14	4			I					H
15	1	D							H

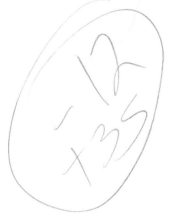

Question #	Answer #	Nursing Process				Client Needs			
		D	P	I	E	S	P	M	H
16	1	D							H
17	3		P						H
18	4			I			P		
19	1	D					P		
20	3				E		P		
21	1		P			S			
22	4	D							H
23	4			I					H
24	1			I					H
25	4	D					P		
26	3			I				M	
27	1	D							H
28	1		P						H
29	3			I			P		
30	3			I				M	
31	1			I		S			
32	1	D				S			
33	2		P						H
34	1			I		S			
35	3			I					H
36	2			I					H
37	4		P						H
38	1			I					H
39	3				E				H
40	4			I					H
41	3			I					H
42	2			I					H
43	1	D							H
44	4				E		P		
45	2			I			P		
46	4				E		P		
47	1			I					H

Question #	Answer #	Nursing Process				Client Needs			
		D	P	I	E	S	P	M	H
48	4			I					H
49	3			I					H
50	4	D					P		
51	1				E	S			
52	4			I			P		
53	1			I			P		
54	2				E				H
55	1			I					H
56	3			I					H
57	1			I					H
58	4			I				M	
59	2			I		S			
60	1			I		S			
61	3			I				M	
62	1			I		S			
63	3	D					P		
64	4		P				P		
65	4				E		P		
66	1			I			P		
67	1			I				M	
68	3			I			P		
69	1			I			P		
70	2			I				M	
71	2			I				M	
72	1				E			M	
73	2			I				M	
74	1			I					H
75	2			I					H
76	2				E				H
77	3			I					H
78	4				E				H

Question #	Answer #	Nursing Process				Client Needs			
		D	P	I	E	S	P	M	H
79	3			I					H
80	3			I					H
81	3			I					H
82	1			I					H
83	2			I					H
84	3				E	S			
85	3				E		P		
86	2			I			P		
87	4				E				H
88	1			I					H
89	2			I					H
90	3				E				H
91	1			I					H
92	2			I					H
93	1			I					H
94	2	D							H
95	3	D							H
96	2				E				H
97	4			I					H
98	3				E				H
99	2	D					P		
100	1			I			P		
101	2			I			P		
102	1				E				H
103	1	D							H
104	4			I		S			
105	2			I			P		
106	2			I			P		
107	4	D					P		
108	4			I					H
109	1	D					P		

Question #	Answer #	Nursing Process				Client Needs			
		D	P	I	E	S	P	M	H
110	2	D					P		
111	2	D					P		
Number Correct	7 9	16	4	47 12		6	25	8	41
Number Possible	111	23	7	63	18	11	28	11	61
Percentage Correct	71	70	57	75	67	55	89	73	67

Unit III

The Nursing Care of Children

The Nursing Care of Infants, Toddlers, and Preschool Children

Directions: With a pencil, blacken the circle in front of the option you have chosen for your correct answer.

NORMAL GROWTH AND DEVELOPMENT OF INFANTS AND TODDLERS

The nurse in a well-baby clinic assesses the growth and development of healthy infants and toddlers and uses that information as a basis for teaching.

1 Which of the following findings would the nurse consider *abnormal* for a 3-month-old?
- ○ 1. Unable to hold bottle
- ◉ 2. Unable to lift head
- ○ 3. Unable to roll from back to abdomen
- ○ 4. Unable to sit with support

2 Which of the following instructions would the nurse include when teaching the parents about introducing solid foods to a 4-month-old?
- ○ 1. Begin introduction with plain strained fruits and vegetables.
- ○ 2. Do not breast- or bottle-feed until after solid food has been given.
- ◉ 3. Introduce one food at a time at an interval of every 4 to 5 days.
- ○ 4. Postpone introduction if the infant pushes food out of its mouth with its tongue.

3 Which of the following findings would the nurse consider *abnormal* for an 18-month-old?
- ◉ 1. Vocabulary of about 6 words
- ○ 2. Uses a spoon when eating
- ○ 3. Walks with support
- ○ 4. Shows readiness for toilet training

4 Which of the following observations by the nurse indicates that the parents of a toddler need additional teaching on safety?
- ○ 1. Household cleaners are in their original containers.
- ○ 2. Medicines are stored on a high shelf out of the child's reach.
- ◉ 3. The hot water heater thermostat is set at 120°F.
- ○ 4. The number for the poison control center is posted by the telephone.

NURSING CARE OF PREMATURE INFANTS

A nurse in a high-risk nursery cares for several preterm infants.

5 Which nursing observation would be *essential* for preventing retrolental fibroplasia in the preterm infant?
- ○ 1. Monitoring the oxygen saturation level
- ◉ 2. Monitoring the bilirubin level
- ○ 3. Checking the infant's hemoglobin level
- ○ 4. Checking the infant's pupil response

6 When feeding the preterm infant, the *best* routine for the nurse to follow is to
- ○ 1. feed the infant every hour.
- ○ 2. give 3 to 4 ounces in each feeding.
- ○ 3. feed by the nasogastric route.
- ○ 4. give glucose feedings for the first month.

The parents of a preterm infant ask the nurse why the infant is being monitored for signs of infection.

7 The nurse explains that the infant is at risk to develop infections *primarily* because the infant
- ○ 1. has fragile skin.
- ○ 2. lacks antibody protection from the mother.
- ○ 3. is exposed to numerous sources of bacterial organisms.
- ○ 4. undergoes many invasive procedures.

8 Which of the following actions by the nurse will *best* ensure that thermoregulation needs of the preterm infant are met?
- ○ 1. The infant is wrapped in a blanket.
- ○ 2. Nursery temperature is between 75° and 79°F.
- ○ 3. The infant is placed in an isolette.
- ○ 4. The crib is positioned away from sources of drafts.

NURSING CARE OF AN INFANT WITH HEMOLYTIC DISEASE

A gravida II para I female, in her 38th week of pregnancy, presents in the emergency room in active labor. She delivers an Rh positive infant with congenital hemolytic disease caused by Rh incompatibility.

9 Which of the following findings would be *most* indicative of the presence of Rh incompatibility?
- ○ 1. A slow and irregular respiratory rate
- ○ 2. Absence of newborn reflexes
- ○ 3. Limited movement in lower extremities
- ○ 4. Jaundice within 24 to 36 hours after birth

A direct Coombs test is ordered to confirm the diagnosis of hemolytic disease.

10 The nurse should be prepared to assist with the collection of a blood specimen from the
- ○ 1. infant's father.
- ○ 2. infant's mother.
- ○ 3. infant's sibling.
- ○ 4. umbilical cord.

The direct Coombs test is positive and the infant's bilirubin level is elevated. The physician leaves orders to begin phototherapy.

11 When initiating phototherapy treatment, the nurse should

- ○ 1. place protective eye shields over the infant's eyes.
- ○ 2. monitor the vital signs every 15 minutes for the first hour.
- ○ 3. catheterize the infant and place on strict intake and output.
- ○ 4. place the infant on n.p.o. status until therapy is completed.

NURSING CARE OF AN INFANT WITH MYELOMENINGOCELE

An infant born with spina bifida with a myelomeningocele high in the spinal column is being cared for in the high-risk nursery.

12 Which of the following actions is *most* important for the nurse to include during the preoperative period?
- ○ 1. Keep diaper area clean in order to prevent contamination of the myelomeningocele.
- ○ 2. Position the infant so that there is no pressure on the myelomeningocele.
- ○ 3. Keep the infant's myelomeningocele clean by washing it with antiseptic soap.
- ○ 4. Encourage the parents to cuddle and hold the infant to promote bonding.

The infant is scheduled for surgery on the day after admission to the nursery. The parents ask, "Why is the surgery being performed so soon?"

13 The nurse is *correct* in explaining that the surgery for this disorder is performed as soon as possible to
- ○ 1. prevent paralysis.
- ○ 2. restore bowel function.
- ○ 3. prevent infection.
- ○ 4. restore respiratory function.

14 Unless the physician orders otherwise, in what position should the nurse place the infant during the postoperative period?
- ○ 1. Supine position
- ○ 2. Prone position
- ○ 3. Right or left side-lying position
- ○ 4. Position most comfortable for infant

15 The plan for home care will be based on the assumption that the infant will
- ○ 1. be unable to walk without crutches.
- ○ 2. have a 50% chance of eventually walking alone.
- ○ 3. have a 95% chance of eventually walking alone.
- ○ 4. someday be able to walk without crutches.

16 In the future, the parents of the infant with myelomeningocele can *best* be prepared to manage their child's urinary incontinence by being taught how to

1. care for a retention catheter.
2. insert a straight catheter.
3. reapply a ureterostomy appliance.
4. attach an external catheter.

NURSING CARE OF AN INFANT WITH HYDROCEPHALUS

An infant who was born with hydrocephalus is now 1 week old and is scheduled for surgery.

17 The *most* prominent finding during the data collection process would be
1. increased head size.
2. paralysis of the lower extremities.
3. absence of the sucking reflex.
4. marked depression of the anterior fontanel.

The parents ask the nurse to explain to them why the child has hydrocephalus.

18 The nurse is *correct* in explaining that hydrocephalus is probably due to
1. absence of the dura mater.
2. blockage of cerebrospinal fluid circulation.
3. an increased amount of cerebrospinal fluid.
4. blockage in the cerebral arteries.

19 After feeding the infant, the nurse should place the infant in which of the following positions?
1. Sitting position
2. Supine position
3. Prone position
4. Side-lying position

20 Which measure would be *most appropriate* to reduce the potential for developing a pressure ulcer?
1. Place a sheepskin under the infant's head.
2. Massage the circumference of the infant's skull.
3. Support the infant's head on two pillows.
4. Apply a padded helmet to the infant's head.

21 If a shunting device is placed on the right side of the infant's head, the postoperative position of choice for the infant is on
1. the right side, to increase absorption of cerebrospinal fluid.
2. the abdomen, to prevent obstruction in the shunt catheter.
3. the left side, to avoid pressure on the operative site.
4. the back, to promote ventricular drainage.

22 Postoperatively, which sign is the *best* indication that the infant is developing increased intracranial pressure?

1. Depression of the fontanel
2. Decreased pulse and respiratory rate
3. Change frequency of bowel movements
4. Sudden increase in weight

23 Which of the following actions is *most* appropriate if the nurse observes that the infant's anterior fontanel is sunken?
1. Document the finding and take no further action.
2. Place the infant in the flat position.
3. Elevate the infant's head.
4. Notify the charge nurse or physician immediately.

NURSING CARE OF AN INFANT WITH CLEFT LIP

An infant with bilateral cleft lip is admitted to the newborn nursery.

24 During the initial data collection process, the nurse palpates the roof of the infant's mouth in order to
1. assess the infant's ability to suck.
2. check for the infant's gag reflex.
3. assess for an opening in the palate.
4. check the position of the uvula.

25 When taking the infant to the parents for the first visit, the *priority* nursing action would be to
1. teach parents how to feed the infant.
2. display acceptance of the infant.
3. discuss plans for surgical repair of the defect.
4. show the parents how to use the bulb syringe.

26 Which of the following utensils is *best* for the nurse to use when feeding the infant?
1. A gavage tube
2. A plastic spoon
3. A rubber-tip syringe
4. A firm rubber nipple

27 Which of the following observations by the nurse indicates that the parents understand how to decrease the risk of aspiration?
1. The infant is burped frequently during feedings.
2. The infant is placed in the prone position.
3. The infant is fed formula thickened with rice cereal.
4. The infant is not fed until after surgical repair of the defect.

NURSING CARE OF AN INFANT WITH PYLORIC STENOSIS

The nurse is caring for a 3-week old infant who has been admitted to the hospital for surgical correction of pyloric stenosis.

28 Which of the following findings would be *most* significant during the data collection process?
- ○ 1. The infant is eager to suck.
- ○ 2. The anterior fontanel is flat.
- ● 3. The gastric peristaltic waves are visible.
- ○ 4. The mucous membranes are dry.

The physician orders an intravenous infusion of dextrose 5% in 0.225 normal saline.

29 The nurse would be *correct* in telling the parents that
- ○ 1. the infant's head may be shaved at the IV site.
- ● 2. the infant will be n.p.o. during IV therapy.
- ○ 3. the infant may be restless during IV therapy.
- ○ 4. the area around the IV site will swell slightly.

30 After surgical correction of the defect, the nurse would be *correct* in instructing the parents to position the infant on the
- ○ 1. abdomen after feedings.
- ○ 2. right side after feedings.
- ○ 3. back after feedings.
- ● 4. left side after feedings.

NURSING CARE OF AN INFANT WITH BILATERAL CLUBFOOT

A newborn infant with bilateral talipes equinovarus (bilateral clubfoot) is admitted to the newborn nursery.

31 If the nurse obtains all of the following data during the admission assessment, which one *best* indicates that the infant has true clubfoot?
- ○ 1. The infant was born in the breech position.
- ○ 2. The heels are drawn in and the feet turned inward.
- ● 3. The feet cannot be corrected to a neutral position.
- ○ 4. Both of the infant's feet are affected.

Bilateral leg casts are applied.

32 Which of the following techniques is *best* for the nurse to use when handling the wet cast?
- ○ 1. Move the cast using the fingertips.
- ○ 2. Move the cast using gloves on both hands.
- ○ 3. Move the cast using a sling made of gauze.
- ● 4. Move the cast using the palms of the hands.

33 Which of the following outcomes indicates that the infant is experiencing neurovascular complication?
- ○ 1. The infant cries 4 hours after the last feeding.
- ○ 2. The infant's toes are wiggling.
- ● 3. The infant's toes are pale and cold.
- ○ 4. The pedal pulse is 110 and regular.

34 Which of the following actions would the nurse implement to minimize swelling of the infant's feet?
- ● 1. Elevate the legs and feet on a pillow.
- ○ 2. Place the infant in the prone position.
- ○ 3. Petal the edges of the cast.
- ○ 4. Apply ice packs over the cast.

35 It would be *correct* for the nurse to tell the parents that initially the infant's cast will be changed every
- ● 1. 3 to 7 days.
- ○ 2. 1 to 2 weeks.
- ○ 3. month.
- ○ 4. other month.

At 8 weeks of age the infant is seen in the doctor's office for a routine cast change. The nurse uses this opportunity to teach the parents ways to promote normal growth and development.

36 The nurse would be *correct* in instructing the parents to
- ○ 1. encourage the infant to crawl about in the crib.
- ○ 2. play peek-a-boo with the infant's favorite blanket.
- ○ 3. encourage the infant to reach for cuddly toys.
- ● 4. place a brightly colored mobile over the crib.

The parents tell the nurse that they can barely feel the soft spot in the back of the infant's head. They ask the nurse if this is normal.

37 The nurse is correct in explaining that this finding is
- ● 1. normal, because the posterior fontanel usually closes between 2 and 3 months.
- ○ 2. abnormal, because the posterior fontanel usually closes between 9 and 18 months.
- ○ 3. abnormal, because the posterior fontanel usually remains open longer in children.
- ○ 4. normal, because the posterior fontanel usually closes earlier in children with congenital skeletal defects.

NURSING CARE OF AN INFANT WITH OTITIS MEDIA

A 6-month-old infant is examined by the physician and found to have otitis media.

38 Which of the following observations by the nurse would *best* indicate the presence of ear pain?
- ○ 1. The infant refuses to suck a bottle.
- ◉ 2. The infant pulls on one ear.
- ○ 3. The infant's temperature is elevated.
- ○ 4. There is drainage from the infant's ear.

The physician prescribes an oral antibiotic to be given for 10 days. The first dose is to be given in the doctor's office.

39 When preparing to give medications, which of the following actions by the nurse will *best* ensure that the infant receives a safe dose of the prescribed medication?
- ◉ 1. Read the doctor's orders carefully.
- ○ 2. Determine the child's weight.
- ○ 3. Determine medication allergies.
- ○ 4. Read the medication label

40 When explaining the prescribed antibiotic treatment, the nurse would be *correct* in instructing the parents to
- ○ 1. position infant on side after giving the antibiotic.
- ◉ 2. give the antibiotic with feedings.
- ○ 3. store the antibiotic at room temperature.
- ○ 4. give the antibiotic for the full 10 days.

NURSING CARE OF AN INFANT WITH A CONGENITAL HEART DEFECT

A 2-day-old infant with a diagnosis of coarctation of the aorta is being cared for in the high-risk nursery.

41 On admission, if the nurse obtains all of the following data, which one *best* indicates the presence of coarctation of the aorta?
- ○ 1. Generalized cyanosis, especially when the infant cries
- ○ 2. Clubbing of the fingers and toes
- ◉ 3. Bounding brachial pulses and weak femoral pulses
- ○ 4. Rapid and irregular apical heartbeat

42 The nurse would be *correct* in telling the parents that the optimal time for surgical correction is
- ○ 1. as soon as the child's condition has be stabilized.
- ○ 2. when the child is 6 months old.
- ◉ 3. when the child is 1 year old.
- ○ 4. when the child is between 2 and 4 years of age.

43 Which of the following actions is *most important* for the nurse to perform before giving Lanoxin?
- ◉ 1. Check the apical pulse for 1 minute.
- ○ 2. Position the infant with the head slightly elevated.
- ○ 3. Check the expiration date on the medication label.
- ○ 4. Monitor the infant's urinary output.

44 The nurse can *best* facilitate reduction of the workload of the heart by
- ○ 1. limiting the amount of holding and cuddling by the infant's parents.
- ◉ 2. organizing nursing care so that the child has longer rest periods.
- ○ 3. giving all feeding by the nasogastric route.
- ○ 4. keeping the child mildly sedated at all times.

The nurse is providing discharge instructions in preparation for when the infant goes home with the parents.

45 Which of the following statements by the parents indicate a need for additional teaching about administering digoxin (Lanoxin)?
- ○ 1. If a dose is missed, the next dose should be given at the regularly scheduled time.
- ○ 2. The apical pulse should be checked before each dose of the medication is given.
- ◉ 3. Each dose of the medication should be mixed in a small amount of formula.
- ○ 4. The dose should be increased or decreased only when ordered by the doctor.

NURSING CARE OF AN INFANT WITH AN INFECTIOUS DISEASE

A 7-month-old infant with chickenpox is seen in the emergency room. The physician admits the infant to the hospital because of moderate dehydration. An intravenous infusion of dextrose 5% in 0.225 normal saline is begun.

46 Which of the following isolation categories is *most appropriate* for the child who has chickenpox?
- ◉ 1. Respiratory isolation
- ○ 2. Strict isolation
- ○ 3. Contact isolation
- ○ 4. Enteric isolation

47 Which of the following actions by the nurse would be *incorrect* when implementing the prescribed isolation precautions?
- ◉ 1. A supply of clean masks is placed in the infant's room.
- ○ 2. Specimens are sent to the lab in a zip-closure biohazard bag.
- ○ 3. The patient is assigned to a private room.
- ○ 4. A thermometer and holder are placed in the infant's room.

48 If the nurse obtains all of the following data, which one is *most* important to report to the nurse in charge?
○ 1. The infant sleeps for short intervals during the day.
○ 2. There is an increase in the frequency and amount of urine.
○ 3. The infant occasionally cries when disturbed by noise.
● 4. There is an increase in the intravenous infusion.

NURSING CARE OF AN INFANT OF AN HIV-POSITIVE MOTHER

An infant is born at 32 weeks gestation to a gravida I para I HIV-positive mother.

49 When providing care for this infant, the nurse would follow
○ 1. strict isolation precautions.
○ 2. respiratory isolation precautions.
● 3. universal precautions.
○ 4. contact isolation precautions.

The mother asks the nurse when the child will be tested for HIV and how long it usually is before HIV-positive babies develop AIDS.

50 The nurse would be *correct* in telling the mother that the infant
● 1. will not be tested because babies of HIV-positive mothers are HIV-positive.
○ 2. will be tested immediately for anti-HIV antibodies to facilitate early treatment.
○ 3. will not be tested for anti-HIV antibodies until after the infant is 3 months of age.
○ 4. will be tested for anti-HIV antibodies for 4 years or until test results are positive.

51 It would be *correct* for the nurse to explain that most children who contract the human immunodeficiency virus *in utero* have symptoms of AIDS
○ 1. at birth.
○ 2. by 6 months of age.
○ 3. by 1 year of age.
● 4. by 2 years of age.

The mother asks if she can breast-feed the infant.

52 The nurse would be *correct* in explaining that
○ 1. it is OK to breast-feed the infant if the anti-HIV test results are positive.
○ 2. it is OK to breast-feed the infant as long as the infant is symptom-free.
● 3. the infant cannot breast-feed if the mother is known to be HIV-positive.
○ 4. the infant cannot breast-feed if the mother has developed symptoms of AIDS.

The infant is discharged home with the mother at 4 weeks of age. At 2 months of age the infant is seen in the doctor's office for a routine checkup.

53 If the nurse obtains all of the following data, which one would be considered a high-risk factor for developing AIDS?
○ 1. The infant has pinpoint white spots on the nose.
● 2. The mother states that the child has had thrush twice.
○ 3. The respirations have an irregular pattern.
○ 4. The mother states that the child has 6 wet diapers per day.

NURSING CARE OF AN INFANT WITH ATOPIC DERMATITIS

A 2-year-old child is seen in the clinic and diagnosed with atopic dermatitis. The mother asks what caused the child's skin condition and why the physician asks many questions about the home environment.

54 The nurse would be *correct* in explaining that the probable cause of atopic dermatitis is
○ 1. poor nutrition.
○ 2. a premature birth.
● 3. an allergic reaction.
○ 4. a hormone imbalance.

55 The nurse should be prepared to give the mother suggestions concerning care measures that will help to relieve the child's
○ 1. nausea.
○ 2. vomiting.
● 3. itching.
○ 4. drowsiness.

The mother is instructed to use hydrocortisone ointment on the child's skin lesions and to give the child colloid baths.

56 On a subsequent visit, the nurse judges that the ointment has been effective if
○ 1. weeping of the skin has subsided.
○ 2. there is no spread of the skin lesions.
● 3. inflammation of the skin has decreased.
○ 4. the child's white blood cell count is increased.

57 The nurse would be *correct* in explaining that a typical colloid bath consist of tepid water and
● 1. cornstarch or baking soda.
○ 2. mineral oil.
○ 3. liquid glycerin soap.
○ 4. salt.

NURSING CARE OF A TODDLER WITH SICKLE CELL CRISIS

An acutely ill, 21-month-old child is admitted to the hospital with vaso-occlusive sickle cell crisis. The child has a 6-year-old sibling who also has sickle cell disease.

58 When admitting the child, the nurse should be prepared to use nursing measures to relieve the child's
- 1. pain.
- 2. diarrhea.
- 3. hemorrhaging.
- 4. bradycardia.

59 The nurse also should anticipate and develop a plan of care that will
- 1. include transfusion of plasma.
- 2. include measures to decrease the hemoglobin level.
- 3. include administration of large doses of iron.
- 4. include measures to rehydrate the child.

The mother informs the nurse that she has the sickle cell trait and the child's father has sickle cell disease.

60 Which of the following statements by the mother indicates that she understands the transmission of sickle cell disease?
- 1. The mother states that all of her offspring will be born with sickle cell disease.
- 2. The mother states that there is a 50% chance that each pregnancy will result in an offspring with sickle cell disease.
- 3. The mother states that if she conceives again, the infant will be born with sickle cell trait.
- 4. The mother states that there is a 75% chance that each pregnancy will result in an offspring with sickle cell disease.

NURSING CARE OF A TODDLER WITH CYSTIC FIBROSIS

An 18-month-old toddler with a diagnosis of cystic fibrosis is admitted to the hospital because of increasing respiratory difficulty and repeated respiratory infections.

61 Which of the statements by the parents describe a typical finding in the child with cystic fibrosis?
- 1. The child rarely cries.
- 2. The child has gained a lot of weight.
- 3. The child tastes salty when kissed.
- 4. The child has poor head control.

62 Which of the following assessment findings would the nurse expect to be present in the child with cystic fibrosis?
- 1. Poor appetite
- 2. Excessive perspiration
- 3. Low urine output
- 4. Bulky, foul-smelling stools

63 Which of the following is the *priority* goal for the child with cystic fibrosis?
- 1. The child will consume appropriate nutrients to meet body needs.
- 2. The child will maintain an effective breathing pattern.
- 3. The child will consume an adequate amount of fluids to meet body needs.
- 4. The child will demonstrate a decreased level of anxiety.

A bronchodilator is prescribed for the child.

64 The nurse would determine that this type of therapy has been successful if
- 1. there is decreased mucus in the stools.
- 2. the serum sodium level decreases.
- 3. the breathing pattern improves.
- 4. excess fat is excreted from the body.

After collecting additional data, the nurse determines that the child has not been receiving the recommended diet. The parents also ask if the physician can prescribe a larger dose of Pancrease given twice daily, instead of the current dose given with each meal.

65 The nurse is *correct* in explaining that the child should receive a diet that is
- 1. high in fat.
- 2. low in protein.
- 3. low in salt.
- 4. high in calories.

66 The nurse is *correct* in explaining that Pancrease has to be given with meals in order to
- 1. prevent gastrointestinal upset.
- 2. increase absorption of nutrients.
- 3. prevent salt depletion.
- 4. increase the child's desire to eat.

67 The nurse is *correct* in explaining to the parents that the child's fluid intake should be increased in order to
- 1. prevent kidney failure.
- 2. increase cardiac function.
- 3. reduce pain and discomfort.
- 4. liquefy secretions in the lung.

68 The parents demonstrate a *correct* understanding of the child's needs if they state that it is most important to protect the child against exposure to
- 1. airborne pollen.
- 2. infections.
- 3. pet dander.
- 4. bright sunlight.

NURSING CARE OF A TODDLER WITH ASTHMA

A 3-year-old toddler has been diagnosed as having asthma. The physician has determined that the child has allergic (extrinsic) asthma. At present the child has an upper respiratory infection.

69 If the nurse collects all of the following data, which one *best* indicates that the child is having an acute asthma attack?
- ● 1. Presence of expiratory wheezing
- ○ 2. Respiratory rate between 20 and 30
- ○ 3. Thoracic breathing pattern
- ○ 4. Clear, watery nasal drainage

70 Which of the following nursing actions is *most* appropriate for relieving the child's acute episode of respiratory distress?
- ○ 1. Distract the child with age-appropriate toys.
- ○ 2. Position a steam vaporizer at the bedside.
- ○ 3. Give antibiotics as ordered.
- ● 4. Place the child in semi-Fowler's position.

The child responds to treatment and is scheduled to be discharged home. The doctor has prescribed breathing exercises for the child.

71 Which of the following activities will *best* facilitate the child's performance of breathing exercises?
- ○ 1. Promise to give the child a treat after the exercises.
- ○ 2. Have the parents assist the child with the exercises.
- ○ 3. Demonstrate the exercise, then have the child do the exercise.
- ● 4. Instruct the parents to have the child blow bubbles.

72 Which of the following instructions is *most* appropriate for the nurse to include during discharge teaching?
- ○ 1. Instruct the parents to give breathing treatments every 2 hours.
- ○ 2. Instruct the parents to eliminate vegetables from the child's diet.
- ○ 3. Instruct the parents to limit the amount of fluid intake.
- ● 4. Instruct the parents to remove area rugs from the home.

NURSING CARE OF A TODDLER WHO HAS SWALLOWED A TOXIC SUBSTANCE

The mother of a 15-month-old toddler calls the doctor's office and reports that the child swallowed a lye-based cleaner.

73 Which of the following instructions should be given *initially*?

- ○ 1. Begin cardiopulmonary resuscitation on the child immediately.
- ○ 2. Induce vomiting with syrup of ipecac immediately.
- ○ 3. Give the child water to drink in order to dilute the substance.
- ● 4. Take the child and substance to the nearest emergency room.

The child is taken the emergency room of the nearest hospital. After examination, the doctor decides to admit the child for further observation.

74 If the nurse collects all of the following data on admission, which one indicates that the child needs to be monitored with a pulse oximeter?
- ● 1. Substernal and intercostal retractions
- ○ 2. Lips red and swollen
- ○ 3. Thin, clear mucus drooling from lips
- ○ 4. Pulse rate 105

75 In addition to monitoring the child with a pulse oximeter, the nurse also would anticipate
- ● 1. performing gastric lavage.
- ○ 2. implementing pain-relieving measures.
- ○ 3. maintaining the child on n.p.o. status.
- ○ 4. performing neurovascular checks.

After 2 days the child is discharged home.

76 Which of the following statements by the mother *best* indicates that she understands how to prevent the child from ingesting poison substances in the future?
- ○ 1. The mother states that she will remove all toxic substances from the home.
- ○ 2. The mother states that she will not let the child out of her sight.
- ○ 3. The mother states that she will place all toxic substances out of the child's reach.
- ● 4. The mother states that she will keep all toxic substances in a locked cabinet.

NURSING CARE OF A TODDLER WITH CROUP

A 2½-year-old toddler is seen in the doctor's office because of coughing and difficulty breathing during the previous night. The physician makes a diagnosis of laryngotracheobronchitis (croup).

77 The nurse would be *correct* in telling the parents that this disorder
- ● 1. is most often caused by a virus.
- ○ 2. occurs in children with asthma.
- ○ 3. occurs in children who have whooping cough.
- ○ 4. is most often caused by underdeveloped lungs.

78 The nurse would expect the child to present with a cough that is
  - ○ 1. moist.
  - ◉ 2. barky.
  - ○ 3. muffled.
  - ○ 4. wheezy.

79 The nurse would be *correct* in explaining to the parents that laryngeal spasms often can be relieved by placing the child in
  - ○ 1. a room with central heating.
  - ○ 2. an air-conditioned room.
  - ◉ 3. a room with a humidifier.
  - ○ 4. a dust-free room.

80 The nurse would be *correct* in telling the parents to contact the physician immediately if the child
  - ○ 1. develops a fever.
  - ◉ 2. becomes extremely anxious.
  - ○ 3. coughs during the night.
  - ○ 4. sleeps during the day.

81 Which of the following statements by the parents indicates a need for further teaching?
  - ○ 1. The parents state that the child may have recurrent episodes of croup for one or two more nights.
  - ◉ 2. The parents state that they will give children's aspirin if the child's temperature is greater than 101°F.
  - ○ 3. The parents state that they will place a cool mist humidifier at the head of the child's bed.
  - ○ 4. The parents state that they will offer the child small sips of clear liquids at frequent intervals.

The child develops acute respiratory distress during the night and is taken to the hospital emergency room. The physician admits the child for further treatment.

82 In order to prevent aggravation of the child's respiratory distress, the nurse should
  - ○ 1. medicate the child with a sedative.
  - ◉ 2. encourage the parents to remain at the child's beside.
  - ○ 3. give the child an age-appropriate toy to play with.
  - ○ 4. postpone unpleasant procedures until the child stabilizes.

83 Which of the following medications would the nurse expect a child with croup to receive?
  - ○ 1. Ampicillin
  - ○ 2. Ferrous sulfate
  - ○ 3. Reglan
  - ◉ 4. Racemic epinephrine

NURSING CARE OF A TODDLER WITH PNEUMONIA

A 2½-year-old toddler is admitted to the hospital with a diagnosis of pneumococcal pneumonia. On admission the child has an intermittent, nonproductive cough. The parents report that the child has been lethargic and anorexic for several days.

84 In addition to the above manifestations, the nurse would expect to find which of the following?
  - ○ 1. Clubbing of the fingers
  - ○ 2. Synchronized chest movement
  - ○ 3. Slow pulse rate
  - ◉ 4. Rapid and shallow respirations

85 Which of the following methods is *most* appropriate for determining the child's hydration status?
  - ◉ 1. The child's urinary output
  - ○ 2. The pH of the urine
  - ○ 3. The child's blood pressure
  - ○ 4. The child's respiratory rate

86 If pulse oximetry is ordered, the nurse should report values that consistently
  - ◉ 1. remain below 95.
  - ○ 2. remain above 95.
  - ○ 3. remain below 100.
  - ○ 4. remain above 100.

87 Which of the following medications would the nurse expect to give to the child who has a nonproductive moist cough?
  - ○ 1. Antibiotic
  - ○ 2. Bronchodilator
  - ◉ 3. Expectorant
  - ○ 4. Suppressant

The child's temperature remains above 103°F. The physician leaves orders to give the child a sponge bath for a temperature greater than or equal to 103°F rectally. The parents ask the nurse if it is OK for them to do the bath.

88 The nurse would be *correct* in explaining, to the parents, that the bath
  - ○ 1. should be given for at least 1 hour.
  - ○ 2. water temperature should be cool.
  - ◉ 3. should be discontinued if the child begins to shiver.
  - ○ 4. should be given until the temperature is below 101°F.

After 3 days of treatment, the child's condition improves significantly. The physician writes discharge orders that include instructions for home care. The parents speak a little English but their primary language is Spanish.

89 Which of the following actions will *best* ensure that the parents understand the discharge instructions?
- 1. Give the parents a copy of the instructions written in Spanish.
- ○ 2. Have an interpreter present when instructions are given.
- ○ 3. Have the physician give the instructions.
- ○ 4. Instruct parents to call if questions arise once they get home.

NURSING CARE OF A PRESCHOOLER WITH SEIZURE DISORDER

A 4½-year-old preschooler is admitted to the hospital with a tentative diagnosis of grand mal seizures.

90 Of all the following data the nurse collects, which one *best* indicates that the child had a grand mal seizure?
- ○ 1. The parents state that the child had a high fever.
- ○ 2. The parents state that the child has begun wetting the bed.
- ○ 3. The parents state that the child suddenly dropped to the floor.
- 4. The parents state that the child's whole body was jerking.

91 Which of the following actions is *most* appropriate when preparing the hospital room for the child's admission?
- 1. Pad the side rails on the bed.
- ○ 2. Keep Phenobarbital at the bedside.
- ○ 3. Place the bed in the Trendelenberg position.
- ○ 4. Follow strict isolation protocols.

92 Which of the following equipment is *least* important to have at the beside?
- ○ 1. Suction equipment
- ○ 2. Oral airway
- ○ 3. Oxygen sources
- 4. Cool mist humidifier

The child has a grand mal seizure while the nurse is at the bedside.

93 Which of the following should be the *first* action taken by the nurse?
- ○ 1. Call for assistance.
- 2. Place the child in a side-lying position.
- ○ 3. Insert a padded tongue blade in the child's mouth.
- ○ 4. Administer oxygen.

The child is placed on phenytoin (Dilantin). After several days on the medication the child has no more seizure activity. The physician writes discharge orders. The child will continue on phenytoin (Dilantin) at home.

94 The nurse would be *correct* in explaining to the parents that an adverse effect of long-term use of phenytoin (Dilantin) is
- ○ 1. a poor appetite.
- ○ 2. urinary incontinence.
- ○ 3. painful joints.
- 4. gum overgrowth.

95 Which of the following statements by the parents indicates that teaching has been effective?
- ○ 1. The parents state that phenytoin (Dilantin) should be given on an empty stomach.
- 2. The parents state that the child should not be restrained during seizure activity.
- ○ 3. The parents state that the child will develop mental retardation.
- ○ 4. The parents state that child should no longer attend preschool.

96 Which of the following statements would be *most* appropriate when communicating with the child about the disorder?
- ○ 1. Tell the child that the pain will stop eventually.
- ○ 2. Tell the child the the seizures are not a punishment.
- ○ 3. Tell the child that the medication must be taken.
- 4. Tell the child that other children also have seizures.

NURSING CARE OF A PRESCHOOLER WITH LEUKEMIA

A 5-year-old child suspected of having leukemia is admitted to the hospital for diagnosis and treatment.

97 The nurse would be *correct* in explaining to the parents that the *most* accurate test for confirming a diagnosis of leukemia is
- 1. the Complete Blood Count (CBC).
- ○ 2. spinal fluid examination.
- ○ 3. bone marrow aspiration.
- ○ 4. x-ray of long bones.

Tests confirm that the child has acute lymphoblastic leukemia (ALL). Induction therapy is begun. The child is started on vincristine sulfate, prednisone, and asparaginase (Elspar). The physician also places the child under protective isolation precautions.

98 Which of the following instructions should be given to those visiting the child who is on protective isolation?

○ 1. Only washable toys should be taken into the patient's room.

● 2. Children under 12 years of age should not be taken into the room.

○ 3. Fresh fruit should not be taken into the room.

○ 4. Only an immediate family member may visit.

99 Which of the following routes of temperature assessment would be contraindicated in the child with leukemia?

○ 1. Axillary

● 2. Oral

○ 3. Rectal

○ 4. Tympanic

100 Which of the following medications should the nurse have on hand when asparaginase (Elspar) is being given?

● 1. Epinephrine (Adrenalin)

○ 2. Calcium gluconate

○ 3. Sodium bicarbonate

○ 4. Furosemide (Lasix)

The child receives a transfusion of packed red blood cells.

101 Which of the following statements by the child *best* indicates that the child is having a transfusion reaction?

○ 1. The child complains of being thirsty.

● 2. The child complains of feeling chilly.

○ 3. The child complains of feeling tired.

○ 4. The child complains of being hungry.

102 If the child experiences a transfusion reaction, the *most* appropriate nursing action would be to *initially*

○ 1. administer oxygen and be prepared to start cardiopulmonary resuscitation.

○ 2. check the temperature and give acetaminophen (Tylenol).

● 3. stop the transfusion but keep the intravenous line opened with normal saline.

○ 4. notify the charge nurse and blood bank.

The child asks the nurse, "Am I going to die?"

103 What would be the *most* appropriate response by the nurse?

● 1. "Are you feeling especially bad today? Tell me more about how you feel."

○ 2. "You shouldn't worry about things like that. You are only a little girl."

○ 3. "We are all going to die someday. Usually we die when we get old."

○ 4. "Let's talk about something else. What is your favorite television program?"

104 Which of the following statements by the parents indicates a need for additional teaching?

● 1. The parents state that the child should receive only passive forms of immunity.

○ 2. The parents state that the child should avoid high-contact play activities.

○ 3. The parents state that the child should receive small but frequent high-protein meals.

○ 4. The parents state that the child should not be around individuals with infections.

NURSING CARE OF A PRESCHOOLER WITH STRABISMUS

A 4-year-old child is to be admitted to an ambulatory surgical center for the correction of strabismus (crossed eyes). On the day before the surgery, the child and parents go to the surgical center for preoperative teaching.

105 Which of the following instructions is *most* important for the nurse to give the parents in preparation for the surgical procedure?

○ 1. Clean the child's eyelid with betadine at bedtime.

○ 2. Give the child a Fleet's enema at bedtime.

● 3. Do not give the child anything by mouth after midnight.

○ 4. Give the child a dose of acetaminophen (Tylenol) at bedtime.

The child asks if the surgery will be painful.

106 Which of the following statements would be the *most* appropriate response to the child's question?

○ 1. "Don't think about that now."

○ 2. "No you will not have any pain."

○ 3. "I don't know, ask the doctor."

● 4. "Your eye may be sore after surgery."

The child is admitted the following morning and undergoes surgery.

107 Which of the following types of restraints would be *most* appropriate for the nurse to apply if the child requires restraints.

○ 1. Elbow restraints

● 2. Clove hitch restraints

○ 3. Mummy restraint

○ 4. Body jacket restraint

108 Which of the following statements by the parents indicate a need for additional teaching?

○ 1. "The child can be up and about after the anesthesia wears off."

○ 2. "We will give the child a regular diet after nausea has ceased."

● 3. "We will not allow the child to play with toys for at least 4 weeks."

○ 4. "The restraints can be removed when we are holding the child."

NURSING CARE OF A PRESCHOOLER HAVING A TONSILLECTOMY AND ADENOIDECTOMY

A 5-year-old child who is scheduled for a tonsillectomy and adenoidectomy arrives in the outpatient department the morning of surgery. The nurse admitting the child assesses the vital signs.

109 Which of the following results should be reported *immediately* to the nurse in charge or the physician?
- ○ 1. Blood pressure of 96/60 mm Hg
- ◉ 2. Temperature of 101°F (38.3°C)
- ○ 3. Respiratory rate of 20 per minute
- ○ 4. Pulse rate of 110 beats per minute

The surgery is completed and the child is admitted to a room in the pediatric unit. The physician leaves orders for pain medication and a clear liquid diet.

110 The nurse would be *correct* in giving the child which of the following?
- ○ 1. Orange juice
- ◉ 2. Apple juice
- ○ 3. Ice cream
- ○ 4. Cream of chicken soup

111 If the nurse observes all of the following behaviors, which one should be *corrected*?
- ○ 1. The ice collar is removed from the child's neck.
- ◉ 2. The child is sucking liquids through a straw.
- ○ 3. The parents are holding the child.
- ○ 4. The child is using the bedpan.

112 If the nurse collects all of the following data, which one indicates that the child may have postoperative complications?
- ○ 1. Small amount of dark red emesis
- ○ 2. Respiratory rate 30 breaths per minute
- ○ 3. Complaint of throat pain
- ◉ 4. Frequent swallowing

113 Which of the following instructions should be given to the parents during discharge teaching?
- ◉ 1. The child should be kept quiet for a few days after discharge.
- ○ 2. The child's fluid intake should be limited for the next 48 hours.
- ○ 3. The child should be given aspirin for discomfort and fever.
- ○ 4. The child should resume a regular diet after nausea subsides.

114 The nurse would also be *correct* in telling the parents that the child
- ○ 1. probably will have a great deal of pain for the first 7 days.
- ◉ 2. will have difficulty swallowing for about 3 weeks.
- ○ 3. may expectorate bright red blood for about 1 week.
- ○ 4. may experience a transient earache for about 1 to 3 days.

Directions: Two numbers appear in parentheses following each rationale. The first number identifies the textbook listed in the references, page 512, and the second number identifies the page(s) in that textbook on which the correct answer can be verified. Occasionally two textbooks are given for verifying the correct answer.

NORMAL GROWTH AND DEVELOPMENT OF INFANTS AND TODDLERS

1 2. The 3-month-old, when in the prone position, should be able to raise the head and shoulders to 45–90 degrees. The other observations in question occur later in development. (22:415; 14:338)
　　Nursing Process—Data collection
　　Client Need—Health promotion/maintenance

2 3. Introducing one food at a time makes it easier to identify food tolerances and allergies. Infants will push food out of the mouth because of the extrusion reflex. Cereals should be the first solid food introduced. It may be necessary to breast- or bottle-feed a hungry infant prior to giving solid food. (14:34; 11:170)
　　Nursing Process—Implementation
　　Client Need—Health promotion/maintenance

3 3. The 18-month-old should be able to walk without support and climb stairs while holding on to a railing. The other observations in question are normal for the toddler of this age. (16:413)
　　Nursing Process—Data collection
　　Client Need—Health promotion/maintenance

4 2. Medicine should be kept in a locked cabinet. The child might be able to climb higher than anticipated. The other observations are correct safety measures. (11:240)
　　Nursing Process—Evaluation
　　Client Need—Health promotion/maintenance

NURSING CARE OF PREMATURE INFANTS

5 1. Oxygen given to a premature infant in high concentrations makes the infant especially vulnerable to developing blindness due to hemorrhage of the blood vessels of the eyes, followed by a detachment of the retina. This called retrolental fibroplasia. Frequent monitoring of the concentration of oxygen being administered is necessary to be sure excessive amounts are not being given. Assessment of the bilirubin level, hemoglobin level, and pupillary response will not assist the nurse in preventing retrolental fibroplasia. (16:338)
　　Nursing Process—Implementation
　　Client Need—Safe, effective care environment

6 3. A weak or absent sucking and swallowing reflex may be seen in preterm infants. These infants may require nasogastric feeding or feeding by an umbilical catheter or peripheral vein. The normal interval between feedings is 2 to 3 hours. The amount fed depends on the size of the infant but may be as small as 1 to 5 mL for each feeding. If glucose is tolerated, the physician may order a formula similar to that fed to normal-sized newborns. (11:119; 16:337)
　　Nursing Process—Implementation
　　Client Need—Physiological integrity

7 2. The primary reason that the preterm infant is at risk for developing infections is the lack of antibodies that are normally supplied by the mother during the third trimester of pregnancy and the inability of the infant to produce antibodies independently. Care is taken to prevent exposure to bacterial and viral infections; procedures are done using strict asepsis. The preterm infant does have fragile skin, but measures are taken to prevent skin breakdown. (16:338)
　　Nursing Process—Implementation
　　Client Need—Physiological integrity

8 3. The preterm infant is kept in an isolette because of the increased risk for cold stress secondary to the immaturity of the temperature regulating centers of the brain and other preterm characteristics. The other actions are appropriate actions to maintain thermoregulation in the full-term newborn but will not ensure that the temperature is adequately regulated in the preterm infant. (11:115; 16:338)
　　Nursing Process—Implementation
　　Client Need—Physiological integrity

NURSING CARE OF AN INFANT WITH HEMOLYTIC DISEASE

9 4. Jaundice within 24 to 36 hours after birth indicates congenital hemolytic disease (erythroblastosis fetalis). Physiological jaundice, which occurs in some newborns, is seen 3 to 4 days after birth. Alterations in the respiratory rate, newborn reflexes, and movement of the extremities are not usual manifestations associated with Rh incompatibility. (11:125; 16:356)
Nursing Process—Data collection
Client Need—Physiological integrity

10 4. The direct Coombs test requires a sample of the infant's blood. The usual procedure is to obtain a specimen from the umbilical cord after the infant is delivered and the cord is cut. An indirect Coombs test is performed using a specimen of maternal blood. The paternal blood and sibling blood are not used when a direct or indirect Coombs test is to be performed. (11:125; 16:484)
Nursing Process—Implementation
Client Need—Safe, effective care environment

11 1. Infants with congenital hemolytic disease are placed on phototherapy to reduce the amount of circulating bilirubin. The infant's eyes are covered to protect the retina from damage. Vital signs are monitored every 4 hours. Fluids are given p.o. to maintain hydration and promote excretion of bilirubin via urine and feces. A small covering is also placed over the genitalia to serve the same purpose as a diaper. (14:270)
Nursing Process—Implementation
Client Need—Physiological integrity

NURSING CARE OF AN INFANT WITH MYELOMENINGOCELE

12 2. The most important nursing measure would be to avoid pressure on and prevent injury to the sac. This is important because a break in the sac could lead to serious infection. Washing the area would not be appropriate because of the danger of injury to the sac. Preventing skin breakdown is important but not as important as preventing injury to the sac. (16:345)
Nursing Process—Implementation
Client Need—Physiological integrity

13 3. Infants with spina bifida and myelomeningocele are prone to infection; therefore surgical repair is performed as soon as possible. (14:265)
Nursing Process—Implementation
Client Need—Health promotion/maintenance

14 2. The prone position (lying on the abdomen) is used after surgical repair of a myelomeningocele. This position is maintained until the operative site heals. It is important to keep the operative site clean and free of pressure in order to prevent infection. (16:345)
Nursing Process—Implementation
Client Need—Physiological integrity

15 1. A child born with spina bifida with myelomeningocele located high in the spinal column has a poor prognosis in terms of being able to walk alone. The child may be able to use a wheelchair or possibly braces and crutches. When the myelomeningocele is low in the spine (in or near the sacral area, for example), only minimal weakness of the lower extremities may be seen. (16:345)
Nursing Process—Planning
Client Need—Safe, effective care environment

16 2. Urinary and bowel control problems usually are seen in those with spina bifida and myelomeningocele. Intermittent catheterization is required in most cases. Parents are taught how to perform catheterization using clean technique. During the early school years the child also will be taught how to perform this procedure. The infant with myelomeningocele usually does not require a ureterostomy. (16:345)
Nursing Process—Implementation
Client Need—Health promotion/maintenance

NURSING CARE OF AN INFANT WITH HYDROCEPHALUS

17 1. An increase in head size is the most prominent symptom of hydrocephalus. Some hydrocephalus infants also have spina bifida with a myelomeningocele and may have lower extremity paralysis, but this neurologic deficit is not a prominent symptom of hydrocephalus. The presence or absence of the sucking reflex is not considered a prominent sign. Usually there is bulging of the fontanel instead of depression. (16:342)
Nursing Process—Data collection
Client Need—Physiological integrity

18 2. The cause of hydrocephalus in most infants is a blockage (obstruction) that prevents proper circulation of cerebrospinal fluid. This is known as the noncommunicating type of congenital hydrocephalus. Absence of the dura mater, increased cerebrospinal fluid, and blockage in the cerebral arteries are not known causes of hydrocephalus. (16:342; 11:1460)
Nursing Process—Implementation
Client Need—Psychosocial integrity

19 4. The side-lying position is the position of choice after feeding an infant with hydrocephalus. Infants with hydrocephalus are at risk for vomiting because of increased intracranial pressure. By placing the infant in the side-lying position, vomitus can escape easily from the mouth, and the chance of aspiration of vomitus is reduced. Each of the positions identified in the remaining options may result in aspiration. (4:1421)

Nursing Process—Implementation
Client Need—Safe, effective care environment

20 1. The head and ears of an infant with hydrocephalus are especially prone to the development of pressure ulcers. The primary reason for using a sheepskin in this situation is to help relieve pressure on the head and ears. The client's position also should be changed frequently to prevent complications due to inactivity. The other options are incorrect because they will not relieve pressure on the infant's head. (4:1421)

Nursing Process—Implementation
Client Need—Safe, effective care environment

21 3. The position of choice after installing a shunting device in an infant with hydrocephalus is on the side opposite the site of the surgical incision. This position prevents damage to the shunt valve. The infant described in this question should be placed on the left side postoperatively because the surgical site of entry was on the right side of the head. (16:343)

Nursing Process—Implementation
Client Need—Safe, effective care environment

22 2. Signs of increased intracranial pressure in an infant include bulging or tense fontanels, a decrease in pulse and respiratory rate, irritability, and vomiting. Changes in weight and bowel elimination are not usual indicators of increased intracranial pressure. (16:343)

Nursing Process—Data collection
Client Need—Physiological integrity

23 2. If the fontanel is sunken, the child is kept in the flat position. This position will prevent a rapid decrease in intracranial pressure. If the fontanel is bulging, the head is elevated. The charge nurse and/or physician may be notified, but not prior to placing the infant in a flat position. (11:146; 16:343)

Nursing Process—Implementation
Client Need—Physiological integrity

NURSING CARE OF AN INFANT WITH CLEFT LIP

24 3. Cleft palate occurs with about 50% of cleft lips, especially bilateral cleft lip. Palpating the roof of the mouth will identify a cleft palate but will not elicit the gag reflex, nor will it assist in assessment of the infant's sucking ability and the position of the uvula. (11:131)

Nursing Process—Data collection
Client Need—Physiological integrity

25 2. A major problem encountered when caring for the child with cleft lip is the parent's reaction to the appearance of the child. Demonstrating acceptance of the child, encouraging expression of feeling, and acknowledging appropriateness of feelings are ways in which the nurse can facilitate parental adjustment. Feeding, surgical repair, and use of the bulb syringe are important, but the parents first must begin to adjust to the child's appearance before they can deal with these issues. (16:349; 11:132)

Nursing Process—Implementation
Client Need—Psychosocial integrity

26 3. Of the four options, a rubber-tip syringe is the best method of feeding the infant with cleft lip. A small medicine dropper or specially designed nipple are other methods that are sometimes used. Feeding the infant with a plastic spoon or firm rubber nipple may still result in aspiration through the opening in the palate. Gavage feeding is not usually necessary because the remainder of the gastrointestinal tract is intact. (16:349; 11:133)

Nursing Process—Implementation
Client Need—Physiological integrity

27 1. Infants with cleft lip swallow more air than usual; therefore they should be burped frequently to decrease the chance of emesis and subsequent aspiration. The prone position should be avoided. The infant is fed regular formula prior to surgery. (16:350)

Nursing Process—Evaluation
Client Need—Health promotion/maintenance

NURSING CARE OF AN INFANT WITH PYLORIC STENOSIS

28 4. Dry mucous membranes are an indication of dehydration. The infant must be rehydrated and electrolytes must be within normal limits prior to going to surgery. The anterior fontanel is normally flat. Hunger and visible gastric peristaltic waves are present with pyloric stenosis but do not indicate the same level of threat to health as does dehydration. (11:260; 14:591)

> Nursing Process—Data collection
> Client Need—Physiological integrity

29 1. The site of choice for IV therapy in infants is the scalp vein because of the supply of superficial veins. Use of scalp veins requires that the infant's hair be shaved. Restlessness and swelling are not usual findings, so they should be reported immediately because they may indicate IV infiltration. IV therapy does not require that the infant be n.p.o., and the infant with pyloric stenosis may be given feedings of thickened formula prior to going to surgery. (11:59; 14:430)

> Nursing Process—Implementation
> Client Need—Health promotion/maintenance

30 2. After feeding, the infant should be placed on the right side or in an infant seat. These positions aid in emptying the stomach and preventing aspiration. The left side does not facilitate gastric emptying. The prone position is not recommended because of its association with the occurrence of sudden infant death syndrome (SIDS). Placing the infant on his or her back creates a greater risk for aspiration of the contents of the stomach. (16:759)

> Nursing Process—Implementation
> Client Need—Health promotion/maintenance

NURSING CARE OF AN INFANT WITH BILATERAL CLUBFOOT

31 3. The infant should be evaluated carefully because the feet may appear to be clubbed but actually be the result of *in utero* positioning. True clubfeet are fixed and cannot be corrected to the neutral or natural position. One or both feet may be involved. The heels may be drawn in and the feet turned inward in both the infant with true clubfoot and the infant with false clubfoot. Not all children who are born breech develop clubfoot. (16:358; 14:268)

> Nursing Process—Data collection
> Client Need—Physiological integrity

32 4. Newly applied casts should be handled with the palms of the hands. Using this technique decreases the likelihood of indentations in the cast, which could cause tissue injury and disturbances in circulation. Using the fingertips may cause indentation of the cast. Gloves and a sling usually are not required when handling the wet cast. (16:704; 22:682)

> Nursing Process—Implementation
> Client Need—Physiological integrity

33 3. Pale, cold extremities are signs of impaired circulation to the extremities caused by pressure of the cast. This problem must be reported immediately. Crying 4 hours after last feeding is normal because the infant is likely to be hungry, but unexplained crying may indicate pain or discomfort. Wiggling the toes is a sign that the nervous system has not been compromised by application of a cast. A pulse rate of 110 is normal. (16:708; 22:684)

> Nursing Process—Evaluation
> Client Need—Physiological integrity

34 1. After a cast is applied to the lower extremities, the extremities are elevated on pillows to improve circulation and prevent swelling. Position is usually changed every 2 hours to promote even drying. Petaling the edges is performed to prevent skin breakdown. Ice packs are not used to decrease swelling associated with casting. (16:705)

> Nursing Process—Implementation
> Client Need—Physiological integrity

35 1. The purpose of casting is to gradually correct the defect without causing trauma; therefore the casts are changed every few days initially, then every 1 to 2 weeks. Correction is usually achieved in approximately 6 to 8 weeks. (16:358; 22:677)

> Nursing Process—Implementation
> Client Need—Health promotion/maintenance

36 4. An infant develops the ability to look at surroundings during the first month of life. By 2 months, the infant is able to follow an object with both eyes. The mobile is an appropriate amusement for a 2-month-old infant. By 4 months of age the infant normally can reach for objects, and by 7 to 9 months the infant is able to crawl and play peek-a-boo. Also, it would not be appropriate to encourage an infant in a cast to crawl. (16:405)

> Nursing Process—Implementation
> Client Need—Health promotion/maintenance

37 1. The posterior fontanel normally closes between 2 and 3 months of age. All of the other options give inaccurate information. (11:168)

> Nursing Process—Implementation
> Client Need—Health promotion/maintenance

NURSING CARE OF AN INFANT WITH OTITIS MEDIA

38 2. The infant with otitis media usually pulls at or rubs the ear that is affected because of the pain that occurs secondary to the pressure of the fluid on

the tympanic membrane. The other options may be present with otitis media but are not caused by or related to the pain. (14:624)
> Nursing Process—Data collection
> Client Need—Physiological integrity

39 2. The physician prescribes the amount of medication to be given. However, the nurse has the responsibility of determining if the prescribed dose is within the recommended safe dosage range. The most reliable method of determining the recommended safe dosage range requires use of the child's weight. The other options are important steps in medication administration but do not relate specifically to determining the safe dose. (14:427; 16:542)
> Nursing Process—Planning
> Client Need—Physiological integrity

40 4. The parents should be instructed to complete the full course of antibiotics even though the child's condition may improve after 2 to 3 days of treatment. Failure to complete the full course of antibiotics may lead to recurrent infection and other associated complications. Whether or not the antibiotic is given with food and how the antibiotic is stored varies, depending on the specific antibiotic. The position of the child after the antibiotic is given normally is not significant; if the medication was an ear drop, however, the position would be significant. (11:213)
> Nursing Process—Implementation
> Client Need—Health promotion/maintenance

NURSING CARE OF AN INFANT WITH A CONGENITAL HEART DEFECT

41 3. In the child with coarctation of the aorta, the pulses are bounding in the upper extremities and are weak in the lower extremities. Also, the blood pressure is higher in the upper extremities than in the lower extremities. This occurs because of the narrowing of the aorta that occurs with coarctation. The other choices may at some point develop, but also can be associated with other defects. (16:744)
> Nursing Process—Data collection
> Client Need—Physiological integrity

42 4. Initially the child may be given prostaglandin E to dilate the narrowed aorta. The corrective treatment is surgical repair, however, which usually is performed when the child is between 2 and 4 years of age. If correction is not performed, the child may developed life-threatening complications. (14:511)
> Nursing Process—Implementation
> Client Need—Health promotion/maintenance

43 1. The apical pulse should be checked for 1 full minute before giving Lanoxin. If the pulse is less than the normal lower limit, the medication should not be given and the doctor should be notified. When giving any medication, not just Lanoxin, the infant should have the head slightly elevated. The expiration date should be checked prior to giving any medication. Kidney function should be adequate, since medications are primarily excreted by the kidneys; these factors are not unique to Lanoxin, however. (11:153)
> Nursing Process—Implementation
> Client Need—Physiological integrity

44 2. Organizing nursing care so that there are longer periods of rest decreases the energy demands; the workload of the heart therefore is decreased. Parents are encouraged to hold and cuddle the child. The child is fed by nasogastric route only when the child has a poor suck reflex or if the feedings are taking too long, because these increase energy expenditure. The child is not routinely sedated. (11:153)
> Nursing Process—Implementation
> Client Need—Physiological integrity

45 3. Lanoxin should not be mixed in the infant's formula or food. The infant may not take all of the formula or food, and thus may not get the correct amount of medication. All of the other statements are correct and indicate that instructions were understood by the parents. (14:514)
> Nursing Process—Evaluation
> Client Need—Health promotion/maintenance

NURSING CARE OF AN INFANT WITH AN INFECTIOUS DISEASE

46 2. Children who are hospitalized with chickenpox are placed in strict isolation because this disease is highly contagious. The other isolation procedures identified in this question do not prevent transmission of chickenpox. (22:558)
> Nursing Process—Implementation
> Client Need—Safe, effective care environment

47 1. The client's room is considered contaminated; the mask and other personal protective equipment (PPE) should be kept outside of the client's room. All of the other actions are consistent with isolation procedures for a client in strict isolation. (18:604)
> Nursing Process—Implementation
> Client Need—Safe, effective care environment

48 4. It is important to monitor the infusion rate carefully to prevent circulatory overload. Voiding frequently,

sleeping, and crying when disturbed by noise are considered normal behaviors for an infant. (16:535)
Nursing Process—Data collection
Client Need—Physiological integrity

NURSING CARE OF AN INFANT OF AN HIV-POSITIVE MOTHER

49 3. Nursing care of the HIV-positive client should include universal precautions. Universal precautions were developed by the Centers for Disease Control in an effort to prevent blood-borne infections such as hepatitis and human immunodeficiency virus (HIV). The other forms of isolation are not necessary and are not used unless additional protection is needed for a specific disorder. (14:273; 18:603)
Nursing Process—Implementation
Client Need—Safe, effective care environment

50 3. From 30% to 50% of children who are HIV-positive contracted the virus via perinatal transmission. Infants of HIV-positive mothers are not tested for anti-HIV antibodies before 3 months of age because the mother's antibodies may be present in the baby's blood for at least that long; thus the HIV antibody test may give a false positive reading. Infants of HIV-positive mothers are usually tested periodically for at least 2 years. (14:531)
Nursing Process—Implementation
Client Need—Health promotion/maintenance

51 4. Infants who are HIV-positive are usually asymptomatic at birth but usually develop symptoms of AIDS by 2 years of age. (11:127; 16:252)
Nursing Process—Implementation
Client Need—Health promotion/maintenance

52 3. The human immunodeficiency virus (HIV) can be transmitted via breast milk; therefore HIV-positive mothers are instructed not to breast-feed the newborn because of the possibility of transmission. Transmission of the human immunodeficiency virus can occur even if the mother is not exhibiting signs and symptoms of acquired immunodeficiency syndrome (AIDS). An infant whose test result is positive for the anti-HIV antibodies may have maternal anti-HIV antibodies; thus the infant actually may not have the virus even though the test result is positive. Because of this the infant should not be breast-fed, regardless of whether the anti-HIV antibody test is positive or not. Absence of symptoms in the newborn would be more indicative of the absence of the HIV than its presence; therefore breast-feeding this infant would possibly expose an uninfected infant to the virus. (11:126)
Nursing Process—Implementation
Client Need—Health promotion/maintenance

53 2. Infants who are HIV-positive and develop AIDS often present with thrush, mouth sores, and severe diaper rashes. It also is not uncommon for these children to develop bacterial infections and *Pneumocystis carinii* pneumonia. The other options are examples of normal behaviors or characteristics of the infant. (11:126)
Nursing Process—Data collection
Client Need—Physiological integrity

NURSING CARE OF AN INFANT WITH ATOPIC DERMATITIS

54 3. Infantile eczema is thought to be caused, at least in part, by allergic reactions to some irritant(s), which is why the physician asked questions about the home environment. Also, it appears that hereditary factors may play a role. The other options have not been identified as causes of infantile eczema. Poor nutrition, premature birth, and hormone imbalances are not associated with the development of atopic dermatitis. (11:229)
Nursing Process—Implementation
Client Need—Health promotion/maintenance

55 3. An infant with eczema experiences severe itching of the skin lesions. The nurse must be prepared to teach home caretakers about measures that will help relieve itching so that the child does not scratch the skin and introduce microorganisms into the lesions, which will cause secondary infection to develop. Nausea, vomiting, and drowsiness are not usual symptoms of atopic dermatitis. (11:229)
Nursing Process—Implementation
Client Need—Health promotion/maintenance

56 3. Hydrocortisone is an anti-inflammatory drug. It helps to reduce inflammation and its symptoms, such as swelling, redness, heat, and discomfort. This medication does not influence weeping of lesions, the spread of the disease, or the white blood cell count. (11:229)
Nursing Process—Evaluation
Client Need—Physiological integrity

57 1. Colloid baths have been found effective for their soothing effects on the irritated and itching skin of an infant with eczema. The most commonly used type of colloidal bath preparations is a mixture of baking soda and cornstarch added to tepid water. Other colloid bath preparations include cooked oatmeal and commercial bath preparations. Mineral oil, liquid glycerin soap, and salt are not components of a colloidal bath. (11:229)
Nursing Process—Implementation
Client Need—Health promotion/maintenance

NURSING CARE OF A TODDLER WITH SICKLE CELL CRISIS

58 1. The sickle-shaped cells tend to clump together in vessels and obstruct the normal blood flow. A thrombus may form and cause death of tissue because of poor blood circulation. The characteristic symptom when tissue is denied normal blood circulation is severe pain in the affected parts of the body. Diarrhea, bradycardia, and hemorrhage usually are not associated with sickle cell crisis. (11:208)
Nursing Process—Implementation
Client Need—Physiological integrity

59 4. The child with sickle cell crisis is prone to dehydration. The child is encouraged to drink fluids. It is helpful to offer the child appealing fluids such as juices, Popsicles, and gelatins. It may be necessary during the acute stage to rehydrate the child with IV fluids. Whole-blood transfusions may be given to increase hemoglobin levels. Iron is of no value in the treatment of this blood disorder. (11:209)
Nursing Process—Planning
Client Need—Physiological integrity

60 2. Sickle cell disease occurs when the child inherits the trait from both parents. If one parent has the disease and one parent has the trait, then all offspring will have at least the trait. Furthermore, there is a 50% chance that the offspring will have sickle cell disease. Providing information about the probability of offspring having sickle cell disease or trait can be given only in terms of each conception. The only instance in which it is possible to predict that all offspring will definitely have the disease is the situation in which both parents have sickle cell disease. (11:207)
Nursing Process—Evaluation
Client Need—Health promotion/maintenance

NURSING CARE OF A TODDLER WITH CYSTIC FIBROSIS

61 3. Many times, caretakers of children with cystic fibrosis become aware of a typical sign of the illness when they report that a child tastes salty when they kiss the child. The perspiration, tears, and saliva contain abnormally high concentrations of salt. Sweat analysis is an important diagnostic tool when children are examined for cystic fibrosis. These children are typically underweight. Infrequent crying, weight gain, and poor head control are findings that may be associated with the presence of other disorders as well. (16:721)
Nursing Process—Data collection
Client Need—Physiological integrity

62 4. Typically, the stools of a child with cystic fibrosis are large, sticky, and foul-smelling; the condition is due to diminished or absent flow of pancreatic enzymes, which leads to faulty absorption of nutrients, especially fat-soluble vitamins. Other signs include malnutrition despite a hearty appetite, chronic coughing, and distended abdomen. Children with cystic fibrosis usually eat very well but fail to gain weight, do not usually perspire excessively, and usually do not have a low urine output. (16:720)
Nursing Process—Data collection
Client Need—Physiological integrity

63 2. The cause of death in children with cystic fibrosis most often is related to respiratory or cardiac failure; thus the priority goal would be maintenance of an effective breathing pattern. All of the other goals are appropriate for the child with cystic fibrosis, but address threats to sustaining life that are not as great as that addressed by altering respiratory function. (16:722)
Nursing Process—Planning
Client Need—Physiological integrity

64 3. The air passages of the lungs of those with cystic fibrosis become clogged with mucus, thus decreasing the amount of oxygen reaching the lungs. A bronchodilator increases the diameter of the bronchi, thereby allowing more air to enter the lungs, and breathing is improved. Characteristics of the stool, serum sodium levels, and fat excretion by the body are not affected by bronchodilator. (14:487)
Nursing Process—Evaluation
Client Need—Physiological integrity

65 4. A child with cystic fibrosis may need 1½ to 2 times the normal caloric intake to meet caloric needs. The diet should be high in protein and carbohydrates. No restrictions on fat intake are necessary if the child is taking the Pancrease as prescribed. However, the child should not consume excessive amounts of fat. The child may require an increase in the intake of salt, especially during summer months when there is excessive sweating. (11:258; 14:487)
Nursing Process—Implementation
Client Need—Health promotion/maintenance

66 2. Commercially prepared pancreatic enzymes should be given with meals and snacks in order to facilitate absorption of nutrients. Pancreatic enzyme preparations have no relationship to the child's appetite, prevention of salt depletion, or prevention of gastric upset. (14:487)
Nursing Process—Implementation
Client Need—Health promotion/maintenance

67 4. In children with cystic fibrosis, sodium and chloride become trapped in the cells of the lining of the lungs. The salt draws liquids from the airways and causes the mucus in the airways to be thick and sticky. Maintaining adequate fluid intake will help to liquefy secretions in the airways, which ultimately will improve breathing. The goal of increased fluid intake for the child who has cystic fibrosis is not to prevent kidney failure, improve cardiac function, or reduce pain and discomfort. (14:486; 16:724)

> Nursing Process—Implementation
> Client Need—Health promotion/maintenance

68 2. Children with cystic fibrosis are very susceptible to infections, especially infections of the respiratory tract. The parents should be taught to guard against exposing the child to infections to the greatest extent possible. Immunization against childhood diseases is highly recommended, especially those that may place the respiratory tract at risk. Airborne pollen and pet dander are usually avoided when there is a history of respiratory symptoms secondary to environmental allergies. Avoiding exposure to bright sunlight is not of great importance unless there is the possibility of excessive sweating, which would result in excessive loss of sodium. Protection from exposure to infection takes priority over preventing exposure to bright sunlight. (11:261)

> Nursing Process—Evaluation
> Client Need—Health promotion/maintenance

NURSING CARE OF A TODDLER WITH ASTHMA

69 1. Wheezing and a dry, hacking cough are major manifestations of an acute asthma attack. The normal respiratory rate for a 3-year-old is 20 to 30 breaths per minute. Also, children begin to assume a thoracic breathing pattern around 3 years of age. Clear, watery nasal drainage is usually seen in upper respiratory tract disorders. (11:348)

> Nursing Process—Data collection
> Client Need—Physiological integrity

70 4. The most effective method of relieving the child's acute respiratory distress is placing the child in the semi-Fowler's position. The older child may be more comfortable leaning forward on a pillow on an over-bed table. Cool mist humidifiers are used, as opposed to steam vaporizers. Antibiotics will not relieve the acute respiratory distress. Distracting the child with age-appropriate toys is not an effective strategy when the child is experiencing acute distress. (11:352)

> Nursing Process—Implementation
> Client Need—Physiological integrity

71 4. If the breathing exercises are incorporated into play activities, the child is more likely to enjoy them and will thus practice the exercises more. Promises of treats, parental assistance with the exercise, and demonstrations and return demonstrations are not likely to be as effective as incorporating the exercises into play activities. (11:351)

> Nursing Process—Implementation
> Client Need—Health promotion/maintenance

72 4. When a client has asthma due to an allergy to one or more environmental factors, general control of the environment is necessary to reduce chances of future asthma attacks. A generous fluid intake is recommended because fluid is lost through sweating and an increased respiratory rate. A well-balanced diet is necessary, especially for the growing child. Asthma cannot be cured, but often it can be controlled. (11:353; 16:735)

> Nursing Process—Implementation
> Client Need—Health promotion/maintenance

NURSING CARE OF A TODDLER WHO HAS SWALLOWED A TOXIC SUBSTANCE

73 3. When a caustic substance is ingested, water or milk should be given to dilute the substance. Vomiting should not be induced because the substance may cause additional injury when coming back up. There also is a danger of respiratory complications secondary to aspiration of vomitus. The threat to life or health should be addressed before the child is taken to the emergency department. Cardiopulmonary resuscitation may or may not be necessary, depending on the injury incurred. (16:467)

> Nursing Process—Implementation
> Client Need—Physiological integrity

74 1. Substernal and intercostal retractions indicate that the child is experiencing respiratory distress; this child therefore should have the oxygen saturation level monitored in order to assist in determining the child's need for additional therapy to relieve or minimize respiratory distress. The child possibly will have all of the other manifestations, but they do not indicate respiratory distress. (14:477)

> Nursing Process—Data collection
> Client Need—Physiological integrity

75 2. The child may experience pain secondary to burns on the lips and in the mouth from the lye-based substance. Gastric lavage is not performed when caustic substances have been ingested. A gastrostomy may be necessary with severe damage. The child is given liquids by mouth as tolerated. Neurovascular checks are not usually required. (11:263)

> Nursing Process—Implementation
> Client Need—Physiological integrity

76 4. All poisonous substances should be placed in locked compartments or cabinets. Children often can climb and reach areas that they might not be thought capable of reaching. It would be very difficult to remove all poisonous substances from the home, or to keep a constant eye on the child. (16:470)

>Nursing Process—Evaluation
>Client Need—Health promotion/maintenance

NURSING CARE OF A TODDLER WITH CROUP

77 1. Laryngotracheobronchitis (LTB) most often is caused by a virus. It is not related to whooping cough or inadequate development of the lungs. LTB may occur in those with or without a history of asthma. (14:482)

>Nursing Process—Implementation
>Client Need—Health promotion/maintenance

78 2. The child with croup has a cough that sounds hoarse, much like a loud, barking, metallic sound. The cough is not usually dry instead of moist and loud instead of muffled. Wheezing is a term used to describe breath sounds, not cough characteristics. (14:483)

>Nursing Process—Data collection
>Client Need—Physiological integrity

79 3. To help liquefy secretions and reduce laryngeal spasms, the child with croup should breathe air that is high in humidity. A mist tent or a cool mist vaporizer may be used for this purpose. A dust-free environment would be required for children who are allergic to dust. Dry or hot air does not provide relief for children with croup. (16:726)

>Nursing Process—Implementation
>Client Need—Health promotion/maintenance

80 2. Extreme anxiousness is a sign of respiratory difficulty and may indicate more serious involvement of the trachea and bronchial tree. The physician should be contacted immediately in this case. Fever, coughing during the night, and sleeping during the day are not considered signs of more serious involvement. (16:726).

>Nursing Process—Implementation
>Client Need—Health promotion/maintenance

81 2. Aspirin, a salicylate, is contraindicated in young children with a fever, flu-like symptoms, or chickenpox; aspirin use has been associated with Reye's syndrome. All of the other options identify appropriate statements about croup. (14:483)

>Nursing Process—Evaluation
>Client Need—Health promotion/maintenance

82 2. The parents are encouraged to remain close to the child because emotional upset can cause an increase in respiratory distress. The child with croup is not usually sedated. Age-appropriate toys usually do not interest the child during the acute stage. Sometimes it is necessary to perform procedures that may be unpleasant for the child in order to stabilize or improve the child's condition. (16:726)

>Nursing Process—Implementation
>Client Need—Psychosocial integrity

83 4. Nebulized racemic epinephrine may be utilized to reduce edema and obstruction of the airway. Laryngotracheobronchitis is usually caused by a virus; thus antibiotics would not be routinely given to this child. The other two medications are also not routinely given to children with croup. (22:628)

>Nursing Process—Implementation
>Client Need—Physiological integrity

NURSING CARE OF A TODDLER WITH PNEUMONIA

84 4. The respiratory pattern in children with pneumonia is usually rapid and shallow. The rapid respiratory rate is the body's way of compensating for the decreased ventilation in the lungs. The pulse is usually elevated in the child with pneumonia. Clubbing of the fingers is seen in chronic illnesses that have associated chronic lack of oxygen. Synchronized breathing is characteristic of a normal breathing pattern. (16:717)

>Nursing Process—Data collection
>Client Need—Physiological data

85 1. Recording the child's urinary output will assist in determining fluid needs. Fluid loss because of high fever, vomiting, and increased respiratory rate are common in the child with pneumonia. As a result of fluid loss, the urinary output decreases. The urine is dark in color and the specific gravity is high. The nurse should measure the fluid intake as well. The pH of the urine will indicate if the urine is acidic or alkalotic; it will not indicate hydration status. The child's blood pressure may be normal and the child still may be dehydrated. A drop in blood pressure occurs with circulatory collapse, but this would be a late sign. An increased respiratory rate may result in an increased insensible fluid loss, which indicates a risk for dehydration, but this does not tell about the hydration status of the child. (16:719)

>Nursing Process—Planning
>Client Need—Physiological integrity

86 3. Pulse oximetry is utilized to determine the oxygen saturation in the blood. A value less than 95 indicates that the saturation level may not be sufficient to meet the oxygen demand of the client. In this case the nurse in charge or physician should be notified. (18:631).

> Nursing Process—Evaluation
> Client Need—Physiological integrity

87 3. Expectorants help loosen secretions so that the client can raise and get rid of mucus that has accumulated in the airways. Suppressants prevent the child from coughing. If there is a moist cough, then secretions are in the airway and they need to be removed. Antibiotics and bronchodilators have no effect on the cough. (16:719)

> Nursing Process—Implementation
> Client Need—Physiological integrity

88 3. If the child is observed to be shivering, the bath should be stopped immediately because shivering will further increase the core body temperature. The bath should not be given for more than 30 minutes. Tepid water is used for the bath. The temperature should fall, but may not fall below 101°F. (11:45)

> Nursing Process—Implementation
> Client Need—Safe, effective care environment

89 2. Having an interpreter present when instructions are given will allow the nurse to give clear instructions, as well as validate the parents' understanding of the instructions. Providing a copy of the instructions in Spanish should be used as a reinforcement, but it will not guarantee that the parents understand the instructions. Having the physician give the instructions will be the same as the nurse giving the instructions if the physician does not speak Spanish. Parents are encouraged to call if questions arise after discharge, but they first must have some basic understanding of instructions prior to being discharged. (18:404)

> Nursing Process—Evaluation
> Client Need—Health promotion/maintenance

NURSING CARE OF A PRESCHOOLER WITH SEIZURE DISORDER

90 4. Generalized involuntary movement of the body is characteristic of grand mal seizures. A child may have seizures associated with fever, but not all children who have a fever have seizures. The child also could drop to the floor with other disorders, such as muscle weakness and unconsciousness. The child may wet the bed after a seizure has ceased, but bedwetting could occur for other reasons. (11:345)

> Nursing Process—Data collection
> Client Need—Physiological integrity

91 1. The priority nursing action for a child experiencing a generalized seizure is protection from injury. Padding the side rails is one means of protecting the child. Phenobarbital may be given to a child who has grand mal seizures, but it is not usually kept in the child's room. The other options are not routinely used in caring for the child with grand mal seizures. (16:663)

> Nursing Process—Planning
> Client Need—Safe, effective care environment

92 4. It is not necessary to have a cool mist humidifier at the bedside of a child subject to seizure activity. Suction equipment may be required to remove mucus from the child's mouth. An oral airway and oxygen may be needed in the case of respiratory arrest, which can occur with generalized seizures. (16:664)

> Nursing Process—Planning
> Client Need—Safe, effective care environment

93 2. Placing the child in the side-lying position establishes a patent airway and prevents aspiration of saliva. Inserting a padded tongue blade is no longer recommended because injury to the mouth and teeth may occur. The nurse should be prepared to administer oxygen after the seizure if it is required. Calling for assistance is not an appropriate first action because the nurse should first implement actions that will minimize injury to the child. (16:663)

> Nursing Process—Implementation
> Client Need—Physiological integrity

94 4. Phenytoin (Dilantin), when used over time, tends to cause an overgrowth of gum tissues. Poor appetite, urinary incontinence, and painful joints are not associated with the use of Dilantin. (11:345)

> Nursing Process—Implementation
> Client Need—Health promotion/maintenance

95 2. The child should not be restrained during seizure activity because this may result in injury to child instead of protection. The parents should be encouraged to maintain as normal a lifestyle as is possible for the child. Mental retardation does not always occur with seizure disorder. Dilantin should be given with food or immediately after meals to reduce stomach irritation. (16:664)

> Nursing Process—Evaluation
> Client Need—Health promotion/maintenance

96 2. The preschool child often thinks that illness or painful treatments are a punishment for having done something bad. It is important to explain to the child that the seizure activity is not a punishment. The nurse must always be honest with the child. The child might be told that the medication must be taken and that other children have seizures, but communicating this information could be necessary for children in any developmental period. (14:376)

> Nursing Process—Implementation
> Client Need—Health promotion/maintenance

NURSING CARE OF A PRESCHOOLER WITH LEUKEMIA

97 3. The test most often used to confirm a diagnosis of leukemia is bone marrow aspiration. The bone marrow of the client with leukemia is characterized by being hypercellular, lacking fat globules, and having blast cells (immature white cells). The CBC and spinal fluid examination also are part of the battery of tests a client may have when leukemia is suspected, but they do not confirm the diagnosis. (16:807)
Nursing Process—Implementation
Client Need—Health promotion/maintenance

98 3. Fresh fruits should not be taken into the child's room because they may harbor organisms that can cause life-threatening illnesses in the child with leukemia. The risk of contracting a life-threatening illness relates to the child's compromised immune system. Washable toys are recommended for children who are in isolation because they are contagious and to prevent the spread of infection to other individuals, whereas the child in protective isolation has a greater chance of contracting an infection than spreading an infection to someone else. Visitation requirements vary from facility to facility. Family members and children under 12 years of age may be permitted to visit as long as they do not have any type of active infectious disease process. (18:607)
Nursing Process—Implementation
Client Need—Safe, effective care environment

99 3. Rectal temperatures should not be taken in children with leukemia because there is a possibility that the child will develop a perirectal abscess. This can lead to a life-threatening situation because of the child's immunosuppressed state. An axillary, oral, or tympanic temperature may be obtained from the child who has leukemia. (16:811)
Nursing Process—Planning
Client Need—Physiological integrity

100 1. Oxygen and epinephrine should be on hand when giving asparaginase (Elspar) because there is an increased risk of the child having an anaphylactic reaction. The other medications are not required. (14:527)
Nursing Process—Planning
Client Need—Physiological integrity

101 2. Signs of transfusion reaction include feeling cold and having chills, fever, and a rapid pulse rate. The client also may complain of itching and low back pain. If a feeling of chilliness occurs very early in a blood transfusion, it may be the result of the cold transfused blood entering the body. Nevertheless, a transfusion reaction should be suspected until proven otherwise. Complaints of hunger, thirst, and tiredness are not usual indicators of a blood transfusion reaction. (18:1133)
Nursing Process—Data collection
Client Need—Physiological integrity

102 3. If a client is having a reaction to blood, the nurse should *first* clamp the tubing to stop the blood flow. The clamp on the second bottle (normal saline) then should be immediately opened in order to maintain intravenous access. The temperature is taken and acetaminophen (Tylenol) may be given if ordered and if necessary. The charge nurse should be notified, but not before the infusion is stopped. (18:1133)
Nursing Process—Implementation
Client Need—Physiological integrity

103 1. "Am I going to die?" is a question that can be answered in many different ways. However, the nurse's response should encourage the child to ventilate feelings about dying. The nurse should avoid responses that would either make the child feel guilty or discourage the child from talking about anxieties experienced. The nurse's response also should not reinforce denials and unrealistic perceptions of the child's prognosis. When dealing with children, it is important that answers to questions be honest and based on the child's level of understanding. (16:836)
Nursing Process—Implementation
Client Need—Psychosocial integrity

104 1. Children who have leukemia should postpone live-virus vaccines for 6 to 12 months after chemotherapy has been discontinued. The child's blood count values also should be within normal ranges. All of the other statements by the parents are consistent with the recommended treatment plan. (14:528)
Nursing Process—Evaluation
Client Need—Health promotion/maintenance

NURSING CARE OF A PRESCHOOLER WITH STRABISMUS

105 3. Foods and fluids generally are withheld for 6 to 12 hours before surgery to reduce the risk of aspirating vomitus when the client is under anesthesia and when recovering from anesthesia. Preparation of the eyelids is usually carried out in the healthcare setting. A Fleet's enema is not routinely needed for eye surgery. Acetaminophen is not usually given as a preparation for eye surgery. (18:1083)
Nursing Process—Implementation
Client Need—Safe, effective care environment

106 4. Some soreness may occur after this type of eye surgery. The child's question should not be ignored or minimized. The nurse should answer the child's question honestly. The explanation also should be developmentally appropriate. (11:252)

> Nursing Process—Implementation
> Client Need—Psychosocial integrity

107 1. If restraints are necessary and are ordered by the physician, elbow restraints are usually preferred because they accomplish the goal, which is to prevent injury to the operative site, and at the same time allow the child to have the maximum possible level of mobility. The other restraint choices will prevent injury to the operative site but also restrict the child's movement more than is necessary. (18:900)

> Nursing Process—Implementation
> Client Need—Safe, effective care environment

108 3. Unless the physician orders otherwise, a regular diet can be given once nausea has ceased and the child can be up and about. Unless both eyes are bandaged, the child can play with toys with adult supervision. Reading to a child of this age is appropriate. (11:252; 18:900)

> Nursing Process—Evaluation
> Client Need—Health promotion/maintenance

NURSING CARE OF A PRESCHOOLER HAVING A TONSILLECTOMY AND ADENOIDECTOMY

109 2. It is important to report promptly an elevated temperature of a preoperative client, along with any other signs of infection, such as a sore throat, cough, or excessive nasal discharge. Surgery will be canceled if the child has an infection. The other vital signs in this question are normal for a child of this age. (11:313)

> Nursing Process—Data collection
> Client Need—Safe, effective care environment

110 2. Clear liquids include clear broth, gelatin, synthetic juices, water, and ice chips. Natural juices, such as orange juice, are irritating to the throat. When a full liquid diet can be tolerated, ice cream, puddings, creamed soups, and custards (which are examples of full-liquid foods) can be added to the diet. (11:314)

> Nursing Process—Implementation
> Client Need—Physiological integrity

111 2. The child should not be allowed to drink from a straw because sucking can dislodge clots and stitches and lead to hemorrhage. An ice collar is applied to promote comfort. If the child is more comfortable without the ice collar, then it can be removed. The child may prefer to use the bedpan or urinal during the immediate preoperative period; it also may be safer for the child to use a urinal or bedpan if the chid has received pain medication. It is appropriate for the parents to hold the child. (18:904)

> Nursing Process—Data collection
> Client Need—Physiological integrity

112 4. Signs of excessive bleeding following a tonsillectomy include frequent swallowing (which may be due to blood trickling down the back of the throat), a rapid pulse rate, restlessness, and vomiting of bright red blood. Vomiting dark old blood is to be expected and would not cause concern unless there is a large amount of emesis. Throat pain is a usual finding in the child who has had a tonsillectomy. A respiratory rate of 30 per minute is within normal range for a 5-year-old child. (14:496)

> Nursing Process—Data collection
> Client Need—Physiological integrity

113 1. It is recommended the child be kept quiet for a few days to discourage bleeding at the operative site. Fluids and soft foods can be taken as desired, but a regular diet usually is not recommended for several days because some of the food included in a regular diet may cause irritation and bleeding of the operative site. Aspirin is contraindicated for a child of this age because its use has been associated with Reye's syndrome. Aspirin also may affect the ability of the blood to clot and therefore increase bleeding tendencies. (11:314; 18:904)

> Nursing Process—Implementation
> Client Need—Health promotion/maintenance

114 4. A transient earache for 1 to 3 days following a tonsillectomy and adenoidectomy is common. The discomfort is due to pain referred from the throat to the ear. A nurse should advise parents of the possibility of earache while giving discharge instructions. Difficulty swallowing for 3 weeks, severe pain for the first 7 days after surgery, and expectorating bright red blood are not normal and should be brought to the attention of the physician. (11:314)

> Nursing Process—Implementation
> Client Need—Health promotion/maintenance

Classification of Test Items

Unit **III**   Review Test **13**

The Nursing Care of Infants, Toddlers, and Preschool Children

Directions: After each question the correct answer is given, as well as a classification of each test question. Compare the correct answer with your answer. If a question has been answered *incorrectly*, draw a line to the end of all the columns. When finished, add up the number of your correct answers in each column and place that number in the respective box at the end in the area identified as *Number Correct*.

To determine the percentage of questions you answered correctly and your performance in each of the test plan categories, divide the *Number Correct* in each column by the *Number Possible* in each column. Then multiply the decimal by 100. For example:

$$\frac{\text{Number Correct: } 90}{\text{Number Possible: } 112} = 0.803 \times 100 = 80\%$$

Any score that is less than 75% indicates an area where further review would be beneficial.

NURSING PROCESS

D = Data collection
P = Planning
I = Implementation
E = Evaluation

CLIENT NEEDS

S = Safe, effective care environment
P = Physiological integrity
M = Psychosocial integrity
H = Health promotion/maintenance

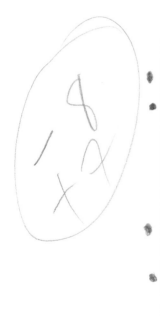

Question #	Answer #	Nursing Process				Client Needs			
		D	P	I	E	S	P	M	H
1	2	D							H
2	3			I					H
3	3	D							H
4	2				E				H
5	1			I		S			
6	3			I			P		
7	2			I			P		
8	3			I			P		
9	4	D					P		
10	4			I		S			
11	1			I			P		
12	2			I			P		
13	3			I					H
14	2			I			P		
15	1		P			S			

365

Question #	Answer #	Nursing Process				Client Needs			
		D	P	I	E	S	P	M	H
16	2			I					H
17	1	D					P		
18	2			I				M	
19	4			I		S			
20	1			I		S			
21	3			I		S			
22	2	D					P		
23	2			I			P		
24	3	D					P		
25	2			I				M	
26	3			I			P		
27	1				E				H
28	4	D					P		
29	1			I					H
30	2			I					H
31	3	D					P		
32	4			I			P		
33	3				E		P		
34	1			I			P		
35	1			I					H
36	4			I					H
37	1			I					H
38	2	D					P		
39	2		P				P		
40	4			I					H
41	3	D					P		
42	4			I					H
43	1			I			P		
44	2			I			P		
45	3				E				H
46	2			I		S			
47	1			I		S			

Question #	Answer #	Nursing Process				Client Needs			
		D	P	I	E	S	P	M	H
48	4	D					P		
49	3			I		S			
50	3			I					H
51	4			I					H
52	3			I					H
53	2	D					P		
54	3			I					H
55	3			I					H
56	3				E		P		
57	1			I					H
58	1			I			P		
59	4		P				P		
60	2				E				H
61	3	D					P		
62	4	D					P		
63	2		P				P		
64	3				E		P		
65	4			I					H
66	2			I					H
67	4			I					H
68	2				E				H
69	1	D					P		
70	4			I			P		
71	4			I					H
72	4			I					H
73	3			I			P		
74	1	D					P		
75	2			I			P		
76	4				E				H
77	1			I					H
78	2	D					P		
79	3			I					H

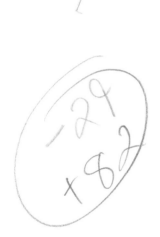

Question #	Answer #	Nursing Process				Client Needs			
		D	P	I	E	S	P	M	H
80	2			I					H
81	2				E				H
82	2			I				M	
83	4			I			P		
84	4	D					P		
85	1		P				P		
86	3				E		P		
87	3			I			P		
88	3			I		S			
89	2				E				H
90	4	D					P		
91	1		P			S			
92	4		P			S			
93	2			I			P		
94	4			I					H
95	2				E				H
96	2			I					H
97	3			I					H
98	3			I		S			
99	3		P				P		
100	1		P				P		
101	2	D					P		
102	3			I			P		
103	1			I				M	
104	1				E				H
105	3			I		S			
106	4			I				M	
107	1			I		S			
108	3				E				H
109	2	D				S			
110	2			I			P		
111	2	D					P		

-30
84

Question #	Answer #	Nursing Process				Client Needs			
		D	P	I	E	S	P	M	H
112	4	D					P		
113	1			I					H
114	4			I					H
Number Correct	84	21	6	46	11	10	42	4	28
Number Possible	114	23	9	67	15	16	51	5	42
Percentage Correct	74	91	67	69	73	63	82	80	67

2 3 21 4 6 9 1 14

Directions: With a pencil, blacken the circle in front of the option you have chosen for your correct answer.

NURSING CARE OF A CHILD WITH APPENDICITIS

An 8-year-old child is seen in the emergency department with an elevated temperature and complaint of generalized abdominal pain. The physician suspects appendicitis, and the child is admitted for observation and possible appendectomy.

1 If the nurse collects all of the following data, which one should be reported *immediately*?
- ○ 1. Child refuses to eat.
- ○ 2. Child complains of nausea.
- ● 3. Bowel sounds are absent.
- ○ 4. Temperature is 101°F orally.

2 During preoperative preparation the nurse would be *correct* to
- ○ 1. give analgesics.
- ● 2. give nothing by mouth.
- ○ 3. give an enema.
- ○ 4. apply heat to the abdomen.

Surgery was performed and the appendix was removed intact. The child was returned to the pediatric unit with an intravenous infusion in progress and an abdominal dressing in place. The physician left orders to continue the intravenous infusion at a rate of 1000 mL in 8 hours.

3 The nurse would be *correct* to set the mL/hr rate on the infusion pump at
- ○ 1. 50 mL.
- ○ 2. 75 mL.
- ○ 3. 100 mL.
- ● 4. 125 mL.

4 Which of the following actions is *most* appropriate for prevention of respiratory complications during the postoperative period?
- ○ 1. Give a bronchodilator by inhalation.
- ○ 2. Administer oxygen by nasal cannula.
- ○ 3. Give the child a corticosteroid.
- ● 4. Have the child use an incentive spirometer.

The physician visits on the second postoperative day and leaves an order to ambulate the child t.i.d. The nurse enters the child's room and begins to assist the child to ambulate. The child begins to cry and states, "I'm scared."

5 Which of the following is the *most* appropriate response by the nurse to the child's behavior?
- ○ 1. "There's nothing to be scared of. This will not hurt."
- ● 2. "The stitches are strong. They will not come out."
- ○ 3. "I know you are scared, but you must be brave."
- ○ 4. "Let's do this later, when you are better prepared."

The parents are visiting the child and ask the nurse how long the child will be hospitalized.

6 The nurse is *correct* to tell the parents that the child who has an uncomplicated appendectomy is usually discharged home within
- ● 1. 3 days.
- ○ 2. 5 days.
- ○ 3. 10 days.
- ○ 4. 14 days.

NURSING CARE OF A CHILD WITH RHEUMATIC FEVER

A 7-year-old child is admitted to the hospital with possible rheumatic fever. The child appears to be acutely ill.

7 If the parents report all of the following, which one indicates a high risk for rheumatic fever?
- ○ 1. The child was exposed to measles within the last 4 weeks.
- ● 2. The child had a severe sore throat within the last 2 weeks.
- ○ 3. The child is no longer interested in school work.
- ○ 4. The child received a bump on the head while playing.

8 Which of the following observations by the nurse is *most* indicative of rheumatic fever?
- ○ 1. Slow, irregular heartbeat
- ○ 2. Generalized erythema
- ○ 3. Decreased ASO titer
- ● 4. Migrating joint tenderness

The child is placed on bed rest and started on penicillin V (Pen-Vee-K) and acetylsalicylic acid (aspirin).

9 Which of the following diversional activities would be *most* appropriate for the child during the acute phase of rheumatic fever?
- ○ 1. Playing with action figures
- ○ 2. Playing Nintendo games
- ● 3. Reading an adventure story
- ○ 4. Pounding wooden pegs with mallet

10 The nurse should withhold the penicillin V (Pen-Vee-K) and notify the physician if the child has had a previous allergic reaction to a medication in which of the following drug groups?
- ○ 1. Amino glycosides
- ○ 2. Cephalosporins
- ○ 3. Macrolides
- ● 4. Sulfonamides

The parents ask why the child is receiving acetylsalicylic acid (aspirin) instead of acetaminophen (Tylenol).

11 The nurse would *best* respond by telling the parents that acetylsalicylic acid (aspirin) is given to the child with rheumatic fever instead of acetaminophen (Tylenol) because it
- ○ 1. controls fever better.
- ○ 2. prevents infections.
- ○ 3. relieves joint inflammation.
- ● 4. prevents cardiac enlargement.

12 Which of the following statements by the parents indicates that teaching has been effective?
- ● 1. Parents state that the penicillin (Pen-Vee-K) should be taken for the full 10 days.
- ○ 2. Parents state that the child should not be allowed to play in bright direct sunlight.
- ○ 3. Parents state that the child should take seizure medication every day.
- ○ 4. Parents state that the doctor will be notified if child has a sore throat.

NURSING CARE OF A CHILD WITH DIABETES MELLITUS

A 9-year-old child is admitted to the hospital with a tentative diagnosis of insulin-dependent diabetes mellitus. The parents state that the child has been complaining of feeling bad for several days. The physician states that the child has signs and symptoms of diabetic ketoacidosis. The physician leaves orders for an intravenous infusion of insulin, hourly blood sugars, and urine checks every 8 hours.

13 Which of the following findings by the nurse *best* indicates that the child is experiencing diabetic ketoacidosis?
- ○ 1. Blood sugar of 120 mg/dL
- ● 2. Fruity-smelling breath
- ○ 3. Pale-colored face
- ○ 4. Excessive perspiration

14 When testing the urine of a child experiencing diabetic ketoacidosis, the nurse would be *correct* to check for
- ○ 1. blood in the urine.
- ○ 2. bilirubin in the urine.
- ● 3. ketones in the urine.
- ○ 4. white blood cells in the urine.

15 When giving insulin intravenously, the nurse would be *correct* to give
- ● 1. regular insulin (Humulin R).
- ○ 2. isophane insulin suspension (Humulin N).
- ○ 3. insulin zinc suspension (Humulin L).
- ○ 4. insulin zinc suspension, extended (Humulin U).

After further tests, the diagnosis of insulin-dependent diabetes mellitus is confirmed. The child's condition improves. The physician leaves orders to discontinue the intravenous infusion and to begin subcutaneous insulin. A dietary consultation also is ordered.

16 The nurse would be *correct* to administer the child's morning dose of regular insulin
- ● 1. 30 minutes before breakfast is served.
- ○ 2. 15 minutes before breakfast is served.
- ○ 3. 30 minutes after breakfast is served.
- ○ 4. 15 minutes after breakfast is served.

17 Which of the following findings best indicates that the child is having a hypoglycemic reaction?
- ○ 1. Child complains of being thirsty.
- ○ 2. Labored prolonged breathing.
- ○ 3. Urine positive for glucose.
- ● 4. Child complains of feeling shaky.

18 If a conscious child develops hypoglycemia, the nurse would be *correct* to *first*
- ● 1. give the child orange juice to drink.
- ○ 2. give the child 10% glucose intravenously.
- ○ 3. notify the physician immediately.
- ○ 4. administer a second dose of insulin.

The child's parents ask the nurse why the child cannot receive the insulin in the form of a pill.

19 The nurse would be *correct* in explaining that insulin must be given subcutaneously because
- ○ 1. the oral form of insulin can lead to the development of birth defects.
- ● 2. the insulin would be destroyed by digestive enzymes if given by mouth.
- ○ 3. the insulin would cause vomiting and dehydration if given by mouth.
- ○ 4. the oral form of insulin is not effective in treating children with diabetes.

The child has completely recovered from the ketoacidosis and is now receiving regular insulin (Humulin R) and isophane insulin suspension (Humulin N) subcutaneously. The blood sugars have stabilized and the physician has requested that diabetic home care teaching be started.

20 The nurse would be *correct* in explaining to the child and parents that the insulin injection sites should be rotated in order to
- ○ 1. slow the absorption of insulin from the subcutaneous tissue.
- ○ 2. prevent accumulation of insulin in the subcutaneous tissue.
- ○ 3. decrease the duration of the action of insulin.
- ● 4. prevent lipodystrophy of subcutaneous tissue.

21 Which of the following statements by the child indicates that teaching has been effective?
- ○ 1. "If I eat more food, my need for insulin will decrease."
- ● 2. "If I increase my activity, my need for insulin will decrease."
- ○ 3. "If I get an infection, my need for insulin will decrease."
- ○ 4. "If I get real upset, my need for insulin will decrease."

22 The nurse would be *correct* to instruct the parents and child to check the blood sugar
- ● 1. twice daily, 30 minutes before eating.
- ○ 2. 15 minutes before eating.
- ○ 3. at least 8 times a day.
- ○ 4. only when a hypoglycemic reaction occurs.

The parents state that the child is very active in sports and likes to swim, play basketball, and soccer. The parents ask the nurse if the child will be able to continue these activities.

23 The nurse can *best* respond by telling the parents that
- ○ 1. the child's interest should be redirected to activities that require less energy expenditure.
- ○ 2. the child can swim because it lowers the metabolism, but the child should not play basketball or soccer.
- ● 3. the child can continue these activities but should be accompanied by a responsible person when swimming.
- ○ 4. the child can play basketball and soccer but should not swim because swimming will increase insulin needs.

NURSING CARE OF A CHILD WITH PARTIAL- AND FULL-THICKNESS BURNS

An 8-year-old child is hospitalized for treatment of extensive partial- and full-thickness burns on his face, neck, anterior chest, and left arm.

24 The nurse would be *correct* to place the child in
- ○ 1. enteric isolation.
- ● 2. protective isolation.
- ○ 3. respiratory isolation.
- ○ 4. contact isolation.

25 The nurse should keep which of the following equipment in the child's room in case an emergency situation arises?
- ○ 1. A footboard or bed board
- ● 2. An endotracheal tube and oxygen supply
- ○ 3. Equipment to administer pain medication
- ○ 4. Extra pillows and sheets

26 During early postburn care it would be *most* important for the nurse to closely monitor the child's
- ○ 1. unburned skin.
- ○ 2. bowel elimination.
- ● 3. intravenous fluid therapy.
- ○ 4. pupillary response to light.

The physician orders hourly measurement of the child's urinary output.

27 The nurse would be *correct* to notify the physician or nurse in charge *immediately* if the urine output was

7) 803 - 7652

1. 1 mL/kg/hr.
2. 1.5 mL/kg/hr.
3. 2.0 mL/kg/hr.
4. 2.5 mL/kg/hr.

28 Which of the following observations by the nurse would *best* indicate that the intravenous meperidine hydrochloride (Demerol) was effective?
1. The respiratory rate is within normal limits.
2. The child no longer complains of nausea.
3. The child no longer complains of pain.
4. The urinary output is 30 mL/hr.

29 Which of the following actions would *best* prevent the development of foot-drop?
1. Apply braces to the feet and ankles.
2. Keep the child in the side-lying position.
3. Keep sheets tucked in at the foot of the bed.
4. Rest the child's feet against a footboard.

30 Which of the following findings, by the nurse, would be *most* indicative of the presence of a Curling's ulcer?
1. Absence of bowel sounds
2. A positive hemoccult test
3. An elevated hematocrit
4. A distended abdomen

After the child's condition stabilizes, the child is placed on a high-protein diet.

31 If all of the following snacks were available, which one would the nurse serve to *best* meet the child's need for protein?
1. Strawberry milk shake
2. Apple sprinkled with cinnamon
3. Character-shaped flavored gelatin
4. Chocolate candy bar

32 Which of the following diversional activities will *best* meet the child's developmental needs?
1. Reading the newspaper
2. Coloring simple designs
3. Playing with a coin collection
4. Playing a solitaire card game

NURSING CARE OF A CHILD WITH JUVENILE RHEUMATOID ARTHRITIS

A 10-year-old child who has juvenile rheumatoid arthritis is being seen in the joint disorders specialty clinic 2 weeks after an acute episode of the disorder. The nurse is discussing home care with the child and parents.

33 Which of the following statements by the child indicates teaching about acetylsalicylic acid (aspirin) use has been effective?

1. "I take acetylsalicylic acid (aspirin) daily to control my joint inflammation."
2. "I take acetylsalicylic acid (aspirin) when my temperature is 101°F or greater."
3. "I take acetylsalicylic acid (aspirin) only when I am having muscle spasms."
4. "I take acetylsalicylic acid (aspirin) daily to increase my prothrombin time."

34 The nurse would be *correct* in explaining that the side effects of aspirin include
1. constipation, weight gain, and fluid retention.
2. ringing in the ears, nausea, and difficulty hearing.
3. anorexia, weight loss, and double vision.
4. headache, dry mouth, and dental cavities.

35 Which of the following activities would be *most* appropriate for the child with juvenile rheumatoid arthritis?
1. Skipping rope
2. Softball
3. Gymnastics
4. Swimming

36 Which of the following statements by the parents indicates a *correct* understanding of home care instructions given by the nurse?
1. "We have made arrangements for a homebound teacher."
2. "We put ice packs on the joints during inflammation."
3. "We serve meals that prevent excess weight gain."
4. "We keep the child in bed most of the time."

37 The nurse would be *correct* in telling the parents that to detect possible complications of juvenile rheumatoid arthritis, the child should have periodic
1. chest x-rays.
2. dental exams.
3. hearing exams.
4. eye exams.

NURSING CARE OF A CHILD WITH A HEAD INJURY

A 9-year-old child is admitted to the hospital for observation after falling off a bicycle. The parents state that the child's head hit the pavement during the fall.

38 If the nurse collects the following data, which one *best* indicates the presence of increased intracranial pressure?
1. Rapid bilateral pupillary response to light
2. Tympanic temperature 97.9°F
3. Blood pressure 150/90
4. Deep tendon reflexes 2+

39 Which of the following findings should be immediately reported to the nurse in charge or to the physician?
- ● 1. Clear watery nasal drainage
- ○ 2. Glasgow Coma Scale score of 15
- ○ 3. Child not knowing the time of day
- ○ 4. Radial pulse 80

The child is monitored overnight and no complications are observed. The physician discharges the client. Prior to discharge, the nurse reviews safety needs with the child and parents.

40 Which statement by the child indicates a need for further teaching on bicycle safety?
- ○ 1. "I will wear my helmet whenever I ride my bicycle."
- ● 2. "I will ride my bicycle in the opposite direction of traffic flow."
- ○ 3. "I will stop at all intersections and look both ways before proceeding."
- ○ 4. "I will not ride my bicycle after dark."

NURSING CARE OF A CHILD WITH A BRAIN TUMOR

An 11-year-old child is admitted to the hospital with complaints of headaches, dizziness, and vomiting. The physician orders x-rays of the head and an MRI (magnetic resonance imaging) scan is scheduled for the next day.

41 If the parents report all of the following data, which one *best* indicates a high risk for the presence of a brain tumor?
- ● 1. The child vomits when first getting out of bed.
- ○ 2. The child complains of nausea frequently.
- ○ 3. The child does not like going to school anymore.
- ○ 4. The child's head tilts toward the side when sleeping.

42 Which of the following statements by the nurse will *best* prepare the child for the MRI test?
- ● 1. "You will be placed in a tunnel-like scanner with a special call button."
- ○ 2. "You will experience a slight headache when the dye is injected."
- ○ 3. "You will be given medicine that will make you sleep during the test."
- ○ 4. "You will have little electrodes placed on your head with a special gel."

The results of the MRI show that the child has a brain tumor. The child goes to surgery. A craniotomy is performed and the tumor is partially removed. When the child returns from surgery the nurse observes a moderate amount of clear drainage on the head dressing.

43 The *most* appropriate action by the nurse would be to
- ○ 1. change the dressing, then notify the physician or nurse in charge.
- ○ 2. remove the dressing and monitor for active drainage.
- ○ 3. reinforce the dressing until the physician can change it.
- ● 4. leave the dressing intact and document findings.

The oncologist visits and leaves orders for the child to begin chemotherapy.

44 Which one of the following actions by the nurse will best help the child to cope with the effects of the chemotherapy?
- ○ 1. Serve the child a well-balanced meal before beginning the chemotherapy.
- ● 2. Give the child an antiemetic before beginning the chemotherapy.
- ○ 3. Encourage the child to get plenty of rest before beginning the chemotherapy.
- ○ 4. Give the child an enema before beginning the chemotherapy.

The child is crying and makes the statement, "Everybody is going to laugh at me. I never want to go to school again!"

45 Which of the following actions, by the nurse, will *best* facilitate the child's reestablishment of friendships with peers?
- ○ 1. Encourage the child to make friends with children who have a similar problem.
- ○ 2. Tell the child that real friends don't care how you look on the outside.
- ● 3. Encourage the child's friends to visit while the child is still in the hospital.
- ○ 4. Tell the child that the appearance changes will not be that bad and are temporary.

The child's parents express their feelings of helplessness and anxiety to the nurse after they learn of the child's diagnosis.

46 Which one of the following statements by the nurse would *best* help the parents to cope with their feelings?
- ○ 1. "Perhaps you would feel better if you visited the child for shorter periods of time."
- ○ 2. "Don't worry, you're doing a great job and everything will work out for the best."
- ● 3. "This is painful for you. Let's identity things you can do that make the child feel good."
- ○ 4. "It's sad that you feel helpless. What do you usually do to take your mind off your worries?"

NURSING CARE OF A CHILD IN TRACTION

A 9-year-old child is admitted to the pediatric unit with a fractured right femur. The child is in 90-90 skeletal traction.

47 The nurse would be *correct* to include which of the following interventions for the child in skeletal traction?
- ○ 1. Maintain child in the prone position.
- ◉ 2. Clean the pin site every 8 hours.
- ○ 3. Perform range-of-motion exercises on legs.
- ○ 4. Release weights on traction every 2 hours.

48 The nurse would be *correct* to check for evidence of skin breakdown
- ○ 1. over the calves.
- ◉ 2. over the scapulae.
- ○ 3. on the knees.
- ○ 4. on the buttocks.

49 Which one of the following findings should the nurse *immediately* report to the physician or to the nurse in charge?
- ○ 1. The pin protrudes through the skin on both sides.
- ○ 2. The foot of the bed is elevated on blocks.
- ○ 3. The weights of the traction are hanging freely.
- ◉ 4. A traction rope is out of the pulley groove.

50 Which of the following interventions will *best* prevent complications associated with traction?
- ◉ 1. Offer the child fluids on a frequent basis.
- ○ 2. Assist the child to select low-fiber foods.
- ○ 3. Assist the child with right leg exercises daily.
- ○ 4. Reposition the child onto side every 2 hours.

51 Which of the following findings should the nurse *immediately* report to the nurse in charge or to the physician?
- ○ 1. Pulse palpable in the right foot.
- ○ 2. Toes of both feet cool to touch.
- ◉ 3. Child unable to wiggle the toes of the right foot.
- ○ 4. Capillary refill in toes of right foot is 2 seconds.

NURSING CARE OF AN ADOLESCENT WITH DYSMENORRHEA

A 16-year-old female is brought by her mother to the pediatric clinic because of recurrent complaints of pain and discomfort during her menstrual cycle. The physician diagnoses her as having primary dysmenorrhea and recommends the use of aspirin or ibuprofen (Advil, Nuprin) for

the pain and discomfort. The physician also asks the nurse to discuss other measures that can be taken to reduce the pain and discomfort.

52 The nurse would be *correct* to suggest which one of the following actions to relieve the pain and discomfort?
- ○ 1. Stay in bed until cramping is relieved, increase your fluid intake, and eat a low-fat diet.
- ○ 2. Drink plenty of cold liquids, add extra salt to your diet, and take a nap in the afternoon.
- ○ 3. Apply ice packs to the abdomen, eat a high-caloric diet, and eat your largest meal at noon.
- ◉ 4. Get at least 8 hours of sleep, eat a well-balanced diet, and apply heat to your abdomen.

53 Which of the following explanations regarding the use of aspirin should the nurse discuss with the client?
- ○ 1. Aspirin should be discarded if not used within 2 years of first being opened.
- ○ 2. Ringing in the ears is a common side effect of aspirin that will go away eventually.
- ○ 3. If aspirin alone does not help, take one or two ibuprofen along with the aspirin.
- ◉ 4. It is best to take aspirin with food in order to prevent gastrointestinal upset.

The adolescent tells the nurse, "One of my friends says she is scared because she has amenorrhea. What does that word mean?"

54 The nurse would be *correct* to explain that amenorrhea means
- ◉ 1. absence of menstruation.
- ○ 2. excessive vaginal bleeding.
- ○ 3. discomfort before menstruation.
- ○ 4. first menstrual period.

NURSING CARE OF AN ADOLESCENT WHO IS ABUSING DRUGS

The parents of a 14-year-old adolescent call for a pediatric clinic appointment because they have discovered amphetamine capsules in the child's room and suspect that the child is abusing the substance.

55 Which of the following symptoms reported by the parents would the nurse consider as the *best* indicator of abuse of amphetamines by the adolescent?
- ○ 1. Watery eyes
- ○ 2. Drowsiness
- ○ 3. Excessive nasal drainage
- ◉ 4. Marked nervousness

56 The nurse would be *correct* in explaining that amphetamines
- ○ 1. are tried by most adolescents and cause no harm.
- ◉ 2. are known to lead to psychological dependence.
- ○ 3. are a central nervous system depressant.
- ○ 4. are only harmful if taken intravenously.

The parents ask the nurse, "What is wrong with my child? Why has this happened?" The parents also tell the nurse that the child likes to hang with a gang that is known to get in trouble and abuse drugs.

57 The nurse would be *correct* to explain that during adolescence, being with and trying out the values of the peer group is a part of the process of developing a sense of
- ◉ 1. identity.
- ○ 2. intimacy.
- ○ 3. integrity.
- ○ 4. idealism.

While the child is talking with the physician, the nurse reviews the child's immunization records and discovers that the last immunization received was when the child was 6 years old.

58 The nurse would be *correct* to explain to the parents that the child is due to receive which of the following immunization boosters?
- ○ 1. Pertussis
- ○ 2. Polio
- ○ 3. Smallpox
- ◉ 4. Tetanus

The parents ask if the child should be forced to enter a drug treatment program.

59 The *best* response the nurse can make to the parents' question is:
- ○ 1. "You should attempt to discuss the dangers of drug abuse with your child before deciding that treatment is necessary."
- ○ 2. "It will be necessary to get a court order before you can force your child to enter a drug treatment program."
- ◉ 3. "The success of the drug treatment program will depend on your child's desire to become drug-free."
- ○ 4. "It is best that you force the child into the treatment program because the child will not participate in the program otherwise."

NURSING CARE OF AN ADOLESCENT WITH A SEXUALLY TRANSMITTED DISEASE

A 16-year-old female has learned that she has been exposed to gonorrhea. She visits the clinic for diagnosis and treatment.

60 When preparing the adolescent for the test, the nurse would be *correct* to explain that
- ○ 1. a blood specimen will be collected.
- ○ 2. a urine specimen will be needed.
- ◉ 3. a vaginal smear will be obtained.
- ○ 4. a biopsy of the cervix will be performed.

The physician confirms the diagnosis of gonorrhea and also informs the client that she has Chlamydia trachomatis, a sexually transmitted disease. Intramuscular ceftriaxone (Rocephin) is given to treat the gonorrhea and a prescription for oral doxycycline is given for treatment of the chlamydia.

61 Which of the following instructions should the nurse give to the client about taking doxycycline (Vibramycin)?
- ○ 1. The medication will normally cause a dark orange discoloration of urine.
- ◉ 2. The medication should be taken 1 hour before or 2 hours after a meal.
- ○ 3. Do not drink water for at least 30 minutes after the medication is taken.
- ○ 4. Report any symptoms of gastrointestinal upset to the health care provider.

Before leaving the clinic, the client ask the nurse, "When can I be certain that I am no longer infectious?"

62 The nurse would be *correct* in explaining that the client will be considered noninfectious
- ○ 1. when she no longer has a vaginal discharge.
- ○ 2. when she no longer experiences discomfort during her menstrual periods.
- ◉ 3. if she has a negative culture after being off antibiotics for at least 7 days.
- ○ 4. 24 hours after receiving the ceftriaxone (Rocephine).

A 17-year-old adolescent is seen in the STD (sexually transmitted disease) specialty clinic and diagnosed with genital herpes (herpes simplex type 2).

63 The nurse would be *correct* to describe the initial lesions observed as
- ○ 1. macules.
- ◉ 2. vesicles.
- ○ 3. papules.
- ○ 4. fistulas.

64 Which of the following statements by the adolescent indicates a need for additional teaching about genital herpes?
- ○ 1. Males who have genital herpes should have a yearly PSA test.
- ◉ 2. Females who have genital herpes should have a Pap test every 6 months.
- ○ 3. Genital herpes is closely associated with the occurrence of sterility.
- ○ 4. Genital herpes is closely associated with Hodgkin's disease.

Oral and topical acyclovir (Zovirax) are prescribed for the adolescent.

65 The nurse would be *correct* to explain that
- ○ 1. if taken as prescribed, ayclovir (Zovirax) will prevent recurrence of lesions.
- ○ 2. sex partners also should be treated for 10 days with oral acyclovir (Zovirax).
- ◉ 3. topical acyclovir (Zovirax) should be applied using a glove or a finger cot.
- ○ 4. oral acyclovir (Zovirax) should be taken even when the disease is in remission.

The nurse discusses sexuality with the client.

66 Which of the following statements by the client indicates that teaching has been effective?
- ○ 1. "Males should use a condom when lesions are present to prevent transmission."
- ○ 2. "Douching after intercourse prevents females from becoming infected."
- ○ 3. "Applying acyclovir (Zovirax) to lesions before intercourse prevents transmission."
- ◉ 4. "Sexual contact should be avoided, especially if lesions or symptoms are present."

The adolescent ask the nurse, "What are the symptoms of AIDS (acquired immunodeficiency syndrome)?"

67 The nurse would be *correct* to tell the adolescent that the symptoms of AIDS include
- ○ 1. increased appetite and night sweats.
- ○ 2. tachycardia, dyspnea, and constipation.
- ◉ 3. fatigue, fever, and persistent yeast infections.
- ○ 4. weight gain, peripheral edema, and jaundice.

The adolescent also asks the nurse if the human immuno-deficiency virus (HIV) can be contracted from a sex partner who has no symptoms of acquired immunodeficiency syndrome (AIDS).

68 The nurse can *best* respond by telling the adolescent that

- ○ 1. in order to be safe, sexual contact with past sex partners should be avoided.
- ◉ 2. an HIV-positive individual may not develop symptoms of AIDS for years.
- ○ 3. the HIV virus can only be transmitted when symptoms of AIDS are present.
- ○ 4. the prescribed medication also will provide protection against HIV.

NURSING CARE OF AN ADOLESCENT WITH SCOLIOSIS

A 14-year-old female adolescent is referred for further evaluation after the school nurse discovers lateral spinal curvature during scoliosis screening.

69 If the child makes the following statements, which one *best* indicates that the child has scoliosis?
- ○ 1. "My friends are getting taller faster than I am."
- ◉ 2. "One of my sleeves is always shorter than the other."
- ○ 3. "I have a difficult time sleeping on my side at night."
- ○ 4. "I always roll crooked when I am doing a forward roll."

70 Which of the following questions is *most* important for the nurse to ask the child when preparing for diagnostic tests that will be performed?
- ◉ 1. "Is there any possibility of your being pregnant?"
- ○ 2. "Have you eaten anything in the past 24 hours?"
- ○ 3. "Have you taken any medications in the past 24 hours?"
- ○ 4. "Are you allergic to iodine or shellfish?"

A diagnosis of structural scoliosis is confirmed and the physician determines that the child has a 35-degree curvature. The parents ask the nurse if treatment is really necessary.

71 The nurse would be *correct* in explaining that
- ○ 1. curvatures of this degree may improve without treatment.
- ○ 2. without treatment the child may develop problems with bladder control.
- ○ 3. without treatment the child may develop problems with bowel control.
- ◉ 4. without treatment the child may develop breathing problems.

The child is to be fitted for a Milwaukee brace. The child asks if the brace has to be worn when she is at school.

72 The nurse would be *correct* in telling the child that the brace has to be worn
    ○ 1. except when taking a bath.
    ● 2. at least 8 hours each day.
    ○ 3. at night while sleeping.
    ○ 4. at all times without exception.

73 To *best* promote the child's compliance with the treatment plan, the nurse should
    ○ 1. tell the parents that they should keep a constant watch on the child.
    ● 2. help the child to identify clothing that is stylish but hides the brace.
    ○ 3. suggest that the parents arrange for a homebound teacher during treatment.
    ○ 4. tell the child that the problem will get worse if the brace is not worn.

INDIVIDUAL TEST ITEMS

74 Which of the following recommendations would be *most* appropriate to give to the mother of a 5-month-old infant with a heat rash?
    ○ 1. Apply baby oil to affected areas.
    ● 2. Avoid overdressing the infant.
    ○ 3. Apply a thin sprinkling of baby powder.
    ○ 4. Avoid strong laundry detergents.

75 Which of the following statements by an adolescent with acne vulgaris indicates that additional teaching about taking tetracycline hydrochloride (Panmycin) is needed?
    ● 1. "I will take the medication with a full glass of water."
    ○ 2. "I will not take any antacids with this medication."
    ○ 3. "I will take this medication with food."
    ○ 4. "I will avoid sun exposure while taking this medication."

76 Which of the following findings would the nurse expect to observe in the child with Down's syndrome?
    ○ 1. Large head and curved index finger
    ○ 2. Long fingers and protruding tongue
    ○ 3. Small head and upward-slanting eyes
    ● 4. Simian creases on the soles of the feet

77 Which of the following statements by a diabetic adolescent indicates a need for additional instructions on how to use an insulin pump?
    ○ 1. "I like the insulin pump because I can wear it under my clothes without anyone noticing I have it on."
    ○ 2. "I like the insulin pump because I only have to change the needle site every 24 to 48 hours."
    ○ 3. "I like the insulin pump because when I need extra insulin, all I have to do is push a button on the pump."
    ● 4. "I like the insulin pump because I don't have to check my blood glucose; the pump checks the glucose for me."

78 When teaching an adolescent male about testicular self-examination, the nurse would be *correct* to explain that
    ○ 1. the examination should be performed after a warm bath or shower.
    ○ 2. a difference in the size of the testicles should be reported to a doctor.
    ○ 3. malignant lumps are usually located on the front side of the testicles.
    ● 4. both testicles should be examined simultaneously to detect differences.

79 A 16-year-old male asks the nurse for instructions on safe condom use. The nurse would be *correct* to explain that
    ○ 1. The condom should be stored in a warm and dry place to prevent damage.
    ○ 2. The condom can be lubricated with mineral oil or petroleum jelly.
    ○ 3. The condom should be put on before the penis becomes erect.
    ● 4. During application, a ½-inch space should be left at the end of the condom.

80 Which of the following findings *best* indicates that a child has acute glomeruli nephritis?
    ● 1. Periorbital edema
    ○ 2. Excessive urination
    ○ 3. Increased appetite
    ○ 4. Low blood pressure

81 Which one of the following diets would be *most* appropriate to suggest for a child with thrush and herpes simplex infections of the oral cavity secondary to AIDS?
    ● 1. High-caloric, bland diet
    ○ 2. Soft, low-protein diet
    ○ 3. Low-residue, low-fat diet
    ○ 4. High-residue, low-cholesterol diet

82 The nurse would be *correct* to instruct the parents of a toddler who has phenylketonuria (PKU) to omit which of the following food groups from the child's diet?
    ○ 1. Vegetables
    ○ 2. Meats
    ● 3. Breads
    ○ 4. Fruits

83 Which one of the following findings during the assessment of a 2-year-old would lead the nurse to suspect child abuse?

  ○ 1. The child protests when approached by the nurse.

  ● 2. The child has varying lengths of hair on the head.

  ○ 3. The child has a fresh bruise on the forehead.

  ○ 4. The child has an abrasion on the right knee.

84 The nurse would be *correct* to instruct the parents of a 15-month-old who has just received routine immunizations to report

  ○ 1. a fever that occurs within 7 to 10 days of the immunization.

  ○ 2. a rash that appears 2 to 4 days following the immunization.

  ○ 3. crying for more than 3 hours, even after comfort measures are taken.

  ● 4. soreness, redness, and swelling at the site of injection.

85 The nurse would be *correct* to instruct the parents of a child who is to be observed at home following a blow to the head to

  ○ 1. return the child for a follow-up visit in 3 to 5 days.

  ○ 2. give the child nothing by mouth for the next 12 hours.

  ○ 3. check the child's pupillary response every 4 hours.

  ● 4. awaken the child every 4 hours during the first night.

86 Which one of the following statements by the parents of a preschool child with tinea capitis indicates that teaching has been effective?

  ○ 1. "I will comb my child's hair with a fine-tooth comb dipped in vinegar to remove the nits."

  ○ 2. "I will give the griseofulvin (Grisactin) with whole milk to increase absorption of the medication."

  ○ 3. "I will give the medication for the full 2 weeks in order to prevent spread of the lesions."

  ● 4. "I will apply the medication to my child's scalp three times a day until the lesions are gone."

87 Which one of the following findings would the nurse expect to be reported by the parents of a child suspected of having pinworms?

  ○ 1. Teeth grinding

  ○ 2. Abdominal pain

  ● 3. Anal itching

  ○ 4. Bulky, greasy stools

88 Which of the following findings by the nurse during a home visit to a family with a 20-month-old would indicate a need for teaching about safety needs of the child?

  ○ 1. Electrical outlets are covered.

  ● 2. The child is eating raw baby carrots.

  ○ 3. Furniture has rounded edges.

  ○ 4. The child is building a tower with large blocks.

89 A 2-year-old is brought in for a wellness checkup. Which of the following sites is considered the *best* site for assessing the pulse for a child this age?

  ○ 1. Apical

  ● 2. Brachial

  ○ 3. Carotid

  ○ 4. Radial

90 Which of the following actions by the parents of an infant indicates that teaching about the administration of oral medications in liquid form was effective?

  ○ 1. The parents add the medication to the bottle of formula.

  ○ 2. The parents pinch the child's nose when giving the medicine.

  ● 3. The parents give the medication with a rubber-tipped medicine dropper.

  ○ 4. The parents place the child in the supine position when giving the medicine.

91 The nurse would be *correct* to tell the parents of a child who has hemophilia to avoid medications containing

  ● 1. aspirin.

  ○ 2. caffeine.

  ○ 3. barbiturates.

  ○ 4. antacids.

92 Which one of the following restraints should the nurse plan to use for a child who has had a cleft lip repair?

  ○ 1. Papoose board

  ○ 2. Leg restraints

  ● 3. Elbow restraints

  ○ 4. Posey belt or jacket

93 The nurse should plan to remove and reapply the restraints at least

  ○ 1. daily.

  ○ 2. every 8 hours.

  ○ 3. every 4 hours.

  ● 4. every 2 hours.

94 Which one of the following findings by the nurse *best* indicates that a child is experiencing hypokalemia?

  ○ 1. Full bounding pulses

  ● 2. Muscle weakness

  ○ 3. Elevated blood pressure

  ○ 4. Hyperactive bowel sounds

95 When assisting with a lumbar puncture, the nurse would be *correct* to place the child in the
○ 1. prone position.
○ 2. Trendelenburg position.
○ 3. supine position.
◉ 4. side-lying position.

96 An infant is brought in for a wellness checkup. The nurse would be *correct* to count the infant's respirations for
○ 1. 10 seconds and multiply by 6
○ 2. 15 seconds and multiply by 4
○ 3. 30 seconds and multiply by 2
◉ 4. 1 minute

97 When giving an infant an enema, the nurse would be *correct* to advance the catheter
◉ 1. 1 inch into the rectum.
○ 2. 2 inches into the rectum.
○ 3. 3 inches into the rectum.
○ 4. 4 inches into the rectum.

98 A preschooler who is recovering from infectious gastroenteritis is advanced to solid foods. The nurse would be *correct* to *initially* serve the child
○ 1. buttered rice.
◉ 2. cereal.
○ 3. applesauce.
○ 4. ice cream.

99 When discussing cerebral palsy with the parents of a newly diagnosed child, the nurse would be *correct* to explain that
◉ 1. cerebral palsy is a nonprogressive disease caused by damage to the brain.
○ 2. brain surgery often can help or cure children with cerebral palsy.
○ 3. physical therapy is of little value to the child with cerebral palsy.
○ 4. cerebral palsy is the result of injury to the sensory areas of the brain.

100 When developing a plan of care for the child with rickets, the nurse would be *correct* to include nutrients that provide a source of vitamin
○ 1. A.
○ 2. B$_{12}$.
○ 3. C.
◉ 4. D.

101 Which of the following findings, during a routine wellness checkup, would *best* indicate that a child has iron-deficiency anemia?
○ 1. Weight gain and hypertension
○ 2. Nervousness and diarrhea
○ 3. Nausea and vomiting
◉ 4. Pallor and listlessness

102 An infant with respiratory syncytial virus is on ribavirin (Virazole) therapy. The nurse would be *correct* to explain that
○ 1. the prescribed medication will be given intravenously.
◉ 2. the child will receive the medication once weekly for 4 weeks.
○ 3. individuals who are pregnant should not visit during treatment.
○ 4. the child will be placed in protective isolation during treatment.

103 When providing care to the child with nephrotic syndrome, the nurse would be *correct* to
◉ 1. restrict the intake of protein.
○ 2. weigh the child daily.
○ 3. monitor for hypotension.
○ 4. measure the head daily.

104 The parents of a 12-year-old with a sprained ankle ask the nurse if there is any danger in applying an ice bag to the child's ankle. The nurse would be *correct* to explain that
○ 1. ice can be applied and left on until the swelling is gone.
◉ 2. ice can be applied but must be removed every 30 minutes to 1 hour.
○ 3. ice should not be used in treating sprains; heat should be used instead.
○ 4. there is no danger associated with the application of ice.

105 The parents of a child with Duchenne's muscular dystrophy are having a difficult time accepting the diagnosis. The nurse can *best* help the parents adjust by
○ 1. recommending that the family place the child in a long-term health care facility.
○ 2. recommending that the family make contact with the local social welfare agency.
◉ 3. recommending that the family talk with other parents who have children with muscular dystrophy.
○ 4. recommending that the family read as much literature as possible about treatment of muscular dystrophy.

106 Which one of the following actions is *most* appropriate for meeting the needs of the infant who has congestive heart failure?
○ 1. Respond quickly to the infant's crying.
◉ 2. Position the infant in the prone position.
○ 3. Avoid holding and cuddling the infant.
○ 4. Use a firm small-hole nipple for feedings.

107 An 8-year-old child has a score of 4 on the faces pain rating scale. Which of the following actions would be *most* appropriate for the nurse to take *initially* in response to this finding?

○ 1. No action is necessary; the child is pain-free.
○ 2. Provide diversional activities to relieve the pain.
○ 3. Document findings and recheck the child later.
◉ 4. Give the prescribed analgesic to relieve the pain.

108 Which one of the following behaviors *best* indicates that an adolescent is at risk to commit suicide?
○ 1. Disregards family rules sometimes
○ 2. Argues with siblings
○ 3. Grades dropped from 92 to 90
◉ 4. Broke up with boyfriend or girlfriend

109 Which of the following statements, by the parents of a toddler, indicates a need for teaching about signs of readiness for toilet training?
◉ 1. Sphincter control is usually not accomplished before 18 to 24 months.
○ 2. Bladder training should be started before bowel training.
○ 3. The child must be able to communicate the need to go to the bathroom.
○ 4. The child should be able to remove clothing (underwear).

110 Which one of the following nursing actions must be *avoided* when giving care to the child diagnosed as having Wilms tumor?
◉ 1. Palpating the child's abdomen
○ 2. Giving the child a book to read
○ 3. Feeding the child
○ 4. Combing the child's hair

111 Which of the following statements by the parents of a 6-year-old child with impetigo would indicate that the parents need additional teaching?
○ 1. Oral antihistamines can be given to decrease inflammation and itching.
◉ 2. Antibiotic treatment in not necessary because the infection is self-limiting.
○ 3. The child's nails must be trimmed to prevent scratching of the lesions.
○ 4. Precautions should be taken to prevent spread of the infection to others.

Directions: Two numbers appear in parentheses following each rationale. The first number identifies the textbook listed in the references, page 512, and the second number identifies the page(s) in that textbook on which the correct answer can be verified. Occasionally two textbooks are given for verifying the correct answer.

NURSING CARE OF A CHILD WITH APPENDICITIS

1 3. Absent bowel sounds should be reported immediately because there is an increased risk of inflammation and obstruction being present, which poses a greater threat to health than the other findings. (11:354; 18:506)
Nursing Process—Data collection
Client Need—Physiological integrity

2 2. Prior to surgery, the child should be kept n.p.o. to decrease the risk of aspiration during surgery. Analgesics are not given prior to surgery in order to avoid masking signs that would be important for making a diagnosis. Enemas and laxatives are avoided because they increase peristalsis, which may cause rupture of the appendix. Heat is avoided because it also may cause the appendix to rupture. (11:354)
Nursing Process—Implementation
Client Need—Physiological integrity

3 4. If a total of 1000 mL is to be given over 8 hours, the amount to be given (1000 mL) is divided by the total number of hours (8). 1000 mL divided by 8 hours is 125 mL per hour. (20:37)
Nursing Process—Implementation
Client Need—Safe, effective care environment

4 4. Incentive spirometry and deep breathing help to prevent respiratory complications that may be experienced by persons having abdominal surgery. A bronchodilator, oxygen, and corticosteroid are used after respiratory complications have occurred and are not preventative measures. (18:634; 22:649)
Nursing Process—Implementation
Client Need—Physiological integrity

5 2. Children and adults are usually afraid the stitches will pull out if they walk or move about too much. The nurse should reassure the client that the sutures are designed to endure movement and walking. Telling the child that walking will not cause discomfort is not true and you must always be honest with the child. It is correct to acknowledge the child's fear, but it also is appropriate to give the child an answer that will help to resolve the fear. (11:354)
Nursing Process—Implementation
Client Need—Psychosocial integrity

6 2. The child who is not experiencing any complications is usually discharged home in 5 days. Those experiencing complications, such as peritonitis, will require longer hospitalization and may receive antibiotics, nasogastric suctioning, and dressing changes. (16:766; 22:649)
Nursing Process—Implementation
Client Need—Health promotion/maintenance

NURSING CARE OF A CHILD WITH RHEUMATIC FEVER

7 2. The exact cause of rheumatic fever is not clearly understood. There is evidence that rheumatic fever may be seen in those with a recent bacterial infection caused by group A beta-hemolytic streptococci. Although not all sore throats are caused by this microorganism, some are; therefore this is brought to the physician's attention. Measles is caused by a virus. A bump on the head and a disinterest in school work probably are not related to a diagnosis of rheumatic fever but should be recorded in the health history. (11:357; 16:750)
Nursing Process—Data collection
Client Need—Safe, effective care environment

8 4. Migrating joint pain is a major manifestation of rheumatic fever. The ASO titer and the pulse rate usually are elevated. The child may have erythema marginatum, which is a distinctive rash found on the trunk and extremities. (11:357; 16:750)
Nursing Process—Data collection
Client Need—Safe, effective care environment

9 3. Reading an adventure story would be the most appropriate activity for the child during the acute phase of the illness. The child will need both physical and emotional rest; therefore quiet, age-appropriate activities are recommended to prevent overexertion as well as to prevent boredom and emotional upset, which may occur if the child is not allowed to have any activity. Play with action figures is usually enjoyed more by preschoolers and also may cause excitement, which will increase energy consumption. Nintendo games also may cause too much excitement. Toy mallets and wooden pegs are more appropriate for the toddler. (16:542; 22:616)

> Nursing Process—Implementation
> Client Need—Safe, effective care environment

10 2. There is a slight cross-sensitivity between medications in the penicillin group and those in the cephalosporin group. Therefore the nurse should practice caution and notify the nurse in charge or the physician before giving the medication. There is no cross-sensitivity between medications in the penicillin group and the other medication categories listed. (18:674)

> Nursing Process—Planning
> Client Need—Physiological integrity

11 3. Aspirin is given instead of acetaminophen (Tylenol) because it not only controls fever but also relieves joint inflammation, which is a major manifestation of rheumatic fever. Acetylsalicylic acid (aspirin) is not necessarily more effective in reducing fever than acetaminophen (Tylenol), and it does not prevent infection or cardiac enlargement. (11:359; 22:616)

> Nursing Process—Implementation
> Client Need—Health promotion/maintenance

12 4. The child who has had rheumatic fever may develop the disease again. Not all sore throats are caused by the streptococci organism, but there is a risk that the causative organism is the streptococci. Therefore any occurrence of a sore throat should be reported promptly in order to facilitate immediate diagnosis and treatment. (11:360)

> Nursing Process—Evaluation
> Client Need—Health promotion/maintenance

NURSING CARE OF A CHILD WITH DIABETES MELLITUS

13 2. Fruity-smelling breath is a manifestation of diabetic ketoacidosis. Excessive perspiration and pale color are signs of hypoglycemia. A blood sugar of 120 mg/dL is within the normal range. (14:685; 16:771)

> Nursing Process—Data collection
> Client Need—Physiological integrity

14 3. The client experiencing diabetic ketoacidosis will have glucose and ketones present in the urine. Blood, white blood cells, and bilirubin are not usually found in the urine of the person experiencing diabetic ketoacidosis. (11:362; 14:687)

> Nursing Process—Implementation
> Client Need—Physiological integrity

15 1. Regular insulin (Humulin R) is the only type of insulin that is given intravenously. Regular insulin also can be given subcutaneously along with insulin zinc suspension (Humulin L), insulin zinc suspension, extended (Humulin U), and isophane insulin suspension (Humulin N). (14:687)

> Nursing Process—Implementation
> Client Need—Physiological integrity

16 1. Regular insulin (Humulin R) is given 30 minutes before a meal because the onset of this type of insulin is 30 minutes to 1 hour. Giving the insulin within a shorter period possibly would result in inadequate coverage because the insulin will not have had a chance to take effect. Giving the insulin after eating will not provide coverage for the food that already has been consumed. (14:682)

> Nursing Process—Implementation
> Client Need—Physiological integrity

17 4. Shakiness is a common sign of hypoglycemia. The remaining items in this questions are signs and symptoms of hyperglycemia. (14:685)

> Nursing Process—Data collection
> Client Need—Physiological integrity

18 1. Hypoglycemia must be corrected immediately. If the child is awake and able to swallow, the nurse should offer a concentrated source of sugar, such as orange juice. Intravenous administration of glucose is reserved for those who have a change in their level of consciousness and are unable to swallow. Insulin would not be given because the child already has too much insulin. The physician should be notified after the problem is corrected. (11:363)

> Nursing Process—Implementation
> Client Need—Physiological integrity

19 2. Persons with insulin-dependent diabetes mellitus require insulin to control the disease. Insulin cannot be given by mouth because it would be destroyed by the digestive enzymes before reaching the site of action. The child is not a candidate for oral hypoglycemic agents because the pancreas has to be able to produce some insulin in order for the child to benefit from the oral hypoglycemics, and this is not the case with the child who has insulin-dependent diabetes mellitus. (18:1067)

> Nursing Process—Implementation
> Client Need—Health promotion

20 4. If insulin sites are not rotated by use of a planned rotation schedule, atrophy (lipodystrophy) of subcutaneous fat may occur. Lipodystrophy can interfere with the absorption of insulin if insulin is given in areas affected by this problem. Rotating the injection sites does not slow the absorption, prevent accumulation, or decrease the duration of insulin. (20:329)

> **Nursing Process—Implementation**
> **Client Need—Health promotion/maintenance**

21 2. Activity requires glucose for energy. Therefore, increasing activity uses up glucose, and the body then requires less-than-usual amounts of insulin. Eating too much, having an infection, and experiencing emotional stress are situations in which the client tends to require more, not less, insulin. (16:772)

> **Nursing Process—Evaluation**
> **Client Need—Health promotion/maintenance**

22 1. Unless the physician orders otherwise, the testing of blood glucose levels is performed at least twice daily. The test is performed 30 minutes before a meal. The physician may request that blood glucose testing be done more frequently, but that usually is tailored to the specific situation and circumstances for a particular client. The blood sugar should be monitored when the client experiences a hypoglycemic response but is routinely observed at other times also. (16:773)

> **Nursing Process—Implementation**
> **Client Need—Health promotion/maintenance**

23 3. The diabetic child can participate in normal activities; certain precautions are necessary in order to promote safety, however, such as swimming with a responsible person, and letting at least one person know that the child is diabetic. The child can participate in activities requiring increased energy expenditure, such as basketball and soccer, as long a this is taken into consideration when planning meals and insulin. Generally the child should consume a snack before engaging in the activity and/or have a simple form of glucose on hand in case a hypoglycemic reaction should occur. (11:368)

> **Nursing Process—Implementation**
> **Client Need—Health promotion/maintenance**

NURSING CARE OF A CHILD WITH PARTIAL- AND FULL-THICKNESS BURNS

24 2. Protective (reverse) isolation techniques are used when caring for a child with severe burns because the child is highly susceptible to infection. The other types of isolation mentioned in this question have as their primary goal preventing a client's microorganisms from being spread to others. (11:263; 18:970)

> **Nursing Process—Implementation**
> **Client Need—Safe, effective care environment**

25 2. It is important for the nurse to know that respiratory distress from a blocked airway may occur following burns to the head, face, neck, and chest. An endotracheal tube and oxygen supply should be kept in the client's room. An oral airway also should be readily available. In this situation, the other devices and equipment stated in the options would not be considered appropriate for treating an emergency arising from respiratory distress. (16:609)

> **Nursing Process—Planning**
> **Client needs—Physiological integrity**

26 3. A burn victim is placed on intravenous fluid therapy during the first 24 hours in order to restore fluid and electrolyte balance and to maintain perfusion of vital organs. During intravenous fluid therapy there is a danger of fluid overload; therefore the nurse should closely monitor the intravenous infusion. (14:665; 18:967)

> **Nursing Process—Implementation**
> **Client Need—Physiological integrity**

27 4. A urinary output of 1.0 to 2.0 mL/kg/hr is considered to be within the normal range. Excessive output requires that the rate of the intravenous infusion be reduced. (16:609)

> **Nursing Process—Data collection**
> **Client Need—Physiological integrity**

28 3. There often is considerable pain associated with severe burns, and a narcotic is used. Meperidine hydrochloride (Demerol) may be prescribed to relieve the pain experienced by the burned client. Meperidine does not prevent nausea, affect the urinary output, or maintain the respiratory rate within the normal range. Instead, nausea and respiratory depression are adverse effects of this drug. (20:134; 11:275)

> **Nursing Process—Evaluation**
> **Client Need—Physiological integrity**

29 4. A footboard is a nursing measure that may be used to prevent foot-drop. Braces cannot be used without a physician's order. Keeping the child in the side-lying position will not prevent foot-drop because this problem can be prevented only when the feet are supported in a normal position. The top sheet should fit loosely over the feet to assist with the prevention of foot-drop. (16:527)

> **Nursing Process—Implementation**
> **Client Need—Physiological integrity**

30 2. Stress ulcers, often called Curling's ulcers, frequently occur in the stomach or duodenum as a complication of burns. If the ulcer bleeds, the client will have blood in the stool, which will be evidenced by a positive hemoccult test and black, tarry stools. The other findings are not usual manifestations of Curling's ulcers. (7:264; 14:668)
   Nursing Process—Data collection
   Client Need—Physiological integrity

31 1. A milk shake has a high protein content. A diet rich in protein is essential for the body to rebuild tissue destroyed by the burns. Apples, candy, and gelatin contain little or no protein. (11:275)
   Nursing Process—Implementation
   Client Need—Physiological integrity

32 3. Of the diversional activities described in this item, an 8-year-old is likely to enjoy playing with a coin collection. Television also may provide diversion. Playing a solitary game of cards, reading the newspaper, or coloring a simple design probably would not appeal to a child of this age. (11:337)
   Nursing Process—Implementation
   Client Need—Safe, effective care environment

NURSING CARE OF A CHILD WITH JUVENILE RHEUMATOID ARTHRITIS

33 1. The primary reason for using aspirin in the treatment of juvenile rheumatoid arthritis is the drug's ability to reduce inflammation. Although acetylsalicylic acid (aspirin) does lower the body temperature, this is not the foremost reason for using this drug. Muscle spasms are not prevented by the administration of aspirin. Acetylsalicylic acid (aspirin) may increase the prothrombin time; however, this is not part of the treatment for rheumatoid arthritis. (14:377; 16:656)
   Nursing Process—Evaluation
   Client Need—Health promotion/maintenance

34 2. Symptoms of aspirin toxicity include tinnitus (ringing in the ears), nausea, vomiting, difficulty in hearing, lassitude, dizziness, diarrhea, and mental confusion. The signs and symptoms identified in the other options are not usual manifestations of aspirin toxicity. (20:125)
   Nursing Process—Implementation
   Client Need—Health promotion/maintenance

35 4. Of the four items in this question, swimming would most likely be the safest form of exercise. When exercise is recommended by the physician, it is most important that this activity be of the type that

would cause the least trauma to the affected joint. (11:378; 22:678)
   Nursing Process—Implementation
   Client Need—Health promotion/maintenance

36 3. Weight gain is to be avoided because extra weight places additional stress on the joint. Thus, serving meals that are well-balanced would be the best response in this item. After the acute phase, the child is encouraged to lead as normal a life as possible, including going to school and participating in age-appropriate activities. Heat is applied to joints during inflammation. (22:678)
   Nursing Process—Evaluation
   Client Need—Health promotion/maintenance

37 4. Uveitis is a complication of juvenile rheumatoid arthritis and can occur without any noticeable symptoms. Therefore, children with juvenile rheumatoid arthritis should have eye exams on a regular basis. Chest x-rays, dental exams, and hearing exams are not recommended any more frequently than they would for the child who does not have juvenile rheumatoid arthritis. (14:641; 16:655)
   Nursing Process—Implementation
   Client Need—Health promotion/maintenance

NURSING CARE OF A CHILD WITH A HEAD INJURY

38 3. The classic signs of increased intracranial pressure are a change in the level of consciousness, a rise in blood pressure, an increase in body temperature, a decrease in the pulse rate, and a widening pulse pressure. Brisk pupillary response to light, tympanic temperature of 97.9°F, and +2 deep tendon reflexes are all indicative of normal central nervous system function. (14:612)
   Nursing Process—Data collection
   Client Need—Physiological integrity

39 1. Cerebrospinal fluid often is noted leaking from the nose of the child who has sustained a basilar skull fracture. The presence of this manifestation should be reported immediately since this is the most serious type of skull fracture. A child who has had a head injury may have lost consciousness and may not remember the time of day. A Glasgow score of 15 and a radial pulse of 80 are within the normal ranges. (22:711)
   Nursing Process—Data collection
   Client Need—Physiological integrity

40 2. When riding a bicycle, the child should travel in the same direction as the flow of traffic. The other options in this item all are correct safety measures that should be followed when riding a bicycle. (11:322)

> Nursing Process—Evaluation
> Client Need—Health promotion/maintenance

NURSING CARE OF A CHILD WITH A BRAIN TUMOR

41 1. The signs and symptoms of a brain tumor usually occur as a result of increased intracranial pressure. Vomiting, especially early in the morning, is one of the signs that is seen in the child with a brain tumor. Nausea is not a usual symptom. The child may not want to go to school, and that should be documented, but this would not be considered a risk factor for the presence of a brain tumor. (16:673)

> Nursing Process—Data collection
> Client Need—Physiological integrity

42 1. The child will be placed in a tunnel-like scanner with a special call button. Sedation is used only if the client is restless or claustrophobic. Gels are not placed on the child's head and headaches do not usually occur during this procedure. (16:498)

> Nursing Process—Implementation
> Client Need—Safe, effective care environment

43 3. The head dressing of a child who has undergone a craniotomy may become damp from cerebrospinal fluid drainage. The nurse should reinforce the dressing until the dressing can be changed by the physician. Intervention is required to prevent the possibility of development of an infection at the operative site; however, complications may occur if the dressing is changed or removed. (16:498)

> Nursing Process—Implementation
> Client Need—Physiological integrity

44 2. Most chemotherapeutic agents cause some degree of nausea and vomiting. To lessen or prevent the occurrence of this side effect, the nurse should give a prescribed antiemetic prior to administering the chemotherapeutic agent. The child should always consume well-balanced meals. Serving the child a meal prior to chemotherapy may cause increased nausea and/or vomiting. The child should get plenty of rest whether receiving chemotherapy or not. Administration of an enema is not usually indicated prior to beginning chemotherapy. (16:811; 20:438)

> Nursing Process—Implementation
> Client Need—Safe, effective care environment

45 3. The nurse should encourage early and consistent visits from the child's friends in order to allow the child to have support when dealing with the reactions of friends. The changes in appearance are usually temporary; however, the nurse should not minimize the distress that the changes cause the child to experience. The other options in this item do not address the concern expressed by the child. (16:810)

> Nursing Process—Implementation
> Client Need—Psychosocial integrity

46 3. The nurse should encourage the parents to express their feelings without concern about being judged by the nurse. The parents need to know that the feelings they are experiencing are normal. In addition to listening, the nurse can suggest ways in which the parents can cope with the feelings they are experiencing. Suggesting that the parents identify things they can do to make the child feel good will assist the parents to cope with their feelings of helplessness. (11:462)

> Nursing Process—Implementation
> Client Need—Psychosocial integrity

NURSING CARE OF A CHILD IN TRACTION

47 2. There is an added risk of infection with skeletal traction. The pin site therefore should be monitored for signs of infection and cleansed as prescribed by the physician. The child would be positioned in the supine position. Range-of-motion exercises cannot be performed on the right leg and the weights should not be released. (22:686; 14:633)

> Nursing Process—Implementation
> Client Need—Physiological integrity

48 2. Pressure areas and skin breakdown are most likely to first develop over bony prominences, such as the heels, elbows, sacrum, ankles, and scapulae. (16:695)

> Nursing Process—Data collection
> Client Need—Physiological integrity

49 4. A traction rope that has slipped out of a pulley should be replaced in the pulley groove. This should be performed by the physician or the registered nurse skilled in orthopedic care. The other findings are appropriate for the child in traction. (16:694)

> Nursing Process—Evaluation
> Client Need—Physiological integrity

50 1. A high fluid intake and a diet high in fiber are recommended to prevent constipation and other complications of immobilization, such as kidney stones. The right leg, which is in traction, is kept immobile. Turning the client is not routinely performed. (16:695)

> Nursing Process—Implementation
> Client Need—Physiological integrity

51 3. The child should be able to move the toes freely. Inability to do so may indicate alteration in neurovascular status. If the toes on both feet are cool, it is probably due to the environmental temperature instead of neurovascular impairment. The other parameters indicate intact neurovascular function. (11:382; 22:686)
  Nursing Process—Evaluation
  Client Need—Physiological integrity

NURSING CARE OF AN ADOLESCENT WITH DYSMENORRHEA

52 4. Proper sleep, a well-balanced diet, warm tub baths or the application of heat to the abdomen, drinking warm liquids, and moderate exercise are some of the recommendations that can be made by the nurse. The other items mentioned are not known to relieve menstrual cramps or pain. (16:59)
  Nursing Process—Implementation
  Client Need—Health promotion/maintenance

53 4. If gastrointestinal distress occurs, aspirin may be taken with food or milk. If gastrointestinal distress persists, the physician should be contacted. Once an aspirin bottle has been opened, it has a short shelf life. Diarrhea is not a common adverse effect of acetylsalicylic acid (aspirin) taken in normal doses. Acetylsalicylic acid (aspirin) should not be taken along with a nonsteroidal anti-inflammatory agent such as ibuprofen (Motrin). (11:415)
  Nursing Process—Implementation
  Client Need—Health promotion/maintenance

54 1. Amenorrhea means the absence of menstruation. Excessive vaginal bleeding is called menorrhagia. Discomfort prior to menstruation is related to premenstrual tension, and the first menstrual period is called menarche. (11:415)
  Nursing Process—Implementation
  Client Need—Health promotion/maintenance

NURSING CARE OF AN ADOLESCENT WHO IS ABUSING DRUGS

55 4. Symptoms of amphetamine abuse include marked nervousness, restlessness, excitability, talkativeness, and excessive perspiration. The remaining items in this question are not characteristic of amphetamine abuse. (20:485)
  Nursing Process—Data collection
  Client Need—Psychosocial integrity

56 2. Amphetamines, which are central nervous system stimulants, do not cause physical abuse but are associated with psychological dependence. Those abusing amphetamines also may be involved with the abuse of other drugs. (11:429; 20:485)
  Nursing Process—Implementation
  Client Need—Health promotion/maintenance

57 1. Adolescents normally try to develop self-identity. It is believed that one way the adolescent gains self-identity is through peer relationships. The search for intimate relationships occurs during the years between 18 and 40. Integrity is a need most often demonstrated by adults rather than adolescents. Idealism is the pursuit of one's ideas or attempting to achieve an idea, and is most likely not related to amphetamine abuse. (11:398)
  Nursing Process—Implementation
  Client Need—Psychosocial integrity

58 4. Booster doses of tetanus toxoid are recommended for the adolescent once every 10 years from that point on. Smallpox vaccination is no longer advised because it is believed that the disease has been essentially eradicated. The last polio vaccine and rubella booster are given between 4 and 6 years of age. (14:410)
  Nursing Process—Implementation
  Client Need—Health promotion/maintenance

59 3. The successful treatment of substance abuse largely depends on the person's desire to become drug-free. When forced to enter a drug rehabilitation program, there is less chance that the person will remain drug-free. Normally, a court order is not necessary for participation in a drug abuse program. Discussing the dangers of drug abuse with a parent is not likely to change the child's pattern of substance abuse. (20:487)
  Nursing Process—Implementation
  Client Need—Psychosocial integrity

NURSING CARE OF AN ADOLESCENT WITH A SEXUALLY TRANSMITTED DISEASE

60 3. A diagnosis of gonorrhea is confirmed when the microorganism is found in the client's vaginal discharge. Diagnosis can be accomplished by microscopic examination of a smear of the vaginal discharge. Cultures of the discharge also may by taken. Cervical biopsy, and blood and urine specimen examination are not used to confirm a diagnosis of gonorrhea. (18:851)
  Nursing Process—Implementation
  Client Need—Safe, effective care environment

61 4. Gastrointestinal upset is one of the adverse reactions to doxycycline (Vibramycin). The client should be advised to notify the physician of any adverse reaction. Potentially serious adverse reactions should be reported to the physician immediately. This medication does not usually discolor the urine. The medication can be taken with food or dairy products, and should be taken with a full glass of water. (20:68)

Nursing Process—Implementation
Client Need—Health promotion/maintenance

62 3. One or preferably two follow-up smears or cultures should be taken after completing therapy on clients who have gonorrhea. If the cultures and smears are negative, the person is considered noninfectious. It is unsafe to assume that a client is no longer infectious when the vaginal discharge ceases, when the menstrual periods are pain-free, or when the patient has received the medication. (18:852)

Nursing Process—Implementation
Client Need—Health promotion/maintenance

63 2. The initial lesions of genital herpes can be described as fluid-filled vesicles. The lesions may become pustules and then, in time, may become crusted over. The other terms in this question do not accurately describe herpes genitalis lesions. (12:365)

Nursing Process—Data collection
Client Need—Physiological integrity

64 3. Genital herpes is currently closely associated with the occurrence of prostate cancer in males and cervical cancer in females. It has also been closely associated with the occurrence of Hodgkin's disease. Females who have genital herpes are advised to have Pap tests performed every 6 months, and males who have genital herpes are advised to have rectal exams and PSA tests done yearly. Genital herpes is not associated with sterility. (18:853)

Nursing Process—Evaluation
Client Need—Health promotion/maintenance

65 3. Topical acyclovir (Zovirax) should be applied with a glove or finger cot to prevent spread. Acyclovir (Zovirax) does not provide protection against or prevent recurrence of the disease; however, it does prolong remission and decrease the pain associated with the presence of the lesions. (20:102)

Nursing Process—Implementation
Client Need—Health promotion/maintenance

66 4. Sexual contact should be avoided, especially during active disease. The herpes virus can cross the condom membrane; therefore wearing a condom does not ensure protection. Douching and taking acyclovir (Zovirax) also do not provide protection against the transmission of the virus. (18:854)

Nursing Process—Evaluation
Client Need—Health promotion/maintenance

67 3. Malaise, fever, and opportunistic infections are some of the common symptoms of acquired immunodeficiency syndrome (AIDS). Females who have acquired immunodeficiency syndrome (AIDS) experience recurrent yeast infections. Other symptoms may include anorexia, weight loss, sore throat, diarrhea, lymph node enlargement, and abdominal cramps. Some people have few or no early symptoms. (22:152)

Nursing Process—Implementation
Client Need—Health promotion/maintenance

68 2. Symptoms of acquired immunodeficiency syndrome (AIDS) may appear months or years after the original infection; therefore the absence of symptoms is no assurance that a sexual partner does not have acquired immunodeficiency syndrome (AIDS). Acquired immunodeficiency syndrome (AIDS) cannot be cured, nor can the spread of acquired immunodeficiency syndrome (AIDS) be controlled with antiviral drugs. The drugs currently in use may slow the progression of the disease in some people. Telling the adolescent to cease sexual activity is rarely effective. (22:152)

Nursing Process—Implementation
Client Need—Health promotion/maintenance

NURSING CARE OF AN ADOLESCENT WITH SCOLIOSIS

69 2. Children with scoliosis often complain of having difficulty with their clothes fitting properly. Common complaints include an uneven hemline and uneven sleeve length. The other options are not usual findings associated with the occurrence of scoliosis. (16:659)

Nursing Process—Data collection
Client Need—Safe, effective care environment

70 1. X-rays are used to confirm the diagnosis of scoliosis. Radiation emitted by x-rays carries a risk of causing genetic mutation that may lead to birth defects in the offspring of those receiving the x-rays. Therefore the nurse should determine if there is a possibility that the client is pregnant prior to the x-ray being performed. Allergies, whether or not the person has taken medication, and whether or not the person has eaten, are not significant when a client is to receive an x-ray. (7:696)

Nursing Process—Data collection
Client Need—Safe, effective care environment

71 4. Curvatures greater than 20 degrees require treatment. If treatment is not implemented, the curvature will continue to increase and the child will be

at risk to develop cardiopulmonary problems. (16:658)
> Nursing Process—Implementation
> Client Need—Health promotion/maintenance

72 1. Curvatures between 20 and 40 degrees usually respond to nonsurgical treatment such as the Milwaukee brace. The brace is worn an average of 22 to 23 hours a day and should be removed only when the child is taking a bath or swimming. (11:372)
> Nursing Process—Implementation
> Client Need—Health promotion/maintenance

73 2. The adolescent child is very concerned about appearance and fitting in with the peer group. Since the Milwaukee brace has to be worn almost all the time, the nurse should discuss ways in which the child can fit in with the peer group and simultaneously comply with the treatment plan. (11:375)
> Nursing Process—Implementation
> Client Need—Health promotion/maintenance

INDIVIDUAL TEST ITEMS

74 2. Avoid overdressing the child in warm weather because this reduces perspiration in areas of the body that are covered with clothes. Fine cornstarch applied to the affected areas may reduce perspiration, but baby powder (which may contain talc) should be avoided because of the asbestos content of talc. Applying baby oil may increase rather than decrease the problem. Strong detergents should be avoided because of the risk of atopic dermatitis, but this will not prevent heat rashes. (11:227)
> Nursing Process—Implementation
> Client Need—Health promotion/maintenance

75 3. Tetracycline hydrochloride should be taken when the stomach is empty. If the medication is taken on an empty stomach, the person must wait 1 hour before eating. The other options in this question are appropriate actions to take when taking tetracycline hydrochloride. (20:68)
> Nursing Process—Implementation
> Client Need—Health promotion/maintenance

76 3. A small head, upward-slanting eyes, protruding tongue, curved little finger, round face, flat nose, and simian crease on the palms are outward signs of Down's syndrome. (11:311; 16:349)
> Nursing Process—Data collection
> Client Need—Health promotion/maintenance

77 4. The child will need to continue to monitor the blood glucose level because the insulin pump only delivers the insulin. It does not monitor the blood glucose level. The other options in this question indi-

cate a correct understanding of the function of the insulin pump. (11:364; 14:682)
> Nursing Process—Evaluation
> Client Need—Health promotion/maintenance

78 1. The testicles should be examined after a warm bath. The testicles should be examined, one at a time. One testicle normally is slightly larger than the other. Lumps are usually found on the side of the testicle. (11:397)
> Nursing Process—Implementation
> Client Need—Health promotion/maintenance

79 4. A ½-inch space should be left at the tip of the condom to allow for collection of the ejaculate and prevent tearing of the condom. The condom should be stored in a cool place because heat can damage the condom. The condom should be applied after the penis is erect, and a water-based lubricant should be used if lubrication is desired and the condom is not prelubricated. (11:398; 16:69)
> Nursing Process—Implementation
> Client Need—Health promotion/maintenance

80 1. Periorbital edema that is worse in the morning, decreased urination, anorexia, and hypertension are all signs of acute glomeruli nephritis. (16:795)
> Nursing Process—Data collection
> Client Need—Physiological integrity

81 1. A high-caloric bland diet served in small amounts at frequent intervals is best for the child for two reasons. The bland foods will not irritate the lesions in the child's mouth, and the additional calories are needed to prevent weight loss, which is a common finding in the child who has acquired immunodeficiency syndrome (AIDS). The other diets mentioned may not provide the nutrients needed or may aggravate other problems found in the child with acquired immunodeficiency syndrome (AIDS). (11:422)
> Nursing Process—Implementation
> Client Need—Health promotion/maintenance

82 2. Phenylketonuria (PKU) is a genetic disorder characterized by the person's inability to metabolize phenylalanine, an amino acid found in natural protein foods such as meats. Accumulation of phenylalanine in the brain tissue leads to mental retardation. If detected early enough, the diet can be modified to prevent this occurrence. Foods low in phenylalanine, such as vegetables, fruits, some cereals, breads, and starches, are recommended. (14:269)
> Nursing Process—Implementation
> Client Need—Health promotion/maintenance

83 2. Hair of varying lengths and/or bald areas may be associated with pulling on the child's hair during

abusive acts. Two-year-olds are very curious and clumsy. It is not unusual to find over bony prominences bruises and abrasions that have been sustained during falls. A bruise over soft tissue such as the abdomen should arouse suspicion. Also, it is not unusual for the 2-year-old to protest when approached by a health care provider, especially if experiences with health care providers in the past have been unpleasant. (14:297)
Nursing Process—Data Collection
Client Need—Psychosocial integrity

84 3. Crying for long periods of time, even after comfort measures have been used, is unusual and should be reported to the health care provider. The other signs and symptoms mentioned are usual side effects of the measles-mumps-rubella (MMR) inoculation, which is given at 15 months, and do not require that the health care provider be notified. (14:324)
Nursing Process—Implementation
Client Need—Health promotion/maintenance

85 4. The person sustaining a head injury should be observed for signs of intracranial bleeding, which can occur even after a "mild" or "slight" head injury. Because signs of bleeding are most likely to occur in the first 24 hours, the parents are instructed to awaken the child every 4 hours during the first night to determine the level of consciousness or other neurological changes. Examples of changes requiring prompt notification of the health care provider include slurred speech, headache, visual problems, or difficulty arousing the child from sleep. (14:316)
Nursing Process—Implementation
Client Need—Health promotion/maintenance

86 2. The preferred treatment for tinea capitis is oral griseofulvin (Grisactin) for a minimum of 6 weeks. It is recommended that the medication be taken with milk or ice cream to increase its absorption. Nits are found in pediculosis capitis, not tinea capitis. Topical medications alone are not effective in the treatment of tinea capitis. (14:662; 20:108)
Nursing Process—Evaluation
Client Need—Health Promotion

87 3. The most common manifestation of pinworms is anal itching. Teeth grinding, abdominal pain, and bulky, greasy stools are not usual findings. (16:764)
Nursing Process—Data collection
Client Need—Physiological integrity

88 2. Raw carrots should not be given to the toddler unless shredded. All of the other observations in

this question indicate that the parents understand the safety needs of the toddler. (14:360)
Nursing Process—Data collection
Client Need—Health promotion/maintenance

89 1. The apical site is preferred when assessing the pulse of a child under 5 years of age. A satisfactory radial pulse cannot be obtained until the child is 2 years of age. The carotid site is not routinely used when assessing children, but is the preferred site when performing child cardiopulmonary resuscitation (CPR). The brachial site is not routinely used when assessing children, but is the preferred site when performing infant cardiopulmonary resuscitation (CPR). (22:484)
Nursing Process—Data collection
Client Need—Health promotion/maintenance

90 3. When an oral medication is added to the infant's formula, there is no guarantee that all of the medication will be taken if the infant does not drink all of the formula. With the infant in an upright position, a rubber-tipped medicine dropper or a small medicine cup may be used to slowly administer a liquid form of the medication. The medication also can be given through the nipple from a bottle. The nose should not be pinched because the child may aspirate on the medication. (16:543)
Nursing Process—Evaluation
Client Need—Health promotion/maintenance

91 1. The salicylates prolong bleeding time by interfering with the ability of the blood to clot. Acetylsalicylic acid (aspirin) is a salicylate and is contraindicated for anyone with a bleeding disorder because it is often extremely difficult to stop the bleeding. Therefore the child might bleed to death from even a relatively small lesion. Caffeine, barbiturates, and antacids are not routinely given to the client who has hemophilia, but they are not contraindicated. (14:527)
Nursing Process—Implementation
Client Need—Health Promotion

92 3. Elbow restraints allow the child to move the arms but prevent the child from touching the face. A papoose board and mummy restraint are restraints that prevent movement of the entire body and normally are not necessary for this type of surgery. A Posey belt or jacket will not prevent the child from touching the face; instead it usually is used to keep the client in bed or in a wheelchair. (14:589)
Nursing Process—Planning
Client Need—Safe, effective care environment

93 4. Unless the physician orders otherwise, most restraints are removed and reapplied at least every 2 hours. (16:524)
Nursing Process—Planning
Client Need—Safe, effective care environment

94 2. Weak pulse, hypotension, muscular weakness, diminished reflexes, loss of peristalsis, and cardiac arrest are signs and symptoms of hypokalemia. (16:531)
Nursing Process—Data collection
Client Need—Physiological integrity

95 4. The side-lying position with the knees drawn up is the position of choice when a lumbar puncture is being performed. This position widens the space between the vertebrae to aid in insertion of the needle. The supine and Trendelenburg positions do not allow exposure of the lumbar region of the back, and thus would not be suitable for this procedure. The prone position will not facilitate widening of the inter-vertebrae spaces. (14:605)
Nursing Process—Implementation
Client Need—Safe, effective care environment

96 4. The infant's respiratory rate is counted for 1 full minute because of normal irregularities. Respirations may be counted for 30 seconds and multiplied by 2 in the older child. (11:41; 14:303)
Nursing Process—Data collection
Client Need—Health promotion/maintenance

97 1. When giving an infant an enema, the catheter is advanced 1 inch into the anal canal. The catheter should never be forced into the anal canal. If resistance is met, the enema should be stopped. (14:582)
Nursing Process—Implementation
Client Need—Safe, effective care environment

98 3. Bananas, rice, applesauce, and toast (BRAT) are usually the first solid foods offered to a child who is recovering from gastroenteritis. Butter should not be put on the rice because of the fat content. The diet is advanced gradually, with milk products being added last. (11:195; 16:762)
Nursing Process—Implementation
Client Need—Physiological integrity

99 1. Cerebral palsy is a nonprogressive neuromuscular disorder caused by an injury to the motor coordinating areas of the brain. Surgery on the brain cannot help or cure those with this disorder. Physical therapy and other disciplines, such as occupational, speech, and recreational therapy, often are of great benefit to those with cerebral palsy. (14:613; 22:695)
Nursing Process—Implementation
Client Need—Health promotion/maintenance

100 4. Rickets is caused by a lack of sufficient vitamin D in the diet. The vitamin is essential for proper calcium and phosphorous use in the body's normal bone and teeth development. Signs of rickets include delayed closure of the fontanels, delayed tooth growth, dental crises, and deformities of the long bones. (14:583)
Nursing Process—Planning
Client Need—Health promotion/maintenance

101 4. Pallor, listlessness, and irritability are observable signs of iron-deficiency anemia. A client history also may reveal anorexia, weight loss, and a decrease in the normal activity of the child. The other signs and symptoms given in this question usually are not related to iron-deficiency anemia. (16:800)
Nursing Process—Data collection
Client Need—Health promotion/maintenance

102 3. Ribavirin (Virazole) is administered through oxygen equipment such as oxyhoods, mist tents, masks, and mechanical ventilators. Caregivers and visitors who are pregnant should not visit during ribavirin treatment because the medication is considered harmful to the unborn child. The treatment usually lasts for at least 3 days but no longer than 7 days. (14:485; 20:102)
Nursing Process—Implementation
Client Need—Safe, effective care environment

103 2. The child with nephrotic syndrome should have daily weighings in order to monitor the amount of edema present. The abdominal circumference is measured also. There is a possibility that the child may develop hypertension. The child usually is given a high-protein, low-sodium diet. (14:551; 16:792)
Nursing Process—Implementation
Client Need—Physiological integrity

104 2. An ice bag can be used safely as long as it is removed every 30 minutes to 1 hour to check the skin and allow the area to return to normal. Continuous application of cold results in vasoconstriction which, if allowed to continue, could result in a loss of blood supply to the part and to gangrene. (18:570)
Nursing Process—Implementation
Client Need—Health promotion/maintenance

105 3. Parents with children having the same disability often are able to provide emotional support. When these parents meet, they share a common bond and a common burden, and learn from one another how obstacles can be overcome. Recommending that the child be placed in a long-term care facility, referring the parents to a social welfare agency, or giving them literature to read probably will not help them cope with their problems as effectively as would talking with someone who has had a similar experience. (16:655)

Nursing Process—Implementation
Client Need—Health promotion/maintenance

106 1. Measures should be taken to minimize crying because excessive crying will increase oxygen demand and thus increase the cardiac workload. The infant should be placed in the semi-Fowler's position. Holding is encouraged to decrease anxiety and the cardiac workload. The infant is fed using a soft nipple with a large hole to decrease the effort required to suck. (14:512; 16:747)

Nursing Process—Implementation
Client Need—Physiological integrity

107 4. A score of 4 indicates that the child is experiencing a lot of pain; therefore the child should be medicated with the prescribed analgesic. Diversional activities can be used in conjunction with analgesics to increase their effectiveness, or alone when the child has mild pain. (22:525; 16:555)

Nursing Process—Implementation
Client Need—Physiological integrity

108 4. Loss of a boyfriend or girlfriend may lead to depression and thoughts of suicide. It is not unusual for the adolescent to challenge rules set by the parents and argue with siblings on occasion. These actions would be of concern only if they were occurring on a frequent basis or if the adolescent's behavior became violent. The drop in the child's grades (2 points) is not significant. (11:430)

Nursing Process—Data collection
Client Need—Psychosocial integrity

109 2. Bowel control is usually easier to accomplish than bladder control and usually is achieved first. The other statements represent appropriate indicators of the child's readiness. (14:363; 11:241)

Nursing Process—Evaluation
Client Need—Health promotion/maintenance

110 1. A Wilms tumor is a congenital, cancerous tumor of the kidney. Feeling, touching, or handling the client's abdomen may result in a rupture of the renal capsule and a spread of cancerous tumor cess. Feeding the client, combing the client's hair, or giving the client a book to read would not exert pressure on the renal capsule. (11:223)

Nursing Process—Implementation
Client Need—Safe, effective care environment

111 2. Impetigo is a contagious disorder caused by a streptococcal or staphylococcal infection of the skin. Both systemic and topical antibiotics usually are prescribed. The lesions are itchy, and oral antihistamines are sometimes ordered to decrease the inflammation and itching. (11:228; 14:659)

Nursing Process—Evaluation
Client Need—Health promotion/maintenance

Classification of Test Items

Unit **III**   Review Test **14**

The Nursing Care of School-Aged Children and Adolescents

Directions: After each question the correct answer is given, as well as a classification of each test question. Compare the correct answer with your answer. If a question has been answered *incorrectly*, draw a line to the end of all the columns. When finished, add up the number of your correct answers in each column and place that number in the respective box at the end in the area identified as *Number Correct.*

To determine the percentage of questions you answered correctly and your performance in each of the test plan categories, divide the *Number Correct* in each column by the *Number Possible* in each column. Then multiply the decimal by 100. For example:

$$\frac{\text{Number Correct: 99}}{\text{Number Possible: 111}} = 0.891 \times 100 = 89\%$$

Any score that is less than 75% indicates an area where further review would be beneficial.

KEY TO ITEM CLASSIFICATION:

NURSING PROCESS

D = Data collection
P = Planning
I = Implementation
E = Evaluation

CLIENT NEEDS

S = Safe, effective care environment
P = Physiological integrity
M = Psychosocial integrity
H = Health promotion/maintenance

Question #	Answer #	D	P	I	E	S	P	M	H
1	3	D					P		
2	2			I			P		
3	4			I		S			
4	4			I			P		
5	2			I				M	
6	2			I					H
7	2	D				S			
8	4	D				S			
9	3			I		S			
10	2		P				P		
11	3			I					H
12	4				E				H
13	2	D					P		
14	3			I			P		
15	1			I			P		

Question #	Answer #	Nursing Process				Client Needs			
		D	P	I	E	S	P	M	H
16	1			I			P		
17	4	D					P		
18	1			I			P		
19	2			I					H
20	4			I					H
21	2				E				H
22	1			I					H
23	3			I					H
24	2			I		S			
25	2		P				P		
26	3			I			P		
27	4	D					P		
28	3				E		P		
29	4			I			P		
30	2	D					P		
31	1			I			P		
32	3			I		S			
33	1				E				H
34	2			I					H
35	4			I					H
36	3				E				H
37	4			I					H
38	3	D					P		
39	1	D					P		
40	2				E				H
41	1	D					P		
42	1			I		S			
43	3			I			P		
44	2			I		S			
45	3			I				M	
46	3			I				M	
47	2			I			P		

Question #	Answer #	Nursing Process				Client Needs			
		D	P	I	E	S	P	M	H
48	2	D					P		
49	4				E		P		
50	1			I			P		
51	3				E		P		
52	4			I					H
53	4			I					H
54	1			I					H
55	4	D						M	
56	2			I					H
57	1			I				M	
58	4			I					H
59	3			I				M	
60	3			I		S			
61	4			I					H
62	3			I					H
63	2	D					P		
64	3				E				H
65	3			I					H
66	4				E				H
67	3			I					H
68	2			I					H
69	2	D				S			
70	1	D				S			
71	4			I					H
72	1			I					H
73	2			I					H
74	2			I					H
75	3			I					H
76	3	D							H
77	4				E				H
78	1			I					H

-16

+62

3 1 9 3 1 4   H

	Question #	Answer #	Nursing Process				Client Needs			
			D	P	I	E	S	P	M	H
	79	4			I					H
	80	1	D					P		
	81	1			I					H
	82	2			I					H
	83	2	D						M	
	84	3			I					H
	85	4			I					H
	86	2				E				H
	87	3	D					P		
	88	2	D							H
	89	1	D							H
	90	3				E				H
	91	1			I					H
	92	3		P			S			
	93	4		P			S			
	94	2	D					P		
	95	4			I		S			
	96	4	D							H
	97	1			I		S			
	98	3			I			P		
	99	1			I					H
	100	4		P						H
	101	4	D							H
	102	3			I		S			
	103	2			I			P		
	104	2			I					H
	105	3			I					H
	106	1			I			P		
	107	4			I			P		
	108	4	D					P		
	109	2				E				H

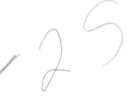

Question #	Answer #	Nursing Process				Client Needs			
		D	P	I	E	S	P	M	H
110	1			I		S			
111	2				E				H
Number Correct	86	20	4	52	11	15	29	6	36
Number Possible	111	24	5	67	15	17	36	6	52
Percentage Correct	77%	83	80	78	73	88	81	100	69

Unit IV

The Nursing Care of Clients with Mental Health Needs

The Nursing Care of Infants, Children, and Adolescents with Mental Health Needs

Mental Health Needs During Infancy
Mental Health Needs During Childhood
Mental Health Needs During Adolescence

Correct Answers and Rationale
Classification of Test Items

Directions: With a pencil, blacken the circle in front of the option you have chosen for your correct answer.

MENTAL HEALTH NEEDS DURING INFANCY

A couple who have been childless for 10 years have just become parents of a newborn with Down syndrome.

1 To help the parents cope with their disappointment, the *best* nursing action *initially* is to
  ○ 1. encourage the parents to verbalize their feelings.
  ○ 2. treat the child as though it is a normal newborn.
  ○ 3. identify community resources for assistance.
  ○ 4. encourage long-term institutional placement.

When the nurse brings the baby with Down syndrome to the mother's room, the father of the infant says, "These doctors don't know anything. We're going to consult specialists."

2 The *best response* from the nurse at this time is,
  ○ 1. "The physicians here are very well qualified."
  ● 2. "This diagnosis is difficult for you to accept."
  ○ 3. "Why do you feel you need a second opinion?"
  ○ 4. "It's not as bad as it may seem right now."

3 After gathering all of the following information, which is the *best evidence* that the mother is bonding with her infant with Down's syndrome?
  ● 1. She smiles and talks to the infant.
  ○ 2. She asks questions about baby care.
  ○ 3. She wants to see visitors who come.
  ○ 4. She gets an adequate amount of rest.

The nurse observes that the mother of the infant with Down syndrome is nervous when he cries as she bathes him.

4 The *most helpful* nursing response *at this time* is to
  ○ 1. take over for the mother briefly.
  ○ 2. advise the mother to discontinue the bath.

  ○ 3. give all future baths in the nursery.
  ● 4. point out the good job she is doing.

A nurse is assigned to care for several infants in the newborn nursery.

5 If an infant born to a mother who used heroin during her pregnancy shows signs of withdrawal, the nurse is *most likely* to observe that the baby manifests
  ○ 1. unresponsiveness.
  ○ 2. dilated pupils.
  ● 3. persistent crying.
  ○ 4. impaired sucking.

6 When caring for an infant experiencing narcotic withdrawal, a *priority* in the plan for care is to
  ● 1. reduce environmental stimuli.
  ○ 2. touch the infant frequently.
  ○ 3. stroke the infant's skin gently.
  ○ 4. leave the baby unwrapped.

7 To ensure optimum mental health for an infant born with a congenital defect like myelomeningocele, it is *best* to emphasize that the caregivers meet the child's need for
  ○ 1. autonomy.
  ● 2. love.
  ○ 3. respect.
  ○ 4. identity.

A teenage mother has brought her female infant, who is 6 months old, for a checkup. She tells the nurse that her baby cries a lot, and she is concerned that the baby is ill.

8 The *most important* information for the nurse to obtain *at this time* is
  ● 1. the infant's weight and length.
  ○ 2. the infant's lung and heart sounds.
  ○ 3. the infant's head and chest circumference.
  ○ 4. the infant's sucking and grasp reflex.

Upon examination of the teenager's infant, no signs of illness are identified.

9 What information is *most helpful* for the nurse to obtain *next*?
- ○ 1. The mother's expectations of an infant's behavior.
- ○ 2. How many more children the mother wants to have.
- ○ 3. Whether the mother plans to finish high school.
- ○ 4. The kind of toys the mother has for the baby.

The infant's teenage mother says she doesn't want to spoil the baby, so she frequently puts her in the crib when she cries.

10 The *best advice* the nurse can give the teenage mother is that
- ○ 1. holding will not result in spoiling.
- ○ 2. grandparents usually spoil babies.
- ○ 3. babies need to be spoiled.
- ○ 4. toddlers are more likely to be spoiled.

11 Which one of the following actions is *most important* for the nurse to recommend to the teenage mother for parenting her infant?
- ○ 1. Give the baby a pacifier whenever she cries.
- ○ 2. Turn on a radio in the room with the baby.
- ○ 3. Cuddle and talk to the baby frequently.
- ○ 4. Place a brightly colored mobile above the crib.

12 When the teenage mother expresses that she feels inexperienced and inadequate in caring for her baby, the *best resource* for referral is
- ○ 1. Project Head Start.
- ○ 2. Planned Parenthood.
- ○ 3. Parent-Teacher Association.
- ○ 4. parenting classes.

13 The nurse is *most accurate* in assuming that without adequate nurturing during infancy, the child of the teenage mother is at risk for developing which of the following psychosocial characteristics?
- ○ 1. Inferiority
- ○ 2. Mistrust
- ○ 3. Doubt
- ○ 4. Isolation

A public health nurse assesses a 24-month-old female at the immunization clinic.

14 Of all the assessment findings gathered at this time, which one is *most indicative* that this child is developmentally delayed?
- ○ 1. The child is being bottle-fed.
- ○ 2. The child is not toilet-trained.
- ○ 3. The child has no language skills.
- ○ 4. The child began crawling at 6 months.

15 One of the *best tools* the nurse can use to more objectively assess the toddler's overall development is the
- ○ 1. Denver II screening test.
- ○ 2. Minnesota Multiphasic Personality Inventory.
- ○ 3. Stanford-Binet test.
- ○ 4. Weber's test.

16 If the mother of the 24-month-old toddler asks the nurse how to appropriately discipline a child of this age, the *best suggestion* is to
- ○ 1. pre-identify the consequences of unacceptable behavior.
- ○ 2. show disapproval immediately after an unacceptable act.
- ○ 3. administer some form of moderate physical punishment.
- ○ 4. explain why certain behavior is undesirable.

A nursing assistant consults a pediatric nurse because she is frustrated by a 2-year-old's persistent response of "no" whenever she asks him to do something.

17 The nurse is *most correct* in explaining that this is normal behavior for toddlers who are developing the psychosocial characteristic of
- ○ 1. integrity.
- ○ 2. identity.
- ○ 3. autonomy.
- ○ 4. generativity.

18 The *best suggestion* the nurse can give the nursing assistant caring for the 2-year-old *at this time* is to
- ○ 1. let the child choose from two acceptable alternatives.
- ○ 2. withhold something the child desires until he complies.
- ○ 3. identify what is expected of the child, rather than asking.
- ○ 4. tell the child that his parents will be told of his refusal.

MENTAL HEALTH NEEDS DURING CHILDHOOD

A 3-year-old-child is frequently treated in the emergency department for sudden, acute episodes of illnesses with vague symptoms. The child also has had multiple hospital admissions. The health care team is beginning to suspect Munchausen syndrome by proxy.

19 If this diagnosis is accurate, it is important for the nurse to assess for evidence that the mother is
- ○ 1. obsessed with the fear that her child will die.
- ○ 2. ignorant of normal health patterns among children.
- ○ 3. responsible for creating the child's symptoms.
- ○ 4. overreacting to minor variations in her child's health.

A 3-year-old is scheduled for cardiac surgery.

20 Which one of the following strategies is *best* for the nurse to implement to help the child overcome the fear of being in the unfamiliar environment of the hospital?
○ 1. Bringing a favorite blanket from home
○ 2. Providing age-specific toys, like a stuffed animal
○ 3. Having one or both parents nearby at all times
○ 4. Placing the child in a room with a same-aged child

21 What is the *best explanation* when the parents ask why their 3-year-old child who will undergo cardiac surgery has resumed sucking his thumb—an activity that has not occurred for over a year?
○ 1. Sucking is a primitive form of self-stimulation.
○ 2. The regressive behavior has a comforting effect.
○ 3. It substitutes for the postoperative restriction of fluids.
○ 4. It satisfies the child's increased need for touch.

22 After explaining the purpose and procedure for starting an intravenous (IV) infusion in language the child can understand, which additional action is *most beneficial* for reducing the 3-year-old child's anxiety?
○ 1. Telling the child that the pain will be minimal.
○ 2. Offering the child a reward for good behavior.
○ 3. Letting the child handle some of the equipment.
○ 4. Showing the child others who have IV infusions.

23 If the 3-year-old child exhibited all of the following behaviors, which one is the *most severe reaction* to prolonged hospitalization?
○ 1. Clinging to the parents
○ 2. Shaking the crib frantically
○ 3. Throwing himself about
○ 4. Ignoring the parents

A 3-year-old child is brought to the emergency department by his mother for the treatment of a fractured femur.

24 What other information is *most suggestive* that the trauma is the result of a nonaccidental injury (i.e., child abuse)?
○ 1. There is evidence of healed fractures.
○ 2. Only the mother witnessed the injury.
○ 3. The child is not fully immunized yet.
○ 4. The child is underweight for his height.

25 The *best strategy* for developing a positive relationship with the injured child at the time of assessment is for the nurse to
○ 1. make an effort to have prolonged eye contact with the child.
○ 2. maintain a body position at the same level as the child.
○ 3. separate the child from the mother during the interview.
○ 4. ask the child direct questions about his mother's parenting.

26 If all of the following facts are present in the social history of an alleged perpetrator of child abuse, which one is *most similar* to the profile of other child abusers?
○ 1. The person grew up in a divorced household.
○ 2. The person's income is at or below poverty level.
○ 3. The person was the victim of child abuse.
○ 4. The person became a parent after the age of 25.

27 If the nurse suspects that a child is the victim of physical abuse, which one of the following actions is *most appropriate* to take *first*?
○ 1. Refer the parent(s) to Parents Anonymous.
○ 2. Recommend that the child be made a ward of the court.
○ 3. Contact a relative to care for the child.
○ 4. Report the facts to child protective services.

28 When interacting with a person suspected of committing child abuse, which attitude is *most conducive* for facilitating a referral to a support group?
○ 1. An impersonal attitude
○ 2. An indifferent attitude
○ 3. A sympathetic attitude
○ 4. A nonjudgmental attitude

A mother who is distressed by the fact that her 3-year-old male child has been publicly masturbating asks a nurse for advice.

29 Which one of the following suggestions is *most helpful* for preventing the child from feeling guilty about masturbating?
○ 1. Interrupt the child casually as soon as masturbation is observed.
○ 2. Explain to the child that this is an unacceptable practice.
○ 3. Tell the child that the genitals can be touched when urinating.
○ 4. Relate that touching the genitals is something that is done privately.

A nurse observes a 4-year-old child with her mother and infant sibling.

30 Which one of the following is the *best example* that the 4-year-old child is going through the developmental process called *identification?*
   ○ 1. The child recognizes animals correctly.
   ○ 2. The child calls her sibling by name.
   ◉ 3. The child pretends to feed her doll.
   ○ 4. The child accurately points to colors.

A pediatric office nurse is helping to prepare a 4-year-old for his preschool physical examination. The child's mother also has brought her newborn for his first immunization.

31 Which one of the following statements is *most indicative* that the preschooler is experiencing anxiety in relation to his new sibling?
   ○ 1. The child wants to use his father's tools.
   ○ 2. The child is taking shorter naps in the afternoon.
   ○ 3. The child cries when his toys become broken.
   ◉ 4. The child has been wetting and soiling himself.

32 The nurse is *most correct* in explaining that the behavior the preschooler is demonstrating is based on a need to feel
   ○ 1. powerful.
   ◉ 2. secure.
   ○ 3. confident.
   ○ 4. dependent.

33 The *best advice* the nurse can give the preschooler's mother for relieving her 4-year-old child's anxiety *at this time* is to
   ○ 1. give him some new toys to play with.
   ○ 2. let him stay up later at night.
   ○ 3. invite the grandparents to visit.
   ◉ 4. spend more time alone with him.

The mother of the 4-year-old child asks the nurse what is most helpful in preparing her preschooler for kindergarten.

34 Which one of the following suggestions is likely to be *most beneficial?*
   ◉ 1. Give him simple responsibilities to perform.
   ○ 2. Teach him to print his first and last name.
   ○ 3. Buy a set of children's encyclopedias.
   ○ 4. Have him watch daytime television programs.

The mother says that when her 4-year-old asks her to buy candy at the grocery store and she refuses, he throws a

temper tantrum. She resorts to buying the candy so he stops kicking and screaming.

35 The *most appropriate* recommendation for eliminating the tantrums when the 4-year-old child does not get his way is to
   ○ 1. give him candy before entering the store.
   ◉ 2. ignore the unacceptable behavior.
   ○ 3. explain to him that his behavior is childish.
   ○ 4. remind him that he's a big boy now.

The parents of a 3-year-old with infantile autism bring their child to a mental health clinic on a regular basis. Today a care conference is planned with the mental health team and the family.

36 When the social worker, who has not had experience with autistic children, asks the nurse to identify typical characteristics of the disorder, the nurse is *most accurate* in identifying
   ◉ 1. repetitive body movements.
   ○ 2. intense attachment to one parent.
   ○ 3. early sexual development.
   ○ 4. profound mental retardation.

37 If the 3-year-old child is typical of other autistic children, the nurse is *most correct* in expecting that the child's response to his parents will be one of
   ◉ 1. indifference.
   ○ 2. friendliness.
   ○ 3. submissiveness.
   ○ 4. impatience.

38 Based on the nurse's knowledge of autistic behavior, which one of the following nursing diagnoses is *most likely* a priority problem for discussion at the team conference?
   ○ 1. Altered Health Maintenance
   ○ 2. Chronic Low Self-Esteem
   ○ 3. Risk for Activity Intolerance
   ◉ 4. Risk for Self-Directed Violence

During the care conference the mother of the autistic child says that he helps dress himself, but he will not eat unless he is fed.

39 The *best suggestion* that the nurse can offer at this time is to
   ○ 1. continue to feed the child until he tries to pick up food.
   ○ 2. try giving the child finger foods while he is dressing.
   ◉ 3. leave the food until he becomes hungry enough to eat it.
   ○ 4. demonstrate how to use a spoon every time it is time to eat.

40 If and when the autistic child actually makes an effort at self-feeding, it is *most appropriate* for the nurse to recommend that the mother
○ 1. note if the self-feeding effort is repeated.
○ 2. stop feeding the child thereafter.
◉ 3. demonstrate approval in some way.
○ 4. offer food more often during the day.

41 The nurse teaches the autistic child's parents that the *best* home environment is one that is
○ 1. stimulating, with a variety of sensory experiences.
◉ 2. consistent, with a minimum amount of physical change.
○ 3. creative, with freedom to develop artistic talents.
○ 4. strict, with narrow limits for acceptable behavior.

The parents express a desire to leave their autistic child with a responsible person for a few hours occasionally so they can have relief from the constant care and supervision that is required.

42 Which one of the following is the *most appropriate* community resource for the nurse to recommend for respite services?
◉ 1. Aid to Dependent Children
○ 2. Association on Mental Deficiency
○ 3. A children's day care facility
○ 4. A home health care agency

A school nurse is training teachers' aides to help assess the development of 6- and 7-year-olds who are nearing the completion of the first grade.

43 When describing the developmental characteristics of school-aged children, the nurse is *most accurate* in saying
○ 1. they are developing long-lasting friendships.
○ 2. they are working beside and with others.
○ 3. they are finding a sense of purpose in life.
◉ 4. they are striving for independence from others.

The school nurse meets with a 7-year-old and his parents to follow up on the child's progress since being diagnosed with attention deficit hyperactivity disorder (ADHD). The child is being treated with the drug, methylphenidate hydrochloride (Ritalin).

44 When the parents of the child with ADHD ask the nurse to tell them what kind of drug their child is taking, the *best answer* is that methylphenidate hydrochloride is a(n)

◉ 1. central nervous system depressant.
○ 2. central nervous system stimulant.
○ 3. antidepressant.
○ 4. tranquilizer.

45 The nurse explains further that the *best evidence* that methylphenidate hydrochloride is achieving its desired effect is
○ 1. their child is more alert and active.
◉ 2. their child is less easily distracted.
○ 3. their child does not feel fatigued now.
○ 4. their child's moods are more stable.

The parents of the child with ADHD ask the nurse to identify the side effects associated with the drug methylphenidate hydrochloride.

46 The nurse is *most accurate* in listing the following cluster of signs and symptoms:
○ 1. Nausea, vomiting, and diarrhea
○ 2. Fatigue, drowsiness, and dry mouth
○ 3. Insomnia, tachycardia, and anorexia
◉ 4. Hypotension, bradycardia, and constipation

47 The nurse tells the parents who administer methylphenidate hydrochloride that to avoid potentiating its effects, it is *best* if their child refrained from consuming
○ 1. dairy products.
◉ 2. cola beverages.
○ 3. processed meats.
○ 4. saturated fats.

An 8-year-old female is tentatively diagnosed with leukemia. A bone marrow puncture is part of the diagnostic work-up.

48 If this child is typical of others her age with a serious illness, which one of the following concepts is the *most commonly* held belief about being ill?
○ 1. Illness is not life-threatening; recovery is assured.
○ 2. Significant others can prevent serious consequences.
◉ 3. Discomfort is a punishment for some wrongdoing.
○ 4. Failure to comply results in parental rejection.

49 To minimize the child's apprehension about the bone marrow puncture, which one of the following nursing strategies is *best*?
○ 1. Explain the procedure shortly before it is done.
◉ 2. Give the child information as soon as the test is scheduled.
○ 3. Postpone teaching until the child asks specific questions.
○ 4. Wait for the physician to explain the procedure to the child.

50 Whenever a school-aged child is prepared for a procedure, test, or medical treatment, the *most essential* information for children this age is
○ 1. when the procedure will take place.
○ 2. who will perform the procedure.
○ 3. where the procedure will be performed.
● 4. what will be experienced during the procedure.

51 The outcome that is *most likely* to develop from providing honest explanations to a school-aged child who is ill, even if it includes unpleasant experiences, is one of
● 1. confidence in caregivers.
○ 2. perseverance in hardship.
○ 3. courage in crises.
○ 4. hope in suffering.

A single parent consults the school nurse for help in dealing with her 8-year-old daughter, who has been diagnosed with a learning disability.

52 If the nurse offers all of the following suggestions, which one is *most important* for preserving the child's self-esteem?
● 1. Set realistic, achievable goals.
○ 2. Obtain professional tutoring.
○ 3. Help the child with homework.
○ 4. Offer rewards for good grades.

It has been called to the attention of the school nurse that a 9-year-old student frequently is absent from school. Even when he attends school, he talks out of turn, fights with classmates, moves about in the classroom during a lesson, and does not complete his in-class assignments or homework. His current grades are not consistent with his past performance. The nurse plans to speak with the student to determine if he has a health problem that has been causing these recent changes in school attendance and academic performance.

53 Which one of the following is the *most appropriate* approach when the nurse speaks with the 9-year-old child about his health status?
● 1. Sitting down at the lunch table with him
○ 2. Arranging to see him in the nursing office before school
○ 3. Calling him aside in the hallway on the way to his classroom
○ 4. Meeting with him on the playground during recess

54 If the 9-year-old student who has been acting out in school tells the nurse all of the following, which one is *most likely* affecting his recent behavior?
● 1. His parents are involved in divorce proceedings.

○ 2. His pet dog just had a litter of puppies.
○ 3. He just acquired a neighborhood paper route.
○ 4. He plans to visit his out-of-state grandparents.

The nurse meets with the teacher of the 9-year-old who disrupts the class.

55 Which one of the following approaches is *best* for the nurse to recommend for helping the child maintain acceptable behavior in school?
○ 1. Send him to the principal's office when he misbehaves.
○ 2. Suspend him until a family conference occurs.
○ 3. Have the school counselor see him on a daily basis.
● 4. Consistently enforce reasonable limits for behavior.

A school nurse observes four students who are all approximately 10 years old.

56 According to socialization patterns, which 10-year-old is demonstrating behavior *most associated* with first-born children?
○ 1. Child A, who has a low tolerance for frustration
○ 2. Child B, who tends to compromise willingly
● 3. Child C, who conforms to adult expectations
○ 4. Child D, who is flexible when given choices

A 10-year-old female is brought to the emergency department in ketoacidosis secondary to undiagnosed Type I diabetes mellitus.

57 If all of the following are observed as the child improves, which one is *most indicative* that she is having difficulty accepting her diagnosis?
○ 1. She stays up later than usual watching television.
● 2. She makes angry remarks to the nurse and her mother.
○ 3. She avoids completing her homework assignments.
○ 4. She talks on the phone for long periods of time.

58 If the nursing care plan included all of the following client activities, which one provides the newly diagnosed diabetic child with the *most sense of control* over her disease?
○ 1. Being informed of laboratory test results
○ 2. Receiving calorie-controlled dietary instructions
● 3. Testing her own capillary blood glucose levels
○ 4. Learning the parts of an insulin syringe

A 12-year-old child is being treated for Tourette's syndrome.

59 Besides helping the client and family cope with the child's repetitive, purposeless movements, which other problem associated with Tourette's syndrome is *essential* for the nurse to address?
- ◉ 1. Verbal obscenities
- ○ 2. Social withdrawal
- ○ 3. Pathologic lying
- ○ 4. Mood swings

Haldoperiodol (Haldol) is prescribed for the child with Tourette's syndrome.

60 It is *most appropriate* for the nurse to teach the client and his family to report side effects of haldoperiodol such as involuntary tremors and muscle
- ◉ 1. spasms.
- ○ 2. weakness.
- ○ 3. atrophy.
- ○ 4. shortening.

The parents are concerned that the self-esteem of their child with Tourette's syndrome may be jeopardized by peer ridicule.

61 The *best suggestion* the nurse can offer the parents is to
- ○ 1. try home-schooling this child.
- ◉ 2. praise deserved accomplishments.
- ○ 3. avoid discussing peer comments.
- ○ 4. show disapproval of negative labels.

MENTAL HEALTH NEEDS DURING ADOLESCENCE

A 13-year-old student takes a gun to school and murders a teacher.

62 Based on the principles of crisis intervention, when is the *best time* to provide assistance to those most affected by this incident?
- ○ 1. After the funeral
- ○ 2. Within 6 months
- ◉ 3. Immediately
- ○ 4. Six weeks later

63 If the adolescents who witnessed the violence at school are typical of others who experience crises, they are *most likely* feeling
- ◉ 1. helpless.
- ○ 2. depressed.
- ○ 3. angry.
- ○ 4. fortunate.

64 When crisis intervention is provided, which action is *most important* for the nurse who is part of the crisis team to take first?

- ○ 1. Explain the benefits of professional counseling.
- ◉ 2. Encourage the survivors to talk about the event.
- ○ 3. Reassure the survivors that they will adapt.
- ○ 4. Advise consulting a physician for drug therapy.

A 15-year-old female is assessed in the emergency department and admitted to the hospital after she fainted at school. She is more than 25% below the normal weight for her height. She is believed to be suffering from anorexia nervosa.

65 During a physical assessment, if the client has anorexia nervosa, the nurse is *most likely* to find
- ◉ 1. growth of fine body hair.
- ○ 2. bruises over her upper torso.
- ○ 3. hyperactive bowel sounds.
- ○ 4. club-shaped fingertips.

The nurse obtains a nursing history on admission of the client with anorexia nervosa.

66 Which of the following data *best correlates* with the profile of a person with anorexia nervosa?
- ○ 1. The client is the middle child of three siblings.
- ◉ 2. The client is a high achiever in school and activities.
- ○ 3. The client thinks her classmates do not like her.
- ○ 4. The client experienced many illnesses during childhood.

The nursing team meets for a conference to plan the anorectic client's care.

67 Which of the following goals has the *highest priority* at this time?
- ○ 1. Improving her distorted body image
- ○ 2. Helping her use healthier coping techniques
- ◉ 3. Restoring normal nutrition
- ○ 4. Developing assertiveness

The anorectic client's mother visits at suppertime. She is overheard to say, "Look at you, you're so thin. Please eat something."

68 Which of the following is *most therapeutic* for the nurse to say privately to the mother of the 15-year-old with anorexia nervosa?
- ○ 1. "All children know how to frustrate parents."
- ◉ 2. "You need to stop pleading with her to eat."
- ○ 3. "You're concerned that she's starving herself."
- ○ 4. "I know how you're feeling; I'm a mother too."

The nursing assistant is frustrated and angry when she sees the anorectic client rearranging the food on her tray but not eating any of it.

69 The *best advice* the nurse can give the nursing assistant caring for the anorectic client is to
○ 1. blend the food, and administer it by tube feeding.
○ 2. remind the client that her intake is being recorded.
○ 3. review the treatment goals with the client again.
● 4. remove the food without making any comments.

Just before it is time for the anorectic client to be weighed, the nursing assistant tells the nurse that she observed her drink a full pitcher of water.

70 The *best nursing action* at this time is to
○ 1. postpone weighing the client until later.
● 2. confront the client about what was observed.
○ 3. say nothing and weigh the client as usual.
○ 4. subtract 2 lb from the client's weight.

A 16-year-old with moderate retardation is admitted for treatment of a ruptured appendix. His mother reports that the client has an IQ in the range of 35 to 50, or that which approximates a 5- to 7-year-old. A temporary colostomy is necessary.

71 If this developmentally disabled client is typical of others his mental age, it is *most appropriate* for the nurse to assess the client for
● 1. distress when separated from his mother.
○ 2. an exaggerated response to pain.
○ 3. difficulty making his needs known.
○ 4. concern over the change in body image.

72 If the nurse who admitted the retarded adolescent notes all of the following maternal behaviors, which one is *most likely* to suppress this child's ability to reach his maximum potential for development?
● 1. The mother dresses and undresses the child.
○ 2. The mother answers all the medical questions.
○ 3. The mother exaggerates her child's abilities.
○ 4. The mother blames herself for her child's condition.

A nursing assistant assigned to care for the young man who is mentally retarded reports that he struck her while she was attempting to help him out of bed.

73 Which one of the following is the *best explanation* for the retarded adolescent's behavior?
○ 1. Aggression is a common behavior manifested by mentally retarded people.
● 2. Aggression is a response that occurs when a person feels threatened.
○ 3. Aggression is an indication that the client has a poor opinion of his care.
○ 4. Aggression is one way that children communicate they are experiencing pain.

The nursing assistant consults the nurse as to how to document the incident in which the retarded adolescent struck her.

74 Which one of the following examples of documentation is *best?*
○ 1. Became angry for no reason and an assault occurred.
○ 2. Hit caregiver unexpectedly even though not provoked.
● 3. Struck nursing assistant when being helped from bed.
○ 4. Attacked nursing assistant without prior warning.

The retarded adolescent's behavioral outburst is discussed at a team conference.

75 If all of the following suggestions are made, which one is *best* for preventing nursing personnel from being injured during future care?
○ 1. Apply soft wrist restraints before ambulating.
○ 2. Ask the mother to ambulate the client.
● 3. Explain steps in care before touching the client.
○ 4. Medicate the client immediately before ambulating.

A 16-year-old male is brought to the emergency department for treatment of a stab wound following a gang-related fight. The 16-year-old eventually is ordered by the court to receive counseling at the community mental health clinic.

76 Which of the following areas of the adolescent's social history is *most appropriate* for the clinic nurse to assess?
● 1. Peer relationships
○ 2. School performance
○ 3. Church attendance
○ 4. Employment records

77 If the nurse obtains all of the following data, which factor has the *strongest influence* on teenagers developing antisocial behavior?
● 1. Parental discipline is inconsistent.
○ 2. There are more than three siblings.
○ 3. The family relies on public welfare.
○ 4. Role models do not value education.

78 Which one of the following is *most important* to communicate each time the adolescent attends a group meeting?
○ 1. The date and time of the next meeting
○ 2. The qualifications of the therapists
○ 3. That everyone should use first names only
● 4. That client information is kept confidential

79 If the adolescent who is involved in gang activities demonstrates all of the following behaviors during group meetings, which one is *most indicative* that he is resisting the therapy?
○ 1. The adolescent borrows cigarettes from others.
○ 2. The adolescent laughs inappropriately.
● 3. The adolescent keeps checking his watch.
○ 4. The adolescent fidgets in his chair.

Family therapy is added to the counseling plan for the adolescent gang member. The client's father arrives late and is intoxicated.

80 If the adolescent is typical of others who have grown up in an alcoholic family, it is *most appropriate* for the nurse to observe for problems with
● 1. low self-esteem.
○ 2. managing stress.
○ 3. long-term learning.
○ 4. fear of authority.

81 The *most appropriate* community resource to which the nurse can refer the adolescent with the alcoholic parent is
● 1. Alcoholics Anonymous
○ 2. Al-Anon
○ 3. Alateen
○ 4. The Substance Abuse Council

82 If this adolescent benefits from therapy that focuses on growing up in an alcoholic household, the nurse is *most likely* to observe that he is developing the ability to
○ 1. keep promises.
● 2. trust others.
○ 3. solve problems.
○ 4. honor commitments.

A 16-year-old has been selected to play on the junior varsity football team. He spends several hours a day in a weight training facility.

83 When the owner of the gym asks the teenager if he would like a drug to help him "bulk up," which of the following factors *most likely* will influence the adolescent to accept?
● 1. Several of his teammates are taking this drug.
○ 2. The team currently is having a winning season.

○ 3. His parents support his interest in football.
○ 4. He can afford to pay for a substantial supply.

After taking the unidentified drug for some time, the high school athlete's weight increases dramatically, and his muscles become more massive and well defined.

84 If the unprescribed drug is an anabolic steroid, which other physical effect is common?
○ 1. Decreased lung capacity
○ 2. Bronzed skin
● 3. Occurrence of or worsened acne
○ 4. Brittle nails

85 A behavioral effect of anabolic steroids is
● 1. aggression and rage.
○ 2. confusion and doubt.
○ 3. friendliness and humor.
○ 4. elation and excitement.

After being suspended from the team for taking anabolic steroids, the teenager tells his mother, "I might as well be dead. My football career is over."

86 What advice is *most appropriate* to give the mother of the teenager at this time?
○ 1. Disregard her son's behavior; he's acting normal.
○ 2. Tell her son to snap out of it; his life is not over.
○ 3. Suggest transferring her son to another school.
● 4. Ask her son if he is having any thoughts of suicide.

A 17-year-old female has been dating a classmate secretly because the relationship is a constant source of parental conflict. She also has stopped attending church, started smoking cigarettes—something her parents strongly dislike—and she has had sexual intercourse. She has not had a menstrual period for 2 months.

87 When the teenager makes an appointment at a birth control clinic, which one of the following qualities is *most important* for the nurse to communicate during the first meeting?
○ 1. Efficiency
○ 2. Intelligence
○ 3. Dexterity
● 4. Acceptance

88 What is the *best approach* for conveying that the nurse is interested in this client?
● 1. Make frequent eye contact with her.
○ 2. Provide her with free clinic literature.
○ 3. Write down information the client provides.
○ 4. Avoid long pauses between questions.

As the adolescent talks with the clinic nurse, she reveals that her parents disapprove of her friends, ideas, and actions.

89 The nurse is *most correct* in sharing that it is normal for adolescents to test previously accepted values to establish their own
  ○ 1. ingenuity.
  ● 2. identity.
  ○ 3. intuition.
  ○ 4. insight.

The nurse is called out of the room by the receptionist, who tells her that the teenager's mother is on the phone and wants to know why her daughter is being seen.

90 The *best advice* for the receptionist is to inform the client's mother that
  ● 1. the clinic cannot release that information.
  ○ 2. her daughter will return her phone call shortly.
  ○ 3. she can talk to her daughter in a few minutes.
  ○ 4. clients come to the clinic for birth control.

A pregnancy test is performed before prescribing a method of birth control for the adolescent client. The test result is positive.

91 Which one of the following is *most beneficial* to the pregnant adolescent at this time?
  ○ 1. A positive mothering instinct
  ○ 2. Making plans for marriage
  ○ 3. Financial support from her boyfriend
  ● 4. Emotional support from her family

The question arises among the clinic personnel as to why the pregnant adolescent asked for contraceptive assistance when she probably suspected she was pregnant already.

92 The *best explanation* is that this client's behavior is an example of the psychological defense mechanism called
  ○ 1. displacement.
  ○ 2. regression.
  ● 3. denial.
  ○ 4. compensation.

The parents of an 18-year-old female bring their daughter to a mental health clinic after she reports hearing voices that tell her she is a bad person.

93 When the parents ask if their daughter is psychotic, the nurse who is performing the initial interview is *most correct* in explaining that psychotic people are those who

  ○ 1. adjust poorly to new situations.
  ○ 2. have difficulty in relationships.
  ● 3. cannot differentiate reality from fantasy.
  ○ 4. feel helpless in resolving problems.

94 As the nurse performs a brief assessment of the client's mental status, which question is *most appropriate* for assessing the client's orientation?
  ● 1. What is today's date?
  ○ 2. How did you get here?
  ○ 3. Where were you born?
  ○ 4. Who is the president?

The 18-year-old client who experiences hallucinations asks to read the form on which the nurse is writing.

95 The *best action* the nurse can take in this situation is to
  ○ 1. ask why she is so suspicious.
  ○ 2. put the clipboard away.
  ● 3. hand her the form to read.
  ○ 4. tell her it is illegal.

The 18-year-old client who experiences hallucinations tells the nurse that she refuses to be admitted to the psychiatric unit of the local hospital.

96 Which one of the following nursing responses is *most accurate*?
  ○ 1. The client cannot be committed involuntarily unless she is uncooperative at this time.
  ● 2. The client cannot be committed involuntarily unless she may harm herself or others.
  ○ 3. The client cannot be committed involuntarily unless she will not keep office appointments.
  ○ 4. The client cannot be committed involuntarily unless she refuses to take medications.

The psychiatrist prescribes the antipsychotic drug haloperidol (Haldol) for the client who hears voices that others do not hear.

97 Which of the following is the *most appropriate* health teaching when a client self-administers Haldol?
  ○ 1. Take the pills on an empty stomach.
  ○ 2. Don't skip meals while taking the drug.
  ○ 3. Stop taking the drug if sedation occurs.
  ● 4. Rise slowly from a sitting position.

98 Which of the following is the *best indication* that haloperidol is achieving a therapeutic effect?
  ● 1. The client no longer hears voices.
  ○ 2. The client sleeps more than before.
  ○ 3. The client thinks of herself as a good person.
  ○ 4. The client feels more energetic and rested.

99 When the client calls and reports all of the following physical changes, which one is a *serious side effect* of haloperidol (Haldol) that needs to be reported to the prescribing physician immediately?
○ 1. Frequent diarrhea
● 2. Severe sore throat
○ 3. Gradual weight loss
○ 4. Ringing of the ears

A 17-year-old is not responding to drug therapy for leukemia and eventually becomes terminal. The parents are unsure of how or if to tell their child.

100 Which one of the following reasons is the *best justification* for openly discussing their child's prognosis with him?
○ 1. The adolescent eventually will guess that he is dying.
● 2. Sharing prevents the teen from dealing with fears alone.
○ 3. It is difficult for everyone to conceal the truth.
○ 4. Being less than honest is immoral and unethical.

Directions: Two numbers appear in parentheses following each rationale. The first number identifies the textbook listed in the references, page 512, and the second number identifies the page(s) in that textbook on which the correct answer can be verified. Occasionally two or more textbooks are given to verify the correct answer.

MENTAL HEALTH NEEDS DURING INFANCY

1 1. Verbalizing feelings is an appropriate step to processing emotional trauma. Emphasizing normal emotional needs, regardless of the infant's cognitive ability, and referring the parents to agencies that provide early intervention techniques eventually are appropriate, but not necessarily before the parents react emotionally themselves. Institutionalization may not be the parents' first choice in how they will care for their child. (4:1426)
   Nursing Process—Implementation
   Client Need—Psychosocial integrity

2 2. An effective communication technique, called reflecting, involves responding to both the feelings and the content of what is said. The empathy that it communicates facilitates further therapeutic interaction. Defending, the first example, is a nontherapeutic technique that implies to clients that their feelings or actions are unnecessary and foolish. Asking a question using the word "why" is referred to as "demanding an explanation." It, too, is nontherapeutic because most people are not able to verbalize their rationale. The last choice is another example of a nontherapeutic communication technique called disagreeing. Disagreeing with the client indicates that the clients have no right to feel as they do. (9:150–151; 10:92)
   Nursing Process—Implementation
   Client Need—Psychosocial integrity

3 1. Evidence of bonding includes eye contact, skin contact, smiling and talking to the infant, and cuddling. The other behaviors are normal and appropriate, but they are not the best evidence of bonding. (22:306; 9:172)
   Nursing Process—Evaluation
   Client Need—Health promotion/maintenance

4 4. Allowing the mother to provide basic care promotes bonding. A mother's self-concept and self-confidence are increased when the nurse offers supportive encouragement. Interfering with parenting

skills contributes to the mother's feelings of insecurity. (9:173; 22:306)
   Nursing Process—Implementation
   Client Need—Psychosocial integrity

5 3. Withdrawal from heroin and other abused drugs, whether it occurs in infants or adults, is characterized by symptoms that are somewhat opposite those of the drug's action. For example, in heroin withdrawal infants are hyperactive, irritable, and cry constantly. (16:371; 18:840)
   Nursing Process—Data collection
   Client Need—Psychosocial integrity

6 1. Because narcotic withdrawal is characterized by central nervous system stimulation, reducing environmental stimuli is a priority when caring for an infant experiencing the effects of narcotic withdrawal. Touching and stroking are more appropriate when caring for normal newborns. Most infants, including those experiencing narcotic withdrawal, are comforted by being wrapped snugly in a blanket. (16:371; 18:840)
   Nursing Process—Planning
   Client Need—Physiological integrity

7 2. Meeting an infant's need for love is one of the best foundations for future mental health, regardless of the child's physical or mental status. The needs for autonomy, respect, and identity also are important, but they represent higher-level needs. (4:1426)
   Nursing Process—Implementation
   Client Need—Health promotion/maintenance

8 1. Infantile anxiety is manifested by excessive crying. Severe anxiety leads to weight loss and stunted growth, commonly referred to as a failure to thrive. Listening to the lung and heart sounds and measuring the head and chest are appropriate, but they do not indicate as readily how this child's growth compares to norms for infants her age. Assessing the sucking and grasp reflex is more appropriate for a newborn infant. (9:42; 17:860, 895)
   Nursing Process—Data collection
   Client Need—Physiological integrity

9 1. A certain amount of crying is normal for an infant. It is the only means a baby has for communicating distress. Finding out the mother's expectations helps the nurse determine if her perception of the infant's behavior is realistic. The other selections do not provide significant additional data needed to analyze the basis for the young mother's observation. (9:43)

Nursing Process—Data collection
Client Need—Health promotion/maintenance

10 1. Neglecting and isolating an infant promotes stress and affects normal development. Babies, like anyone else, cannot develop negative effects from being held and touched in an affectionate manner. Infants are extremely sensitive to the attitudes and actions of those caring for them. All humans, not just babies or toddlers, need physical and social contact with other humans for adequate nurturing. (9:43)

Nursing Process—Implementation
Client Need—Health promotion/maintenance

11 3. Touching and hearing a parent's voice are essential for optimal emotional growth during infancy. When an infant receives affectionate sensory stimulation, it helps promote a feeling of trust, the major developmental task during infancy. Inanimate sensory stimulation is appropriate, but physical human interaction is a priority. (9:41; 10:86)

Nursing Process—Planning
Client Need—Health promotion/maintenance

12 4. Parenting classes are taught by one or more people who have expertise in successful child-rearing techniques. Participants learn by imitating the modeled behavior of others in the group. Members of the group support one another by sharing common experiences. Project Headstart is for preschool children. Planned Parenthood is concerned with family planning. The Parent-Teacher Association is for parents of school children. (16:281, 398)

Nursing Process—Implementation
Client Need—Health promotion/maintenance

13 2. Mistrust is the characteristic most likely to develop if infants are not nurtured adequately. The other characteristics—inferiority, doubt, and isolation—are negative attributes that are acquired at later stages of unfulfilled development. (18:84; 22:410)

Nursing Process—Evaluation
Client Need—Health promotion/Maintenance

14 3. A 24-month-old child uses at least single words, like "no" and "me" to make their ideas understood.

The other behaviors are not necessarily an indication of developmental delay. (4:93)

Nursing Process—Evaluation
Client Need—Health promotion/maintenance

15 1. The Denver II screening test measures four major areas of development and is able to identify developmental delays from infancy through preschool ages. The Minnesota Multiphasic Personality Inventory is administered to adults to identify psychological characteristics. The Stanford-Binet test is an IQ (intelligence) test. The Weber's test is a hearing assessment. (16:433)

Nursing Process—Planning
Client Need—Health promotion/maintenance

16 2. It is appropriate to demonstrate disapproval immediately after unacceptable behavior. This helps the child associate the undesirable behavior with negative consequences. Toddlers are too young to control their impulses just by identifying potential consequences or explanations for behavioral expectations. Physical punishment tends to teach impressionable youngsters that it is appropriate to be physically violent. (4:93)

Nursing Process—Planning
Client Need—Health promotion/maintenance

17 3. To exercise autonomy, toddlers often become defiant and refuse to cooperate with requests, routines, and regulations. The psychosocial characteristics of integrity, identity, and generativity are acquired at later stages of development. (2:103)

Nursing Process—Evaluation
Client Need—Health promotion/maintenance

18 1. To avoid a power struggle, it is best to give the child an opportunity to choose between two acceptable alternatives. Withholding something that is desirable is not likely to meet with success since a child this age tends to be quite oppositional when challenged. The child is too young to comprehend abstract explanations. Threatening the child is not a therapeutic approach to gaining cooperation. (9:45)

Nursing Process—Implementation
Client Need—Safe, effective care environment

MENTAL HEALTH NEEDS DURING CHILDHOOD

19 3. Munchausen syndrome by proxy is characterized by causing symptoms in a dependent child. Consequently, the victims of this illness are subjected to a variety of medical procedures. This condition is considered a form of child abuse and reported to the authorities. (14:296)

>   Nursing Process—Data collection
>   Client Need—Psychosocial integrity

20 3. Having one or both parents within sight and touch helps to prevent separation anxiety and provides one of the best coping strategies for dealing with the pain and suffering that the child may experience. The other alternatives also have secondary therapeutic value. (9:181)

>   Nursing Process—Implementation
>   Client Need—Health promotion/maintenance

21 2. Regressive behavior, like thumb-sucking, is considered a coping mechanism that relieves anxiety. Given the child's circumstances and behavioral observations among others who have experienced stressful situations, it is the most credible explanation for the phenomenon. (16:510)

>   Nursing Process—Implementation
>   Client Need—Health promotion/maintenance

22 3. Handling equipment, whenever that is possible, helps children overcome some of their initial fears. It is important to be honest with children when procedures involve pain. However, the term "minimal" is relative and, from a child's perspective, the pain may be more than minimal. Bribing a child by offering a reward is not a therapeutic technique for gaining cooperation. Seeing others who have IVs does not necessarily diminish the unique feelings and perceptions of the child who is about to have this procedure performed. (18:863)

>   Nursing Process—Implementation
>   Client Need—Psychosocial integrity

23 4. Ignoring the parents is the most severe reaction that occurs among toddlers as hospitalization is prolonged. It is characteristic of detachment, the third stage in what has been described as typical hospital adjustment. The other choices are associated with the protest stage that occurs initially. The second stage, called despair, is characterized by apathy and withdrawal. (16:511; 18:862–863)

>   Nursing Process—Evaluation
>   Client Need—Psychosocial integrity

24 1. One of the classic signs of physical abuse is evidence of scars, bruises, and fractures in various stages of healing. Being underweight and not fully immunized is cause to suspect neglect or that the family is financially needy, but in and of itself is not as strongly suggestive of abuse. And it is possible

for injuries to occur without an adult witness. (16:472; 18:894)

>   Nursing Process—Data collection
>   Client Need—Physiological integrity

25 2. Positioning oneself at a young child's level, regardless of the purpose of an interaction, reduces the potential for feeling threatened. Prolonged eye contact tends to heighten anxiety. Victims of child abuse often protect their abusers. Separation and asking direct questions are not appropriate techniques for promoting a positive nurse-client relationship. (4:1349)

>   Nursing Process—Planning
>   Client Need—Psychosocial integrity

26 3. Child abusers frequently have been victims of child abuse themselves. There are significant stressors for those who are raised by a single parent or those who are not financially secure, but these factors are not uniquely contributory to child abuse. Those who abuse their children are more often young and immature at the time the violence begins. (16:472; 18:894)

>   Nursing Process—Data collection
>   Client Need—Psychosocial integrity

27 4. Nurses are among those who are required by law to report suspected child abuse. To not do so is considered a crime. It is the responsibility of the child protective services agency to find a temporary, safe environment, such as foster care, for the child who is in future danger. Parents Anonymous is an organization that provides support to those who wish to break the cycle of child abuse. However, the priority at this time is for the child's safety. (16:473; 18:895)

>   Nursing Process—Implementation
>   Client Need—Safe, effective care environment

28 4. Perpetrators of child abuse, as well as those with other social problems, are more likely to be receptive to seeking help if the nurse conveys a nonjudgmental attitude during the interaction. The other examples are not necessarily negative, but are not more likely to motivate clients toward self-help. (9:178; 23:531)

>   Nursing Process—Planning
>   Client Need—Psychosocial integrity

29 4. Giving the child permission to masturbate privately sets limits as to where this is done, but does not imply that it is a deviant behavior. Interrupting the practice or providing the child with another alternative temporarily stops the activity, but the child does not understand the purpose for the diversion. The other choices imply that experiencing pleasure from touching oneself is objectionable. (2:100)

    Nursing Process—Implementation
    Client Need—Health promotion/maintenance

30 3. Feeding a doll is most suggestive of the process of identification. Identification is behavior that imitates the same-sex parent or other adult. The other behaviors are examples of the child's cognitive development. (2:70)

    Nursing Process—Evaluation
    Client Need—Health promotion/maintenance

31 4. A toddler who is not accustomed to sharing attention may feel that the new child is taking his place. He may behave like an infant to regain attention, or he may resort to behavior manifested during an earlier period of development to feel more secure. It is normal for a 4-year-old to begin identifying with and imitating the same-sex parent at this age. Preschoolers begin to need less daytime sleep. At this age, crying is a natural emotional response to disappointing events. (9:45, 71)

    Nursing Process—Data collection
    Client Need—Health promotion/maintenance

32 2. Anxiety occurs when a person perceives himself or herself in a threatening situation. The perceived threat creates a feeling of insecurity. Mental mechanisms, such as regression, are unconsciously or subconsciously used to eliminate or reduce conflict, protect one's self-image, and resolve an emotional dilemma. (10:32, 428–429)

    Nursing Process—Implementation
    Client Need—Health promotion/maintenance

33 4. Anxiety that results from competing for attention is diminished if some time is spent alone with the child. The other choices in this item are not inappropriate, but they will not necessarily relieve the child's anxiety. (9:46)

    Nursing Process—Implementation
    Client Need—Health promotion/maintenance

34 1. A school-aged child must learn to follow directions and carry out a task. Providing the preschooler with activities that are within his level of accomplishment promotes success and a positive feeling about his own competence. Children may become confused and frustrated if a parent's instructions are different from the teacher's. A preschooler has no immediate use for a children's encyclopedia. Daytime television programs are not necessarily educational. (9:47)

    Nursing Process—Implementation
    Client Need—Health promotion/maintenance

35 2. Children learn how to manipulate others through certain types of behavior. When a child realizes that a tantrum will not obtain the desired result, the behavior likely will be extinguished. Giving candy beforehand does not support the principle that candy is not allowed at this time. A young child is more likely to behave based on his emotions rather than on intellectual logic. Therefore, the toddler is not likely to accept an explanation about the inappropriateness of his behavior or the plea that he act differently. (9:105)

    Nursing Process—Implementation
    Client Need—Health promotion/maintenance

36 1. Autistic children tend to display bizarre body movements. For example, they rock their bodies or touch their hands to their faces in peculiar mannerisms. None of the other items describes characteristics of autism. (23:489)

    Nursing Process—Implementation
    Client Need—Safe, effective care environment

37 1. Autistic children tend to show little or no ability to relate to other humans, including their parents. All the remaining examples require that the individual interact with and respond to one or more people. This is not a characteristic of a person with autism. (23:488)

    Nursing Process—Data collection
    Client Need—Psychosocial integrity

38 4. One of the common behaviors among autistic people is a tendency to cause self-harm by head banging, biting, and pulling out hair and fingernails. The autistic client is not capable or responsible for maintaining his own health. Self-esteem is established on the basis of receiving approval or disapproval from others. Because an autistic client is indifferent to the physical presence and the opinion of others, low self-esteem is not a likely problem. An autistic person's general physical health is not affected by his mental disorder. Therefore, if the client cannot tolerate activity, it is due to another, unrelated condition. (2:200; 23:489)

    Nursing Process—Planning
    Client Need—Safe, effective care environment

39 1. People with autism have varying levels of impairment and require full assistance with some or all activities of daily living. When the child demonstrates an attempt at self-feeding, it is appropriate to encourage him to participate in this aspect of his self-care. Learning takes place when a person is ready. Until an autistic child demonstrates some

interest, attempts to gain his cooperation are likely to be frustrating. (18:938; 2:200)
    Nursing Process—Planning
    Client Need—Physiological integrity

40 3. Rewards, even in the form of praise, tend to promote repetition of a desired behavior. Noting if the behavior is repeated is not inappropriate, but it is not the best technique to use first. It is too much to expect that a child will continue self-feeding after only one attempt. Giving the child more food does not necessarily encourage the self-feeding behavior; if it does, obesity is a possible consequence. (18:952; 23:115)
    Nursing Process—Implementation
    Client Need—Health promotion/maintenance

41 2. If autistic individuals' possessions, routines, or environment are altered, they are likely to become very upset and combative toward others or themselves. A stimulating environment creates chaos and distress for a person with autism. Autistic people often have limited artistic potential. Limit-setting is important, but a rigid, inflexible atmosphere can be distressing. (2:00; 23:489)
    Nursing Process—Planning
    Client Need—Psychosocial integrity

42 4. Private home health care agencies employ various levels of health practitioners. An agency of this type selects the surrogate caregiver most appropriate for the type of client and level of care that is needed. Aid to Dependent Children is a social welfare agency that provides economic assistance to a parent who is unable to financially support the care of one or more children. The Association on Mental Deficiency is concerned with people who are mentally retarded, not mentally ill. Most day care facilities do not provide evening care and perhaps would not accept a child with special needs. (18:953, 1376)
    Nursing Process—Implementation
    Client Need—Safe, effective care environment

43 2. Children between the ages of 6 and 11 are acquiring *industry*, which is characterized by learning to work beside and cooperatively with others. The other characteristics are associated with later stages of development. (2:104)
    Nursing Process—Implementation
    Client Need—Health promotion/maintenance

44 2. Methylphenidate hydrochloride is a central nervous system stimulant that acts primarily on the cerebral cortex. Its action appears to be similar to amphetamines. (10:639; 20:212)
    Nursing Process—Implementation
    Client Need—Health promotion/maintenance

45 2. Some of the chief characteristics of attention deficit disorder include distractibility, difficulty following directions and remaining focused on a task, and sustaining attention. Relief of these symptoms indicates a therapeutic response. Despite the fact that methylphenidate hydrochloride is a central nervous system stimulant, it should not cause a child to be more alert, active, or less fatigued than he was prior to being treated with the drug. In fact, overstimulation indicates a nontherapeutic or adverse response to the drug. Methylphenidate may cause a child to be less irritable and aggressive, but the primary reason for administering this drug is not to alter a child's moods. (17:332)
    Nursing Process—Evaluation
    Client Need—Physiological Integrity

46 3. Because methylphenidate hydrochloride is a central nervous system stimulant, side effects reflect overstimulation. Some people experience an intense degree of these symptoms even with low dosages. The remaining choices are not associated with this particular drug. (17:333; 10:639)
    Nursing Process—Implementation
    Client Need—Health promotion/maintenance

47 2. Caffeine is present in ¾ of all soft drinks. It is an ingredient in all cola products unless they are labeled caffeine-free. Caffeine is a stimulating drug that contributes to overstimulation in a child taking methylphenidate hydrochloride. (6:279)
    Nursing Process—Implementation
    Client Need—Health promotion/maintenance

48 3. School-age children tend to view disease and its treatment as a form of punishment even though the transgression is not specifically identifiable. Although school-age children consider adults quite powerful, they are aware that serious illnesses have unpredictable outcomes. (9:179; 16:511)
    Nursing Process—Evaluation
    Client Need—Health promotion/maintenance

49 1. School-age children tend to fantasize and exaggerate a potentially unpleasant experience. Therefore it is best to avoid providing information far in advance. However, the child may be totally unprepared if the teaching is postponed until questions are asked or if the nurse assumes that the physician

will provide all the information the child needs to know. (16:511–512; 18:953)
Nursing Process—Planning
Client Need—Psychosocial integrity

50 4. Most children are primarily concerned with how they will be affected by a diagnostic test, procedure, or medical treatment. The other information is secondary to this. (16:512)
Nursing Process—Implementation
Client Need—Psychosocial integrity

51 1. Confidence and trust result when the reality of an experience correlates with the preteaching that is done. The other characteristics may be acquired, but not as a consequence of an honest nurse-client relationship. (16:512–513)
Nursing Process—Evaluation
Client Need—Psychosocial integrity

52 1. Setting achievable goals allows the child the potential for success. Success instills a sense of pride in accomplishment and motivation for improvement. The other suggestions are not inappropriate; however, they are not the best techniques for supporting the self-esteem of the child. (18:937)
Nursing Process—Implementation
Client Need—Psychosocial integrity

53 2. Privacy is an essential component of a therapeutic environment. Selecting a location where the person cannot be observed or overheard by others facilitates open communication and a therapeutic relationship. (10:100)
Nursing Process—Planning
Client Need—Safe, effective care environment

54 1. In addition to the death of a parent, divorce is one of the most disruptive events a child can experience. Changes in family structure jeopardize a child's sense of security. Acting out is a behavioral manifestation of conflict. Even positive experiences, such as a dog having puppies, acquiring a paper route, and visiting grandparents, can be stressful. However, they do not have as intense an emotional impact as parental divorce. (2:142, 10:632)
Nursing Process—Data collection
Client Need—Health promotion/maintenance

55 4. Discipline that is delivered immediately, fairly, and consistently helps a child understand the limits of acceptable and unacceptable behavior. Anxious people need reassurance that someone will enforce limitations if they are unable to remain in control. Sending the child to the principal indicates that the teacher is evading personal responsibility for controlling classroom behavior. Suspension isolates the child from any resource for help and is likely

to contribute to continued low academic performance. Sending the child to the counselor on a daily basis is premature and severe for the behavior manifested at this time. (9:50)
Nursing Process—Planning
Client Need—Psychosocial integrity

56 3. The oldest child in a family tends to be one who conforms to the expectations of adults, is more affected by criticism, more responsible, and more behaviorally rigid. The youngest child is likely to be less tolerant of frustration and more dependent on others. Middle children are more flexible and independent. (2:80–81)
Nursing Process—Evaluation
Client Need—Health promotion/maintenance

57 2. Making angry remarks suggests that this child is demonstrating displacement. Displacement is a psychological defense mechanism in which a person releases feelings onto someone or something else other than the true object of the anger, in this case, the illness. The other behaviors are more indicative of normal behavior for a child this age, especially one whose usual routine is unstructured due to unusual circumstances. (4:1352; 10:34)
Nursing Process—Evaluation
Client Need—Psychosocial integrity

58 3. Taking an active role in one's own care is the most effective way to acquire a sense of control over a disease. Thus, actually performing self-testing of blood glucose levels is therapeutic. The other activities are important, but they are less effective in promoting a sense of control. (22:654)
Nursing Process—Evaluation
Client Need—Psychosocial integrity

59 1. Persons with Tourette's syndrome tend to utter verbal obscenities and make other vocal sounds that are embarrassing to all concerned. The bizarre symptoms, which are not easily self-controlled, tend to make the client an object of ridicule or avoided by those who are unfamiliar with the condition. If any of the other symptoms in the alternative options occur, they are secondary or unique to the individual client. (18:938; 23:486–487)
Nursing Process—Planning
Client Need—Psychosocial integrity

60 1. Antipsychotic drugs cause a cluster of side effects known as extrapyramidal symptoms (EPS). Parkinsonian-like tremors and sudden strong muscle spasms, especially about the neck, are two types of EPS. (17:311; 20:212)

> Nursing Process—Implementation
> Client Need—Health promotion/maintenance

61 2. Self-esteem develops as a consequence of experiencing deserved praise from those whom the child respects. Positive reinforcement is preferable to focusing on negative behavior. Praise is considered a far healthier approach than sheltering and protecting the child physically or emotionally from peers. (2:87)

> Nursing Process—Planning
> Client Need—Psychosocial integrity

MENTAL HEALTH NEEDS DURING ADOLESCENCE

62 3. The best outcomes are obtained when crisis intervention is initiated immediately after the precipitating event. Although crises tend to become resolved, even without professional support, the outcomes are less than optimum as time passes. (2:313)

> Nursing Process—Planning
> Client Need—Psychosocial integrity

63 1. Most people who experience a crisis have an overwhelming feeling of helplessness. This feeling is a direct consequence of having inadequate coping strategies. The other emotional responses may occur among some individuals, but they are not ones that are characteristic of the majority of individuals experiencing crises. (10:105; 23:130)

> Nursing Process—Data collection
> Client Need—Psychosocial integrity

64 2. The first step toward resolving a crisis is to have survivors process the event from their own perspective. Some individuals require professional counseling, but most do not if crisis intervention is initiated soon after the event. Reassuring survivors that they will adapt may be appropriate, but it is not the most important action to take initially. Drug therapy in the form of minor tranquilizers usually is unnecessary, and in fact, may be detrimental since they tend to interfere with processing the reality of the crisis. (23:133)

> Nursing Process—Implementation
> Client Need—Psychosocial integrity

65 1. People with anorexia nervosa manifest lanugo, a growth of fine downy hair similar to that seen on newborn infants. It is thought that this occurs to promote or maintain normal body temperature on people who have little or no body fat. Bruises may indicate a vitamin deficiency, but they would not be limited to the upper torso. Generally, bowel

sounds are normal in anorectic people. Clubbing of the fingers is characteristic of conditions causing chronic hypoxia. (23:510)

> Nursing Process—Data collection
> Client Need—Safe, effective care environment

66 2. Generally, anorectics are characterized as being perfect children with above-average scholastic achievement, perhaps owing to a fear of failure. None of the other characteristics listed is unique to clients with anorexia nervosa. (23:510)

> Nursing Process—Data collection
> Client Need—Psychosocial integrity

67 3. Initial treatment of a client with anorexia nervosa focuses on meeting physiological needs. Once nutrients, fluids, vitamins, and electrolytes are administered, attention shifts to the client's psychosocial problems. (4:369; 6:375)

> Nursing Process—Planning
> Client Need—Physiological integrity

68 3. Validation is a therapeutic communication technique in which the nurse interprets what he or she perceives to be the underlying meaning of the words. If the interpretation is correct, it increases rapport and forms a basis for future collaboration. The techniques of generalizing, giving advice, and responding with a stereotypical statement are all examples of nontherapeutic communication techniques. (9:152–153)

> Nursing Process—Implementation
> Client Need—Psychosocial integrity

69 4. Controlling the desire to eat is a nonverbal technique the client with anorexia nervosa uses to demonstrate power and control. Getting attention as a result of this behavior reinforces its effectiveness. Until a client's malnutrition becomes life-threatening, forced feeding is unethical and inappropriate. Recording intake is not is an incentive for eating. The fear of becoming fat often is greater than a prior commitment to collaborated goals. (23:516)

> Nursing Process—Implementation
> Client Need—Psychosocial integrity

70 2. Confrontation is a therapeutic communication technique that is useful in pointing out differences between an expected behavior and the actual action. Postponing weighing is likely to result in more accurate assessment data. However, this choice of action, as well as saying nothing or subtracting 2 lb, avoids the greater issue of dealing with the behavior. (9:154)

> Nursing Process—Implementation
> Client Need—Psychosocial integrity

71 1. Separation anxiety is a common response when there is a change in caretakers in an unfamiliar environment. Pain is a subjective experience; it is erroneous to assume that a person with this diagnosis will respond any differently than others with normal intelligence. A person with this cognitive capacity is able to communicate his or her basic needs. An adolescent with normal cognitive ability is concerned about changes in his or her body image, but that is not likely for someone at this developmental level. (4:171)
   Nursing Process—Data collection
   Client Need—Psychosocial integrity

72 1. Assuming responsibility for skills that can be performed independently, like dressing and undressing, tend to interfere with the ability to achieve maximum levels of self-care. It is normal for a parent to be the medical historian for nonadult children. Exaggerating the child's abilities and self-blame are indications that the mother is not coping well with the child's condition. (18:942)
   Nursing Process—Evaluation
   Client Need—Psychosocial integrity

73 2. An aggressive response is a defensive reaction, not unlike that displayed by much younger children when they perceive themselves in threatening situations. It is overgeneralizing to say that all mentally retarded people are physically aggressive. One incidence of striking out is not sufficient to conclude that the client has a poor opinion of his care. The most common way for children to demonstrate they are in pain is by crying or moaning. (10:126; 18:942)
   Nursing Process—Implementation
   Client Need—Psychosocial integrity

74 3. Facts, not opinions, are documented. Although the best example requires more elaboration, it is better than any other. It is inaccurate to state that the aggression was a consequence of feeling angry or that the act was spontaneous. The word "attacked" is an emotionally charged term that suggests something more violent than actually occurred. (25:99; 23:63)
   Nursing Process—Implementation
   Client Need—Safe, effective care environment

75 3. To avoid misperceptions, it is best to offer explanations before physically touching a client. Entering a client's personal space without warning is interpreted as a threatening act. Restraints are unjustified in this situation. The mother should not be asked to assume total responsiblity for ambulating the client. Medication, assuming it is an analgesic, is

justified if the client experiences pain, but it is best to administer it at least 20 to 30 minutes before an activity. (18:862–863)
   Nursing Process—Planning
   Client Need—Psychosocial integrity

76 1. The attitudes and behavior of adolescents are influenced much more by peers than school, religion, or employment—although all of these affect the dynamics of each individual. (22:426)
   Nursing Process—Data collection
   Client Need—Psychosocial integrity

77 1. Inconsistency in setting limits or imposing consequences when limits are violated weaken adolescents' ability to recognize that there are boundaries for behavior. Discipline provides security, even though restrictions are not appreciated at the time. (23:497)
   Nursing Process—Data collection
   Client Need—Psychosocial integrity

78 4. Reassuring clients that the information they divulge will remain confidential is perhaps the most important concept to stress. Most therapy meetings are scheduled on a day and at a time that repeats on a regular basis. It is understood that someone who leads a group is qualified to do so. Using first names is common, but indicating this is a practice to follow is less important than stressing confidentiality. (23:89
   Nursing Process—Implementation
   Client Need—Psychosocial integrity

79 3. Persistently checking a wristwatch is a nonverbal way of saying that one would rather be someplace else. Borrowing cigarettes demonstrates irresponsibility. Laughing inappropriately suggests insensitivity. Fidgeting is a sign of anxiety. (2:57)
   Nursing Process—Evaluation
   Client Need—Health promotion/maintenance

80 1. Children who have grown up with an alcoholic parent commonly have a problem with low self-esteem. The other problems may be present in any person exposed to alcoholism, but they are not commonly shared characteristics. (10:633)
   Nursing Process—Data collection
   Client Need—Psychosocial integrity

81 3. All of the resources listed are helpful in some way to a person growing up in an alcoholic family. However, the one best suited for an adolescent is Alateen. (2:231; 10:160)
   Nursing Process—Implementation
   Client Need—Psychosocial integrity

82 2. Learning to trust others is a major sign of accomplishment for children of alcoholic parents. The other psychosocial skills are positive accomplishments, but they are not commonly associated with those who have grown up in an alcoholic household. (14:296; 18:950)

    Nursing Process—Evaluation
    Client Need—Psychosocial integrity

83 1. The peer group becomes more influential than parents in determining how adolescents behave. Peer behavior is used as a model for establishing what activities are acceptable or unacceptable. The fact that the team is winning is no more a motivation for taking controlled substances than if the team were losing. Affordability is not necessarily a factor in compromising values. (4:99)

    Nursing Process—Evaluation
    Client Need—Health promotion/maintenance

84 3. Acne occurs frequently in all age groups and both sexes who take anabolic steroids. The other physical changes are not related to the use of anabolic steroids. (20:367)

    Nursing Process—Data collection
    Client Need—Physiological integrity

85 1. Anabolic steroids are synthetic drugs chemically related to androgens like testosterone. Androgens and anabolic steroids are associated with aggressive behavior. Severe mental changes, such as uncontrolled rage ("roid rage") and personality changes, are not uncommon. The other emotional changes are unrelated to steroid use. (20:367)

    Nursing Process—Data collection
    Client Need—Physiological integrity

86 4. The described signs indicate depression. Adolescents are likely to attempt suicide impulsively when they are unable to cope with a significant loss. It is appropriate to ask overtly about suicidal feelings. Talking or asking about suicide does not make a person more likely to act on his feelings; in fact, just the opposite is true. A dramatic change in behavior is never disregarded. When dealing with crises, adolescents lack the perspective of life experiences to understand that their problems will be resolved. Establishing new peer relationships at another school may be equally traumatic for a depressed adolescent. (9:56)

    Nursing Process—Implementation
    Client Need—Psychosocial integrity

87 4. The basis for developing a therapeutic relationship is acceptance. This attitude indicates that the client is unique and worthy of respect. Trust develops once a client feels accepted. All of the other qualities are desirable but are not as likely to facilitate building trust. (2:47)

    Nursing Process—Planning
    Client Need—Safe, effective care environment

88 1. Eye contact communicates that the nurse is paying attention. Giving away free literature does not communicate a sincere, personal regard for the client. Writing information is a job-related task. Avoiding pauses could be interpreted as disinterest. (9:147)

    Nursing Process—Implementation
    Client Need—Psychosocial integrity

89 2. It is normal for teenagers to go through a period during which they reject the standards and ideals of their parents and other adults. By experimenting with new behaviors, often opposite those of the parents, the adolescent emerges with a unique identity and a lasting set of values. Adolescent rebellion is not likely to facilitate ingenuity, intuition, or insight. (2:105)

    Nursing Process—Implementation
    Client Need—Health promotion/maintenance

90 1. Treatment of a client is a confidential matter. Neither the nurse nor any other clinic personnel may reveal the identity of a client or the purpose for their treatment without the client's consent. All the other actions overtly or covertly divulge a relationship between the clinic and the client and violate the principle of confidentiality. (2:90)

    Nursing Process—Implementation
    Client Need—Safe, effective care environment

91 4. One of the most important elements in resolving a crisis is the emotional support of significant others. The client's mothering instinct, marriage plans, and financial support are not as beneficial as a family's unconditional love and encouragement. (2:308)

    Nursing Process—Evaluation
    Client Need—Psychosocial integrity

92 3. Denial is a form of behavior that protects one's consciousness from dealing with a catastrophic situation. By denying a situation exists, anxiety is kept to an acceptable level. Displacement involves discharging angry feelings onto an unrelated person or object. Regression occurs when a person resorts to behavior associated with a younger age. Compensation is characterized by pursuing an activity that ensures success to make up for feeling inadequate. (10:33)

    Nursing Process—Evaluation
    Client Need—Psychosocial integrity

93 3. People who are psychotic generally have thoughts that are unrealistic and irrational. Yet these thoughts

seem real and logical to the psychotic person. Many people who are mentally healthy experience difficulty in relationships, have problems adjusting to new situations, and feel helpless in resolving some problems. (2:243; 9:22)
> **Nursing Process—Implementation**
> **Client Need—Health promotion/maintenance**

94 1. Orientation is the person's ability to identify who and where she is and the day, month, and year. Asking how the client arrived assesses short-term memory. Identifying one's place of birth assesses long-term memory. Knowing the current president assesses the client's fund of knowledge. (2:127)
> **Nursing Process—Data collection**
> **Client Need—Psychosocial integrity**

95 3. The American Hospital Association identifies the fundamental right to review one's medical records. Also, the Mental Health Systems Act, passed by the United States Congress in 1980, contains a model for the mental health client's bill of rights. It states that a client has the right to access his or her mental health care records, except for information provided by third parties and information deemed by a mental health professional to be detrimental to the client's health. Asking a "why" question is a nontherapeutic communication technique called demanding an explanation. Putting the clipboard away is a nonverbal method of denying her request. It is not illegal for clients to read their own medical records. (25:40)
> **Nursing Process—Implementation**
> **Client Need—Safe, effective care environment**

96 2. The most essential criterion for an involuntary commitment is that the person is a "clear and present" danger to herself or to others. Commitment criteria have been established to protect the right of the client to appropriate treatment in the least restrictive setting. There are other methods for assessing a client other than involuntary commitment. Failure to keep office appointments is not a criterion for commitment. All competent adults have the right to refuse treatment, which includes taking medications. (10:51)
> **Nursing Process—Evaluation**
> **Client Need—Safe, effective care environment**

97 4. Postural hypotension is a side effect associated with this category of drugs. Cautioning a client to rise slowly helps moderate the drop in blood pressure, thus minimizing the potential for dizziness, fainting, or falling. Taking the medications on an empty stomach or skipping meals does not affect the drug's therapeutic action. This category of drugs is likely to make the client feel drowsy when treatment is first initiated. The client should never omit or discontinue a drug without collaborating with her physician. (20:210, 212)
> **Nursing Process—Implementation**
> **Client Need—Safe, effective care environment**

98 1. Antipsychotics are likely to reduce or eliminate psychotic symptoms, such as delusions and hallucinations. However, they do not generally relieve symptoms of apathy or withdrawal. Increased drowsiness is an undesirable side effect. It is doubtful that the client will feel more energetic and rested because a common side effect is sedation. The drug does not alter the client's self-concept. (10:232; 20:211)
> **Nursing Process—Evaluation**
> **Client Need—Physiological integrity**

99 2. Antipsychotic drugs can depress the bone marrow's production of blood cells. A severe sore throat suggests that the client does not have sufficient white blood cells to fight off microorganisms. A complete blood count is needed to assess the possibility of this adverse effect. This drug is likely to cause constipation and weight gain. Tinnitus is not associated with haloperidol. (10:244)
> **Nursing Process—Planning**
> **Client Need—Physiological integrity**

100 2. Although all of the reasons for discussing the prognosis with the dying teen are basically true, the best rationale for encouraging open communication is that it facilitates coping and emotional support. (18:954)
> **Nursing Process—Implementation**
> **Client Need—Psychosocial integrity**

Classification of Test Items

Unit **IV**   Review Test **15**

The Nursing Care of Infants, Children, and Adolescents with Mental Health Needs

Directions: After each question the correct answer is given, as well as a classification of each test question. Compare the correct answer with your answer. If a question has been answered *incorrectly*, draw a line to the end of all the columns. When finished, add up the number of your correct answers in each column and place that number in the respective box at the end in the area identified as *Number Correct*.

To determine the percentage of questions you answered correctly and your performance in each of the test plan categories, divide the *Number Correct* in each column by the *Number Possible* in each column. Then multiply the decimal by 100. For example:

$$\frac{\text{Number Correct: } 75}{\text{Number Possible: } 100} = 0.750 \times 100 = 75\%$$

Any score that is less than 75% indicates an area where further review would be beneficial.

KEY TO ITEM CLASSIFICATION:

NURSING PROCESS	CLIENT NEEDS
D = Data collection	S = Safe, effective care environment
P = Planning	P = Physiological integrity
I = Implementation	M = Psychosocial integrity
E = Evaluation	H = Health promotion/maintenance

Question #	Answer #	Nursing Process				Client Needs			
		D	P	I	E	S	P	M	H
1	1			I				M	
2	2			I				M	
3	1				E				H
4	4			I				M	
5	3	D						M	
6	1		P				P		
7	2			I					H
8	1	D					P		
9	1	D							H
10	1			I					H
11	3		P						H
12	4			I					H
13	2				E				H
14	3				E				H
15	1		P						H

	Question #	Answer #		Nursing Process				Client Needs		
			D	P	I	E	S	P	M	H
	16	2		P						H
	17	3				E				H
	18	1			I		S			
	19	3	D						M	
	20	3			I					H
	21	2			I					H
	22	3			I				M	
	23	4				E			M	
	24	1	D					P		
	25	2		P					M	
	26	3	D						M	
	27	4			I		S			
	28	4		P					M	
	29	4			I					H
	30	3				E				H
	31	4	D							H
	32	2			I					H
	33	4			I					H
	34	1			I					H
	35	2			I					H
	36	1			I		S			
	37	1	D						M	
	38	4		P			S			
	39	1		P				P		
	40	3			I					H
	41	2		P					M	
	42	4			I		S			
	43	2			I					H
	44	2			I					H
	45	2				E		P		
	46	3			I					H
	47	2			I					H

		Nursing Process				Client Needs			
Question #	Answer #	D	P	I	E	S	P	M	H
48	3				E				H
49	1		P					M	
50	4			I				M	
51	1				E			M	
52	1			I				M	
53	2		P			S			
54	1	D							H
55	4		P					M	
56	3				E				H
57	2				E			M	
58	3				E			M	
59	1		P					M	
60	1			I					H
61	2		P					M	
62	3		P					M	
63	1	D						M	
64	2			I				M	
65	1	D				S			
66	2	D						M	
67	3		P				P		
68	3			I				M	
69	4			I				M	
70	2			I				M	
71	1	D						M	
72	1				E			M	
73	2			I				M	
74	3			I		S			
75	3		P					M	
76	1	D						M	
77	1	D						M	
78	4			I				M	
79	3				E				H

Question #	Answer #	Nursing Process				Client Needs			
		D	P	I	E	S	P	M	H
80	1	D						M	
81	3			I				M	
82	2				E			M	
83	1				E				H
84	3	D				P			
85	1	D					P		
86	4			I				M	
87	4		P			S			
88	1			I				M	
89	2			I					H
90	1			I		S			
91	4				E			M	
92	3				E			M	
93	3			I					H
94	1	D						M	
95	3			I		S			
96	2				E	S			
97	4			I		S			
98	1				E		P		
99	2		P				P		
100	2			I				M	
Number Correct	89	19	16	34	20	11	9	41	28
Number Possible	100	19	19	42	20	13	10	44	33
Percentage Correct	89	100	84	81	100	85	90	93	85

Mental Health Needs During Young Adulthood
Mental Health Needs During Middle Age (35–65)
Mental Health Needs During Late Adulthood (Over 65)

Correct Answers and Rationale
Classification of Test Items

Directions: With a pencil, blacken the circle in front of the option you have chosen for your correct answer.

MENTAL HEALTH NEEDS DURING YOUNG ADULTHOOD

A nurse works in a substance abuse clinic where most of the clients are ages 18 to 35.

1 When a 24-year-old with a record of multiple convictions for driving while intoxicated (DWI) claims he is not an alcoholic, which is the *most pertinent* assessment question the nurse can ask?
- ○ 1. "When you drink, do you only drink beer?"
- ○ 2. "Did you begin drinking before or after you were of legal age?"
- ○ 3. "Do you prefer to drink alcohol rather than soft drinks?"
- ● 4. "Have you ever been unable to recall events that occurred while drinking?"

2 The nurse is *most correct* in explaining to the alcoholic's family that the *first step* in recovering from alcoholism is
- ● 1. admitting an inability to control drinking.
- ○ 2. eliminating nutritional deficiencies.
- ○ 3. resuming some form of religious affiliation.
- ○ 4. developing more willpower to stay sober.

3 One of the *best resources* to which the nurse can refer family members of alcoholics is
- ● 1. Alcoholics Anonymous.
- ○ 2. Recovery Anonymous.
- ○ 3. Al-Anon.
- ○ 4. Synanon.

4 When an anonymous phone caller asks how to tell if someone has been smoking marijuana within the last few hours, the nurse is *most accurate* in identifying a physical sign of recent use as
- ○ 1. shivering.
- ○ 2. inflamed eyes.
- ○ 3. rapid breathing.
- ● 4. restlessness.

5 The nurse is *most correct* in telling the caller that the *most likely* effect of marijuana is
- ● 1. drowsiness.
- ○ 2. hyperactivity.
- ○ 3. apprehension.
- ○ 4. suspiciousness.

6 If one of the nurse's clients believes all of the following are true about smoking marijuana, which one is *most accurate*?
- ○ 1. It suppresses motivation.
- ○ 2. It is physically addicting.
- ○ 3. It can cause lung cancer.
- ● 4. It can inhibit respiration.

7 If the nurse observes all of the following in an otherwise healthy young adult client who is known to use illegal drugs, which one is *most suggestive* that the client is a chronic user of marijuana?
- ○ 1. The client has difficulty sleeping.
- ○ 2. The client's memory is impaired.
- ○ 3. The client drinks large volumes of liquids.
- ● 4. The client has low tolerance for frustration.

Twenty-year-old parents accompany their infant son who is dead on arrival in the emergency department. Sudden infant death syndrome (SIDS) is the tentative cause of death.

8 When resuscitation efforts are unsuccessful, what is *most important* for the nurse to do *next*?
- ○ 1. Ask the parents for permission to perform an autopsy.
- ○ 2. Inquire about the possibility of harvesting organs for transplant.
- ○ 3. Check on the parents' choice for the funeral arrangements.
- ● 4. Take the parents to a room where they can be with the baby.

9 Which emotional response are the parents *most likely* to experience *immediately* following the sudden death of their infant son?
○ 1. Anger
● 2. Guilt
○ 3. Fear
○ 4. Depression

10 The *most important* concept for the nurse to convey to the parents *as soon as possible* after they have been informed of their infant's death is that
○ 1. the staff did all they could to resuscitate the infant.
○ 2. the infant would have been brain damaged if he had survived.
● 3. they did not cause, nor could they have prevented, the death.
○ 4. there are grief support groups available in the community.

While making a home visit, a nurse suspects that a 20-year-old female is the victim of domestic assault.

11 Which one of the following is the *best technique* for determining if abuse is taking place?
○ 1. Ask directly if domestic abuse is occurring.
○ 2. Arrange a second visit to validate suspicions.
● 3. Assess the young children for signs of injury.
○ 4. Make inquiries among relatives or neighbors.

12 If incidences of domestic abuse are occurring, it is *best* for the nurse to
○ 1. offer the victim her personal phone number.
● 2. identify resources for shelter and safety.
○ 3. recommend that she end the abusive relationship.
○ 4. suggest joint counseling with a therapist or clergyman.

13 If the 20-year-old female is typical of other victims who remain in an abusive relationship, she is *most likely* to believe that
○ 1. she is not in any serious danger.
○ 2. she can turn to her family for protection.
● 3. she can prevent the battering behavior.
○ 4. she is free to leave at any time.

A nurse is a volunteer at a crisis center answering telephone calls on a hotline.

14 When the nurse responds to a call from a 20-year-old rape victim, which instruction is *most important* before referring the woman to the emergency department of the local hospital?
● 1. Do not bathe or shower.
○ 2. Make a sketch of the rapist.

○ 3. Write down what happened.
○ 4. Call a 911 operator.

15 When the rape victim arrives at the emergency department, which nursing action is *best* for relieving the client's anxiety?
○ 1. Determining the victim's last date of menstruation
○ 2. Collecting evidence for criminal prosecution
○ 3. Assessing the extent of the client's injuries
● 4. Staying with the client at all times

16 Which one of the following is the *highest nursing priority* during the *immediate care* of a rape victim?
● 1. Documenting the circumstances of the rape
○ 2. Keeping contact with strangers to a minimum
○ 3. Offering the victim a choice of sedatives
○ 4. Contacting the victim's own clergyman

The emergency department nurse describes procedures and their purpose to the rape victim before they are implemented.

17 The *best rationale* for the nurse's action is that this approach
● 1. diminishes feelings of powerlessness.
○ 2. tends to reduce the client's anxiety.
○ 3. is a policy of the emergency department.
○ 4. meets the client's need for teaching.

18 If a rape victim desires medical treatment, but objects to having evidence collected for criminal prosecution, the nurse is *most correct* in
○ 1. persuading her to change her mind.
● 2. proceeding because it is required.
○ 3. accepting the rape victim's wishes.
○ 4. advising her to use better judgment.

Before being discharged, the rape victim is referred to a rape support counselor who also is a nurse.

19 If the rape victim reports all of the following, which is *most indicative* of a *severe* adjustment reaction?
○ 1. The victim reports feeling somewhat anxious.
● 2. The victim describes having sporadic nightmares.
○ 3. The victim has no appetite, but eats out of habit.
○ 4. The victim has occasional doubts about her self-worth.

The counselor invites the rape victim to attend a group meeting of others who have been raped.

20 Which is the *most desired* outcome of a self-help group consisting of rape victims?
- ◉ 1. Obtaining mutual assistance with similar problems
- ○ 2. Receiving authoritative information about rape trauma
- ○ 3. Establishing new friendships with other victims
- ○ 4. Developing additional social skills for the future

A public health nurse must inform a 26-year-old male homosexual that he is HIV-positive.

21 If the man who is HIV-positive is typical of others who receive bad news, the nurse can expect that *initially* he will be
- ○ 1. angry.
- ○ 2. shocked.
- ○ 3. resentful.
- ◉ 4. depressed.

22 If the HIV-positive client does all of the following, which one is *most suggestive* that he is denying his illness?
- ○ 1. He conceals the information from his family.
- ○ 2. He avoids contact with his homosexual friends.
- ○ 3. He confronts some of his former sexual partners.
- ◉ 4. He has intercourse without using condoms.

23 If the HIV-positive client has all of the following strengths, which one is *most important* for coping with the diagnosis?
- ○ 1. Acceptance by religious leaders
- ◉ 2. A sustained network of support
- ○ 3. Acquiring many social acquaintances
- ○ 4. Sexual tolerance within the community

24 If an otherwise symptom-free HIV-positive client makes all of the following remarks, which one might the nurse interpret as *most potentially suicidal*?
- ○ 1. "I've had recurring dreams about dying."
- ○ 2. "How many people do you know who died from HIV?"
- ○ 3. "Will I be alert when I'm near death?"
- ◉ 4. "Everyone would be better off without me."

A 20-year-old female is being treated for bulimia.

25 When the client's assessment data is reviewed, which one of the following can the nurse *most expect* to find?
- ○ 1. Extremely low body weight
- ◉ 2. Erosion of dental enamel
- ○ 3. Cessation of menstruation
- ○ 4. Patchy loss of hair

The nurse has been working with the bulimic client on selecting measures to control her eating disorder.

26 If the following measures are considered, which one is likely to be *most effective* for a client with bulimia?
- ◉ 1. Staying out of the bathroom after meals
- ○ 2. Taking a daily inventory of the unit's food
- ○ 3. Avoiding meals in fast-food establishments
- ○ 4. Recording all the calories she consumes

The bulimic client has been taking fluoxetine (Prozac) for several weeks.

27 The *most desired* therapeutic effect for this client is evidenced by a report that she is
- ○ 1. feeling less depressed.
- ○ 2. eating more nutritiously.
- ◉ 3. having fewer food binges.
- ○ 4. feeling less suicidal.

At a group meeting for people with eating disorders, the client with bulimia says to another member who is very emaciated, "You're a real weirdo if you think you've got a weight problem."

28 Which nursing action is *most appropriate* at this time?
- ○ 1. Criticize the nature of the bulimic's rude behavior.
- ○ 2. Support the emaciated person targeted by the remark.
- ◉ 3. Invite others in the group to respond to the situation.
- ○ 4. Embarrass the bulimic client with a similar comment.

A 25-year-old male who abuses dextroamphetamine (Dexedrine) occasionally attends the eating disorder group meetings.

29 Which sign is *most suggestive* that he is taking dextro-amphetamine at this time?
- ○ 1. He stares blankly into space.
- ○ 2. He monopolizes the discussions.
- ◉ 3. He wears sunglasses indoors.
- ○ 4. He slurs his words as he speaks.

30 If the history of the amphetamine abuser includes all of the following, which one is *most indicative* that he has *not* achieved the developmental characteristics for this stage in the life cycle?
- ◉ 1. He drifts in and out of relationships.
- ○ 2. He worries about his financial security.
- ○ 3. He questions his sexual identity.
- ○ 4. He hesitates to assert himself.

31 When discussing his problems with obesity, which one of the following comments is *most suggestive* that the amphetamine abuser is using the coping mechanism of *rationalization*?
- ○ 1. "I have many health risks from being obese."
- ○ 2. "I have real difficulty resisting ice cream."
- ○ 3. "I know you don't like me because I'm fat."
- ◉ 4. "I can't help being overweight, it's in my genes."

A 27-year-old foreign immigrant is admitted with abdominal pain. The client is apprehensive and speaks very little English.

32 If four health agency employees speak the client's language, which one is *most appropriate* to contact for translating information?
- ◉ 1. The one who is the same gender as the client
- ○ 2. The one with a similar marital status
- ○ 3. The one who is older than the client
- ○ 4. The one who has lived longest in America

The sister of the non-American client places a knife beneath the client's pillow to "cut" the client's pain.

33 Which nursing action is *most appropriate* at this time?
- ○ 1. Explain through a translator that analgesic drugs will be administered.
- ○ 2. Explain through a translator that sharp objects pose a safety hazard.
- ◉ 3. Explain through a translator that a form must be signed relieving the agency of responsibility.
- ○ 4. Explain through a translator that the staff will leave the knife in place as long as necessary.

A 30-year-old male with a history of substance abuse is assessed prior to having a colonoscopy in the ambulatory care department.

34 If the client snorts cocaine on a regular basis, which physical assessment is *most appropriate* to perform?
- ○ 1. Examine the oropharynx.
- ◉ 2. Inspect the nasal mucosa.
- ○ 3. Listen to lung sounds.
- ○ 4. Assess olfactory function.

35 If a drug screen is positive for cocaine, it is *most appropriate* for the nurse to advise a staff person to monitor the client closely for
- ○ 1. cardiac arrhythmias.
- ◉ 2. depressed respirations.
- ○ 3. low blood pressure.
- ○ 4. elevated blood sugar.

A home health nurse monitors several young adults who have been diagnosed with schizophrenia, but who are able to function for extended periods of time in the community.

36 During a home visit, which of the following is *most suggestive* that a client with schizophrenia is experiencing auditory hallucinations?
- ○ 1. The client sings a song as he walks about the room.
- ○ 2. The client quickly changes the topic of conversation.
- ○ 3. The client repeats a sentence over and over again.
- ◉ 4. The client cocks his head as if listening to someone.

A schizophrenic client says, "Wing ding, the world is a ring."

37 The *best response* by the nurse is
- ○ 1. "How clever, you've made up a poem."
- ○ 2. "I don't understand what you mean."
- ○ 3. "Earth does orbit in a circle."
- ◉ 4. "Tell me more about the world."

38 Which nursing assessment is *most indicative* that a community-based client with schizophrenia needs to be rehospitalized temporarily?
- ◉ 1. The client neglects eating, hygiene, and sleep.
- ○ 2. The client has missed some counseling appointments.
- ○ 3. The client is hesitant about applying for work.
- ○ 4. The client wants to live with his relatives.

MENTAL HEALTH NEEDS DURING MIDDLE AGE (35–65)

A nurse is assigned to care for a brain-injured client who is 35 years old.

39 When the client purposely spits at the nurse during the course of being fed, which action is *most appropriate* to take *first*?
- ○ 1. Leave the client's room immediately.
- ◉ 2. Indicate the behavior is unacceptable.
- ○ 3. Act like the behavior was accidental.
- ○ 4. Stand as far from the bed as possible.

40 If the brain-injured client's spitting becomes habitual, which plan is *most likely* to reduce or eliminate it?
- ◉ 1. Establish a significant consequence, like no television for 30 minutes.
- ○ 2. Wear a face shield or other form of barrier protection when feeding the client.
- ○ 3. Explain how rude it is to spit at other people.
- ○ 4. Identify the health risks from being spat upon.

A 36-year-old client is undergoing diagnostic tests to determine if he has myxedema (adult-onset hypothyroidism).

41 When performing a mental status assessment on the client with myxedema, which action is *most appropriate* for the nurse to take?
- ○ 1. Ask open-ended questions like, "How have you been feeling lately?"
- ◉ 2. Allow extra time for the client to respond to assessment questions.
- ○ 3. Defer mental status questions to a spouse or significant other.
- ○ 4. Omit the mental status assessment; the results will be abnormal.

A 42-year-old female is assessed in the emergency department to determine the etiology of her chest pain.

42 If the client with chest pain is experiencing a panic attack, the physical assessment data collected by the nurse is *most likely* to reveal
- ◉ 1. tachycardia.
- ○ 2. hypotension.
- ○ 3. increased salivation.
- ○ 4. constricted pupils.

43 If the diagnosis of panic disorder is accurate, the nurse is *most correct* in assuming the chest pain is related to
- ○ 1. unknown causes.
- ○ 2. feigned illness.
- ○ 3. attention seeking.
- ◉ 4. intense fear.

44 When the nurse interacts with the client experiencing a panic attack, which nursing technique is *best* for reducing the anxiety the client is experiencing?
- ○ 1. Stand less than an arm's length from her.
- ○ 2. Wear a laboratory coat and name tag.
- ○ 3. Offer her a cup of coffee or tea.
- ◉ 4. Explain all actions and procedures.

45 Which concept is *most important* for the nurse to convey to a client during a panic attack?
- ○ 1. That the client is safe
- ◉ 2. That the client is believed
- ○ 3. That the client is trusted
- ○ 4. That the client is accepted

46 When the client who is having a panic attack cries and says, "Nurse, I feel like I'm going to die," which response is *most therapeutic*?
- ○ 1. "Don't cry. It won't help matters right now."
- ○ 2. "You don't want the doctor to see you this way."
- ○ 3. "Everyone feels frightened in an emergency."
- ◉ 4. "I'll stay with you until you feel better."

The client who has a panic disorder is given a prescription for alprazolam (Xanax).

47 Which of the following information is *most appropriate* for the nurse to tell the client about alprazolam?
- ◉ 1. Avoid consuming alcohol while taking this drug.
- ○ 2. Long-term use will not cause drug dependency.
- ○ 3. This drug can cause insomnia in some people.
- ○ 4. A blood test will be required periodically.

48 If panic attacks become more and more frequent, which response among affected clients is *most typical*?
- ○ 1. They tend to refer themselves for psychiatric treatment.
- ◉ 2. They fear venturing from their homes and become reclusive.
- ○ 3. They take more than the prescribed amount of medication.
- ○ 4. They become psychotic and require psychiatric admission.

A 48-year-old male client becomes angry and belligerent toward a nurse after talking with his wife on the phone.

49 The nurse is *most correct* in explaining to an unlicensed staff person that this client is using a coping mechanism called
- ○ 1. introjection.
- ◉ 2. projection.
- ○ 3. compensation.
- ○ 4. displacement.

50 Which nursing action is *best* to use *first* when trying to help the angry client maintain self-control?
- ○ 1. Administer a sedating type of medication.
- ○ 2. Get the client involved in an activity.
- ◉ 3. Remain calm and appear nonthreatening.
- ○ 4. Offer to talk to the client's wife.

51 If the angry client continues to escalate to potentially violent behavior, it is *best* to
- ◉ 1. assemble a number of staff together.
- ○ 2. ask the physician to calm the client.
- ○ 3. go alone with the client to his room.
- ○ 4. place restraints in the client's view.

52 If the angry client is out of control and refuses a "stat" sedative medication, *legally* the nurse
- ○ 1. should respect the client's right to refuse.
- ◉ 2. can administer it to protect the safety of others.
- ○ 3. must get permission from a probate court judge.
- ○ 4. ask the hospital's attorney for an opinion.

A nurse prepares to teach a 60-year-old male client who is highly anxious about a heart catheterization that he will undergo next week.

53 Which teaching approach is *most beneficial* when preparing the anxious client?
- ○ 1. Provide detailed explanations.
- ○ 2. Use short, simple sentences.
- ○ 3. Draw elaborate diagrams.
- ● 4. Show a teaching videotape.

54 If the nurse notes all of the following information in a database assessment, which one is the *most significant* source of conflict for a middle-aged adult?
- ● 1. The client is facing forced retirement.
- ○ 2. The client has 12 grandchildren.
- ○ 3. The client is learning to use a computer.
- ○ 4. The client wants to sell his home.

A 38-year-old female consults a nurse about her fear of flying.

55 If this person is typical of others who have phobias, the *most common* coping mechanism they share is
- ○ 1. suppression.
- ○ 2. compensation.
- ● 3. avoidance.
- ○ 4. undoing.

The phobic person asks the nurse to explain cognitive therapy, the type of treatment that she is receiving.

56 The *most correct* nursing explanation is that cognitive therapy involves
- ● 1. changing people's irrational beliefs.
- ○ 2. exposing people to things they fear.
- ○ 3. helping people verbalize their feelings.
- ○ 4. rewarding people's altered behaviors.

A nurse volunteers to participate in a support group for people with post-traumatic stress disorder (PTSD).

57 When asked to identify the characteristics of PTSD, the nurse is *most accurate* in saying that a common finding among people with this disorder is
- ● 1. recurring nightmares.
- ○ 2. auditory hallucinations.
- ○ 3. rapidly changing emotions.
- ○ 4. anger that erupts easily.

58 One of the *most therapeutic* interventions the nurse can implement when caring for clients with PTSD is to
- ○ 1. administer antianxiety medications.
- ○ 2. monitor their physical symptoms.
- ● 3. encourage the expression of feelings.
- ○ 4. explore current family interactions.

59 When a counselor asks the members of the PTSD group to draw a picture of their traumatic experience, the nurse is *most correct* in assuming that the primary purpose for drawing is to help members
- ● 1. deal consciously with painful memories.
- ○ 2. bond with other members in the group.
- ○ 3. receive approval from group members.
- ○ 4. justify their participation in the group.

A military veteran with PTSD asks why he is startled and fearful when he attends Fourth of July fireworks displays.

60 The *best explanation* from the nurse is that
- ○ 1. he was frightened of them as a child.
- ○ 2. he has lost his spirit of patriotism.
- ● 3. he associates the sound with gunfire.
- ○ 4. he is worried he may be drafted again.

Someone asks if anyone other than military veterans acquires post-traumatic stress disorder.

61 The *most accurate* statement by the nurse is that PTSD can occur in anyone who
- ○ 1. has experienced multiple failures.
- ● 2. has survived a catastrophic event.
- ○ 3. was abandoned or unloved as a child.
- ○ 4. has inherited a genetic tendency.

A 40-year-old female has multiple symptoms that do not resemble any specific disease. The client is anxious and worried because no definite diagnosis has been made.

62 When the anxious client summons the nurse and says she feels weak and dizzy, the *most appropriate* nursing action at this time is to
- ○ 1. help the client to relax.
- ○ 2. give the client something to eat.
- ○ 3. administer oxygen by cannula.
- ● 4. take the client's vital signs.

The undiagnosed client shares that she regrets never going to college or having children.

63 The *best explanation* for the basis of her statement is that during the middle years of life, adults generally
- ● 1. assess their accomplishments.
- ○ 2. set unreasonable goals.
- ○ 3. envy others' achievements.
- ○ 4. doubt their own judgments.

One day the client with multiple symptoms says to the nurse, "Do you think they'll ever be able to find out what's wrong with me?"

64 Which is the *best nursing response?*
- ○ 1. "That's something to discuss with your doctor."
- ● 2. "It sounds like you are feeling discouraged."
- ○ 3. "Let us worry about your lack of progress."
- ○ 4. "You need to practice a little more patience."

A co-worker says, "The undiagnosed client sounds just like any other hypochondriac to me."

65 It is important for the nurse to point out that the *most damaging consequence* of this type of attitude is that it
- ○ 1. violates the client's right to treatment.
- ● 2. disregards a client's individuality.
- ○ 3. interferes with continuity of client care.
- ○ 4. disrupts good staff relationships.

The pastor of the client with puzzling symptoms asks to see the client's chart.

66 The *most appropriate* nursing action in this case is to
- ● 1. tell him to ask the client for permission.
- ○ 2. ask him if he is a certified hospital chaplain.
- ○ 3. inform him that he cannot read the chart.
- ○ 4. check the policy with the nursing supervisor.

The nursing team holds a conference concerning a 38-year-old male who has been admitted with ulcerative colitis, a psychophysiologic disease.

67 When a nursing assistant asks if "psychophysiologic" means that the client is not really sick, the *most accurate* response from the nurse is that a client with this type of illness
- ○ 1. pretends to be sick when he needs a rest.
- ○ 2. thinks he is sick, but tests are all negative.
- ○ 3. would rather be hospitalized than have to work.
- ● 4. has an illness that is influenced by his emotions.

At the team conference, the assessments that are important in the care of the client with ulcerative colitis are discussed.

68 If all of the following are identified, which one is of *highest* priority?
- ● 1. The number and characteristics of his bowel movements
- ○ 2. How much the client knows about colostomy care
- ○ 3. What coping mechanisms he uses for handling stress
- ○ 4. The types of relationships he has with peers

The conference discussion turns toward exploring ways to maintain the self-esteem of the client with ulcerative colitis.

69 If all of the following are suggested, which is the *best approach* for managing the client's care?
- ○ 1. Use a nonjudgmental manner when cleaning the client of stool.
- ○ 2. Ask the client's mother to help clean him when possible.
- ○ 3. Hold the client responsible for all of his hygiene.
- ● 4. Assign only male nurses to care for the client.

A 35-year-old male is scheduled for a hemorrhoidectomy. He also is a chronic alcoholic, but he has not identified this problem to his physician or the nurse.

70 If the nurse makes all of the following postoperative assessments, which one is *most indicative* of current alcoholism?
- ○ 1. The blood pressure is generally lower than normal.
- ● 2. Pain is unrelieved with usual dosages of analgesics.
- ○ 3. Bowel sounds are absent in the right upper quadrant.
- ○ 4. Pulse rates are slow, weak, and irregular.

Approximately 24 hours after his admission, the client who abuses alcohol becomes very restless and shouts that he must "kill all the bugs" in his room.

71 In this situation it is *essential* for the nurse to
- ○ 1. place restraints on his arms and legs.
- ● 2. reassure him that he is not seeing bugs.
- ○ 3. remain at the bedside with the client.
- ○ 4. close his door so others are not alarmed.

72 Based on the change in the alcohol abusing client's condition, which of the following nursing actions is *most appropriate* to perform next?
- ○ 1. Schedule a team conference.
- ○ 2. Call the supervisor.
- ● 3. Notify the physician.
- ○ 4. Chart the assessed data.

73 During the next 24 hours, the nurse is *most correct* in continuing to monitor the client who is acutely withdrawing from alcohol for which additional complication?
- ○ 1. Hypothermia
- ● 2. Seizures
- ○ 3. Bleeding
- ○ 4. Jaundice

At the beginning of the shift, a team member says in reference to the client in alcohol withdrawal, "Don't expect me to take care of that good-for-nothing."

74 When the nurse counsels the team member privately, it is generally agreed that the *first step* in understanding and accepting the behavior of clients is
○ 1. understanding one's own behavior.
◉ 2. analyzing what motivates clients' behavior.
○ 3. becoming familiar with abnormal behavior.
○ 4. taking courses in counseling.

A home health nurse changes an abdominal dressing every day on a 45-year-old female client with a history of bipolar disorder.

75 While reviewing the psychiatric history of the client with bipolar disorder, the nurse can expect to find that a *major problem* the client experiences is
○ 1. ritualistic behavior.
○ 2. symbolic aggressiveness.
◉ 3. cyclic mood swings.
○ 4. periodic amnesia.

The client with bipolar disorder takes lithium carbonate (Lithane).

76 What is *most important* for the nurse to monitor to determine if the current dose is appropriate for the client?
○ 1. Vital signs
○ 2. Urine volumes
◉ 3. Blood levels
○ 4. Brain scans

77 If the nurse collects all of the following data, which is *most suggestive* that the client is experiencing an exacerbation of the bipolar disorder?
○ 1. The client has been spending money extravagantly.
○ 2. The client wants to become a hospice volunteer.
◉ 3. The client has been methodically cleaning her house.
○ 4. The client has been staying up late to read.

MENTAL HEALTH NEEDS DURING LATE ADULTHOOD (OVER 65)

A nurse performs a home assessment on a reasonably healthy older adult who chooses to live in a supervised retirement community.

78 If the older adult's sons and daughters are present, which action is *most appropriate* before beginning the assessment?

○ 1. Encourage them to offer their comments at any time.
○ 2. Ask the client where she and the nurse might be alone.
◉ 3. Identify the names and relationships of those present.
○ 4. Offer to share the assessment results with them.

79 When interviewing the older adult, which question or statement made by the nurse is likely to generate the *most information*?
◉ 1. "Tell me about your family."
○ 2. "Are you currently married?"
○ 3. "Who is your nearest relative?"
○ 4. "Give me a list of your family."

80 Which of the following questions is *best* for assessing the older adult's long-term memory?
○ 1. "What is your current age?"
○ 2. "What is today's date?"
◉ 3. "What is your date of birth?"
○ 4. "What occurred last January?"

81 Which action is *best* for determining if the older adult's inappropriate responses to several questions are due to miscommunication or to impaired cognition?
◉ 1. Ask the client to repeat the question before answering it.
○ 2. Ask questions that require only a "yes" or "no" response.
○ 3. Ask the client's next of kin for answers to the questions.
○ 4. Ask questions to which the client is sure to know the answers.

82 Which assessment finding is *most atypical* for an adult who is 65 years old?
○ 1. The person makes errors in copying a line drawing.
◉ 2. The person forgets names of longstanding neighbors.
○ 3. The person is slow at retrieving information.
○ 4. The person can name two of the last three presidents.

83 If the older adult is typical of others her age, the nurse is *most correct* is assuming she shares the age-related problem of
◉ 1. dealing with losses.
○ 2. becoming cynical.
○ 3. losing patience.
○ 4. developing hostility.

A 68-year-old male who currently is being treated for major depression is transferred to a medical unit following an episode of acute abdominal pain.

84 If all of the following rooms are available, in which one is it *best* to locate the depressed client?
○ 1. In a private room where stimuli are reduced
○ 2. In a semi-private room with a cheerful roommate
○ 3. In an empty room at the end of the hallway
● 4. In a room within view of the nursing station

85 After gathering the following data on the depressed client, which one indicates the *highest risk* for suicide?
○ 1. The client feels hopeless about the future.
● 2. The client has a plan in mind for suicide.
○ 3. The client states that he'd be better off dead.
○ 4. The client says he can't stand the pain anymore.

86 If amitriptyline hydrochloride (Elavil) is prescribed for the depressed client, the nurse is *most correct* in questioning its administration if the client has
○ 1. diabetes mellitus.
○ 2. pernicious anemia.
● 3. prostatic hypertrophy.
○ 4. chronic emphysema.

87 If the client indicates after 3 days of taking amitriptyline hydrochloride (Elavil) that he continues to feel depressed, which of the following responses is *most accurate*?
● 1. "Drug therapy may not be effective for 14 or more days."
○ 2. "You are probably not as aware of its therapeutic benefit as staff."
○ 3. "You may have to make various dietary changes as well."
○ 4. "Drug therapy is the least effective method of treating depression."

88 Which nursing action is *especially important* when administering medications to the depressed client?
○ 1. Encourage him to drink a full glass of water.
● 2. Check that the oral medication is swallowed.
○ 3. Give the medication on an empty stomach before meals.
○ 4. Have the client take each medication separately.

89 When the depressed client is scheduled for a series of electroconvulsive therapy (ECT) treatments, which is he *most likely* to experience in the *immediate* recovery period?
○ 1. Brief episodes of absence seizures
○ 2. Sensitivity to light and double vision
● 3. Short-term memory loss and headaches
○ 4. Periods of unexplained fear and anxiety

A nurse who is employed in a nursing home observes that a romantic relationship is developing between two residents.

90 If the nurse discovers the older couple having sexual intercourse, which action is *most appropriate*?
○ 1. Report it to their adult children.
○ 2. Restore a measure of privacy.
○ 3. Suggest they become roommates.
● 4. Censure their sexual activity.

An older adult client with chronic mental illness is transferred from a state psychiatric hospital to a nursing home for custodial care.

91 If the client with chronic mental illness develops all of the following after the physician discontinues haldoperiodol (Haldol), which one is a *consequence* of the drug therapy?
● 1. The client develops facial tics.
○ 2. The client becomes depressed.
○ 3. The client loses patches of hair.
○ 4. The client has daytime lethargy.

A nurse refers her 66-year-old home care client to a mental health clinic to evaluate if there is a co-existing depressive disorder.

92 If the home health nurse observed all of the following, which one is *most suggestive* that the client is depressed?
○ 1. The client is irritable after her grandchildren visit.
● 2. The client has multiple unrelated physical complaints.
○ 3. The client takes lengthy naps in the late afternoon.
○ 4. The client cries when talking about her dead spouse.

93 If the nurse notes that all of the following develop after the depressed client begins taking sertraline (Zoloft), which one is *most likely* drug-related?
○ 1. Polyuria
○ 2. Diplopia
○ 3. Drooling
● 4. Insomnia

A 70-year-old female client with dementia removes her clothes and walks naked through the halls of a nursing home.

94 Which action is *most appropriate* for the nurse to take *first*?
○ 1. Remind her that she can be seen by others.
○ 2. Tell her to put her clothes back on.
● 3. Give her directions to the nearest toilet.
○ 4. Escort her to a vacant room nearby.

A client at a care facility who has had a stroke struggles to manage his own activities of daily living.

95 If the client with the stroke frequently comes to meals with soap on his face or an unbuttoned shirt, the course of action that is in the client's *best emotional interest* is to
- ○ 1. send him back to his room to finish.
- ○ 2. bathe, shave, and dress him daily.
- ○ 3. schedule his hygiene for after meals.
- ◉ 4. comment on how self-reliant he is.

A nurse joins a group of older adult clients during reminiscence therapy.

96 Which of the following activities is *most helpful* in facilitating reminiscence therapy among older adult clients?
- ○ 1. Discussing a current event topic
- ◉ 2. Singing popular songs from the 1940s
- ○ 3. Reading an article from the newspaper
- ○ 4. Making decorations for a future holiday

97 When one of the older adults at reminiscence therapy says, "If I had it to do all over again, I wouldn't change a thing," the nurse is *most accurate* in interpreting this to mean that the client has acquired the developmental characteristic of
- ○ 1. trust.
- ◉ 2. integrity.
- ○ 3. intimacy.
- ○ 4. autonomy.

A group of nurses in a long-term care facility attend an in-service program on documentation.

98 When asked to critique a chart entry that says, "States, 'I feel unwanted.' Appears to be confused," which statement *best describes* why this entry is unsatisfactory?
- ○ 1. The nurse who made the entry failed to interpret the significance of feeling "unwanted."
- ○ 2. The nurse who made the entry failed to indicate the importance of the client's statement.
- ○ 3. The nurse who made the entry failed to substantiate that the quote was made by the client.
- ◉ 4. The nurse who made the entry failed to describe the evidence of the confused behavior.

A nurse is employed on a special unit for clients with dementia.

99 When an older client with Alzheimer's disease seems confused about how to use a fork, the *best nursing action* for prolonging her ability to maintain self-care is to
- ○ 1. ask the physician to order a liquid diet.
- ◉ 2. position her so she can mimic other clients.
- ○ 3. serve her first so she has more time to eat.
- ○ 4. seat her alone so no one will see her mess.

100 What is the *best approach* for managing a confused client who wanders and mistakenly goes into other clients' rooms?
- ◉ 1. Place a large sign with the client's name on her door.
- ○ 2. Keep the room doors on the unit locked at all times.
- ○ 3. Restrain her in a wheelchair when unattended.
- ○ 4. Speak to her about invading others' privacy.

101 The *most therapeutic* technique for helping clients with dementia remain oriented is to
- ○ 1. call each client by their first name.
- ○ 2. ask clients to identify a goal for the day.
- ○ 3. assign clients to greet visitors each day.
- ◉ 4. post large calendars with the current date.

102 The *best technique* for reducing confusion among clients with dementia is to
- ○ 1. wear an employee name tag when caring for clients.
- ◉ 2. adhere to a consistent routine of unit activities.
- ○ 3. provide diversional activities, like field trips.
- ○ 4. distribute a list of the day's scheduled events.

103 What is the *best response* to the daughter of a client with Alzheimer's disease who says, "I'm not sure Mother knows who I am."
- ○ 1. "This is probably the beginning of the end for her."
- ◉ 2. "You're distressed that she does not respond to you."
- ○ 3. "Don't worry. We're taking very good care of her here."
- ○ 4. "Behind every cloud there's a silver lining."

At a team conference, the nurses explore ways to help a client with dementia understand verbal communication.

104 The *best intervention* for communicating with the demented client is to
- ○ 1. speak loudly to get his attention.
- ◉ 2. use short sentences when speaking.
- ○ 3. use written forms of communication.
- ○ 4. let him listen to news programs.

The family of a client with Alzheimer's disease wants to take him home for a day.

105   Which of the following is *essential* to assess for ensuring the client's well-being during the home visit?
  ○ 1. The caregiver's understanding of the symptoms he manifests
  ○ 2. The caregiver's understanding of when the client must return
  ● 3. The caregiver's understanding of when to administer medications
  ○ 4. The caregiver's understanding of how to provide hygiene measures

106   When a client with dementia says, "I want to go home," it is *best* for the nurse to respond by saying
  ● 1. "You are at home."
  ○ 2. "You are staying here."
  ○ 3. "You must not like us."
  ○ 4. "You need to call your family."

107   When a nurse notes that the wife who regularly visits her spouse with dementia is demonstrating signs of exhaustion and self-neglect, it is *most therapeutic* to
  ○ 1. suggest that she make an appointment for a physical examination.
  ● 2. discuss modifying the amount of time she is devoting to caretaking.
  ○ 3. remind her of the scheduled times for visiting clients on the unit.
  ○ 4. explain that there are many staff who can care for her husband.

An older adult is dying of a terminal illness. The dying client has an advance directive indicating that he does not want any heroic measures used to prolong his life.

108   What is the *most appropriate* nursing action when the terminally ill client's death is imminent?
  ● 1. Sit quietly and hold the dying client's hand.
  ○ 2. Move him into the hall where he can be observed.
  ○ 3. Place him in a room by himself near the nurse.
  ○ 4. Tell him to use his signal if he needs anything.

Following the death of the terminally ill client, a nursing assistant is extremely distraught.

109   What nursing approach is *most beneficial* for helping the nursing assistant at this time?
  ○ 1. Being sent home for the rest of the shift
  ○ 2. Being terminated from this type of work
  ● 3. Being allowed to express how he or she feels
  ○ 4. Being asked to perform postmortem care

Family members of the deceased client are referred to a grief support group.

110   When a new member to the group tells the nursing leader that she "senses" her dead husband's presence in their home, it is *best* for the nurse to
  ○ 1. recommend more professional counseling.
  ○ 2. assure her that it is wishful thinking.
  ● 3. let her be comforted by the experience.
  ○ 4. encourage her to stay with relatives.

Directions: Two numbers appear in parentheses following each rationale. The first number identifies the textbook listed in the references, page 512, and the second number identifies the page(s) in that textbook on which the correct answer can be verified. Occasionally two or more textbooks are given to verify the correct answer.

MENTAL HEALTH NEEDS DURING YOUNG ADULTHOOD

1 4. Although an affirmative answer to all of the questions is significant, one of the most suggestive signs of alcoholism is the occurrence of "blackouts." Blackouts are a form of amnesia for actions and events that take place when a person is drinking. Alcoholism is not related to the amount of time over which it is consumed. Alcoholism occurs among individuals who consume alcohol in any form. A preference for alcohol is just that, a personal choice. The consequences of consuming alcohol, however, are substantial criteria for alcoholism. (2:230–231; 10:236; 23:347)
    Nursing Process—Data collection
    Client Need—Psychosocial integrity

2 1. Denial is one of the major barriers to recovery from alcoholism. The first step of Alcoholics Anonymous (AA) and other treatment programs is to help the alcoholic give up his or her denial. Most alcoholics are malnourished, but improving the alcoholic's dietary intake does not necessarily help him or her stop drinking. Alcoholism is not a consequence of weak willpower. AA does emphasize belief in a higher power, but participating in an organized religion is not promoted. (10:535)
    Nursing Process—Implementation
    Client Need—Health promotion/maintenance

3 3. Al-Anon is an organization specifically for family members of alcoholics who may or may not be involved in recovery. Alcoholics Anonymous is for recovering alcoholics. Recovery is a support group for persons with mental disorders. Synanon is a private organization involved in drug rehabilitation. (10:538)
    Nursing Process—Implementation
    Client Need—Psychosocial integrity

4 2. Inflammation of the eyes is almost always present after smoking marijuana. The pulse rate is likely to be rapid. Other signs include euphoria, drowsiness, lightheadedness, and hunger. Shivering accompan-

ies opiate withdrawal. Rapid breathing and restlessness are observed in abrupt alcohol withdrawal or use of a central nervous system stimulant. (20:484)
    Nursing Process—Data collection
    Client Need—Psychosocial integrity

5 1. The most likely effect of marijuana from among those listed is drowsiness. Abused drugs that are more likely to cause hyperactivity, apprehension, and suspiciousness are those that are central nervous system stimulants, such as cocaine and amphetamines. (20:484)
    Nursing Process—Data collection
    Client Need—Psychosocial integrity

6 1. Marijuana is known to produce apathy among those who use it. Consequently, many chronic users become disinterested in school, work, or other social responsibilities. As a result, they fail to reach their potential for success. Marijuana is more likely to be psychologically addicting. Most do not use this drug often enough or long enough to show a statistical relationship with lung cancer. Breathing may be impaired, but the respiratory center in the brain is not usually suppressed as it is in heroin or morphine abuse. (20:484)
    Nursing Process—Data collection
    Client Need—Psychosocial integrity

7 2. Chronic use of marijuana may cause problems with memory, which is also an effect associated with chronic alcohol abuse. The other behaviors are not common among those who use marijuana. (20:484)
    Nursing Process—Data collection
    Client Need—Psychosocial integrity

8 4. The most immediate need for the parents whose child has died from SIDS is to experience the reality of their loss. Facilitating an opportunity to have personal contact with the infant promotes the grieving process. (22:546–547)
    Nursing Process—Implementation
    Client Need—Psychosocial integrity

9 2. Most parents feel guilty immediately after the death of a previously healthy infant. They need reassurance that they are in no way to blame for the child's death. Later, parents who have experienced the loss of a child from sudden infant death syndrome (SIDS) may need professional or support group help in resolving their anger, fear, and depression. (2:546–547)
　　Nursing Process—Implementation
　　Client Need—Psychosocial integrity

10 3. It is important to relieve parents of any self-blame after the unexpected death of an infant. Unfortunately, many parents are suspected of child abuse in cases like this. Informing them of the staff's efforts and where grief support may be obtained are appropriate nursing actions, but they are secondary to relieving undeserved guilt. Indicating that the child may have had brain damage is little consolation immediately after the infant's death. (22:546)
　　Nursing Process—Implementation
　　Client Need—Psychosocial integrity

11 1. Candidly asking if the person is being abused is the most straightforward way to obtain information. Although many victims of abuse protect their abuser, they are not apt to reveal their abuse unless they sense that someone is concerned enough to ask. It is appropriate to assess the children for signs of abuse, but this is done secondarily. Checking with relatives or friends may damage the nurse-client relationship or jeopardize the safety of the victim if the spouse is made aware of the inquiry. (10:620)
　　Nursing Process—Data collection
　　Client Need—Psychosocial integrity

12 2. More than anything else, knowing where there is a safe place to go for help empowers the victim to protect herself when exposed to future violence. Giving out a personal phone number is never appropriate. Many women stay in abusive relationships because they think the abuser will change. Trying to terminate an abusive relationship also may escalate the frequency or severity of violence. Most male batterers are resistant to change and are unlikely to participate in joint counseling. (10:619, 621)
　　Nursing Process—Implementation
　　Client Need—Psychosocial integrity

13 3. Many victims of family violence believe that if they behave in an ideal way, they can prevent the cycle of abuse. Some even blame themselves or believe that they deserve the abuse. Most know that the abuse is serious or even life-threatening, that they may be murdered if they attempt to terminate the

relationship, and that their family most likely will be unsupportive. (10:617–621)
　　Nursing Process—Data collection
　　Client Need—Psychosocial integrity

14 1. Bathing or showering can destroy evidence that may be essential for convicting the rapist. Although a sketch of the rapist or written description of the crime may be helpful, rape victims are not usually capable of completing these activities independently. If the victim is in no immediate danger, it is inappropriate to recommend calling 911. However, it is appropriate to advise the victim to call a support person. (10:603; 23:552)
　　Nursing Process—Implementation
　　Client Need—Safe, effective care environment

15 4. The most supportive nursing activity is to remain present with a rape victim at all times. Stress for crime victims is often increased when they must interact with physicians or police officers who are both strangers and males. The other nursing actions are important to the care of rape victims, but they are not as likely to reduce anxiety as the continuous presence of an empathetic nurse. (10:605; 23:554)
　　Nursing Process—Implementation
　　Client Need—Psychosocial integrity

16 2. Victims of violent crimes are likely to perceive strangers as a threat to their safety. Therefore, a priority for nursing care is to limit the number of contacts with people with whom the victim is unfamiliar, even though the strangers are well-meaning staff. The nurse assesses for physical and emotional trauma; the police document the circumstances of the rape. Sedation is generally avoided, if at all possible, because it interferes with crisis resolution. The victim's permission is obtained before contacting anyone. To not do so violates the client's right to privacy and confidentiality. (10:604–605)
　　Nursing Process—Implementation
　　Client Need—Psychosocial integrity

17 2. Providing explanations helps to reduce anxiety. It is especially important for those clients who are trying to manage the stress of a traumatic experience. Powerlessness is diminished by giving clients opportunities to make choices. Although giving information does support standards for care and provides teaching, that is not the primary principle underlying this situation. (10:604–605)
　　Nursing Process—Evaluation
　　Client Need—Safe, effective care environment

18 3. Competent adult clients always have the right to make decisions regarding their treatment. Although

a nurse may not feel that the decision is in the client's best interests, the client's right to refuse must be respected. Coercion in any form is inappropriate. (23:554; 25:40)
    Nursing Process—Implementation
    Client Need—Safe, effective care environment

19 3. Eating out of habit or hardly eating anything at all are indications that a rape victim is not recovering readily from the assault. The other behavioral symptoms are more characteristic of a mild reaction to the rape trauma and are likely to be relieved with short-term support. (10:606–607)
    Nursing Process—Evaluation
    Client Need—Psychosocial integrity

20 1. Although all of the options are possible outcomes of the group process, the most desired outcome for a self-help group is that the group members obtain mutual support from one another. (9:130; 10:138)
    Nursing Process—Evaluation
    Client Need—Psychosocial integrity

21 2. For an instant, most people are shocked after receiving bad news. This is followed by disbelief or denial. Later, common emotional responses include anger, depression, and acceptance, generally in that order. (23:561)
    Nursing Process—Data collection
    Client Need—Psychosocial integrity

22 4. The need to deny may be so overwhelming that it interferes with a person's good judgment to implement safer sex practices. Concealing the information, avoiding contact with, or confronting others are more indicative of depression and anger. (23:562)
    Nursing Process—Evaluation
    Client Need—Psychosocial integrity

23 2. A crisis is diminished and subsequent coping is promoted by having a social network of supportive friends and relatives. Acceptance by religious leaders, sexual tolerance, and new social acquaintances do not provide the same quality of emotional support. (23:562)
    Nursing Process—Planning
    Client Need—Psychosocial integrity

24 4. Some people entertain thoughts of suicide as their only means of relieving others and themselves from the hopelessness of living with a terminal disease. Signs of despair indicate that a client deserves close observation to ensure safety. Dreams may be an indication that a client is fearful of dying. The

other remarks are more suggestive of requesting information. (10:407)
    Nursing Process—Evaluation
    Client Need—Psychosocial integrity

25 2. Repeated contact between gastric acid and teeth from self-induced vomiting results in deterioration of dental structures. Bulimics usually are of normal weight. They control their weight by a cycle of purging after eating binges. Anorectics are more likely to cease menstruating when their body fat is depleted. Loss of hair also is correlated more with the malnutrition of anorexia nervosa. (9:290)
    Nursing Process—Data collection
    Client Need—Psychosocial integrity

26 1. Binging and purging take place privately. If the client stays out of the bathroom following a meal, it interferes with the opportunity to induce vomiting and use laxatives or enemas to stimulate bowel elimination. Taking an inventory of food may precipitate an uncontrollable urge to go on an eating binge. The bulimic food binges are not isolated to fast-food establishments. Recording calories only increases the anxiety bulimics experience when their eating is out of control. (6:376)
    Nursing Process—Planning
    Client Need—Psychosocial integrity

27 3. A reduction in binging is the best therapeutic effect for this client since it breaks the binge-purge cycle. The problem with bulimics is not that they do not eat nutritious food, but that they eat too much food. Although fluoxetine is an antidepressant, it works equally as well in controlling the symptoms of bulimics who are not clinically depressed. (10:566)
    Nursing Process—Evaluation
    Client Need—Physiological integrity

28 3. Peer censure is much more therapeutic than disapproval from the group leader. If the therapist or members of the treatment team react positively or negatively to the individuals involved in the conflict, it is likely to divide the group members and jeopardize group work. (23:161)
    Nursing Process—Implementation
    Client Need—Psychosocial integrity

29 2. Being overly talkative is a suggestive sign of amphetamine use. Dextroamphetamine is a stimulant; staring into space and slurring words are side effects from using depressant types of drugs. Sunglasses are sometimes worn to disguise the inflamed eyes that occur with marijuana use. (20:485)
    Nursing Process—Data collection
    Client Need—Psychosocial integrity

30 1. Young adults who have not acquired the developmental characteristic of *intimacy* will tend to have superficial relationships that are temporary in nature. Worrying about financial security is more common during the middle years of adulthood. A person's sexual identity is established much earlier in life. Assertiveness is more a unique personality characteristic than one that is commonly acquired at a particular stage in life. (2:310; 9:39)

> **Nursing Process—Evaluation**
> **Client Need—Health promotion/maintenance**

31 4. Rationalization is a coping mechanism in which a person fails to take responsibility for something by offering some acceptable explanation for it. Indicating that there are health risks from being overweight is an example of intellectualization. Projection is used when accusing others of one's own feelings that are too painful to acknowledge. The failure to resist ice cream demonstrates insight into behavior. (10:33; 23:13)

> **Nursing Process—Data collection**
> **Client Need—Psychosocial integrity**

32 1. Non–English-speaking clients or those who speak very little English feel more comfortable communicating with and through a translator that is their same gender. This reduces embarrassment when there are questions that pertain to genitourinary functions, bowel elimination, reproductive history and other sensitive issues. (25:68)

> **Nursing Process—Implementation**
> **Client Need—Safe, effective care environment**

33 4. As long as a health belief has no detrimental effect, it is best to integrate it within the plan of care. Rejecting an otherwise neutral cultural practice interferes with a therapeutic nurse-client relationship. (10:171)

> **Nursing Process—Implementation**
> **Client Need—Safe, effective care environment**

34 2. Snorting cocaine is most likely to ulcerate and erode the nasal mucosa and septum. Rapid respirations are due to systemic effects of the drug, but the lung sounds should be clear. The oropharynx may show some signs of irritation and the ability to smell may be damaged, but these signs are not the most appropriate assessments to perform first. (20:484)

> **Nursing Process—Data collection**
> **Client Need—Psychosocial integrity**

35 1. Cocaine abuse can result in cardiac dysrhythmias and death. Toxicity can occur any time and with any dose. Cocaine is a central nervous system stimulant. As such, it increases respirations and raises blood pressure. Blood glucose may be lowered ow-ing to the use of calories during periods of hyperactivity. (20:484)

> **Nursing Process—Planning**
> **Client Need—Psychosocial integrity**

36 4. Hallucinations are sensory experiences of which only the client is aware. An auditory hallucination involves hearing a voice or sound that no one else perceives. The person rarely volunteers his or her altered perceptions. The observant nurse draws inferences based on the client's nonverbal cues. The first three examples are not associated with the behavior of an hallucinating client. (10:375)

> **Nursing Process—Data collection**
> **Client Need—Psychosocial integrity**

37 2. As a result of the schizophrenic's disordered thoughts, he or she may have difficulty putting thoughts into words. The nurse never pretends to understand the meaning of a client's illogical statement. (10:375; 23:95)

> **Nursing Process—Implementation**
> **Client Need—Psychosocial integrity**

38 1. Hospitalization is indicated when a client is a danger to others or himself, as in this case of self-neglect. The other options suggest that the client is having problems with socialization skills, but none that are improved with hospitalization. (23:445, 452)

> **Nursing Process—Evaluation**
> **Client Need—Psychosocial integrity**

MENTAL HEALTH NEEDS DURING MIDDLE AGE (35–65)

39 2. Regardless of the cause or the client's level of dementia, it is important to establish that there are limits for the client's behavior. Leaving the room first is not sufficient to establish a relationship between the nurse's response and the unacceptable behavior. Ignoring the behavior is more likely to communicate permission to repeat it. The same is true for trying to avoid being a repeat target. (10:127)

> **Nursing Process—Implementation**
> **Client Need—Psychosocial integrity**

40 1. One of the best ways to modify behavior is to impose a significant consequence which has been previously communicated to the client. Wearing protective garments will not stop the behavior, although it is appropriate hygienically. Clients with impaired cognition are not likely to be persuaded to change behavior as a result of intellectual explanations. (23:116)

> **Nursing Process—Planning**
> **Client Need—Psychosocial integrity**

41 2. To obtain the most valid results from a mental status assessment of a client who is most likely to demonstrate cognitive impairment, it is best to allow extra time for responding to questions. A certain number of open-ended questions are necessary during a mental status examination. It violates standards of care to omit the assessment or to defer the entire assessment to someone else. (4:954–955; 9:221)

> Nursing Process—Data collection
> Client Need—Psychosocial integrity

42 1. Panic attacks are one type of anxiety disorder. The physical symptoms are generally a consequence of sympathetic nervous system stimulation. The release of adrenaline causes an increase in the heart rate. Clients may think they are having a heart attack or even dying. Sympathetic nervous system stimulation also is associated with a dry mouth, dilated pupils, and hypertension. (2:276; 10:432)

> Nursing Process—Data collection
> Client Need—Physiological integrity

43 4. Panic attacks are due to an interplay of both biological and physiological factors. Once the person begins to experience the symptoms, he or she fears the symptoms are life-threatening. The combination of symptoms followed by fear, followed by intensified symptoms, creates a vicious circle. (10:432)

> Nursing Process—Data collection
> Client Need—Psychosocial integrity

44 4. Anxiety is heightened during situations in which there have been no prior experiences. Providing explanations and instructions diminishes insecurity. Standing within an arm's length invades a client's personal space and heightens anxiety. Wearing a laboratory coat may nonverbally upset a client, depending on what it represents from past experiences. Wearing a name tag and introducing oneself are always appropriate. Coffee and tea contain stimulating chemicals that are avoided. (10:434)

> Nursing Process—Planning
> Client Need—Physiological integrity

45 1. Being reassured about safety helps more than the other actions to reduce the client's feelings of fear and loss of control. (10:434)

> Nursing Process—Implementation
> Client Need—Psychosocial integrity

46 4. Staying with a frightened client communicates genuine concern. The presence of a caring person tends to reduce anxiety. The first choice is an example of giving advice, which is a nontherapeutic communication technique. Trying to shame the client with the possibility that the out-of-control behavior may be seen by the physician is inappropriate. The third nontherapeutic example is one of generalizing. It disregards this client's right to be considered unique. (10:434; 23:290)

> Nursing Process—Implementation
> Client Need—Psychosocial integrity

47 1. Antianxiety drugs produce a calming effect. If alcohol is consumed with this medication, it is likely to potentiate the drug's action and endanger the client's safety from profound sedation. Drug dependency is related to this drug's dosage and length of administration. The drug causes sedation. Blood levels are not commonly monitored when benzodiazepines are prescribed. (20:207, 216)

> Nursing Process—Planning
> Client Need—Physiological integrity

48 2. Many clients who experience panic attacks go on to develop *agoraphobia*, a fear of being someplace where help may be unavailable. Some patients who experience panic attacks seek psychiatric treatment and some take more than the prescribed amount of medication, but these are not characteristic of the majority of individuals with this anxiety disorder. Persons with panic disorder rarely develop psychotic symptoms. (10:432)

> Nursing Process—Evaluation
> Client Need—Psychosocial integrity

49 4. Displacement is a coping mechanism in which a person transfers his angry feelings for one person onto someone else who is less likely to retaliate with significant consequences. Introjection involves taking on the characteristics of another. Projection is characterized as accusing someone of one's own weaknesses. Compensation is demonstrated by overcoming some inadequacy by excelling at another. (23:13–15)

> Nursing Process—Implementation
> Client Need—Psychosocial integrity

50 3. By remaining calm the nurse models the type of behavior that is expected and reduces stimuli that the client may interpret as threatening. It is appropriate to encourage the client to discuss what triggered his anger, but it is inappropriate to suggest talking to the client's wife. Using additional medication relieves the client of responsibility for managing his feelings. Physical activity is a way of dissipating anger, but it does not supersede discussing his feelings. (9:91; 10:128)

> Nursing Process—Implementation
> Client Need—Psychosocial integrity

51 1. Gathering staff is referred to as a "show of force." It is sometimes all that is needed to convince a client that it is best to regain control. Asking a physician to intervene implies that nurses are unable to effectively manage a disruptive client's behavior. It is unsafe to go anywhere alone with a client who is beyond anger and in danger of losing self-control. It is unethical to display restraints as an implied threat for controlling the client's behavior. (10:128)

Nursing Process—Implementation
Client Need—Psychosocial integrity

52 2. It is legal to administer medications against a client's will when the circumstances indicate danger to the client or others. To avoid liability, documentation must objectively describe the evidence of danger and the *lack* of success when alternative measures were attempted. (10:58, 130)

Nursing Process—Implementation
Client Need—Safe, effective care environment

53 2. Using short, simple sentences is best when teaching anxious clients who have short attention spans and therefore difficulty concentrating. Anxious clients are overwhelmed by detailed explanations or elaborate diagrams. Videotapes are not as effective as person-to-person instruction. The nurse can assess the client's comprehension periodically and repeat information that is unclear. (10:426; 25:87)

Nursing Process—Implementation
Client Need—Health promotion/maintenance

54 1. Middle-aged adults who may be forced into retirement are likely to experience a great deal of stress since this is the stage in life when adults are most concerned with their future financial security. The other events are challenging, but they probably are not major sources of conflict as adults achieve *generativity*. (9:39; 10:38; 23:219)

Nursing Process—Evaluation
Client Need—Health promotion/maintenance

55 3. Phobic people *avoid* what they perceive as the cause of their discomfort. Suppression is a coping mechanism in which a person chooses to refrain from thinking about something that is a source of conflict. Compensation is characterized by pursuing an activity that ensures success to make up for feeling inadequate. Undoing is a coping mechanism in which one makes amends for having offended someone. (9:279; 10:34)

Nursing Process—Data collection
Client Need—Psychosocial integrity

56 1. Cognitive therapy involves confronting irrational thoughts and behaviors. The expected outcome is that people recognize the flaws in their thinking and ultimately change their behavior. The other

options describe desensitization therapy, assertiveness training, and behavioral modification, in that order. (23:114–116)

Nursing Process—Implementation
Client Need—Psychosocial integrity

57 1. People with PTSD generally reexperience their respective traumatic event in some way, such as in upsetting dreams, nightmares, or flashbacks. A few have visual hallucinations, but not generally auditory hallucinations. Most have a "numbed" or blunted emotional response to others with whom they interact. (10:440)

Nursing Process—Implementation
Client Need—Health promotion/maintenance

58 3. Those who are able to recall their precipitating traumatic event use a tremendous amount of energy to control their feelings or to suppress the memory of it. Giving clients permission to let the "demons" out can be very therapeutic. Many PTSD clients abuse drugs and alcohol to help "numb" their consciousness; antianxiety drugs are likely to do the same. Improving damaged relationships is a goal of therapy, but it is not the primary focus of treatment. (10:443)

Nursing Process—Implementation
Client Need—Psychosocial integrity

59 1. Art is used as a therapeutic tool to promote expression of thoughts or feelings that are too difficult to verbalize. Although the other outcomes in the remaining options may occur, they are not the primary purpose underlying the intervention. (10:433)

Nursing Process—Implementation
Client Need—Psychosocial integrity

60 3. A stimulus that evokes a memory of the original traumatic event can trigger the anxiety from the prior experience. If the person had been frightened of fireworks as a child, he probably would have manifested a continued fear response prior to his military experience. The startle response is not associated with a loss of patriotism or a fear of being drafted. (2:279)

Nursing Process—Implementation
Client Need—Health promotion/maintenance

61 2. Post-traumatic stress disorder can occur in anyone who is involved in an uncommon event outside the realm of usual human experience. This can involve natural disasters like earthquakes, or situational disasters like being raped. None of the other situations plays a role in developing post-traumatic stress disorder. (2:278)

Nursing Process—Implementation
Client Need—Health promotion/maintenance

62 4. Assessment is the first step in the nursing process. Vital signs are taken before any further action is implemented. (18:382; 25:18)
   Nursing Process—Data collection
   Client Need—Safe, effective care environment

63 1. Middle adulthood is characterized as a period of generativity or stagnation. It is common for people to assess their accomplishments during this stage in the life cycle. People who do not see themselves as counting for much can experience what is known as a midlife crisis. Goals generally are established at an earlier age. Middle-aged people may regret their judgments, but they do not doubt them. (9:62)
   Nursing Process—Implementation
   Client Need—Health promotion/maintenance

64 2. Therapeutic communication requires that the nurse perceive hidden meanings within a client's statements or questions. It is then appropriate to verbalize the feeling or tone for validation. Deferring discussion to the physician is a form of scapegoating in which the nurse chooses to remain uninvolved. Telling the client to let the staff worry or to practice more patience are forms of giving advice. Giving advice is a nontherapeutic form of communication. (10:92; 23:95)
   Nursing Process—Implementation
   Client Need—Psychosocial integrity

65 2. Emotional care involves a sincere respect, interest, and concern for people. Nurses demonstrate emotional care when they accept individual differences in people and treat each client as a unique person. Although all of the other outcomes can occur, the most detrimental effect is to the client. A health worker's biases and prejudices, if unchallenged, can interfere with objective care. (23:90–91; 25:77)
   Nursing Process—Evaluation
   Client Need—Safe, effective care environment

66 3. Only hospital employees who are immediately involved in the care of a client may have access to a client's health record. A signed written release from the client must be obtained before divulging confidential information. The nurse must take all necessary measures to safeguard health information contained in the client's medical record. (10:55; 25:39–40)
   Nursing Process—Implementation
   Client Need—Safe, effective care environment

67 4. A client with ulcerative colitis has an inflamed bowel and experiences severe diarrhea. Endoscopic examinations and x-rays confirm the pres-

ence of pathology. The exact cause of the disease is unknown, but emotional stress is one of many cofactors. Most clients with psychophysiologic diseases would rather work than experience their symptoms. (21:103, 697)
   Nursing Process—Implementation
   Client Need—Safe, effective care environment

68 1. Meeting physiological needs always takes precedence over other needs, such as security, love and belonging, and so forth. The most important information needed at this time concerns his bowel elimination and the impact it is having on his fluid status, nutrition, and electrolyte balance. (21:698–699)
   Nursing Process—Planning
   Client Need—Physiological integrity

69 1. A nonjudgmental attitude conveys to the client that help is being provided without holding the client personally responsible. Cleaning stool is never pleasant, but the nurse avoids making the client feel that he is an offensive person. When a client is treated with dignity, it sustains his self-esteem. It would not promote this client's self-esteem if he were cleaned by his mother or male nurses or if he were required to do that task himself. (21:699; 23:87)
   Nursing Process—Planning
   Client Need—Psychosocial integrity

70 2. A consequence of alcohol abuse is a cross-tolerance to all sedative drugs. A need for a higher dosage or more frequent administration can indicate that the client abuses alcohol or some other central nervous system depressant drug. An alcoholic's blood pressure and pulse become abnormally high during withdrawal from alcohol. There is no cause and effect relationship between the absence of bowel sounds and the abuse of alcohol. (17:659)
   Nursing Process—Data collection
   Client Need—Psychosocial integrity

71 3. Visual hallucinations occur in advanced withdrawal from alcohol. These are real and terrifying experiences for the alcoholic. To maintain safety and reduce the client's fear and anxiety, it is essential that a nurse remain with the client. Restraints are not used unless there is no other alternative for maintaining the client's or staff's safety. In the client's mind the hallucination is real. Telling him that he is not seeing "bugs" is illogical and untrue. Closing the client's door is unsafe and likely to heighten his fear. (10:516–517)
   Nursing Process—Implementation
   Client Need—Safe, effective care environment

72 3. It is always best to notify the physician first whenever there is a sudden change in a client's condition. Alcohol withdrawal generally is treated with one of the minor tranquilizers such as lorazepam (Ativan), or a central nervous system depressant such as phenobarbital, which is prescribed by a physician. (10:516–517)
Nursing Process—Implementation
Client Need—Physiological integrity

73 2. Seizures occur from rebound central nervous system stimulation as the depressant drug, alcohol, is metabolized from the client's system. Seizures occur in some people as early as the first 24 hours of withdrawal. Bleeding and jaundice are the results of liver damage from chronic alcohol abuse. Hyperthermia occurs during alcohol withdrawal. (20:486)
Nursing Process—Data collection
Client Need—Physiological integrity

74 1. Staff members are better able to understand client behavior by increasing their own self-understanding. Nurses who are generalists are not academically prepared to analyze a client's motivation or provide psychotherapy. A knowledge of abnormal behavior is important, but it is not the first step in understanding the behavior of others. (2:49)
Nursing Process—Implementation
Client Need—Safe, effective care environment

75 3. People with bipolar disorder, formerly called manic-depressive disorder, have cycles during which they display a marked change in mood. The exaggerated mood is followed or preceded by an interval of normal mood. None of the other behaviors is symptomatic of bipolar disorder. (2:259)
Nursing Process—Data collection
Client Need—Psychosocial integrity

76 3. Toxic reactions occur with lithium carbonate therapy when blood levels reach more than 1.5 mEq/L. Blood levels usually are drawn during therapy and the dosage of lithium adjusted according to the results. The client who takes lithium may develop polyuria, but the volume of urine eliminated is not used to monitor the lithium level. Neither vital signs nor brain scans are used to evaluate the client's ability to metabolize his or her lithium dose. (20:214)
Nursing Process—Evaluation
Client Need—Physiological integrity

77 1. Spending money extravagantly is a sign that a client with bipolar disorder is having difficulty using good judgment. Although wanting to become a hospice volunteer, being physically active, and staying up late may be signs of grandiose ideas and hyperactivity that often accompany a manic phase of bipolar disorder, they are not as suggestive of a loss of control as spending money extravagantly. (10:341)
Nursing Process—Data collection
Client Need—Psychosocial integrity

MENTAL HEALTH NEEDS DURING LATE ADULTHOOD (OVER 65)

78 2. Privacy is important whenever information of a personal nature is gathered. Regardless of the environment, clients have the right to expect that what they reveal will be kept private and confidential—even from well-meaning family members. (1:304)
Nursing Process—Planning
Client Need—Safe, effective care environment

79 1. An indirect leading statement or open-ended question is purposely general and nonspecific. It allows the client to give as much information as he or she wants. Close-ended questions or statements, exemplified in the other three options, provide facts or sometimes one-word replies. (9:156)
Nursing Process—Planning
Client Need—Psychosocial integrity

80 3. Asking the client to identify his or her birth date is a standard technique for assessing long-term memory. The nurse should know the answer to the question that is asked to evaluate the client's response. Asking the client his or her current age and today's date helps in the assessment of short-term memory and orientation. Asking what occurred in January is too vague a question for a valid assessment. (23:61)
Nursing Process—Data collection
Client Need—Safe, effective care environment

81 1. Asking a client to repeat the question helps to rule out a hearing deficit or possible dementia. A client has a 50% chance of being right when having to respond only with a "yes" or "no." Asking the next of kin is appropriate if the client is not a reliable historian. Asking questions only the client can answer does not provide comprehensive data. (9:190, 194)
Nursing Process—Data collection
Client Need—Safe, effective care environment

82 2. Being unable to provide the names of longstanding neighbors is the most significant sign of mental deterioration from among the options provided. The other assessment findings are normal or typical for an older adult who is 65 years old. (3:359)
Nursing Process—Evaluation
Client Need—Health promotion/maintenance

83 1. Late adulthood is a time when most deal with multiple losses. The characteristics in the incorrect options reflect myths about aging that many younger people believe are true. (1:306; 2:106; 3:435)
Nursing Process—Evaluation
Client Need—Health promotion/maintenance

84 4. In the interests of client safety, it is best to locate a depressed client where he or she can be frequently and closely observed by the nursing staff. Placing the depressed client alone or at the end of the hallway increases the potential opportunity for attempting suicide. Being in a room with a cheerful person and being placed in a nonstimulating environment are not considered therapeutic modalities for relieving depression. (2:270; 10:409–410)
Nursing Process—Planning
Client Need—Psychosocial integrity

85 2. A plan for suicide indicates that the client has given serious thought to ending his life. Once a plan has been developed, the client is much more likely to act on his feelings. The remaining examples are characteristic of passive suicide ideation, which is not associated with as much lethal risk as an active suicide plan. (2:270–271)
Nursing Process—Data collection
Client Need—Psychosocial integrity

86 3. Tricyclic antidepressants like amitriptyline hydrochloride (Elavil) have anticholinergic effects. Therefore they are likely to increase the potential for urinary retention, which may already be a problem for a client with prostatic hypertrophy. Neither diabetes mellitus, pernicious anemia, nor chronic emphysema are contraindications for administering anticholinergic drugs.(28:105; 17:324)
Nursing Process—Implementation
Client Need—Physiological integrity

87 1. Tricyclic antidepressants take as long as 2 to 3 weeks to produce a therapeutic effect. Improvement in mood may be subtle, but the client is likely to feel better after an appropriate trial of drug therapy. Dietary changes are not necessary with tricyclic drug therapy. Drug therapy is a major treatment modality for depression, but electroconvulsive therapy (ECT) sometimes produces improvement more rapidly. (17:314)
Nursing Process—Implementation
Client Need—Health promotion/maintenance

88 2. The nurse checks that depressed clients have swallowed their medication. Some clients "cheek" the medications and then use them as a method of suicide when a quantity accumulates. Taking medications with a full glass of water is appropriate for clients who are not restricted in their fluid intake. Some medications are absorbed better on an empty stomach; some are better taken with food if they cause stomach upset. Taking one or all of the prescribed drugs at one time is a matter of preference if the client does not have difficulty swallowing them. (10:402)
Nursing Process—Implementation
Client Need—Physiological integrity

89 3. Following electroconvulsive therapy (ECT) it is common for clients to experience headaches and temporary retrograde and antegrade memory loss for events that are nearest in time to the treatment. Proponents of ECT claim that the capacity to remember information eventually returns to the pretreatment level. The effects identified in the other options may occur, but they are not associated effects of ECT. (10:589)
Nursing Process—Data collection
Client Need—Physiological integrity

90 2. Providing privacy is appropriate for preserving the sexually active couple's self-esteem. Reporting their sexual behavior to adult children is not appropriate as long as they are competent and consenting adults. The request to become roommates is better initiated by the residents themselves. Censuring sexuality is not appropriate; even older adults have a need for love and affection. (3:119; 9:339–340)
Nursing Process—Implementation
Client Need—Psychosocial integrity

91 1. Involuntary facial movements indicate the development of *tardive dyskinesia*, a consequence of antipsychotic drug therapy. The condition, once it develops, is usually irreversible even after the drug is discontinued. None of the other assessment findings are linked to antipsychotic drug withdrawal. (10:237–238)
Nursing Process—Evaluation
Client Need—Physiological integrity

92 2. Depression in the elderly is often masked under the guise of multiple physical complaints. It often is easier to seek help for physical problems than to verbalize the need for emotional help. Being irritable after a visit from active grandchildren is normal for some older adults. Sleeping a great deal of time is suggestive of depression, but taking a lengthy nap regularly in the afternoon is not necessarily pathologic. Crying when talking about a dead spouse is normal if the death has been recent. If the crying is brief, it is not interpreted as unresolved grief. (9:224; 10:653)

Nursing Process—Data collection
Client Need—Psychosocial integrity

93 4. Selective serotonin reuptake inhibitors such as sertraline (Zoloft) tend to cause insomnia, nervousness, headache, anxiety, urinary retention, blurred vision, and dry mucous membranes. (28:996; 17:315)

Nursing Process—Data collection
Client Need—Physiological integrity

94 4. It is essential that the nurse treat a client with cognitive impairment with dignity. Shielding her from public view is the most appropriate action for the nurse to take in this situation. The other options are better suited for a client with a higher level of cognitive function. (3:383, 388)

Nursing Process—Implementation
Client Need—Psychosocial integrity

95 4. Self-worth is maintained by experiencing satisfaction in accomplishments. Giving genuine praise promotes a positive self-concept. The longer a person can maintain independence, the less likely that physical deterioration will occur. All of the other choices communicate to the client that he is not able to manage his self-care satisfactorily. (10:317–318)

Nursing Process—Planning
Client Need—Psychosocial integrity

96 2. Some techniques that may facilitate reminiscing include singing songs from an earlier period, looking at picture albums, old catalogs, movies, and magazines. Discussing current events and reading a recent newspaper helps clients remain oriented. Making holiday decorations is more likely to provide diversional therapy and help clients remain oriented. (9:216; 27:278)

Nursing Process—Implementation
Client Need—Psychosocial integrity

97 2. During senescence it is common for people to review their life experiences. If the analysis results in the belief that their lives have been satisfying and worthwhile, they acquire integrity. If the analysis results in regrets, they close their lives with a feeling of despair. Trust is acquired during infancy. Intimacy is established during young adulthood. The toddler stage in the life cycle is associated with autonomy. (2:105–106)

Nursing Process—Evaluation
Client Need—Health promotion/maintenance

98 4. Words may not mean the same thing to all people. Reporting what was observed is a much more accurate and objective method for documenting behav-ior. None of the other critiques identified the vague and subjective quality of the charting. (25:99)

Nursing Process—Evaluation
Client Need—Safe, effective care environment

99 2. Confusion is relieved by providing a client with environmental cues. Repetitious reminders help the confused person maintain or relearn how to function. A liquid diet is unappetizing and unnecessary as long as the client can chew, swallow, and digest food naturally. Serving this client early will not eliminate her confusion. Seating her alone deprives her of any role models to imitate. It also shows disregard for this client's dignity. (18:1366)

Nursing Process—Implementation
Client Need—Psychosocial integrity

100 1. Labeling rooms with easily identifiable words or pictures promotes environmental awareness. Sensory cues restore the confused client's ability to reorient herself. Locking the unit deprives all of the clients of a certain amount of freedom and privacy. If physical restraint is used unnecessarily, it is considered battery. A confused client is not able to process the information about the consequences of her behavior. (9:214; 18:1367)

Nursing Process—Planning
Client Need—Psychosocial integrity

101 4. Displaying a large calendar with easily read words and numbers in a prominent place is one way to help older clients remain oriented. All of the other options have therapeutic benefits, but they are not useful in orienting clients to present reality. (1:347; 9:213–215)

Nursing Process—Implementation
Client Need—Psychosocial integrity

102 2. Consistent repetition in the unit routine helps clients with cognitive impairments stay oriented to the activities in which they are expected to participate. Wearing a name tag is a helpful technique, but it is even better if the same employee is routinely assigned to care for the same clients. Altering a set routine of activities with field trips tends to disorient clients at least temporarily. Clients with dementia are not likely to be able to read and follow a written schedule. (10:475–476)

Nursing Process—Implementation
Client Need—Psychosocial integrity

103 2. Reflection is a therapeutic communication technique in which the receiver conveys to the sender her expressed thoughts and related feelings. One of the greatest stressors for family members of clients with dementia is that they are physically present but emotionally absent. The first and fourth responses are clichés. They probably will not encourage the client's daughter to talk more about her feelings. The third response combines giving advice and a defensive statement, both of which are nontherapeutic techniques of communication. (18:403; 25:79)

> Nursing Process—Implementation
> Client Need—Psychosocial integrity

104 2. To facilitate attention, concentration, and retention, all verbal communication with a client with dementia is brief and simple. Directions are given in understandable language with a minimum of distracting stimuli in the environment. Speaking loudly does not improve memory. Writing some information down helps a client remember oral instructions, but overall it is not the best recommendation of the choices provided. Listening to a news program helps maintain reality orientation, but it does not promote memory. (21:562)

> Nursing Process—Implementation
> Client Need—Psychosocial integrity

105 3. Drugs are potentially unsafe if they are not administered correctly. Information about drug administration is explained verbally. It also is helpful to accompany verbal instructions with written information. Before the client leaves, the nurse determines that he or she has an accurate understanding of the instructions. The family already is familiar with the other types of information. (18:1345)

> Nursing Process—Implementation
> Client Need—Health promotion/maintenance

106 2. It is best to reinforce that the client is in the appropriate place. Trying to convince the client that he is at home may provoke the client or agitate him even more. Treating his request lightly communicates disrespect. Using the family as a scapegoat avoids responsibility for helping the client understand and cope. (18:1363)

> Nursing Process—Implementation
> Client Need—Psychosocial integrity

107 2. Nurses need to be alert to signs of burnout among family members. If a caring staff member encourages longer periods of separation, it can relieve the potential for feeling guilty. The client's wife may benefit from a physical examination, but that is not the most therapeutic action in the list of choices. Clients in a long-term health care facility have a right to see visitors at any time within reason. Indicating that the staff is capable of caring for the client's husband may imply that she is not appreciated or that her presence is an inconvenience. (18:1366)

> Nursing Process—Implementation
> Client Need—Psychosocial integrity

108 1. Dying clients are not abandoned even though they do not want heroic measures taken to keep them alive. Being in the hall or in a room nearby does not guarantee that the dying client will receive support from the nursing staff. Even if a dying client has access to a signal light, it does not replace the sustained presence of another human being. (25:41, 812)

> Nursing Process—Implementation
> Client Need—Psychosocial integrity

109 3. Expressing feelings to an understanding listener helps facilitate the grieving process. Communication helps people deal openly with their emotions and feelings, which is healthier than suppressing the emotional impact of the event. Being sent home or terminated does not help promote grieving. Asking the nursing assistant to perform postmortem care in this emotional state shows a disregard for the trauma he or she is experiencing. (18:1434)

> Nursing Process—Implementation
> Client Need—Psychosocial integrity

110 3. Having a paranormal experience like sensing a deceased person's presence or even reporting seeing or talking to the deceased can be comforting. As long as there is no potential for being financially, emotionally, or physically disadvantaged, the nurse should not dispute the bereaved's experience. (3:438)

> Nursing Process—Implementation
> Client Need—Psychosocial integrity

Classification of Test Items

Unit **IV** Review Test **16**

The Nursing Care of Adult Clients with Mental Health Needs

Directions: After each question the correct answer is given, as well as a classification of each test question. Compare the correct answer with your answer. If a question has been answered *incorrectly*, draw a line to the end of all the columns. When finished, add up the number of your correct answers in each column and place that number in the respective box at the end in the area identified as *Number Correct.*

To determine the percentage of questions you answered correctly and your performance in each of the test plan categories, divide the *Number Correct* in each column by the *Number Possible* in each column. Then multiply the decimal by 100. For example:

$$\frac{\text{Number Correct: } 90}{\text{Number Possible: } 110} = 0.818 \times 100 = 82\%$$

Any score that is less than 75% indicates an area where further review would be beneficial.

KEY TO ITEM CLASSIFICATION:

NURSING PROCESS

D = Data collection
P = Planning
I = Implementation
E = Evaluation

CLIENT NEEDS

S = Safe, effective care environment
P = Physiological integrity
M = Psychosocial integrity
H = Health promotion/maintenance

Question #	Answer #	Nursing Process				Client Needs			
		D	P	I	E	S	P	M	H
1	4	D						M	
2	1			I					H
3	3			I				M	
4	2	D						M	
5	1	D						M	
6	1	D						M	
7	2	D						M	
8	4			I				M	
9	2			I				M	
10	3			I				M	
11	1	D						M	
12	2			I				M	
13	3	D						M	
14	1			I		S			
15	4			I				M	

Question #	Answer #	Nursing Process				Client Needs			
		D	P	I	E	S	P	M	H
16	2			I				M	
17	2				E	S			
18	3			I		S			
19	3				E			M	
20	1				E			M	
21	2	D						M	
22	4				E			M	
23	2		P					M	
24	4				E			M	
25	2	D						M	
26	1		P					M	
27	3				E		P		
28	3			I				M	
29	2	D						M	
30	1				E				H
31	4	D						M	
32	1			I		S			
33	4			I		S			
34	2	D						M	
35	1		P					M	
36	4	D						M	
37	2			I				M	
38	1				E			M	
39	2			I				M	
40	1		P					M	
41	2	D						M	
42	1	D					P		
43	4	D						M	
44	4		P				P		
45	1			I				M	
46	4			I				M	

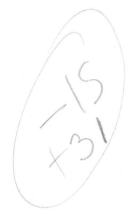

6 1 6 23 12

Question #	Answer #	Nursing Process				Client Needs			
		D	P	I	E	S	P	M	H
47	1		P				P		
48	2				E			M	
49	4			I				M	
50	3			I				M	
51	1			I				M	
52	2			I		S			
53	2			I					H
54	1				E				H
55	3	D						M	
56	1			I				M	
57	1			I					H
58	3			I				M	
59	1			I				M	
60	3			I					H
61	2			I					H
62	4	D				S			
63	1			I					H
64	2			I				M	
65	2				E	S			
66	3			I		S			
67	4			I		S			
68	1		P				P		
69	1		P					M	
70	2	D						M	
71	3			I		S			
72	3			I			P		
73	2	D					P		
74	1			I		S			
75	3	D						M	
76	3				E		P		
77	1	D						M	

Question #	Answer #	Nursing Process				Client Needs			
		D	P	I	E	S	P	M	H
78	2		P			S			
79	1		P					M	
80	3	D				S			
81	1	D				S			
82	2				E				H
83	1				E				H
84	4		P					M	
85	2	D						M	
86	3			I			P		
87	1			I					H
88	2			I			P		
89	3	D					P		
90	2			I				M	
91	1				E		P		
92	2	D						M	
93	4	D					P		
94	4			I				M	
95	4		P					M	
96	2			I				M	
97	2				E				H
98	4				E	S			
99	2			I				M	
100	1		P					M	
101	4			I				M	
102	2			I				M	
103	2			I				M	
104	2			I				M	
105	3			I					H
106	2			I				M	
107	2			I				M	
108	1			I				M	

7 3 14 2 7   18 1

126
84

Question #	Answer #	Nursing Process				Client Needs			
		D	P	I	E	S	P	M	H
109	3			I				M	
110	3			I				M	
Number Correct	*85*	*21*	*10*	*38*	*15*	*9*	*13*	*50*	*12*
Number Possible	110	28	13	52	17	16	13	68	13
Percentage Correct	*77*	*75*	*77*	*73*	*88*	*56*	*100*	*70*	*92*

7   3   14 2   7   18   1

Comprehensive Examination
Parts I and II

Directions: A two-part comprehensive examination that resembles NCLEX-PN as closely as possible is presented next. Each part consists of 120 items.

Follow these instructions for both parts of the comprehensive examination:

Each item consists of 4 possible answers or options. (Items are described more fully on page xix in the *Frequently Asked Questions* section.) Read each item carefully and then select the one correct or best answer for each item.

Indicate your choice for the correct or best answer on the appropriate answer sheets at the end of this book. The answer sheets are perforated and may be removed for convenience.

There is only one correct answer for each item. If you think the correct answer for an item is not among the options, choose the option that you believe is the best possible answer.

Work systematically and proceed steadily. Do not spend too much time on any one item.

Time your progress occasionally so that you know you will finish the entire part in 2 hours.

Correct answers and rationales are provided for both parts of the comprehensive examination so that you can determine how well you scored. If you gave correct answers to about 180 to 190 items or more of the 240 items in the examination (75% to 80%), you probably are prepared for the national licensing examination. If you answered fewer than 180 to 190 items correctly, however, it is suggested that you continue with your reviewing. It is also suggested that you concentrate your review on the subject matter on which you tested poorly in the review tests. The tables that begin on on pages 479 and 507, when completed, will help you identify your areas of strength and weakness.

Proceed to the next page for Part I of the comprehensive examination.

Part I of the
Comprehensive Examination

Time

Directions: Allow yourself 2 hours to complete Part I. Start this part now.

---

1 Which sign is the *best indication* that a client's tracheostomy needs suctioning?
- ○ 1. The client's pulse rate is decreased.
- ○ 2. The client's skin is cool and moist.
- ● 3. The client's respirations are noisy.
- ○ 4. The client is somewhat lethargic.

2 Before suctioning a client with a tracheostomy, which nursing action is *most important* to perform first?
- ○ 1. Insert the suction catheter within the tracheostomy.
- ○ 2. Instill 5 mL of saline within the tracheostomy.
- ● 3. Administer 100% oxygen for 1 to 2 minutes.
- ○ 4. Occlude the vent on the catheter for 15 seconds.

3 When the nurse changes a sterile dressing, which nursing action *violates* principles of asepsis?
- ○ 1. The nurse dons clean gloves to remove the soiled dressing.
- ○ 2. The nurse places the soiled dressing in a moisture-resistant bag.
- ○ 3. The nurse performs handwashing before donning sterile gloves.
- ● 4. The nurse cleans the wound from the outer edge toward the center.

A client with a conduction hearing loss asks the nurse how a hearing aid improves hearing.

4 The nurse is *most accurate* in telling the client that a hearing aid
- ● 1. amplifies what is currently heard.
- ○ 2. makes sounds sharper and clearer.
- ○ 3. produces more distinct, crisp speech.
- ○ 4. eliminates hearing garbled sounds.

The nurse observes a colleague caring for a client who just returned to his room following a bronchoscopy.

5 It is *essential* that the nurse intervene if which of the following actions is observed?
- ○ 1. The nurse giving care takes the client's radial pulse.
- ● 2. The nurse giving care offers the client some water.

- ○ 3. The nurse giving care raises the head of the bed.
- ○ 4. The nurse giving care provides an additional blanket.

A client becomes angry and shouts at the nurse when a meal is not to his liking.

6 The *best nursing response* at this time is to
- ○ 1. say something humorous and promise to call the dietitian.
- ● 2. listen attentively and allow the client to express himself.
- ○ 3. leave the room and allow the client a period of privacy.
- ○ 4. explain that though it is tasteless, it is nutritious.

7 At the time of a retinal detachment, a client is *most likely* to describe which symptom?
- ● 1. Seeing flashes of light
- ○ 2. Being unable to see light
- ○ 3. Feeling discomfort in light
- ○ 4. Seeing poorly in daylight

A nurse observes others administering liquid medication to a 3-month-old infant.

8 Which nurse is using the *best* medication administration technique for a 3-month-old infant?
- ○ 1. Nurse A puts the medication in the infant's bottle and gives it during the next feeding.
- ● 2. Nurse B puts the medication in a needleless syringe and administers it orally.
- ○ 3. Nurse C places the medication in a medicine cup and gives it while pinching the nose closed.
- ○ 4. Nurse D mixes the medication with a small amount of jelly and gives it with a spoon.

9 Which one of the following is the *best indication* that Bryant's traction is applied properly to a small child?
- ○ 1. The child can sit up without experiencing discomfort.
- ○ 2. The child can reach the trapeze hanging above the bed.
- ● 3. The child's buttocks are raised slightly off the mattress.
- ○ 4. The child's legs are pulled toward the bottom of the bed.

10 When the nursing team plans the care of the client in sickle cell crisis, a *chief priority* is to include measures for
○ 1. promoting self-care.
○ 2. preventing immobility.
● 3. relieving discomfort.
○ 4. improving self-esteem.

11 The *best advice* a nurse can give parents for helping a 3-year-old overcome the rivalry created by the birth of a sibling is to
○ 1. enroll the child immediately in a day-long preschool program.
○ 2. arrange extended visits with grandparents for the child.
● 3. find ways that the child can assist with the infant's care.
○ 4. invite other similarly aged children to play with the child.

12 It is *essential* for the nurse to tell a client receiving external radiation therapy that when he or she bathes to
○ 1. avoid getting the irradiated skin wet when bathing.
○ 2. use alcohol instead of soap on the irradiated skin.
○ 3. cover the reddened irradiated area with clear plastic.
● 4. use a soft washcloth to wash the irradiated skin.

The physician writes "Diet as tolerated" in the immediate postoperative orders for a client who has just returned to the nursing unit from surgery.

13 When implementing the physician's order, which diet is *most appropriate* to serve the postoperative client *initially?*
○ 1. Bland diet
○ 2. Soft diet
● 3. Clear liquid diet
○ 4. General house diet

14 If a pregnant client in her third trimester tells the nurse that she has had a severe headache for the past 2 days, the *best plan* of action is to tell the client to
○ 1. increase her rest and leisure activities.
○ 2. eliminate coffee or other sources of caffeine.
○ 3. take 2 aspirin and lie down for an hour.
● 4. be checked today in the physician's office.

The laboratory data of an adult client with Pneumocystis pneumonia indicates that he is immune-suppressed.

15 Which aspect of data collection is *most helpful* in determining why the client is susceptible to an opportu-

nistic infection like Pneumocystis pneumonia?
○ 1. The client's immunization history
○ 2. The client's family history
○ 3. The client's hygiene practices
● 4. The client's sexual practices

16 Which statement made by the parents of a toddler is *most suggestive* that the child has cystic fibrosis?
● 1. "Our child's perspiration is very salty."
○ 2. "Our child vomits immediately after eating."
○ 3. "Our child's stools are soft and bright yellow."
○ 4. "Our child's urine is very light-colored."

17 Which statement is the *best indication* that the client who is taking corticosteroid medication for a prolonged interval understands the danger in their use?
● 1. The client says, "I should never suddenly stop taking my medication."
○ 2. The client says, "My reaction time will be slowed while taking this drug."
○ 3. The client says, "If I forget to take one dose, I should call the physician."
○ 4. The client says, "I should not take this drug for more than 6 months."

18 When monitoring the treatment response of a client with diabetes insipidus, which component of the urinalysis is most important for the nurse to assess?
○ 1. Urinary pH
○ 2. Urinary casts
● 3. Specific gravity
○ 4. Microscopic cells

A home health care nurse visits a client who takes a prescribed diuretic.

19 The *best evidence* for evaluating the drug's effectiveness is obtained by monitoring the client's
● 1. weight.
○ 2. pulse.
○ 3. appetite.
○ 4. reflexes.

20 When applying nitroglycerin ointment, which is the *best technique* for the nurse to use?
● 1. Squeeze a ribbon of ointment on paper.
○ 2. Rub the ointment thoroughly into the skin.
○ 3. Press the mouth of the tube to the chest.
○ 4. Spread the ointment over the heart area.

A nurse is assisting with the development of a teaching plan for the parents of a newborn who is at risk for sudden infant death syndrome (SIDS).

21 The nurse is *correct* to include which of the following instructions regarding rescue breathing for the infant?

○ 1. Cover the nose and mouth; blow as much air as is possible.

○ 2. Cover the nose; blow just enough air to make the chest rise.

● 3. Cover the nose and mouth; blow puffs of air from the cheeks.

○ 4. Cover the mouth and pinch the nose closed; blow puffs of air.

22 When helping to plan the nursing care of a client with an acute respiratory infection, such as pneumonia, the *priority focus* of care involves

○ 1. relieving the cough.

● 2. maintaining oxygenation.

○ 3. providing nourishment.

○ 4. encouraging self-care.

The nurse caring for a client after a subtotal thyroidectomy places the client in a semi-Fowler's position.

23 The *best rationale* for the nurse's action is that it is appropriate for

○ 1. helping the client talk.

● 2. reducing incisional edema.

○ 3. decreasing tissue perfusion.

○ 4. facilitating client comfort.

24 Which question is *most important* to ask *first* when assessing a client who has attempted suicide by taking an overdose of medication?

○ 1. "How many pills were taken?"

○ 2. "Why did you take the pills?"

● 3. "What is the name of the drug?"

○ 4. "Where were the pills obtained?"

A 6-year-old has just had a bilateral myringotomy and placement of polyethylene tubes into the middle ear.

25 The nurse assisting with the development of a discharge teaching plan is *correct* to include which instruction?

● 1. Allow the child to eat only soft and liquid foods.

○ 2. Speak in a louder voice when talking to the child.

○ 3. Insert earplugs whenever the child swims or showers.

○ 4. Irrigate the ears daily while the tubes are in place.

A nurse prepares to withdraw 2 mL of medication from a vial and inject it intramuscularly.

26 Which technique is *most correct* for administering the intramuscular medication?

● 1. The nurse adds 2 mL of air to the vial before withdrawing the drug.

○ 2. The nurse withdraws the medication using a tuberculin syringe.

○ 3. The nurse selects the deltoid muscle for injecting the medication.

○ 4. The nurse inserts a ⅝-inch needle into the muscle at a 45-degree angle.

A nurse prepares to assess the lower extremity of a client who has a freshly applied plaster of paris cast.

27 If the nurse performs all of the following, which assessment is *appropriate* for determining the neurological function of the extremity that is covered with the cast?

○ 1. The nurse asks the client to wiggle his toes.

● 2. The nurse depresses the nailbed and observes the color.

○ 3. The nurse feels the temperature of the toes.

○ 4. The nurse compares the size of the toes bilaterally.

28 During a nursing interview of a teenager with extreme weight loss, which of the following information *best correlates* with the profile of a person with anorexia nervosa?

○ 1. The client is the middle child of three siblings.

● 2. The client is a high achiever in school and activities.

○ 3. The client thinks her classmates do not like her.

○ 4. The client had many illnesses during childhood.

A homeless person has an enlarged, tender liver. A hepatitis B infection is suspected.

29 If the nurse obtains all of the following information in the client's history, which one is the *most likely etiological factor* for the disease?

○ 1. The client eats food that he finds in garbage bins.

○ 2. The client has open skin sores over his lower extremities.

○ 3. The client smokes cigarettes extinguished on the street.

● 4. The client occasionally shares needles to inject heroin.

30 If a nurse collects the following data, which indicates the *greatest risk* for the development of complications for the mother and fetus during pregnancy?

● 1. The client regularly restricts food intake to avoid gaining weight.

○ 2. The client remains sexually active throughout the pregnancy.

○ 3. The client participates regularly in an aerobic exercise program.

○ 4. The client is 25 years old and pregnant for the first time.

A client who weighs 88 lb is to receive 2 mg of a drug per kg of body weight.

31 The nurse is *accurate* in administering
- ○ 1. 0.4 mg of the drug.
- ○ 2. 44 mg of the drug.
- ○ 3. 8 mg of the drug.
- ● 4. 80 mg of the drug.

A nurse massages the uterus of a postpartum client.

32 Which finding is the *best indication* that the intended effect of this nursing action has been achieved?
- ○ 1. Postpartal pain is relieved.
- ● 2. The uterus becomes firm.
- ○ 3. Lactation is suppressed.
- ○ 4. Uterine contractions cease.

33 Which one of the following teaching aids is *developmentally appropriate* when preparing a preschool child for a diagnostic test such as a bone marrow puncture?
- ● 1. Dolls or puppets
- ○ 2. Pamphlets or booklets
- ○ 3. Colored diagrams
- ○ 4. Commercial videotapes

34 When a depressed client says, "No one really cares what happens to me," the *best nursing response* is:
- ○ 1. "You're exaggerating! Lots of people care about you."
- ○ 2. "Talking like that will only make you feel worse."
- ● 3. "Tell me why you think no one cares what happens to you."
- ○ 4. "It sounds like you're feeling ignored or abandoned."

35 Which one of the following physical assessments is best for determining if a client has a fecal impaction?
- ○ 1. Auscultate the bowel sounds.
- ○ 2. Measure the abdominal girth.
- ● 3. Insert a finger within the rectum.
- ○ 4. Inspect the appearance of the anus.

36 When a client who has had a tonsillectomy asks the nurse why his physician told him to avoid taking aspirin or aspirin products, the *best explanation* in this case is that aspirin
- ○ 1. lowers the temperature and therefore can mask a fever.
- ● 2. interferes with clotting and promotes bleeding.
- ○ 3. irritates the stomach and could cause an ulcer.
- ○ 4. reduces inflammation and conceals an infection.

37 The *best evidence* that Kegel exercises are being performed correctly is that the client can
- ○ 1. perform deep knee bends without back discomfort.
- ○ 2. touch the toes without abdominal discomfort.
- ○ 3. sit in a tailor position and fill the lungs deeply.
- ● 4. stop and restart the flow of urine during voiding.

An HIV-positive client is admitted to the hospital in active labor.

38 The nurse is *correct* to assist with which method of fetal assessment for this client?
- ○ 1. Fetal scalp sampling
- ○ 2. Amniocentesis
- ● 3. External fetal monitoring
- ○ 4. Internal fetal monitoring

39 Which behavior can the nurse expect as *typical* when performing a mental status assessment on an adult client with hypothyroidism?
- ○ 1. Quick recall of events
- ○ 2. Rapid response to questions
- ○ 3. Bizarre thought processes
- ● 4. Impaired cognitive function

A nurse assistant is in a toddler's room when the nurse makes rounds.

40 If the nurse observes the assistant do all of the following, which is *most indicative* that the assistant needs additional teaching about the safety of the hospitalized toddler?
- ○ 1. The temperature of the bath water is checked before the child is given a bath.
- ○ 2. The nurse assistant removes all toys that have sharp edges from the child's room.
- ● 3. The side rails are partially raised when the nurse assistant is away from the crib.
- ○ 4. The crib is positioned so that the child cannot reach the electric wall outlets.

41 Which is the *best documentation* for recording that a schizophrenic client claims to be seeing demons in his room?
- ○ 1. Experiencing hallucinations
- ○ 2. Frightened by hallucinations
- ● 3. States seeing "demons in my room"
- ○ 4. Having distorted sensory perceptions

At the time of delivery, a stillborn infant is gestationally small and the cranium is malformed.

42 The *best plan* of action for promoting the parents' grieving process is

1. allowing the parents to see and touch the dead infant before hospital discharge.
2. covering and shielding the dead infant from parental view.
3. describing the positive characteristics of the dead infant.
4. discharging the mother within 24 hours of her delivery.

43 Which action is *most appropriate* for the nurse to take when caring for the school-age child who is experiencing a nosebleed?
1. Tilt the child's head backward and apply an ice pack to the nose.
2. Tilt the child's head forward while gently pinching the nares.
3. Pack the affected nostril with a small amount of clean cotton.
4. Clean the affected nostril and instill saline nose drops.

44 The *best nursing technique* for removing an object that completely obstructs the airway of an unconscious adult is to administer
1. up to 5 abdominal thrusts.
2. 2 quick ventilations of air.
3. 5 chest thrusts and a breath.
4. 15 chest compressions.

45 Which of the following is the *best evidence* that a client with a colostomy is adjusting to his or her change in body image?
1. The client wears loose-fitting garments.
2. The client takes a shower each day.
3. The client empties his or her own appliance.
4. The client avoids foods that form gas.

46 Following an upper gastrointestinal x-ray, sometimes referred to as a barium swallow, which nursing assessment is *essential* to monitor?
1. The ability to eat
2. The passage of stool
3. The color of urine
4. The feeling of hunger

Data is collected from a 17-year-old postpartum client who is being discharged from the hospital.

47 Which assessment finding is *most indicative* of the greatest need for referral for community-based assistance upon discharge.
1. The client is a primipara.
2. The client lives on her own.
3. The client had a previous spontaneous abortion.
4. The client continues to see the newborn's father.

A hospitalized client has a sealed source of radiation inserted into her vagina to treat cancer.

48 What information is *most important* to obtain for ensuring the safety of each nurse that is assigned to care for the client?
1. Is the nurse sensitive to radiation?
2. Could the nurse possibly be pregnant?
3. What medications does the nurse take routinely?
4. Does the nurse have a family history of cancer?

A team conference is held to discuss interventions to use for resolving the inadequate dietary intake of a client with bipolar disorder.

49 If all of the following nursing interventions are suggested, which one is *most likely* to facilitate the desired outcome?
1. Providing high-calorie finger foods every waking hour
2. Serving extra large portions on the dietary tray
3. Giving the client additional time to eat each meal
4. Having relatives bring food from home for each meal

50 The *best assessment technique* the nurse can use for detecting thrombophlebitis in a lower extremity is to
1. have the client dorsiflex his feet.
2. palpate the dorsalis pedis pulses.
3. observe his gait while walking.
4. monitor the client's temperature.

Prior to discharge, a client with a colostomy says, "There is so much to remember about my care. I don't know whom to contact if I have questions or problems."

51 The *best resource person* to refer the colostomy client for assistance with managing future self-care problems is a(n)
1. enterostomal therapist.
2. gastroenterologist.
3. gastronome.
4. entomologist.

When a client who will undergo a subtotal thyroidectomy for Graves disease is admitted preoperatively, the nurse omits palpating the thyroid gland.

52 The *best analysis* of the nurse's action is that it is
1. inappropriate because it eliminates essential information.
2. inappropriate because the data is needed for comparison.
3. appropriate because palpation can cause extreme discomfort.
4. appropriate because palpation can release thyroid hormones.

53 Which statement made by an alcoholic client who takes disulfiram (Antabuse) is *most indicative* of a need for more health teaching?
- ○ 1. "If I miss one dose of the drug, I'll experience nausea, vomiting, and fainting."
- ● 2. "I can get very sick if I consume alcohol in any form while taking this drug."
- ○ 3. "I can have a reaction even 2 weeks after I stop taking this drug."
- ○ 4. "I shouldn't apply aftershave lotion or cologne to my skin while taking this drug."

54 When discontinuing the administration of intravenous fluid, which nursing action is *essential*?
- ○ 1. Pulling the privacy curtain
- ● 2. Donning latex gloves
- ○ 3. Taking vital signs
- ○ 4. Weighing the client

A few days before a client has a malignant growth removed from his colon, he says to the nurse, "I am scared. This operation worries me."

55 The *best nursing response* is
- ○ 1. "There is no need for fear and worry, trust me."
- ● 2. "Tell me more specifically about your concerns."
- ○ 3. "You know as well as I that you have an excellent surgeon."
- ○ 4. "Try to relax. Worrying will only make matters worse."

56 It is *essential* that the nurse have topical anesthesia available when the physician wishes to
- ○ 1. test deep tendon reflexes.
- ○ 2. remove vaginal secretions.
- ○ 3. measure intraocular pressure.
- ● 4. examine the tympanic membranes.

57 When a 10-year-old falls from a bicycle and loses a permanent incisor tooth, the *best action* the nurse can recommend while en route to the dentist is to
- ○ 1. submerge the tooth in water.
- ○ 2. hold the tooth under the tongue.
- ● 3. wrap the tooth in a clean cloth.
- ○ 4. clean the tooth with alcohol.

The nurse monitors a client with a nasogastric (NG) tube who has just returned from the postanesthesia recovery room following gastric surgery.

58 After collecting all of the following data, which finding is *essential* to report to the physician or charge nurse?
- ○ 1. The client says his throat hurts.
- ○ 2. The client indicates he is thirsty.
- ○ 3. There is dried mucus on the NG tube.
- ● 4. There is bright red bloody drainage.

59 When the nurse cares for a middle-aged adult, which client behavior is *most suggestive* of the developmental task of generativity?
- ○ 1. The client expresses fear of having further serious illnesses.
- ○ 2. The client wishes to know the purpose of his medications.
- ● 3. The client wants to resume writing a book about his boyhood.
- ○ 4. The client desires to learn more about using a computer.

60 To plan care with respect to cultural values, the *best method* for determining if a male client of the Jewish faith follows the strict Orthodox customs of his religion is to
- ○ 1. ask if he speaks the Hebrew language.
- ● 2. inquire as to his dietary preferences.
- ○ 3. question if he wears a skullcap.
- ○ 4. see if the client has been circumcised.

61 Which nursing action is *best* when a chest tube is pulled from its insertion site?
- ● 1. Cover the opening to keep out air.
- ○ 2. Reinsert the displaced chest tube.
- ○ 3. Apply suction with a thin catheter.
- ○ 4. Tell the client to hold his breath.

62 If all of the following nursing orders appear on the plan of care for a client with a nasogastric tube used for decompression, which one is *potentially unsafe*?
- ● 1. Encourage liberal fluid intake every hour.
- ○ 2. Irrigate nasogastric tube if drainage stops.
- ○ 3. Offer throat lozenges every 4 hours as needed for discomfort.
- ○ 4. Give oral hygiene every 4 hours during the day and as needed.

63 When giving an enema to an adult client, the *most correct nursing technique* is to insert the enema tip a distance of approximately
- ○ 1. 1 to 2 in (2.5 to 5 cm).
- ● 2. 3 to 4 in (7.5 to 10 cm).
- ○ 3. 6 to 8 in (15 to 20 cm).
- ○ 4. 9 to 10 in (22.5 to 25 cm).

64 When the nursing care plan calls for giving perineal care to an uncircumcised male client, which technique is *correct*?
- ○ 1. The anal area is washed at a separate time.
- ● 2. The foreskin is retracted and the area beneath the foreskin cleansed.
- ○ 3. The foreskin is not retracted except by a physician.
- ○ 4. The scrotum is carefully washed with sterile normal saline.

65 Which of the following information is *most important* for developing a teaching plan to help an adult client reduce the recurrence of low back pain?
- ○ 1. The client's age
- ◉ 2. The client's job
- ○ 3. The client's gait
- ○ 4. The client's energy

66 The *best plan* a nurse can recommend to a young adult male seeking assistance in helping his girlfriend deal with being raped is to
- ○ 1. always act happy and enthusiastic around her.
- ○ 2. prevent her from isolating herself from people.
- ◉ 3. encourage her to talk about her traumatic experience.
- ○ 4. take frequent vacations or do pleasurable activities.

67 A client demonstrates *correct information* about performing breast self-examination (BSE) when stating that
- ○ 1. the entire examination is performed while lying on the back with the arm down at the side.
- ◉ 2. the examination includes standing in front of a mirror to detect any breast changes.
- ○ 3. she should lie on her abdomen to detect any breast pain or tenderness.
- ○ 4. the breasts are examined while lying prone as well as sitting upright.

68 The *best indication* that a client with nephrotic syndrome (acute glomerulonephritis) is experiencing a therapeutic effect from corticosteroid therapy is an increase in the client's
- ○ 1. body weight.
- ○ 2. muscle mass.
- ◉ 3. urinary output.
- ○ 4. blood pressure.

69 When assessing the frequency of a pregnant client's contractions, the nurse is *correct* to count the time interval between the
- ○ 1. beginning of one contraction to the end of the same contraction.
- ○ 2. end of one contraction and the beginning of the next contraction.
- ○ 3. beginning of one contraction and the end of the next contraction.
- ◉ 4. beginning of one contraction and the beginning of the next contraction.

A client is startled and continues to worry about an alarm that sounded from his electronic intravenous infusion pump.

70 The *best plan* the nurse can implement for relieving the patient's anxiety at this time is to
- ○ 1. infuse the solution by gravity.
- ◉ 2. explain why the alarm sounded.
- ○ 3. give a prescribed tranquilizer.
- ○ 4. provide a magazine for reading.

An adolescent brings her 3-month-old infant in for a well baby checkup. She tells the nurse that she is frustrated because she gets little sleep since the baby was born.

71 Which nursing response is *most appropriate?*
- ◉ 1. Explain that this is a normal feeling and suggest that the client ask a family member or friend for occasional relief.
- ○ 2. Explain that parenting is a big responsibility and suggest that the client place the child up for adoption.
- ○ 3. Explain that this feeling usually precedes abusive behavior and inform her that you must report your concern.
- ○ 4. Explain that this feeling is temporary and encourage the client to be patient until the frustration disappears.

One hour after delivery, the nurse notes that a postpartum mother has pronounced vaginal bleeding.

72 Which action should the nurse take first?
- ○ 1. Call the physician.
- ◉ 2. Massage the uterus.
- ○ 3. Count the pulse.
- ○ 4. Elevate the legs.

A surgical client asks the nurse why leg exercises are important to perform.

73 The *best explanation* is that leg movement which involves contracting and relaxing leg muscles helps to prevent
- ○ 1. loss of muscle strength.
- ◉ 2. formation of blood clots.
- ○ 3. swelling of the extremities.
- ○ 4. developing varicose veins.

A child with asthma is receiving aminophylline (Amoline) by intravenous infusion.

74 Which is the nurse *most likely* to observe as an adverse drug effect?
- ○ 1. Bradycardia
- ○ 2. Drowsiness
- ◉ 3. Restlessness
- ○ 4. Hypotension

75 If the nurse observes all of the following, which one is *most suggestive* that an older adult client in a nursing home is depressed?
- ○ 1. The client demands more and more attention.
- ○ 2. The client makes sarcastic remarks about staff.
- ● 3. The client sleeps a great deal of the time.
- ○ 4. The client wants to see her family more often.

76 Which prescribed antibiotic should the nurse question before administering it to a child less than 8 years of age?
- ○ 1. cefazolin (Kefzol)
- ○ 2. amoxicillin (Amoxil)
- ○ 3. oxytetracycline (Terramycin)
- ● 4. gentamicin (Garamycin)

77 Which nursing response is *best* when an older adult female with Alzheimer's disease says she must leave the extended care facility to be home when her children return from school?
- ○ 1. "Nonsense! Your children are adults with their own children."
- ○ 2. "I'm sure a neighbor will take care of them for awhile."
- ○ 3. "I'll call the school and tell them to expect you later."
- ● 4. "You're in a nursing home. I'm your nurse."

78 Which of the following is *avoided* when offering liquids to a child with laryngotracheobronchitis (croup)?
- ○ 1. Ginger ale
- ○ 2. Apple juice
- ● 3. Whole milk
- ○ 4. Cold water

79 When performing cardiopulmonary resuscitation on an unresponsive infant, the nurse is *correct* to assess the pulse at which location?
- ○ 1. Over the radial artery
- ○ 2. Over the femoral artery
- ● 3. Over the brachial artery
- ○ 4. Over the carotid artery

A nurse finds a client who appears to have fallen out of the hospital bed.

80 Which nursing action is *best* to perform first?
- ○ 1. Report the accident to the proper person.
- ○ 2. Help the person back to bed or a chair.
- ○ 3. Make sure the side rails are raised.
- ● 4. Check the client's physical condition.

81 If the nurse observes all of the following behaviors, which one *best* indicates healthy parent-newborn attachment?
- ○ 1. The parents observe the care of their newborn.
- ○ 2. The parents are satisfied with the baby's gender.
- ○ 3. The parents watch and listen to their newborn.
- ● 4. The parents touch and talk to their newborn.

The nursing team meets for a conference to plan the care of a client with anorexia nervosa.

82 Which of the following has the *highest priority* at the time of the client's admission?
- ○ 1. Changing the client's distorted body image
- ○ 2. Improving the client's coping techniques
- ● 3. Correcting nutritional imbalances
- ○ 4. Developing the family's support

83 If a postoperative client is on a clear liquid diet, which food item is *most appropriate* to provide?
- ○ 1. A glass of milk
- ○ 2. A bowl of ice cream
- ● 3. A dish of gelatin
- ○ 4. A cup of creamed soup

The nursing team reviews the effectiveness of interventions being used to promote a confused client's orientation.

84 Which of the client's actions is the *best evidence* of progress in accomplishing the goal?
- ○ 1. The client walks with others to the dining room.
- ○ 2. The client dresses himself without difficulty.
- ● 3. The client locates his room without assistance.
- ○ 4. The client talks on the telephone to his family.

The nurse observes that a school-age child who has rheumatic fever develops shortness of breath when ambulating to the bathroom. The physician's orders state that the client may have bathroom privileges.

85 Which change in the plan of care is *most appropriate* in response to the assessment finding?
- ○ 1. Have the child use a bedside commode for elimination.
- ○ 2. Administer oxygen after the child uses the bathroom.
- ● 3. Instruct the child to call for assistance when ambulating to the bathroom.
- ○ 4. Provide a walker for the child to use when ambulating to the bathroom.

A nurse teaches an asthmatic client how to use a metered-dose aerosol inhaler.

86 The nurse is *most correct* in instructing the client that after inhaling slowly and deeply when the cartridge is depressed, the *next step* is to
- ○ 1. immediately exhale the aerosol.
- ● 2. briefly hold the inhaled breath.
- ○ 3. quickly swallow the bubble of air.
- ○ 4. subsequently cough, then breathe.

87 Which assessment finding is *most indicative* of a 2-year-old having otitis media?
- ○ 1. The child wants to be held.
- ○ 2. The child is cutting teeth.
- ○ 3. The child swallows frequently.
- ● 4. The child tugs at the ear.

88 If all of the following medications are ordered for a client with Ménière's disease, which one is *most appropriate* to administer during an acute attack?
- ○ 1. acetaminophen (Tylenol)
- ● 2. meclizine (Antivert)
- ○ 3. meperidine (Demerol)
- ○ 4. triazolam (Halcion)

89 Following thyroidectomy surgery, it is *most appropriate* for the nurse to monitor the client for signs of
- ○ 1. hypokalemia.
- ○ 2. hyponatremia.
- ○ 3. hypomagnesemia.
- ● 4. hypocalcemia.

90 Assuming that all of the following nursing measures are possible, which one is *best* for helping a postoperative male client void?
- ○ 1. Encourage the client to use a bedpan rather than a urinal.
- ○ 2. Teach the client perineal exercises to improve sphincter tone.
- ● 3. Help the client stand to void into a urinal.
- ○ 4. Increase the client's fluid intake until he voids.

91 When the nurse observes that a client with jaundice is scratching his skin in response to severe itching, which plan is *best* for preventing skin impairment?
- ○ 1. Bathing the client with very warm water
- ○ 2. Dusting the client's body with cornstarch
- ● 3. Trimming the client's fingernails
- ○ 4. Using hypoallergenic bed linen

92 Since a client with hyperparathyroidism is prone to hypercalcemia, the *most appropriate* plan for the client's care is to
- ○ 1. monitor the client's respirations.
- ● 2. provide a high fluid intake.
- ○ 3. offer supplemental nourishment.
- ○ 4. administer frequent skin care.

93 Which physical assessment finding is *most suggestive* that a client has an abdominal aortic aneurysm?
- ● 1. A pulsating mass is felt when palpating the client's abdomen.
- ○ 2. An extra heart sound is heart during chest auscultation.
- ○ 3. Uneven chest movements are noted when observing respirations.
- ○ 4. A hollow sound is heard when percussing the abdomen.

94 If a known substance abuser is experiencing a "racing heart," the *most appropriate* question to ask is
- ○ 1. "When was the last time you used heroin?"
- ● 2. "When was the last time you used cocaine?"
- ○ 3. "When was the last time you used barbiturates?"
- ○ 4. "When was the last time you used marijuana?"

95 Which assessment finding is the *best evidence* that a client remained adequately oxygenated while being suctioned?
- ● 1. The heart rate stays within 88 to 92 beats per minute.
- ○ 2. A moderate amount of tracheal secretions are removed.
- ○ 3. The client remains alert during suctioning.
- ○ 4. The client's skin remains warm and dry.

A friend shares the news that she is engaged to be married. The nurse knows that the friend's fiancé has tested positive for the human immunodeficiency virus (HIV).

96 Which of the following is the nurse *legally obligated* to do?
- ○ 1. Inform the friend of the fiancé's HIV infectious status.
- ○ 2. Recommend that the friend be tested for HIV antibodies.
- ○ 3. Advise the friend to postpone the marriage indefinitely.
- ● 4. Safeguard information in the fiancé's health history.

During the first stage of labor, the nurse finds that the fetal heart rate decreases during a contraction and returns to normal at the end of the contraction.

97 Which action is *most appropriate* for the nurse to take in response to the assessment finding?
- ○ 1. No action is indicated at this time.
- ● 2. Notify the physician immediately.
- ○ 3. Turn the client onto her back in bed.
- ○ 4. Elevate the head of the client's bed.

98 Which one of the following comments made by a client who is taking aspirin is *most likely* due to the effects of the drug therapy?
   ○ 1. "My thoughts are racing."
   ○ 2. "I'm urinating a lot."
   ○ 3. "I've developed diarrhea."
   ◉ 4. "I hear buzzing in my ears."

A client is given a prescription for the benzodiazepine drug alprazolam (Xanax).

99 Which of the following is the *best indication* that the client has understood the nurse's health teaching about taking Xanax?
   ◉ 1. The client says he should not drink alcohol while taking this drug.
   ○ 2. The client says he will need to continue taking this drug for life.
   ○ 3. The client says this drug can cause insomnia in some people.
   ○ 4. The client says a blood test will be required periodically.

100 Which action by parents of a 16-month-old toddler indicates that they understand how to *best minimize* separation anxiety during their child's hospitalization?
   ○ 1. The parents bring the child's favorite toy to the hospital.
   ○ 2. The parents explain all procedures to the child.
   ◉ 3. The parents remain with the child during the hospital stay.
   ○ 4. The parents bring the siblings to visit the child.

101 Which plan of care is *best* for drying a plaster cast?
   ○ 1. Increase the temperature of the room.
   ◉ 2. Turn the client every 1 to 2 hours.
   ○ 3. Fan the wet cast with folded newspaper.
   ○ 4. Take the client outside in the sun.

102 Which of the following statements made by a 38 week gestation primigravida client is *most indicative* that "lightening" has occurred?
   ○ 1. "I'm not as hungry as I used to be."
   ○ 2. "My backaches seem to be relieved."
   ◉ 3. "I can breathe so much easier now."
   ○ 4. "I've noticed slight contractions lately."

103 Which one of the following is the *best evidence* that rescue breathing is being performed appropriately?
   ◉ 1. The chest rises when air is forced in.
   ○ 2. The pupils of both eyes are dilated.
   ○ 3. A carotid pulse is palpated at the neck.
   ○ 4. The rescuer forms a seal over the nose.

After having a rectal tube in place for 20 minutes, a client's abdominal distention remains unrelieved.

104 The *best plan* of action for the nurse to take at this time is to
   ○ 1. rotate the tube several times within the rectum.
   ○ 2. insert the rectal tube farther into the rectum.
   ○ 3. remove the tube and reinsert it in 2 to 3 hours.
   ◉ 4. replace the tube with one of larger diameter.

The nurse observes resuscitation efforts on a six-month-old infant.

105 Cardiac compressions are being administered *correctly* if the rescuer uses
   ○ 1. both hands.
   ◉ 2. two fingers.
   ○ 3. the heel of one hand.
   ○ 4. the palm of one hand.

106 Which one of the following is *most important* to assess to determine if a client taking methylphenidate hydrochloride (Ritalin) is experiencing undesirable side effects?
   ○ 1. Elimination patterns
   ○ 2. Food intolerances
   ◉ 3. Blood pressure
   ○ 4. Skin integrity

107 Which assessment finding is *most likely* to be observed while caring for the newborn of a mother who has heavily consumed alcohol throughout her pregnancy?
   ○ 1. Lethargy
   ◉ 2. Irritability
   ○ 3. Flaccidity
   ○ 4. Apathy

108 At least 30 minutes after administering a minor tranquilizer, which one of the following provides the *best evaluation* of the client's response?
   ◉ 1. Measuring the client's heart rate and arterial blood pressure
   ○ 2. Asking the client to rate the anxiety on a scale of 0 to 10
   ○ 3. Observing the length of time a client sleeps
   ○ 4. Monitoring the client's interactions with others

During the first stump dressing change of a client with a below-the-knee amputation, the client says, "I just can't look at it!"

109 Of the following comments, which one is the *best response* for the nurse to make at this time?
   ◉ 1. "Look away until you feel ready."
   ○ 2. "Maybe you should get counseling."
   ○ 3. "I'd be curious to see how it looks."
   ○ 4. "Come on! It doesn't look that bad."

110 The *best time* for the nurse to plan postural drainage is when the client
1. has an empty stomach.
2. feels short of breath.
3. experiences coughing.
4. says it is necessary.

111 Which is the *earliest indication* that a person is hypoxic?
1. The client is cyanotic.
2. The client is disoriented.
3. The client is restless.
4. The client is hypotensive.

112 Following a perineal prostatectomy for cancer of the prostate, which one of the following nursing actions is *essential* to include on the written plan for care?
1. Perform the Valsalva maneuver during defecation.
2. Maintain in high Fowler's position postoperatively.
3. Administer laxatives to promote bowel elimination.
4. Provide perineal care following each bowel movement.

113 If an older adult describes all of the following home conditions, which one presents the *greatest safety hazard*?
1. The television set is in the bedroom.
2. The client takes showers rather than tub baths.
3. There are throw rugs throughout the house.
4. There are grounded electrical outlets in the kitchen.

114 When informed that a client who tests positive for the human immunodeficieny virus (HIV) is being admitted to a hospital, the nurse is *most correct* in planning to follow guidelines for
1. strict isolation.
2. standard precautions.
3. droplet precautions.
4. contact isolation.

115 When obtaining a health history, which information is the *most likely* contributing factor for the client acquiring an inguinal hernia?
1. The client experiences abdominal cramping when he drinks milk.
2. The client does not get much physical exercise except at work.
3. The client lifts heavy mail bags in his job as a postal worker.
4. The client has been underweight most of his adult life.

The physician orders an immune assay enzyme test to confirm a diagnosis of acute bronchiolitis secondary to the respiratory syncytial virus (RSV).

116 Which type of specimen is it *most correct* for the nurse to collect?
1. Throat swab
2. Nasal secretions
3. Sputum specimen
4. Blood specimen

117 If an older adult client has dry, flaky skin, which of the following instructions on the care plan is *most appropriate* for managing the problem?
1. Offer high-calorie snacks.
2. Bathe the client every 2 days.
3. Use only cotton bed linen.
4. Keep fingernails trimmed short.

The nurse finds a diabetic perspiring, feeling weak, and trembling.

118 After administering orange juice, which of the following is the *best indication* that the nurse has managed the client's symptoms successfully?
1. The client says he is hungry.
2. The client's skin is cool.
3. The blood sugar is normal.
4. The blood pressure is stable.

119 If a young adult female client develops a thrombophlebitis, it is *most appropriate* for the nurse to ask the client if she routinely takes
1. iron supplements.
2. oral contraceptives.
3. nasal decongestants.
4. stomach antacids.

120 Following the physician's explanation of the risks and benefits of a transurethral resection of the prostate (TURP), the *best evidence* that the client understands the effect this surgery will have on his sexual function is the statement
1. "I won't ejaculate normally any more."
2. "I won't have an orgasm any more."
3. "I won't have an erection any more."
4. "I won't desire to have sex any more."

Correct Answers and Rationale

Part I of the Comprehensive Examination

Directions: Two numbers appear in parentheses following each rationale. The first number identifies the textbook listed in the references, page 512, and the second number identifies the page(s) in that textbook on which the correct answer can be verified. Occasionally two or more textbooks are given to verify the correct answer.

1 3. Typical signs indicating that a tracheostomy needs suctioning include noisy respirations, dyspnea, increased respiratory and pulse rates. Auscultation of the chest helps most to determine when suctioning of a tracheostomy should be done. (4:892; 25:779)
  Nursing Process—Data collection
  Client Need—Physiological integrity

2 3. Giving oxygen before suctioning prevents hypoxemia and hypoxia while removing air and debris from the upper airway. Before the catheter is inserted, saline may be instilled to liquefy thick secretions. The catheter is then inserted. Once the tip is at the desired level, usually 6 to 10 in, the vent is occluded and the catheter is twisted as it is removed. The client is then reoxygenated a second time. (25:780)
  Nursing Process—Planning
  Client Need—Physiological integrity

3 4. The most appropriate aseptic technique for cleansing wounds is to clean them in such a way that debris and microorganisms are carried away from the impaired skin. It is appropriate to use a clean glove to remove a soiled dressing, to place the soiled dressing in a container that acts as a barrier against transmitting microorganisms that may be present, and to perform handwashing after removing clean gloves. (25:574)
  Nursing Process—Evaluation
  Client Need—Safe, effective care environment

4 1. A hearing aid amplifies sound waves that are transmitted by air and bone conduction. If a person hears garbled, distorted sound, a hearing aid increases the volume, but it does not improve the quality of the sound. (18:1094–1095; 25:325)
  Nursing Process—Implementation
  Client Need—Health promotion/maintenance

5 2. Food and fluids are withheld temporarily following a bronchoscopy until the gag reflex returns. If the gag reflex is absent, aspiration may occur. Taking the radial pulse and raising the head of the bed are safe actions. Providing a blanket is an appropriate comfort measure. (21:272)
  Nursing Process—Evaluation
  Client Need—Safe, effective care environment

6 2. It is therapeutic to allow an angry person to express his or her feelings within social limits. By remaining neutral, the nurse demonstrates acceptance of the client as an individual. The nurse acts as a role model for assisting clients in regaining control. Using humor, leaving an angry client, or providing an explanation may add to the angry feelings because the client interprets these actions to mean that the circumstances of the anger are unimportant. (10:114)
  Nursing Process—Implementation
  Client Need—Psychosocial integrity

7 1. Most individuals with a retinal detachment describe seeing flashes of light. Only the most profoundly blind cannot see light. Photophobia is associated with many primary and secondary disorders, but it is not generally experienced by someone with a retinal detachment. The client with a retinal detachment generally retains vision in a large portion of the retina. The visual defect is evident only in the area of the tear or separation of the sensory layer from the pigmented layer. Therefore, in the intact retina, vision during daylight is unchanged. (18:1092; 21:630)
  Nursing Process—Data collection
  Client Need—Physiological integrity

8 2. Giving an infant medication using a syringe without a needle helps to reduce the incidence of choking, coughing, and vomiting. Medications are not routinely given in an infant's bottle because the infant may not finish the bottle and thus may not get the prescribed amount of medication. Pinching a child's nose is not recommended because this action increases the chance of aspiration. Solid forms of medication are crushed and mixed with jelly, pudding, or applesauce, but liquid medications are not. (14:428)
  Nursing Process—Evaluation
  Client Need—Safe, effective care environment

466

9 3. When a child is in Bryant's traction, the buttocks just clear the mattress. The ropes that lead to pulleys above the bed keep the child's legs at a 90-degree angle to his trunk. The child should not sit up or use a trapeze. The legs are pulled toward the ceiling. (11:380; 22:685)

  Nursing Process—Evaluation
  Client Need—Safe, effective care environment

10 3. During a sickle cell crisis, the plan of care addresses interventions for relieving discomfort. During a crisis, clients commonly experience severe pain in the chest, joints, and abdomen. Analgesics often are administered routinely. The type of analgesic, the dosage, or its administration schedule may need frequent adjustment, depending upon the response of the client. Activity, including a client's self-care, usually is limited during sickle cell crisis to prevent hypoxia. Although helping a chronically ill client improve his self-esteem is an appropriate nursing goal, it is not a priority during the acute phase of the individual's illness. (4:800; 21:450–451)

  Nursing Process—Planning
  Client Need—Physiological integrity

11 3. Finding age-related tasks that involve nurturing and responsibility tend to promote a feeling that a child's contributions are valued and appreciated. Sending the child to a preschool program or for long visits away from home further reinforces the feeling of abandonment. Although playing with same-age children promotes socialization skills, it does not relieve sibling rivalry. (9:46)

  Nursing Process—Planning
  Client Need—Health promotion/maintenance

12 4. To avoid additional injury to radiated skin, the client is instructed to use gentle washing with warm water and a soft cloth. Water will not harm the skin, but harsh soaps, lotions, alcohol-based cosmetics, and rubbing the skin is avoided. Covering the reddened area with clear plastic will not serve any therapeutic purpose. (4:1197)

  Nursing Process—Implementation
  Client Need—Health promotion/maintenance

13 3. A clear liquid diet generally is offered initially after surgery. A clear liquid diet provides fluid and some energy-supplying calories. It also is least likely to contribute to nausea or vomiting. If tolerated well, the diet can progress to a full liquid, soft, or general diet. (6:53)

  Nursing Process—Implementation
  Client Need—Physiological integrity

14 4. Any pregnant client in the third trimester with a persistent, severe headache needs to be promptly examined by a physician. A persistent headache may be insignificant, but it also is an accompanying sign of pregnancy-induced hypertension, formerly known as toxemia or eclampsia. Any of the other suggestions are appropriate after the client has been medically assessed. (14:133; 16:260)

  Nursing Process—Planning
  Client Need—Physiological integrity

15 4. Acquired immunodeficiency syndrome (AIDS) is suspected when individuals succumb to opportunistic infections. Since homosexual and heterosexual transmission is the most common mode for acquiring the human immunodeficiency virus (HIV), it is important to assess a client's sexual practices. If the client does not indicate any high-risk sexual practices, the nurse may assess the possibility of intravenous drug use and a history of having received blood or blood products. A client's immunization history, family history, and hygiene practices are not likely to provide etiological information about opportunistic infections. (4:1165, 1175)

  Nursing Process—Data collection
  Client Need—Health promotion/maintenance

16 1. Parents of children with cystic fibrosis often report that the child's perspiration tastes very salty. This is attributed to the fact that children with cystic fibrosis lose large amounts of salt in their perspiration. Vomiting immediately after eating is not a usual sign of cystic fibrosis, but it is associated with pyloric stenosis. Soft, bright yellow stools are characteristic of a breast-fed infant. In cystic fibrosis, the stools are large, foamy, and foul-smelling. Very light colored urine usually indicates that the urine is dilute. This characteristic is related to the hydration status and function of the kidneys, and is unrelated to cystic fibrosis. (14:487; 16:721)

  Nursing Process—Data collection
  Client Need—Physiological integrity

17 1. For the person who takes corticosteroids for a prolonged time, abruptly discontinuing the medication can cause life-threatening consequences. Acute adrenal insufficiency can occur. This condition is also called Addisonian crisis or adrenal crisis. Death may occur due to fluid volume depletion, hypotension, and shock. Taking steroid medication does not interfere with a person's reaction time. If a dose is missed, it is not necessary to consult the physician. Although long-term corticosteroid therapy causes

many side effects, individuals can take the medication for long periods of time. (17:239–240)
>Nursing Process—Evaluation
>Client Need—Health promotion/maintenance

18 3. The specific gravity is an indication of the ratio of water to dissolved substances. In diabetes insipidus, the specific gravity is 1.002, little more than water. As the client improves, the specific gravity increases as less water is excreted in the urine. (21:776)
>Nursing Process—Data collection
>Client Need—Physiological integrity

19 1. Daily to weekly weights are a way of monitoring the effectiveness and or compliance of a client who takes a diuretic at home. Other valuable assessments include measuring the client's blood pressure, listening to lung sounds, and inspecting the skin for signs of edema. Pulse rate, appetite, and reflexes are not affected by diuretics. (20:312)
>Nursing Process—Evaluation
>Client Need—Physiological integrity

20 1. To apply topical nitroglycerin ointment, the nurse squeezes a ribbon of the drug onto calibrated application paper. The paper is placed on the chest, back, or arms; not necessarily over the heart area. Applying the ointment over the heart may interfere with the assessment of heart sounds, obtaining an apical pulse rate, or create hazards if the client requires defibrillation. The paper is covered with plastic wrap and taped to hold it in place. The nurse must avoid coming into direct skin contact with the ointment while measuring or applying it. Contact results in the nurse absorbing the medication. The drug is not rubbed into the skin. (25:715)
>Nursing Process—Implementation
>Client Need—Physiological integrity

21 3. An infant is given controlled, gentle breaths of air from a rescuer. The breaths are sometimes described as "puffs" of air. The volume is just large enough to make the chest rise. The rate of rescue breaths for an infant is approximately 20 per minute. (16:580; 18:369)
>Nursing Process—Planning
>Client Need—Health promotion/maintenance

22 2. Maintaining and improving oxygenation is a priority goal when planning the nursing care of a client with an acute respiratory infection. In some circumstances, such as when there are moist secretions in the airways, it is important to promote coughing instead of relieving it. Nourishment is important in the care of any person with an infection. However, impaired breathing is more life-threatening than a brief reduction in caloric intake. Eventually assuming self-care is desirable, but during the acute phase of illness, providing rest and assistance from the nurse is prudent for reducing oxygen requirements. (21:299)
>Nursing Process—Planning
>Client Need—Physiological integrity

23 2. Head elevation tends to relieve edema and the potential for airway obstruction. Controlling edema has secondary benefits of helping the client talk and experience comfort. It is inappropriate to interfere with tissue perfusion. (26:488)
>Nursing Process—Evaluation
>Client Need—Physiological integrity

24 3. The name of the drug is essential in determining the potential effects and what treatment is needed. Secondly, determining the approximate number of pills helps assess the potential lethality of the overdose. It also is important to determine how long ago they were taken. While the client's life is threatened, discussing the reason for the overdose is not a priority. The source of the pills does not affect the client's treatment. (21:255)
>Nursing Process—Data collection
>Client Need—Physiological integrity

25 3. Custom-made ear plugs are used as a barrier against water entering through the tubes used to equalize pressure within the middle ear. Suppurative (producing pus) otitis media is a potential consequence of introducing water from these activities. There are no dietary restrictions while tympanostomy tubes are in place. The child's hearing improves as pressure within the middle ear is relieved. Instilling water is contraindicated for the same reasons that water from swimming and showering are prohibited from entering the ears. (14:625)
>Nursing Process—Planning
>Client Need—Health promotion/maintenance

26 1. Adding a volume of air equal to the amount of drug that will be withdrawn from a vial increases the pressure within the vial and facilitates filling the syringe. A tuberculin syringe holds a maximum volume of 1 mL and thus does not accommodate a 2 mL volume of medication. The deltoid muscle is not used when the volume of the medication exceeds 1 mL. It is appropriate to select a 1½- to 2-inch needle length to reach the depth where muscle is located. The needle is inserted at a 90-degree angle when administering an intramuscular injection. (18:732; 25:729, 739–741)
>Nursing Process—Implementation
>Client Need—Physiological integrity

27 1. Observing if a client can move the fingers or toes of the extremity within a cast is the best method for assessing neurological function. Muscles cannot move unless the nervous system is intact. Monitoring capillary refill, feeling the skin temperature, and inspecting the size of exposed fingers or toes are techniques for assessing the vascular status. (25:523)
   Nursing Process—Data collection
   Client Need—Physiological integrity

28 2. Individuals who develop anorexia nervosa often are described as being perfect children. They perform above average in school and often participate in a variety of extracurricular activities. Anorectics are not uniquely the middle child or sickly during childhood. There is no data suggesting that a characteristic of this disease is a feeling that others dislike them. (9:57–58; 10:493)
   Nursing Process—Data collection
   Client Need—Psychosocial integrity

29 4. Hepatitis B is transmitted from infected blood, serum, semen, and vaginal fluid. Viruses depend on living cells to grow and reproduce. Therefore, it is extremely unlikely that the virus could be transmitted by eating unsanitary food, smoking cigarettes that have long since been extinguished, or by entering open sores from a nonliving source within the environment. (18:1266; 21:743)
   Nursing Process—Data collection
   Client Need—Health promotion/maintenance

30 1. Reasonable weight gain is expected during pregnancy. Poor nutrition due to poverty or lack of knowledge is a leading contributor to high risk during pregnancy. It is important to the health of both mother and infant to eat a variety of foods. Many physicians do not restrict sexual activity during pregnancy unless complications such as uterine bleeding occurs or the amniotic sac ruptures. A certain amount of regular exercise is preferable to sporadic activity. The type and amount of exercise depends upon the health, habits, and obstetrical history of each individual. Pregnancy beyond age 35 is considered a risk factor. (14:115; 16:124)
   Nursing Process—Data collection
   Client Need—Health promotion/maintenance

31 4. A client weighing 88 pounds should receive 80 mg of drug prescribed at 2 mg/kg. There are 2.2 pounds per kilogram; therefore, 88 pounds divided by 2.2 equals 40 kg. Since the client should receive 2 mg for every kg, the nurse multiplies $2 \times 40 = 80$ mg.

Using the ratio-proportion method, the dosage is calculated as follows: (20:38)

Step 1 (known ratio to unknown ratio):

$$\frac{2\,mg}{1\,kg} = \frac{X\,mg}{40\,kg}$$

Step 2 (cross-multiply and solve for X):

$$1X = 80$$

$$X = 80$$

   Nursing Process—Implementation
   Client Need—Physiological integrity

32 2. Massaging the uterus causes the myometrium to contract and occlude blood vessels, thereby controlling postpartum bleeding. The client may experience pain when the uterus is massaged. The discomfort is due to the contraction of the uterus. Massaging the uterus does not suppress lactation. However, lactation is said to assist with involution of the uterus. (14:209; 16:216)
   Nursing Process—Evaluation
   Client Need—Physiological integrity

33 1. Using dolls or puppets as a teaching aid is the most appropriate strategy for a preschooler's cognitive ability. Pamphlets and diagrams are too abstract for the cognitive level of children who are 3, 4, or 5 years of age. The use of a videotape might be confused as a form of entertainment rather than personal instruction. (9:181; 18:863)
   Nursing Process—Planning
   Client Need—Safe, effective care environment

34 4. Paraphrasing the content of the client's statement is a therapeutic communication technique. It helps the client know that the message was heard and how it was interpreted. This technique will likely encourage the client to continue verbalizing. Classifying the statement as an exaggeration is belittling. Telling the client that talking will contribute to sadness indirectly is saying that this line of communication should cease. Demanding an explanation by asking "why" is also a block to therapeutic communication. It requires that the client justify a rationale for the statement and puts the client on the defensive. (10:70; 25:79–80)
   Nursing Process—Implementation
   Client Need—Psychosocial integrity

35 3. The only reliable method for confirming the presence of hard, dry stool within the rectum is digital examination. Auscultating bowel sounds, measuring abdominal girth, and inspecting the anus are all appropriate physical assessment techniques, but

they do not aid in determining if the client has a fecal impaction. (25:670–671)
  Nursing Process—Planning
  Client Need—Physiological integrity

36 2. Acetylsalicylic acid, also known as aspirin, interferes with platelet aggregation. Salicylates are avoided both preoperatively and postoperatively to reduce the potential for hemorrhage. (20:125)
  Nursing Process—Implementation
  Client Need—Health promotion/maintenance

37 4. If the pubococcygeal muscles are being contracted and relaxed properly during the performance of Kegel exercises, the client is able to stop and restart the flow of urine during voiding. Kegel exercises are performed to relieve stress incontinence; they are not effective in relieving back pain, improving posture or breathing. (18:1330; 25:642)
  Nursing Process—Evaluation
  Client Need—Health promotion/maintenance

38 3. External monitoring minimizes the risk of exposing the fetus to the mother's blood. Internal fetal monitoring, fetal scalp blood sampling, and amniocentesis are all invasive techniques that increase the risk of exposing the fetus to the HIV-infected blood of the mother. (14:146)
  Nursing Process—Implementation
  Client Need—Safe, effective care environment

39 4. Persons with hypothyroidism (myxedema) are most likely to demonstrate a general slowing of thought processes. Although they are slow in responding, their thought processes usually are based in reality. Quick recall of events, rapid verbal responses, and bizarre thinking are uncharacteristic of clients with hypothyroidism. (4:954)
  Nursing Process—Data collection
  Client Need—Psychosocial integrity

40 3. The crib's side rails are completely raised when the child is unattended regardless of how short a period of time it may be. Removing toys that have sharp edges, checking the temperature of bath water, and positioning the crib away from electrical outlets are all appropriate safety precautions. (11:35; 16:525)
  Nursing Process—Evaluation
  Client Need—Safe, effective care environment

41 3. Charting must be as clear and objective as possible. Quoting the client is always appropriate. Interpreting or labeling what the nurse suspects is occurring is not the best form of documentation. (25:92)
  Nursing Process—Implementation
  Client Need—Safe, effective care environment

42 1. Having direct contact with a stillborn infant tends to initiate healthy grieving. A verbal description that focuses on the infant's attributes is therapeutic, but not as much as personally seeing and touching the infant. Preventing any interaction between the parents and infant interferes with the grief process. Many postpartum clients are discharged within 24 to 48 hours, but this is not considered a technique for resolving the grief of a perinatal loss. (9:174)
  Nursing Process—Implementation
  Client Need—Psychosocial integrity

43 2. A child experiencing a nosebleed is placed in a sitting position with the head tilted forward while the nares are gently compressed between the thumb and forefinger. Tilting the head backward may lead to nausea, vomiting, and aspiration. Applying ice may or may not help stop the bleeding. If bleeding does not stop, the nose is packed with a small piece of gauze preferably impregnated with petrolatum, or a solution such as aqueous epinephrine (1:1000) is used. (16:728; 18:853)
  Nursing Process—Implementation
  Client Need—Physiological integrity

44 1. To remove an object from the airway of an unconscious, nonpregnant adult, the rescuer administers up to 5 forceful thrusts upward from the abdomen. If the series of abdominal thrusts does not clear the airway, the rescuer performs a finger sweep followed by two breaths. The cycle is repeated until respiration is restored. If the adult is conscious, the abdominal thrusts are repeated until the object is dislodged or the victim becomes unconscious. Ventilating the client is ineffective as long as the airway is obstructed. Chest compressions are performed when the victim no longer has a pulse. (18:372; 25:797)
  Nursing Process—Implementation
  Client Need—Physiological integrity

45 3. Performing self-care indicates that a client has progressed from denial and anger to a stage of acceptance. Wearing loose fitting garments can be an attempt to hide the change in body image. Although showering daily and avoiding gas-forming food are appropriate, they may indicate that the client is self-conscious about possible fecal odor. (4:685–686; 21:725)
  Nursing Process—Evaluation
  Client Need—Psychosocial integrity

46 2. Following any gastrointestinal procedure that uses barium as a contrast medium, the nurse monitors the client's bowel elimination. Retained barium can cause constipation and even bowel obstruction. A laxative or some other method for promoting the passage of the stool is needed if elimination is delayed. The color of the stool will appear to be largely white or chalky. Assessing the color of urine or presence of hunger are data that are unrelated to the consequences of the radiographic procedure. (7:688; 21:651)

Nursing Process—Data collection
Client Need—Physiological integrity

47 2. An adolescent who lives alone has the greatest need for community resources. Provision of financial assistance is important, as is providing for emotional support such as with a teen parenting group. Additional information is needed to determine if a primipara client or client who has had a previous spontaneous abortion has a greater need for community support than the adolescent client living alone. The client who maintains a relationship with the baby's father may or may not have a need for community-based assistance, depending on the nature of the client's relationship. Again, additional information is needed to make that decision. (14:238; 16:281)

Nursing Process—Data collection
Client Need—Safe, effective care environment

48 2. The care of clients with radioactive implants is best assigned to nonpregnant nurses. Acute or chronic exposure to ionizing radiation can cause gene mutation and birth defects. All nurses, male and female alike, pregnant and nonpregnant, are at risk from radiation if policies for time, distance, and shielding are not followed. Taking prescribed medication on a daily basis and having a family history of cancer are not risks in managing the care of a client with an external radioactive implant. (18:1149; 21:152)

Nursing Process—Data collection
Client Need—Safe, effective care environment

49 1. High-calorie finger foods are best for clients with bipolar disorder who find it almost impossible to sit or stand in one location for more than a few minutes. The problem is not the quantity of food, time available for eating, variety, or personal preferences. Rather, the underlying problem for bipolar clients is their limited attention and concentration on any physical task. This problem is generally temporary and becomes resolved once psychotropic medications achieve a therapeutic effect. (10:343, 348)

Nursing Process—Planning
Client Need—Physiological integrity

50 1. To detect the presence of thrombophlebitis, the nurse has the client dorsiflex each foot separately and notes if calf pain is experienced. The presence of calf pain is considered a *positive Homans' sign*

and is reported immediately. Palpating the pedal pulse is a method of assessing distal arterial blood flow. The client may guard the use of a leg with a thrombophlebitis while walking and may even have a slightly elevated temperature. However, these are not the primary assessment techniques for detecting a thrombophlebitis. (21:357)

Nursing Process—Data collection
Client Need—Physiological integrity

51 1. An enterostomal therapist is a health professional who is certified in the specialized care of individuals who have ostomies or other problems with impaired skin. A gastroenterologist is a physician who has specialized in the diagnosis and treatment of pathology occurring in the gastrointestinal system. A gastronome is a person who judges cooking. An entomologist is a person who studies insects. (18:1226; 21:721)

Nursing Process—Implementation
Client Need—Safe, effective care environment

52 4. Palpation of the thyroid increases the postoperative risk for developing thyroid crisis or storm. This complication is a direct result of manipulating the thyroid gland preoperatively or during its surgical removal. None of the other analyses is accurate. (21:783)

Nursing Process—Evaluation
Client Need—Safe, effective care environment

53 1. Missing a dose of disulfiram will *not* cause a drug reaction. The reaction occurs when the client ingests or applies alcohol to his skin. To make sure that a reaction does not occur, the client must abstain from alcohol for at least two weeks or more after the drug is discontinued. (10:452–453; 20:487; 28:403)

Nursing Process—Evaluation
Client Need—Health promotion/maintenance

54 2. Standard precautions are followed whenever there is a potential for direct contact with blood, as when removing a needle from an intravenous site. It is appropriate to pull the privacy curtain, but it is not essential. Taking vital signs and weighing a client help to monitor the effects of fluid replacement therapy, but they are not essential to discontinuing the intravenous fluid. (25:282)

Nursing Process—Implementation
Client Need—Safe, effective care environment

55 2. When a client indicates signs or symptoms of anxiety, it is best for the nurse to help him to express his concerns. Belittling his fears by saying "There is no need for fear," using a reassuring cliché such as "trust me" or "you have an excellent surgeon," and giving advice such as "try to relax," are all nontherapeutic communication techniques. (10:70; 25:79–80)

> Nursing Process—Implementation
> Client Need—Psychosocial integrity

56 3. Topical anesthesia is needed when a tonometer is used to measure the pressure within a client's eyes. The anesthetic, prepared in liquid eyedrop form, makes it possible to apply the tonometer on the cornea without the client feeling as if something is touching the eye. The other assessments are performed with a reflex hammer, a vaginal speculum, and an otoscope—none of which require a topical anesthetic when used. (21:607)

> Nursing Process—Planning
> Client Need—Safe, effective care environment

57 2. The root of a tooth is temporarily preserved by holding it under the tongue or placing the tooth in milk. Water, alcohol, and air-drying damage the root and reduce the potential success of implantation. (18:351)

> Nursing Process—Implementation
> Client Need—Physiological integrity

58 4. Bright red drainage indicates that the client is hemorrhaging. Preventing life-threatening consequences depends on collaboration with the physician. Comfort measures are used to relieve the sore throat, but the client's life is not endangered by the condition. The nurse provides more frequent mouth care or offers the client sips of water or ice chips to relieve thirst. The nurse can independently clean the nose with an applicator or moist face cloth. (18:1238; 21:624)

> Nursing Process—Implementation
> Client Need—Physiological integrity

59 3. Eric Erikson describes generativity as a concern for leaving something of worth to society. Adults over the age of 40 seek to identify a positive contribution for which they will be most remembered. For some, their legacy is having been a good parent, an upstanding citizen, community volunteer, or more tangible activities such as writing, painting, and so on. (21:50)

> Nursing Process—Data collection
> Client Need—Health promotion/maintenance

60 2. Asking about dietary practices is the most direct method among the options provided for determining if the client follows Orthodox Jewish lifestyle. Reform, Conservative, and Orthodox Jewish men may wear a *yarmulke,* or skullcap, especially on the Sabbath or when attending synagogue. Hebrew is commonly spoken by individuals who have im-

migrated from Israel. Many Christian men as well as Jews are circumcised. (6:296–297, 308–309)

> Nursing Process—Data collection
> Client Need—Safe, effective care environment

61 1. Air is prevented from entering the opening from which a chest tube is pulled or there is a potential for recollapsing the lung. Once the tube is out, its sterility is compromised. If replaced, a sterile tube is used. Applying suction is not an effective method for keeping the lung inflated. Holding the breath may help temporarily, but the client cannot sustain this effort. (25:421)

> Nursing Process—Implementation
> Client Need—Physiological integrity

62 1. Fluids are restricted to a few ice chips or small sips of water. This practice prevents electrolyte imbalance. Relieving throat discomfort and providing oral hygiene are appropriate nursing care. Irrigating a nasogastric tube is not unsafe. However, the nurse follows the physician's written order or the agency's standards for care when carrying out this procedure. (25:604)

> Nursing Process—Implementation
> Client Need—Physiological integrity

63 2. The tip of the enema tubing is inserted approximately 3 to 4 in (7.5 to 10 cm) when giving an enema to an adult client. This allows the tube to enter the anal canal and pass the internal sphincter, where the solution is instilled. Introducing the tube farther may injure mucous membranes. Introducing it a shorter distance places the solution in the rectum and causes the client to expel the enema before it has had a chance to be effective. (18:545; 25:679)

> Nursing Process—Implementation
> Client Need—Physiological integrity

64 2. Retracting the foreskin is necessary to remove secretions and prevent infection. The foreskin is replaced after the area is cleansed. The scrotum is washed with plain water or soap; normal saline is not necessary for this procedure. The anal area is washed after the penis and scrotum are cleansed. (25:309)

> Nursing Process—Implementation
> Client Need—Physiological integrity

65 2. Knowing a client's occupation and the type of work that is performed provides valuable information as to whether to include principles of body mechanics in a teaching plan for a client with recurrent back pain. The client's age and energy level affect the strategies selected for providing the health teaching. Observing the client's gait is more medically

diagnostic since a limb that is shorter than another may suggest an alteration in the alignment of spinal vertebrae. (25:467)
Nursing Process—Data collection
Client Need—Health promotion/maintenance

66 3. Talking and dealing with an anxiety-provoking experience is healthier than avoiding or suppressing. Failing to deal with the terror of an event leads to post-traumatic stress disorder. Most victims can detect insincerity when others pretend to be happy in their presence. Although interacting with others who have experienced a similar traumatic event is therapeutic, socializing for the sake of socializing is not. Taking vacations and participating in pleasurable activities are a form of stress management, but they serve as distractions and delay processing the impact of a traumatic event. (10:374–375)
Nursing Process—Planning
Client Need—Psychosocial integrity

67 2. Standing in front of a mirror helps the client detect any physical breast changes, such as redness, changes in the nipple, or dimpling of the skin. Lying on the abdomen, performing the entire examination while lying on the back, or sitting when palpating the breast are not recommended methods of BSE. (18:1319; 25:186)
Nursing Process—Evaluation
Client Need—Health promotion/maintenance

68 3. Corticosteroid therapy reduces the immunologic injury to the nephrons. As the nephrons recover, there is an increase in urinary output. Blood pressure decreases from previously hypertensive levels as renal function improves. Long- and short-term high-dose therapy with corticosteroids is likely to create muscle weakness and atrophy. Weight gain is a nontherapeutic effect of steroids due to altered glucose metabolism and sodium retention. (26:680, 682)
Nursing Process—Evaluation
Client Need—Physiological integrity

69 4. The frequency of contractions is the time between the beginning of one contraction and the beginning of the next contraction. The duration of a contraction is the time between the beginning and the end of a single contraction. It is incorrect to calculate the frequency of contractions by timing from the end of one to the beginning of the next or the beginning of one to the end of the second contraction. (14:157; 16:164)
Nursing Process—Data collection
Client Need—Safe, effective care environment

70 2. One of the best techniques for reducing anxiety is to provide instructions before performing any procedure and to provide explanations when something unexpected, like an alarm sounding, occurs. Hospitalized clients tend to fantasize and exaggerate the significance of what health personnel know is insignificant. Without an explanation, the client's anxiety is not likely to be relieved by switching the infusion to flow by gravity. Anxiety interferes with attention and concentration; reading is not a realistic option. Medication is not given until the results of other nursing interventions are evaluated. (21:106)
Nursing Process—Planning
Client Need—Psychosocial integrity

71 1. It is not unusual for any new mother to feel frustrated and overwhelmed by the demands of parenting. It also is appropriate for the nurse to suggest coping methods. Telling the mother to be patient until the feeling goes away does not help her deal with the situation at hand. Suggesting that the client place the child up for adoption is extreme for the circumstances. The information as presented does not warrant reporting the situation to child protective services. (16:281)
Nursing Process—Implementation
Client Need—Psychosocial integrity

72 2. When vaginal bleeding is noted shortly after delivery, the nurse first massages the uterus. This is often sufficient to cause contraction of the uterus, which may have become relaxed and soft. Normally, with firming of the uterus, bleeding is controlled. If this conservative care is ineffective, the nurse collects more data, such as obtaining a current measurement of vital signs and informs the physician. Intravenous fluids and drugs are required if independent nursing measures do not suffice in controlling blood loss through massage. (16:216; 22:290)
Nursing Process—Implementation
Client Need—Physiological integrity

73 2. The main reason for performing leg exercises is to prevent the formation of blood clots by promoting circulation of venous blood. Leg exercises are used as an alternative when ambulation and activity are less than adequate. Exercise does maintain muscle strength, reduces dependent edema, and relieves congestion of blood in varicosed veins. However, none of these are the primary reason for performing leg exercises postoperatively. (25:551)
Nursing Process—Implementation
Client Need—Health promotion/maintenance

74 3. Aminophylline is likely to produce stimulating effects such as restlessness, insomnia, irritability, tachycardia, and hypertension. It is sometimes difficult to differentiate between the effects of the drug therapy and the manifestations of hypoxia. Lung sounds and respiratory effort are monitored frequently along with vital signs. Blood levels of the drug are monitored to evaluate a person's ability to metabolize the drug. Dosages are adjusted depending on the response. Bradycardia, drowsiness, and hypotension are all opposite of the stimulating effects associated with aminophylline. (20:239)

      Nursing Process—Data collection
      Client Need—Physiological integrity

75 3. Excessive sleeping is one method some depressed clients use to withdraw from others. Demanding attention, making sarcastic remarks, and wanting to see family are not typical signs of depression among older adults. (3:371; 10:395, 404)

      Nursing Process—Data collection
      Client Need—Psychosocial integrity

76 3. Tetracyclines, of which oxytetracycline is one example, are not recommended for children under the age of 8 unless their use is absolutely necessary. This family of antibiotics causes yellow, gray, or brown discoloration to the teeth which is permanent. Penicillins, cephalosporins, and aminoglycosides do not discolor the teeth if given to young children. (16:391; 20:66)

      Nursing Process—Implementation
      Client Need—Physiological integrity

77 4. It is best to first promote reality orientation when any client with dementia becomes confused. Disagreeing may agitate the client and interfere with therapeutic effectiveness. Collaborating in the delusion by offering to call the school or indicating that a neighbor will care for the children contributes to the alteration in thought processes. (9:221)

      Nursing Process—Implementation
      Client Need—Psychosocial integrity

78 3. Milk and milk products are avoided because they increase the production of mucus. Croup is accompanied by a severe cough and often requires expectorants to loosen secretions. Clear liquids, Popsicles, gelatin and other fluids are permitted. (11:255; 16:912)

      Nursing Process—Implementation
      Client Need—Physiological integrity

79 3. The brachial artery is used for assessment during cardiopulmonary resuscitation (CPR) of an infant. The rationale is that an infant's neck is short and fat, which makes it difficult to assess the carotid pulse. The radial and femoral arteries are not routinely used when assessing any age client during CPR. (14:327; 18:369)

      Nursing Process—Implementation
      Client Need—Psychosocial integrity

80 4. The nurse's first concern is to assess the physical condition of the client before attempting any change in the client's position. Once the nurse has examined the client, adequate help is obtained to help the client to a safer and more comfortable place. After all the data is collected and the nurse provides comfort and reassurance to the client, the accident is reported to the supervisor and physician. A written description of the accident and its outcome is recorded and kept on file in the agency's administration office. (25:391)

      Nursing Process—Implementation
      Client Need—Physiological integrity

81 4. The best evidence of parent-newborn attachment is that the parents hold, touch, and talk to their newborn child. Physical contact tends to stimulate the beginning of parental love and protectiveness. It communicates comfort and security to the infant. Observing others caring for the infant or watching from a distance is not as effective as eye-to-eye and direct skin contact in promoting bonding. Being pleased with the baby's gender is a positive sign, but it is not as indicative of the future relationship between parents and an infant. (14:241; 22:306)

      Nursing Process—Evaluation
      Client Need—Health promotion/maintenance

82 3. Physiological needs, such as correcting nutritional imbalances, have a higher priority. Once the client's weight is stabilized and weight gain is progressing, the focus can turn to improving the client's body image and methods of coping. Assertiveness may or may not be a problem among individuals with anorexia nervosa. (6:375)

      Nursing Process—Planning
      Client Need—Physiological integrity

83 3. Gelatin is permitted on a clear liquid diet. Clear liquid diets include fluids and foods that are transparent. Milk and other items containing milk, such as ice cream and creamed soup, are not permitted. (6:53; 25:242)

      Nursing Process—Implementation
      Client Need—Physiological integrity

84 3. A sign that a client is able to orient himself is the ability to find his or her own room without assistance. Walking with others is not evidence that the client can independently find the dining room. The

ability to dress is evidence that the client is able to perform activities of daily living. Talking on the telephone indicates that the client has retained the ability to communicate verbally. (9:213)
  Nursing Process—Evaluation
  Client Need—Psychosocial integrity

85 1. The use of a commode is an appropriate alternative to reduce the workload of the heart. Shortness of breath indicates that the heart is unable to adapt to the demands required during ambulation. Oxygen given after elimination and continuing ambulation, even with the assistance of the nurse or a walker, is not likely to prevent or reduce the effort of the heart in response to activity. (11:359; 16:751)
  Nursing Process—Planning
  Client Need—Physiological integrity

86 2. It is best to hold aerosolized medication in the lungs for a few seconds to maximally disperse the inhaled drug throughout the lungs. Immediately exhaling causes inadequate absorption. Swallowing the inhaled medication fails to distribute the drug to the appropriate location for absorption. Coughing causes the aerosolized medication to be displaced into the upper airways. (25:723)
  Nursing Process—Implementation
  Client Need—Health promotion/maintenance

87 4. A young child may not be able to verbally indicate the location of discomfort. Pulling at the infected ear is a common indication that the symptoms are related to a middle-ear infection. It is normal for a 2-year-old child to want to be held by his mother in a strange environment. Teething and swallowing are not directly associated with a primary infectious process in the oropharynx. (11:211; 22:596)
  Nursing Process—Data collection
  Client Need—Physiological integrity

88 2. Meclizine is an antihistamine drug that is prescribed for motion sickness and vertigo due to vestibular disease. Acetaminophen has antipyretic and analgesic actions. Meperidine is a narcotic analgesic. Triazolam is in the benzodiazepine family of drugs. It is a commonly prescribed drug for promoting sleep. (28:672)
  Nursing Process—Implementation
  Client Need—Physiological integrity

89 4. Following a thyroidectomy, clients are monitored for hypocalcemia since it is possible that the parathyroids may have been accidentally removed. Hypocalcemia is manifested by tingling and numbness

of the extremities and mouth and muscle contractions of the fingers and hand. (4:953; 21:784)
  Nursing Process—Data collection
  Client Need—Physiological integrity

90 3. Standing is the natural position men assume when urinating. A male is psychologically helped to relax his urinary sphincter by simulating normal conditions for urinating as much as possible. Using a bedpan requires sitting. This client is already distended. Increasing fluids would add to his discomfort. Perineal exercises help to control stress incontinence. (25:633)
  Nursing Process—Implementation
  Client Need—Physiological integrity

91 3. The fingernails are cut short to maintain the integrity of the skin. Some also recommend that the client wear cotton gloves to prevent opening the skin in the event that scratching cannot be controlled. Warm water accentuates the itching sensation. Dry cornstarch absorbs perspiration, but does not relieve itching. Since jaundice is not related to an allergic reaction, using specially laundered linen is inappropriate. (21:746)
  Nursing Process—Planning
  Client Need—Physiological integrity

92 2. Clients with hyperparathyroidism are prone to forming kidney stones. Keeping the urine dilute and promoting frequent urinary elimination reduce the potential for stone formation. The diet is limited in calcium. Hypercalcemia also puts clients at risk for hypertension and cardiac arrhythmias. Clients with hyperparathyroidism are not at greater risk for skin breakdown than others. (18:1062)
  Nursing Process—Planning
  Client Need—Physiological integrity

93 1. When the descending aorta develops an aneurysm, an examiner may feel a pulsating abdominal mass. Extra heart sounds are associated with disorders of the conduction system or congestive heart failure. Uneven chest movements are more often a sign of a pneumothorax or flail chest. It is normal to hear a hollow sound when percussing most areas of the abdomen. (4:770; 21:388)
  Nursing Process—Data collection
  Client Need—Physiological integrity

94 2. Cocaine is a central nervous system stimulant. It can increase blood pressure, heart rate, and cause cardiac dysrhythmia. Any or all of these cardiovascular side effects can result in chest pain, tachycardia or palpitations in an otherwise young, healthy person. Opioids such as heroin, barbiturates, and marijuana are central nervous system depressants that are more likely to cause bradycardia and hypotension. (20:485)

Nursing Process—Data collection
Client Need—Physiological integrity

95 1. A heart rate that remains within 60 to 100 beats per minute is a sign that a client is not suffering hypoxia. Tachycardia and irregular cardiac rhythm are warning signs of oxygen deprivation. The volume of secretions and warm, dry skin are not the best assessments for evaluating the oxygenation status of a client. Loss of consciousness is a late sign of hypoxia. (18:1185)

Nursing Process—Evaluation
Client Need—Physiological integrity

96 4. The nurse has an ethical responsibility to protect the confidentiality of the person who is HIV-positive. When persons test positive for HIV, they are provided counseling and education concerning measures for preventing its transmission. Legally, HIV-infected persons are required to divulge their infectious status to any and all potential sexual partners. As long as safe sex practices and blood and body fluid precautions are followed, it is possible to prevent transmission of HIV from an infected person to a noninfected person. (4:1183; 21:346)

Nursing Process—Implementation
Client Need—Safe, effective care environment

97 1. Early decelerations are usually benign and require no intervention. However, the nurse continues to monitor the client to detect the presence of late decelerations, a more serious condition that requires intervention. If late decelerations occur, the nurse turns the client onto her side, elevates the legs, and notifies the physician. (16:172)

Nursing Process—Implementation
Client Need—Health promotion/maintenance

98 4. Buzzing, or tinnitus, is a common side effect experienced by individuals who take large, frequent doses of aspirin. Neither racing thoughts, polyuria, nor diarrhea are side effects associated with aspirin. (20:126)

Nursing Process—Data collection
Client Need—Physiological integrity

99 1. The combination of alcohol and a minor tranquilizer can cause central nervous system and respiratory depression. Many have died accidentally when these two drugs are concerned. Generally minor tranquilizers are given in low doses for a short amount of time while an individual develops other effective coping techniques. Benzodiazepines cause drowsiness rather than insomnia. Blood levels are not generally indicated to monitor the effec-

tiveness of benzodiazepine drug therapy. (17:309; 28:81)

Nursing Process—Evaluation
Client Need—Health promotion/maintenance

100 3. The most effective means for minimizing separation anxiety is that a parent remains with the child during hospitalization. A familiar toy helps the child to deal with the separation, but is not as effective as a parent actually being there. Sibling visitation is not a substitute for the parents' presence. It may or may not assist with minimizing separation anxiety, depending on the child's relationship with the siblings. Explaining a procedure to the child does not decrease separation anxiety. (14:439; 11:20)

Nursing Process—Evaluation
Client Need—Psychosocial integrity

101 2. Turning a client with a wet plaster cast frequently helps to dry the complete circumference of the cast. Increasing the heat in the room high enough to have a significant effect on the cast would more than likely make the client feel uncomfortable. Manually fanning the cast is tedious and time-consuming. It is impractical to take a client outside in the sun to dry a plaster cast. (25:524)

Nursing Process—Planning
Client Need—Physiological integrity

102 3. When a pregnant client indicates that breathing is eased, it is an indication that lightening has occurred. This means that the fetus has settled into the pelvic inlet. Lay persons often remark that "the baby has dropped." Multiparas may not experience this phenomenon until just before or during true labor. Lightening may cause backaches to increase due to the descent of the fetus and relaxation of the pelvic joints prior to delivery. Braxton Hicks contractions are irregular and weak uterine contractions. When these contractions become more noticeable they are a sign of impending labor. Changes in the appetite are not related to the phenomenon of lightening. (14:152; 16:159)

Nursing Process—Data collection
Client Need—Health promotion/maintenance

103 1. Seeing the chest rise is the best evidence that rescue breathing is being performed appropriately. A rising chest indicates that the airway is open and no air is leaking from the victim's nose or mouth. It also indicates that a sufficient volume of air is being administered by the rescuer. Dilated pupils are a sign that the brain is not receiving adequate oxygenation. A pulse indicates that cardiac compressions are not necessary. The rescuer needs to seal or cover both the nose and the mouth. (18:365)

Nursing Process—Evaluation
Client Need—Physiological integrity

104 3. If a rectal tube has not brought relief after about 20 minutes, it is best to remove the tube temporarily and wait to reinsert the tube a few hours later to allow the gas to travel further down the large intestine. Rotating a rectal tube or replacing the tube with one that is larger does not increase its effectiveness. If a rectal tube is inserted correctly beyond the internal rectal sphincter, inserting it further does not improve the potential for relieving intestinal distention. (25:672)

Nursing Process—Planning
Client Need—Physiological integrity

105 2. Because of the disproportionate size of an adult's hand in comparison with an infant's heart and chest, the rescuer uses just one or two fingers to perform the chest compressions on an infant who is 1 year old or less. The rate of compressions for an infant is 100 per minute. The heel of one hand is used on children between 1 to 8 years of age. The interlocked fingers of both hands are used when performing chest compressions on individuals over the age of 8. The palms of the hands are not used during chest compressions regardless of the age of the victim. (25:806)

Nursing Process—Evaluation
Client Need—Physiological integrity

106 3. Methylphenidate hydrochloride is a central nervous system stimulant. Common side effects include tachycardia, hypertension, sleep disturbances, and decreased growth rate. (28:728)

Nursing Process—Data collection
Client Need—Physiological integrity

107 2. Infants who are born with fetal alcohol syndrome tend to be extremely irritable at birth. They may go on to develop disorders characterized by hyperactivity as they mature. Lethargy, flaccidity, and apathy are not exhibited by infants with fetal alcohol syndrome.(14:273)

Nursing Process—Data collection
Client Need—Physiological integrity

108 2. One of the best ways to quantify the client's subjective response to a medication is to use some form of a rating scale. The heart rate and blood pressure may be lowered with antianxiety medication, but that does not help evaluate the client's perception. The other assessment techniques are too vague to be significant. (25:366–367)

Nursing Process—Evaluation
Client Need—Psychosocial integrity

109 1. Although it is therapeutic to involve a client with a change in body image in his or her care, acceptance of the change in body image cannot be rushed. Therefore, it is best for the nurse to accept the client's behavior and choice without judgment. This shows respect for the individual's unique effort to cope. In the early postoperative period, it is premature to suggest that the client needs professional help to adjust. How the nurse would deal with the same circumstance is immaterial. Saying that the stump "doesn't look that bad" is an evaluative statement based on the nurse's standards and experiences. (9:356–357; 21:1010)

Nursing Process—Implementation
Client Need—Psychosocial integrity

110 1. Postural drainage is performed before eating or after consumed food has left the stomach. If done on a full stomach, the positioning, coughing, or expectorating may cause the person to feel nauseated and vomit. Postural drainage is performed according to a scheduled routine to mobilize secretions, not just when individuals feel short of breath or are actively coughing. Although the client is consulted concerning the plan for care, waiting until the client says it is necessary to perform postural drainage is not appropriate. Some may resist this form of therapy because it is tiring and uncomfortable for them. (25:778)

Nursing Process—Planning
Client Need—Physiological integrity

111 3. The earliest signs of hypoxia are manifested by behavioral changes such as restlessness, apprehension, anxiety, decreased judgment, and drowsiness. As hypoxia progresses, the nurse observes dyspnea, tachypnea, and tachycardia. The blood pressure may become elevated due to anxiety. Cyanosis is one of the last signs the nurse is likely to observe in a client who is hypoxic. (25:402)

Nursing Process—Data collection
Client Need—Physiological integrity

112 4. Maintaining cleanliness is of highest priority following a perineal prostatectomy since there is a high risk for wound infection from organisms present in stool. Straining during defecation is contraindicated; therefore, performing Valsalva's maneuver (bearing down against a closed glottis) is inappropriate. A high Fowler's position can contribute to discomfort in the perineal incisional area. Laxatives generally are too harsh for prophylactically maintaining comfortable elimination of stool. (18:1303)

Nursing Process—Planning
Client Need—Physiological integrity

113 3. Throw rugs are the greatest potential hazard. Due to their instability, individuals tend to slip on them. Also, falls occur when a foot trips on a wrinkled portion of rug or a curled edge. Taking a shower is safer than bathing in a tub. Grounded outlets that receive cords with three prongs are safer than the customary two-pronged plug. A television in the bedroom is no more unsafe than in any other room in the house. (25:391)
Nursing Process—Evaluation
Client Need—Safe, effective care environment

114 2. Standard precautions (formerly universal precautions) are followed when caring for *all* clients, even those who are already infected with the HIV virus. Transmission of other infectious diseases are prevented by following either airborne, droplet, or contact precautions. (25:451–452)
Nursing Process—Planning
Client Need—Safe, effective care

115 3. The most common cause of a hernia is performing an activity that increases intra-abdominal pressure, such as lifting heavy objects. When intra-abdominal pressure increases, it causes the intestine to protrude through areas in the abdominal musculature that are structurally weak. Discomfort related to ingesting milk products indicates lactose intolerance. Obesity accompanying inactivity does play a role in weakening abdominal muscles, but this person is reported to be thin. (21:709)
Nursing Process—Data collection
Client Need—Health promotion/maintenance

116 2. An immune assay enzyme test to confirm respiratory syncytial virus (RSV) infection, requires a specimen of nasal secretions. Throat swabs, sputum specimens, and blood specimens cannot be used to perform this particular diagnostic test. (11:212; 14:484)
Nursing Process—Implementation
Client Need—Safe, effective care environment

117 2. To counteract an older client's dry skin, the plan of care is modified to include less frequent bathing, applying an emollient to the skin, and increasing the client's fluid intake. Providing high-calorie snacks contributes to the client's nutrition. Using cotton bed linen promotes comfort, but it does not rehydrate the skin. Keeping the fingernails short promotes skin integrity should the client scratch the skin. (3:155; 25:328)
Nursing Process—Planning
Client Need—Physiological integrity

118 3. The described symptoms are typical of a hypoglycemic reaction. Therefore, A normal blood sugar is the best evidence that hypoglycemia is corrected. The blood pressure is generally within normal limits or increased during hypoglycemia because of anxiety and the secretion of adrenaline. Assessing the blood pressure is not as valuable in determining the client's response to the nursing intervention. (21:806)
Nursing Process—Evaluation
Client Need—Physiological integrity

119 2. Oral contraceptives containing estrogen place individuals who take them at risk for thromboembolic disease. It is estimated that taking oral contraceptives increases the risk for blood clot formation from 3 to 11 times more than women who do not use this form of birth control. A history of having formed a blood clot is generally a contraindication to taking oral contraceptive agents. Iron supplements, nasal decongestants, and antacids do not promote the formation of blood clots. (20:373)
Nursing Process—Data collection
Client Need—Physiological integrity

120 1. Following a TURP, men experience retrograde ejaculation. That is, during orgasm ejaculation is "dry." Semen is deposited into the bladder. The first voiding after intercourse is likely to appear cloudy because it contains the seminal fluid and sperm. Because of this change in physiology, men can expect to be unable to impregnate a sexual partner. Despite retrograde ejaculation, following a TURP males maintain normal libidos, achieve erections during sexual excitement, and experience orgasms. (2:122; 26:680)
Nursing Process—Evaluation
Client Need—Health promotion/maintenance

Classification of Test Items

Part I of the Comprehensive Examination

Directions: After each question the correct answer is given, as well as a classification of each test question. Compare the correct answer with your answer. If a question has been answered *incorrectly*, draw a line to the end of all the columns. When finished, add up the number of your correct answers in each column and place that number in the respective box at the end in the area identified as *Number Correct*.

To determine the percentage of questions you answered correctly and your performance in each of the test plan categories, divide the *Number Correct* in each column by the *Number Possible* in each column. Then multiply the decimal by 100. For example:

$$\frac{\text{Number Correct: 90}}{\text{Number Possible: 120}} = 0.75 \times 100 = 75\%$$

Any score that is less than 75% indicates an area where further review would be beneficial.

KEY TO ITEM CLASSIFICATION:

NURSING PROCESS	CLIENT NEEDS
D = Data collection	S = Safe, effective care environment
P = Planning	P = Physiological integrity
I = Implementation	M = Psychosocial integrity
E = Evaluation	H = Health promotion/maintenance

Question #	Answer #	Nursing Process				Client Needs			
		D	P	I	E	S	P	M	H
1	3	D					P		
2	3		P				P		
3	4				E	S			
4	1			I					H
5	2				E	S			
6	2			I				M	
7	1	D					P		
8	2				E		P		
9	3				E	S			
10	3		P				P		
11	3		P						H
12	4			I					H
13	3			I			P		
14	4		P				P		
15	4	D							H

Question #	Answer #	Nursing Process				Client Needs			
		D	P	I	E	S	P	M	H
16	1	D					P		
17	1				E				H
18	3	D					P		
19	1				E		P		
20	1			I			P		
21	3		P						H
22	2		P				P		
23	2				E		P		
24	3	D					P		
25	3		P						H
26	1			I			P		
27	1	D					P		
28	2	D						M	
29	4	D							H
30	1	D							H
31	4			I			P		
32	2				E		P		
33	1		P			S			
34	4			I				M	
35	3		P				P		
36	2			I					H
37	4				E				H
38	3			I		S			
39	4	D						M	
40	3				E	S			
41	3			I		S			
42	1			I				M	
43	2			I			P		
44	1			I			P		
45	3				E			M	
46	2	D					P		
47	2	D				S			

Question #	Answer #	Nursing Process				Client Needs			
		D	P	I	E	S	P	M	H
48	2	D				S			
49	1		P				P		
50	1	D					P		
51	1			I		S			
52	4				E	S			
53	1				E				H
54	2			I		S			
55	2			I				M	
56	3		P			S			
57	2			I			P		
58	4			I			P		
59	3	D							H
60	2	D				S			
61	1			I			P		
62	1			I			P		
63	2			I			P		
64	2			I			P		
65	2	D							H
66	3		P					M	
67	2				E				H
68	3				E		P		
69	4	D				S			
70	2		P					M	
71	1			I				M	
72	2			I			P		
73	2			I					H
74	3	D					P		
75	3	D						M	
76	3			I			P		
77	4			I				M	
78	3			I			P		
79	3			I				M	

Question #	Answer #	Nursing Process				Client Needs			
		D	P	I	E	S	P	M	H
80	4			I			P		
81	4				E				H
82	3		P				P		
83	3			I			P		
84	3				E			M	
85	1		P				P		
86	2			I					H
87	4	D					P		
88	2			I			P		
89	4	D					P		
90	3			I			P		
91	3		P				P		
92	2		P				P		
93	1	D					P		
94	2	D					P		
95	1				E		P		
96	4			I		S			
97	1			I					H
98	4	D					P		
99	1				E				H
100	3				E			M	
101	2		P				P		
102	3	D							H
103	1				E		P		
104	3		P				P		
105	2				E		P		
106	3	D					P		
107	2	D					P		
108	2				E			M	
109	1			I				M	
110	1		P				P		
111	3	D					P		

−13

	Question #	Answer #	Nursing Process				Client Needs			
			D	P	I	E	S	P	M	H
	112	4		P				P		
	113	3				E	S			
	114	2		P			S			
	115	3	D							H
	116	2			I		S			
	117	2		P				P		
	118	3				E		P		
	119	2	D					P		
	120	1				E				H
	Number Correct	107	31	18	34	24	17	55	15	20
	Number Possible	120	32	23	39	26	19	61	17	23
	Percentage Correct	89%	97	78	87	92	89	90	88	87

1 5 5 2 2 6 2 3

57 min

Part II of the Comprehensive Examination

Directions: Allow yourself 2 hours to complete Part II. Start this part now.

1 If a client takes all of the following nonprescription drugs on a regular basis, which one is most likely related to the client's current complaint of epigastric pain?
○ 1. Milk of magnesia, which the client takes for constipation
● 2. Aspirin, which the client takes for joint discomfort
○ 3. Nyquil®, which the client takes to fall asleep
○ 4. Benadryl®, which the client takes for allergy symptoms

A client who is 3 months pregnant complains of feeling tired.

2 The *best advice* the nurse can give the pregnant client is to
○ 1. do most of her work during the middle afternoon.
○ 2. take two prenatal vitamins daily instead of one.
○ 3. avoid napping during the day.
● 4. rest whenever she feels tired.

3 Which of the following foods is *best* for the nurse to include in a diet plan for a pregnant client who needs additional iron?
○ 1. Potatoes
● 2. Legumes
○ 3. Oranges
○ 4. Cheese

A young adult is brought to the emergency department in an unconscious state.

4 To determine if the adolescent has overdosed on an opiate drug such as heroin, the nurse is *correct* to expect that the physician will order
○ 1. methadone hydrochloride (Dolophine)
○ 2. succinylcholine chloride (Anectine)
● 3. naloxone hydrochloride (Narcan)
○ 4. pancuronium bromide (Pavulon)

5 When performing a physical assessment on an extremely thin adolescent, which assessment finding is *most consistent* with a possible diagnosis of anorexia nervosa?

● 1. There is a fine growth of body hair.
○ 2. There are bruises over the upper torso.
○ 3. The client's bowel sounds are hyperactive.
○ 4. The client has club-shaped fingertips.

A physician's standing orders include administering a laxative to postpartum clients who have not had a bowel movement by the day of discharge.

6 For which client is it *best* for the nurse to collaborate with the physician before implementing the order?
○ 1. A client who has hemorrhoids
● 2. A client who is breast-feeding
○ 3. A client who has a third-degree perineal tear
○ 4. A client who had a vacuum extraction delivery

7 When a client with gallstones asks about treatment with extracorporeal lithotripsy, the *best explanation* is that it eliminates the stones by
○ 1. dissolving them with strong chemicals.
● 2. pulverizing them with shock waves.
○ 3. removing them with a special endoscope.
○ 4. binding them to a sticky resin material.

A client who is 4 months pregnant states that she lives on a limited income and is having a problem purchasing enough meat to supply sufficient protein for her diet.

8 The nurse can *best* respond to the client's needs by recommending that she supplement the meat with which of the following foods?
○ 1. Broccoli
○ 2. Cauliflower
○ 3. Fortified cereal
● 4. Dried beans

9 When teaching a postmenopausal client about breast self-examination, which instruction is *most correct*?
○ 1. Examine your breasts upon awakening from sleep.
● 2. Examine your breasts on the first day of the month.
○ 3. Examine your breasts after you finish your shower.
○ 4. Examine your breasts before your yearly mammogram.

When testing the urine of a client who is 6 months pregnant, the urine tests positive for albumin.

10 The *most accurate* assumption by the nurse is that the pregnant client is developing
  ● 1. preeclampsia.
  ○ 2. liver failure.
  ○ 3. amniotic embolism.
  ○ 4. placenta previa.

A 10-year-old child is admitted to the hospital with endocarditis secondary to rheumatic fever.

11 Which assessment finding is *most consistent* with the expected history of a client with this condition?
  ○ 1. The child had a congenital heart defect at birth.
  ● 2. The child had a recent untreated streptococcal infection.
  ○ 3. The child has consistently had inadequate nutrition.
  ○ 4. The child has failed to receive proper immunizations.

A pregnant client is admitted to the labor and delivery area and is experiencing vaginal bleeding.

12 If the physician's routine admission orders include the administration of an enema, the nurse is *correct* to
  ○ 1. give the client the enema as ordered.
  ● 2. withhold giving the enema at this time.
  ○ 3. give the enema if the client is constipated.
  ○ 4. substitute a laxative for the cleansing enema.

13 When the blood pressure of a client who had a hysterectomy 10 hours earlier falls abruptly, the *best action* for the nurse to take is to
  ○ 1. withhold the administration of analgesic drugs.
  ○ 2. document the information on the client's chart.
  ● 3. inform the surgeon about the client's condition.
  ○ 4. change the client to a Fowler's position.

14 When a postoperative transurethral prostatectomy (TURP) client asks why he must drink so much water, the *best answer* the nurse can provide is,
  ● 1. "It helps keep the catheter unobstructed."
  ○ 2. "It promotes the excretion of toxic wastes."
  ○ 3. "It helps increase your bladder capacity."
  ○ 4. "It promotes postoperative bladder retraining."

The physician performs a vaginal examination on a client in labor and states that the client is completely effaced and fully dilated.

15 At this time, the nurse is *correct* to plan nursing actions that meet the needs of the client who is entering the
  ○ 1. first stage of labor.
  ● 2. second stage of labor.
  ○ 3. third stage of labor.
  ○ 4. fourth stage of labor.

The physician writes an order for the nurse to give ½ ounce of ipecac syrup to a client who has ingested an overdose of a poisonous substance.

16 The nurse is *correct* in administering which one of the following equivalents?
  ○ 1. 30 mL
  ○ 2. 15 mL
  ● 3. 2 teaspoons
  ○ 4. 1 teaspoon

1 oz = 30 ml

A weak nursing home client falls repeatedly by slipping from the seats of various chairs.

17 The *most appropriate* action the nurse can plan to take is to
  ○ 1. use a sheet to tie the client to the chair.
  ○ 2. keep the client in sight at all times.
  ● 3. apply a front-releasing chest harness.
  ○ 4. put the client in a locked geriatric chair.

18 Which assessment finding *best justifies* withholding the continued intramuscular administration of penicillin (Bicillin) until consulting with the prescribing physician?
  ○ 1. The client states that the injection sites are painful.
  ● 2. The client shows the nurse a red, itchy skin rash.
  ○ 3. The client's body temperature has dropped to 100°F.
  ○ 4. The client's stool is dry and difficult to pass.

19 If a client provides the following information in a diet history, which one is the *most likely* contributing cause for the client's constipation?
  ○ 1. The client eats five daily servings of fresh vegetables.
  ○ 2. The client eats breakfast cereal with skim milk daily.
  ● 3. The client drinks an average of four glasses of liquids.
  ○ 4. The client substitutes grains and beans for meat.

20 If the nursing interventions used to reduce a client's anxiety are *effective,* the client will indicate that he or she feels
- ○ 1. less depressed.
- ○ 2. less hopeless.
- ● 3. less worried.
- ○ 4. less resentful.

A colleague asks a nurse to clarify the meaning of the abbreviation o.d. *used in a physician's drug order.*

21 The nurse is *correct* in explaining that the abbreviation stands for
- ○ 1. right ear.
- ○ 2. left ear.
- ● 3. both eyes.
- ○ 4. right eye.

A postoperative client asks the nurse to explain the purpose for the open wound drain, called a Penrose drain.

22 The *best explanation* is that an open wound drain is used to
- ○ 1. decrease the formation of scar tissue.
- ● 2. help fluid escape from the surgical area.
- ○ 3. provide a means for irrigating the wound.
- ○ 4. release accumulating intestinal gas.

During a home visit, the nurse asks a client to describe how be gives his oral medication through a nasogastric tube.

23 If the client reports all of the following, which action is *incorrect,* indicating a need for additional teaching?
- ○ 1. The medication is crushed finely and mixed with 30 mL of warm water.
- ○ 2. Prior to instilling the medication, the tube is flushed with 50 mL of water.
- ● 3. The liquefied medication is mixed into the tube-feeding formula and instilled.
- ○ 4. The tube is flushed after medication administration with 50 mL of water.

24 The *most appropriate* temperature for a cleansing, soapsuds enema solution is
- ○ 1. 70° to 85°F (21° to 30°C)
- ○ 2. 80° to 90°F (26° to 32°C)
- ● 3. 105° to 110°F (40° to 43°C)
- ○ 4. 120° to 130°F (48° to 54°C)

25 The *best nursing action* for enhancing a therapeutic outcome from postural drainage is to
- ○ 1. place the client in a supine position.
- ● 2. encourage the client to cough deeply.
- ○ 3. help the client select nutritional foods.
- ○ 4. instruct the client to breathe slowly.

26 When preparing a client for the insertion of a nasogastric tube, the *best position* for introducing the tube into the nostril is to have the neck
- ○ 1. flexed.
- ○ 2. rotated.
- ○ 3. circumducted.
- ● 4. hyperextended.

A previously healthy client is seen in the emergency department with severe nausea and vomiting within hours of having eaten in a restaurant.

27 Which assessment question is *best* for determining if a food-borne pathogen is the cause of the client's symptoms?
- ● 1. "What foods did you eat?"
- ○ 2. "Do you have a fever?"
- ○ 3. "Did your food look spoiled?"
- ○ 4. "Have you ever had food poisoning?"

28 If a care plan for a client receiving internal radiation therapy includes all of the following, which intervention needs to be revised because it is *potentially unsafe*?
- ○ 1. Maintain a radiation symbol on the outside wall or door to the client's room.
- ○ 2. Inform non-nursing personnel that the client is receiving radiation therapy.
- ○ 3. Wear a radiation monitoring badge when providing care to the client.
- ● 4. Assign the same personnel to consistently care for the client.

29 Following a perineal prostatectomy for cancer, which one of the following nursing actions is *essential* to include on the written plan for care?
- ○ 1. Perform the Valsalva maneuver during defecation.
- ○ 2. Maintain in high Fowler's position postoperatively.
- ○ 3. Administer laxatives to promote bowel elimination.
- ● 4. Provide perineal care following each bowel movement.

30 Which question is *essential* for the nurse to ask before a client undergoes an intravenous pyelogram (IVP)?
- ○ 1. "Are you afraid of needles?"
- ○ 2. "Have you ever had x-rays taken?"
- ● 3. "Do you have any allergies?"
- ○ 4. "When did you last urinate?"

31 Which diversional activity is *best* to include in the plan of care of a client with recent loss of vision?
- ● 1. Arrange for a radio or tapes.
- ○ 2. Promote verbal communication.
- ○ 3. Encourage listening to the TV.
- ○ 4. Provide books set in Braille.

An 8-year-old child is brought to the emergency department after falling from a swing.

32 Which assessment finding provides the nurse with the *best evidence* that the child has a compound fracture?
- ○ 1. Complaint of pain at the site of injury
- ○ 2. Abnormal mobility of the injured extremity
- ○ 3. Grinding sensation over the site of injury
- ◉ 4. Bone protruding at the site of injury

33 If a client is to receive 1000 mL of an intravenous solution in 8 hours, the nurse is *accurate* in checking that the electronic infusion device is administering an hourly volume of
- ○ 1. 50 mL.
- ○ 2. 100 mL.
- ◉ 3. 125 mL.
- ○ 4. 150 mL.

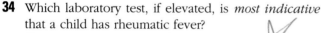

34 Which laboratory test, if elevated, is *most indicative* that a child has rheumatic fever?
- ○ 1. Latex agglutination test
- ◉ 2. Antistreptolysin O titer
- ○ 3. Heterophile antibody titer
- ○ 4. Fluorescent antibody test

35 When assisting with the discharge planning of a client who had a prostatectomy, which information is *most appropriate* to include?
- ○ 1. Avoid eating foods containing roughage.
- ◉ 2. Avoid heavy lifting and strenuous exercise.
- ○ 3. Use an enema if constipation occurs.
- ○ 4. Limit fluid intake to 8 glasses per day.

36 Which of the following nursing interventions is *best* to include in the plan of care for a client with expressive (motor) aphasia?
- ○ 1. Use a louder than normal voice when communicating.
- ○ 2. Write questions and directions for the client to read.
- ○ 3. Speak in short sentences to promote understanding.
- ◉ 4. Give the client time to respond to questions.

37 After assessing a closed water-seal drainage system that was inserted 4 hours previously on a client with a hemothorax, which finding needs to be reported *immediately*?
- ◉ 1. There is approximately 2 cm of water in the water-seal chamber.
- ○ 2. There is continuous bubbling in the water-seal chamber.
- ○ 3. There is dark bloody drainage in the collection chamber.
- ○ 4. There are diminished lung sounds in the lung with the hemothorax.

38 When assessing a femoral pulse, the nurse is *correct* to press his or her fingers
- ○ 1. behind the knee.
- ○ 2. on the dorsum of the foot.
- ◉ 3. into the inguinal area.
- ○ 4. over the lower tibia.

39 Which of the following data is the *best indication* that a pregnant client is in the transition phase of labor?
- ○ 1. The client states that she feels a gush of water coming from her vagina.
- ○ 2. The client states that she feels as if she needs to have a bowel movement.
- ◉ 3. The client tells her coach not to touch her, but also asks not to be left alone.
- ○ 4. The client tells the nurse that she cannot stop shivering and asks for blankets.

40 Which of a client's descriptions is the *best indication* that Kegel exercises are being performed correctly?
- ◉ 1. "I tighten and then alternately relax my perineal muscles."
- ○ 2. "I lie supine, and alternately raise and lower my legs."
- ○ 3. "I tighten my abdominal muscles for 45 seconds and repeat ten times."
- ○ 4. "I roll from side to back to side four to six times an hour."

41 The *best technique* for withdrawing a parenteral drug from a multiple-dose vial is to
- ○ 1. withdraw the entire volume in a syringe and discard the unneeded portion.
- ○ 2. inject 1 mL more of air than the amount of the drug to be withdrawn.
- ○ 3. refrigerate the vial for 10 minutes before withdrawing the drug from the vial.
- ◉ 4. inject the same volume of air into the vial as liquid that will be removed.

42 If all of the following actions are observed when a nurse administers an injection, which one is *potentially unsafe*?
- ○ 1. The nurse wears clean gloves when administering the injection.
- ○ 2. The nurse discards the empty syringe in a biohazard container.
- ◉ 3. The nurse recaps the needle securely before discarding the syringe.
- ○ 4. The nurse uses an alcohol swab to disinfect the injection site.

43 Which of the following assessment findings of a child with hemophilia indicates information that the nurse needs to report to the physician *immediately*?
○ 1. The child is experiencing anorexia.
○ 2. The child has discomfort from joint pain.
○ 3. The child's mood is somewhat depressed.
● 4. The child has developed nasal congestion.

44 Before discharging a client with leukemia, which question is *most important* for the nurse to ask?
○ 1. "Are you glad you are finally going home?"
○ 2. "Is there someone who will drive you home?"
○ 3. "Have you decided what you will do to keep busy?"
● 4. "Do you have any questions about your home care?"

45 When an unlicensed care technician provides care for a 10-month-old infant, which observation indicates the technician *needs additional teaching*?
○ 1. The room temperature is set at 75°F (24°C) during the infant's bath.
○ 2. For oral hygiene, the infant's teeth are swabbed with wet gauze.
○ 3. Prior to bathing, the water temperature is checked with an elbow.
● 4. The infant's chest is sprinkled with baby powder after the bath.

The father of a 4-year-old tells the nurse that he is concerned because his child frequently talks about a make-believe playmate.

46 The *best* nursing response is to
● 1. tell the father that this is normal behavior for a preschooler.
○ 2. help the father identify stressors that may be causing regression.
○ 3. recommend that the child be seen promptly by a child psychologist.
○ 4. recommend that the child be given a timeout when this is observed.

47 If the nurse notes multiple sores that appear like needle punctures on a client's arms, which category of drugs is it *most accurate* to suspect the client of abusing?
○ 1. Opiates
○ 2. Barbiturates
● 3. Amphetamines
○ 4. Hallucinogens

An older adult client is comatose and on life support. The family asks that life support measures be discontinued.

48 Which one of the following is *best* for determining whether it is appropriate to carry out the family's request?

○ 1. Considering the cost of continued life-support measures
○ 2. Checking if the client's insurance covers life-support measures
○ 3. Validating that all immediate relatives are in total agreement
● 4. Examining the specifications in the client's advance directive

49 When a client ingests a toxic substance either intentionally or accidentally, what information is *most important* for the nurse to obtain?
○ 1. The age of the client
○ 2. Who found the client
● 3. The substance involved
○ 4. The past medical history

A nursing assistant voices concern for her own safety when assigned to care for a client with acquired immunodeficiency syndrome (AIDS).

50 What information is *best* for allaying the nursing assistant's fears?
○ 1. The life expectancy for AIDS clients is longer than it once was.
● 2. AIDS is commonly transmitted by contact with blood and body fluids.
○ 3. Mechanical barriers, such as gloves, can prevent viral transmission.
○ 4. If infected, insurance may assist with the cost of care.

51 Immediately after a pregnant client's membranes rupture, the *most appropriate* nursing action is to
● 1. monitor the fetal heart rate.
○ 2. begin the client on antibiotics.
○ 3. put a waterproof pad beneath the client.
○ 4. place the client in Trendelenberg position.

52 When the client with a slow-bleeding cerebral aneurysm asks for assistance to the toilet for a bowel movement, which one of the nursing responses is *most appropriate*?
○ 1. The nurse complies with the client's request.
○ 2. The nurse offers to obtain a bedside commode.
● 3. The nurse places the client on a steel bedpan.
○ 4. The nurse suggests administering a suppository.

53 When performing the initial assessment of a newborn, the nurse collects the following data. Which one is *most important* for the nurse to report?
○ 1. Blue hands and feet
● 2. Flaccid muscle tone
○ 3. Heart rate over 100
○ 4. Loud, vigorous cry

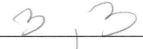

A maintenance worker in a health agency comes to a nurse after receiving a minor burn to a finger.

54 The *most appropriate* first-aid measure is to
○ 1. apply petroleum jelly to the burn.
○ 2. cover the burn with nonallergenic tape.
● 3. immerse the burned area in cool water.
○ 4. immerse the burned area in warm water.

55 Which assessment finding is the *best evidence* that a client with acute angle-closure glaucoma is responding to drug therapy?
○ 1. Swelling of the eyelids is decreased.
○ 2. Redness of the sclera is reduced.
● 3. Eye pain is reduced or eliminated.
○ 4. Peripheral vision is diminished.

56 The *most appropriate* nursing action before instilling ear drops is to
● 1. warm the medication to room temperature.
○ 2. refrigerate the medication for 30 minutes.
○ 3. clean the outer surface of the dropper.
○ 4. fill the dropper with no more than 1 mL.

57 The best reason for advising pregnant women to avoid consuming even as much as 1 ounce of alcohol per day during pregnancy is that its fetal effects might result in
● 1. mental retardation.
○ 2. congenital cataracts.
○ 3. seizure disorders.
○ 4. missing limbs.

58 Which one of the following is the best *initial* nursing response if a child confides information that indicates sexual abuse?
○ 1. Persuade the child to provide details.
○ 2. Examine the child for genital injuries.
● 3. Let the child know he or she is believed.
○ 4. Look for signs of sexually transmitted diseases.

59 When assessing a chronic alcoholic client who has been drinking up to the time of admission, the nurse is *most likely* to observe signs of alcohol withdrawal in
○ 1. 1 to 2 hours.
● 2. 4 to 6 hours.
○ 3. 12 to 72 hours.
○ 4. 3 to 7 days.

60 When caring for a client who has been burned about the face and neck, the *most important* nursing assessment is to observe for
○ 1. hearing deficits.
○ 2. signs of hemorrhage.
○ 3. patchy loss of hair.
● 4. respiratory distress.

61 When adding to the plan of care for a client with extensive burns, which nursing measure is *best* for preventing contractures?
○ 1. Encourage isometric exercises.
● 2. Perform range-of-motion exercise.
○ 3. Elevate extremities on pillows.
○ 4. Use a pressure-relieving mattress.

62 When a 17-year-old confides to the school nurse that she is sexually active, which community health referral is *most appropriate*?
○ 1. Parents Anonymous
○ 2. Parents Without Partners
● 3. Planned Parenthood
○ 4. Parent Action

63 When assessing the client with severe burns, which one of the following is the best evidence that the burn wound is infected?
● 1. The wound has a foul odor.
○ 2. The eschar is quite black.
○ 3. Urine output is increased.
○ 4. Pulse rate is decreased.

A 6-year-old child is recovering from acute noninfectious gastroenteritis. The physician leaves orders to advance the child to solid food.

64 Which one of the following foods is *best* for the nurse to offer the child *initially*?
○ 1. Vanilla pudding
○ 2. Chicken broth
○ 3. Cereal with banana
● 4. Strained applesauce

65 If all of the following activities are possible for a client with generalized anxiety, which one is *most therapeutic* for the nurse to recommend?
○ 1. Playing cards
○ 2. Assembling models
○ 3. Using a treadmill
● 4. Painting pictures

66 Which one of the following behaviors is the nurse *most likely* to find when observing a 2-year-old autistic child?
○ 1. Constant use of the words "I" and "me"
● 2. Preoccupation with repetitive behaviors
○ 3. Inability to separate from the parents
○ 4. Increased interest in others' actions

67 Which one of the following is *most appropriate* to include in the plan of care for an autistic toddler?
○ 1. Interactive play activities
○ 2. Ongoing use of soft restraints
● 3. Care by a consistent caregiver
○ 4. Rocking chair for calming the child

68 When collecting data from the parent of a child who has a tentative diagnosis of rheumatic fever, the nurse demonstrates an *accurate understanding* of the etiology by asking if the child has recently had
- ○ 1. chickenpox.
- ● 2. a sore throat.
- ○ 3. measles.
- ○ 4. mumps.

69 Which of the following signs or symptoms can the nurse *most expect* to find when assessing a child who has rheumatic fever?
- ○ 1. Urticaria
- ○ 2. Hypothermia
- ○ 3. Hypotension
- ● 4. Arthralgia

A 42-week gestation primigravida is having a nonstress test.

70 Which is the *best evidence* of an *unfavorable response* to the test?
- ● 1. Fetal heart rate accelerations of at least 15 beats per minute above baseline
- ○ 2. Fetal movement within 20 minutes of beginning the nonstress test
- ○ 3. More than 2 fetal heartbeat accelerations during a 20- to 30-minute period
- ○ 4. Each fetal heart rate acceleration lasting less than 15 seconds

The radiologist has used a red pencil to mark the skin on a client with cancer where radiation will be administered.

71 Which of the following actions is *essential* to this client's nursing care?
- ○ 1. Remove the marks by using ether or acetone.
- ● 2. Do not rub or use lotion on that area of skin.
- ○ 3. Keep the irradiated skin exposed at all times.
- ○ 4. Use talcum powder to absorb skin perspiration.

A client has been taking aluminum hydroxide gel (Amphogel) for 3 days.

72 If the client reports all of the following symptoms, which one is most likely a *side effect* of the antacid?
- ● 1. "I am constipated."
- ○ 2. "My skin itches."
- ○ 3. "My mouth is dry."
- ○ 4. "I feel tired."

A nursing assistant is assigned to care for a 5-year-old child with acute lymphoblastic leukemia.

73 Which of the nursing assistant's actions is *most indicative* of a need for additional teaching when caring for this child?

- ○ 1. The nurse assistant performs oral care using a sponge-type brush.
- ● 2. The nurse assistant assesses the child's temperature rectally.
- ○ 3. The nurse assistant maintains protective isolation precautions.
- ○ 4. The nurse assistant places a sheepskin under the bony prominences.

The physician prescribes sucralfate (Carafate) for a client with peptic ulcer disease.

74 When the client asks the nurse to explain the action of the medication, the *most accurate* response is that sucralfate
- ○ 1. makes gastric secretions less acidic.
- ● 2. covers the ulcer with a protective barrier.
- ○ 3. inhibits gastric acid production.
- ○ 4. blocks histamine receptors in the stomach.

75 When planning to irrigate a client's colostomy, the *most appropriate* volume of solution to use is
- ○ 1. 50 to 100 mL.
- ○ 2. 100 to 150 mL.
- ○ 3. 250 to 500 mL.
- ● 4. 500 to 1000 mL.

76 When administering eyedrops, the nurse is *correct* to instill them into the
- ○ 1. inner canthus.
- ○ 2. outer canthus.
- ○ 3. upper conjunctival sac.
- ● 4. lower conjunctival sac.

77 To determine the infectious status of a 6-month-old infant whose mother tests positive for the human immunodeficiecy virus (HIV), which laboratory test can the nurse *most likely* expect the physician to order?
- ● 1. Enzyme-linked immunosorbent assay (ELISA)
- ○ 2. Immunoglobulin A (IgA) test
- ○ 3. Western blot blood test
- ○ 4. Rapid plasma reagin (RPR)

78 Which physical assessment is *most appropriate* for the nurse to perform to determine if a homeless adult's unresponsiveness is due to an overdose of heroin?
- ● 1. Checking the size of the client's pupils
- ○ 2. Measuring the client's blood pressure
- ○ 3. Observing the client's response to pain
- ○ 4. Smelling the odor of the client's breath

79 Which position is *best* for the nurse to *avoid* when repositioning a pregnant client in labor who is receiving epidural anesthesia?
- ○ 1. Supine
- ● 2. Semi-Fowler's
- ○ 3. Right side-lying
- ○ 4. Left side-lying

The nursing team is developing a teaching plan for a newly diagnosed 10-year-old diabetic client who also has attention deficit disorder (ADD).

80 Which one of the following is the *most appropriate* teaching strategy for this client?
- 1. Provide individualized teaching in a quiet environment.
- 2. Plan group teaching with other children with ADD.
- 3. Administer penalties for inappropriate behavior.
- 4. Vary the method of instruction for each session.

A widowed person whose husband died 1 month earlier tells a nurse that she plans to sell her home and move into the home of her daughter and son-in-law.

81 Which of the following is the *best nursing response?*
- 1. Encourage the client to move on with her life.
- 2. Congratulate the client on making a hard decision.
- 3. Caution the client to postpone making major changes.
- 4. Suggest the client look into renting an apartment.

82 Which nursing action is *most therapeutic* for helping an older adult resolve her grief after the death of her spouse a month earlier?
- 1. Recommend taking a cruise with other senior citizens.
- 2. Inform her that grieving takes about 6 months.
- 3. Allow her to verbalize her feelings about her loss.
- 4. Refer her to an accountant for financial advice.

A nurse makes a home visit to check on an older adult who has been discharged for a month in the care of her daughter and son-in-law. The nurse observes that the older adult has several bruised areas on her arms.

83 Which of the nurse's assessment findings is *most indicative* that the older adult is a victim of elder abuse?
- 1. The client sleeps on a couch in the living room.
- 2. There are conflicting explanations for the injury.
- 3. The home is in need of being cleaned.
- 4. Perishable food is not refrigerated.

84 The *best evidence* that a client who has had a cancerous breast removed understands why her ovaries also will be excised is the client's explanation that the surgery is being done to
- 1. enhance the action of antineoplastic drugs.
- 2. slow tumor growth and metastasis to other sites.
- 3. prevent adverse reactions of antineoplastic drugs.
- 4. increase blood levels of progesterone.

85 What information about estrogen deficiency is *most appropriate* to include in the discharge teaching of a client who is recovering from having her ovaries removed?
- 1. Hot flashes and a feeling of warmth are common.
- 2. Menstrual periods are accompanied by heavy flow.
- 3. Leg cramps may occur during sleep and inactivity.
- 4. Orgasms may be absent or reduced in the future.

The family of an older adult consult a nurse about relocating their aging mother from her home to a nursing home.

86 Which nursing suggestion is *most therapeutic* for facilitating her transition to the nursing home?
- 1. Identify the costs and services of several facilities.
- 2. Involve the older adult in planning the relocation.
- 3. Consult with the older adult's personal physician.
- 4. Emphasize the positive outcomes of the relocation.

87 When planning the care of a client with an abdominal hysterectomy, which nursing measure is *most helpful* for preventing postoperative complications and facilitating an early discharge?
- 1. Re-establishing oral fluids and nutrition
- 2. Promoting ambulation and movement
- 3. Maintaining accurate intake and output
- 4. Exploring feelings about altered image

88 When a nurse discusses hospice care with the family of a terminally ill client, which statement is *most accurate?*
- 1. Hospice nurses give better care than hospital nurses.
- 2. Hospice nurses give around-the-clock care at home.
- 3. Hospice nurses empower personal end-of-life decisions.
- 4. Hospice nurses help extend predicted life expectancy.

89 Which behavior can the nurse *most expect* to find when observing an 8-year-old child who has attention deficit disorder?
- ○ 1. The child has difficulty understanding instructions.
- ○ 2. The child appears uninterested in the surroundings.
- ○ 3. The child refuses to play with others.
- ● 4. The child often fidgets and squirms.

A newborn infant of a diabetic mother is admitted to the nursery.

90 Which intervention is *most important* to perform *first* when providing initial care for the infant?
- ● 1. Check the infant's blood glucose level.
- ○ 2. Perform a gestational age assessment.
- ○ 3. Administer oxygen via an oxyhood.
- ○ 4. Begin phototherapy immediately.

The goal for the initial treatment of a newly diagnosed client with myasthenia gravis is to determine an effective maintenance dose of pyridostigmine (Mestinon), one of various anticholinesterase medications.

91 The *best evidence* that the client is experiencing an *overdosage* is that the client develops
- ○ 1. drooping eyelids.
- ● 2. muscle rigidity.
- ○ 3. labored breathing.
- ○ 4. extreme weakness.

A 17-year-old client is seen in the dermatology clinic for treatment of acne vulgaris that is affecting her face.

92 When teaching the client about facial skin care, the *most important* instruction for avoiding secondary infections and scarring is to
- ○ 1. avoid wearing cosmetics.
- ○ 2. apply a drying agent nightly.
- ● 3. avoid squeezing blackheads.
- ○ 4. scrub with a mild face soap.

93 It is *essential* that the nurse plan to instruct a client undergoing a repair of an inguinal hernia that postoperatively he must
- ● 1. avoid forceful coughing.
- ○ 2. empty his bladder often.
- ○ 3. turn to the operated side.
- ○ 4. limit early ambulation.

94 Immediately after a physician inserts a mercury-weighted intestinal decompression tube, which nursing action is *correct*?
- ○ 1. The nurse supports the tube so it can advance.

- ○ 2. The nurse connects the tube to mechanical suction.
- ○ 3. The nurse irrigates the tube to keep it patent.
- ● 4. The nurse offers the client sips of ice water.

A client takes ibuprofen (Motrin) for discomfort associated with osteoarthritis.

95 The *best evidence* that the client understands the hazards of taking a nonsteroidal anti-inflammatory drug (NSAID) is the client's ability to name which common side effect?
- ○ 1. Double vision
- ○ 2. Transient dizziness
- ○ 3. Irregular pulse
- ● 4. Upset stomach

96 The *best* emergency nursing treatment of a chemical burn is
- ● 1. irrigating the area with large amounts of water.
- ○ 2. using a towel or cloth to soak up the chemical.
- ○ 3. applying a thick layer of petroleum jelly.
- ○ 4. rubbing the burned skin with crushed ice.

97 Which nursing assessment is *best* for determining if oral-pharyngeal suctioning is necessary?
- ○ 1. Noting the type of cough
- ○ 2. Examining sputum color
- ○ 3. Observing ability to raise sputum
- ● 4. Counting the respiratory rate

98 Which instruction is *most appropriate* for the family of an older adult who struck her head and briefly lost consciousness?
- ○ 1. Give the older adult extra fluids for the next 72 hours.
- ○ 2. Keep the older adult flat in bed for the next several days.
- ● 3. Notify the physician if the older adult is difficult to arouse.
- ○ 4. Check the older adult's eyes, ears, and nose for signs of bleeding.

99 Which assessment finding is *most indicative* that there is an infection under a client's cast?
- ○ 1. There is a long crack in the cast.
- ● 2. There is a foul odor from the cast.
- ○ 3. There is blood on the cast surface.
- ○ 4. There is an indentation in the cast.

100 To avoid the potential for Reye's syndrome, it is *best* for the nurse to recommend that caregivers avoid administering which drug to their children?
- ○ 1. acetaminophen (Tylenol)
- ○ 2. ibuprofen (Nuprin)
- ● 3. aspirin (Anacin)
- ○ 4. naproxen (Naprosyn)

101 The *best evidence* that traction is maintained correctly is that the client's
   ○ 1. legs are parallel to the bed.
   ○ 2. comfort is not compromised.
   ● 3. weights are hanging free of the floor.
   ○ 4. feet are resting against the footboard.

102 Which cluster of assessment findings is *most suggestive* that a client is developing pulmonary edema?
   ○ 1. Bradycardia, transient confusion, mild anxiety
   ● 2. Orthopnea, sudden dyspnea, elevated blood pressure
   ○ 3. Tachycardia, decreased respiratory rate, weak pulse
   ○ 4. Flushed face, hypotension, thick tenacious sputum

A 5-year-old child is scheduled to have a cardiac catheterization at 8 AM.

103 Which of the following is the *best indication* that there has been appropriate preparation for the procedure?
   ○ 1. The child's chest has been cleansed with an antiseptic solution.
   ○ 2. The parents state that the child has had nothing by mouth since 6 AM.
   ● 3. The child has been shown pictures of the cardiac catheterization lab.
   ○ 4. The parents state that the child will not be conscious during the procedure.

104 The *first step* in planning a bladder retraining program for an incontinent client is to
   ○ 1. determine the client's voiding patterns.
   ○ 2. limit the client's oral fluid intake.
   ● 3. develop a regular schedule for urination.
   ○ 4. requisition a portable bedside commode.

105 The *best evidence* that a paraplegic client is correctly performing the Credé method to empty his bladder is that the client
   ● 1. inserts a straight catheter into the urethra.
   ○ 2. takes several deep breaths before trying to void.
   ○ 3. exhales slowly while tensing the abdominal muscles.
   ○ 4. applies light pressure over the bladder area.

The care plan for a 7-year-old child who has partial-thickness burns indicates that the child should be placed in the prone position for 2 hours each shift.

106 If the nursing assistant carries out the plan of care *correctly*, the nurse will observe that the child is positioned
   ○ 1. on his or her back.
   ○ 2. on his or her side.
   ● 3. on his or her abdomen.
   ○ 4. in a sitting position.

The nurse assesses a newborn infant that has just been admitted to the nursery from the delivery room.

107 Which assessment finding *best indicates* that the infant is experiencing respiratory distress?
   ○ 1. The infant has an abdominal breathing pattern.
   ○ 2. The infant has a respiratory rate of 40 per minute.
   ○ 3. The infant has an irregular breathing pattern.
   ● 4. The infant makes grunting sounds on expiration.

A male client who had a radical prostatectomy for advanced cancer is taking diethystilbesterol (DES).

108 Which effect is the client *most likely* to report as a consequence of the drug therapy?
   ○ 1. Increased facial hair
   ● 2. Breast enlargement
   ○ 3. Deepening of the voice
   ○ 4. Significant weight loss

109 Which is the *best plan* of action for reducing the abdominal incisional discomfort a surgical client experiences when coughing postoperatively?
   ○ 1. Tell the client to flex both knees while coughing.
   ○ 2. Have the client lay supine before trying to cough.
   ● 3. Apply light pressure to the incision with a pillow.
   ○ 4. Administer an analgesic soon after forced coughing.

110 What is the *best time* for providing a liquid nutritional supplement to an older adult who is not eating adequately?
   ○ 1. Just preceding the noon meal
   ○ 2. With other food at the noon meal
   ○ 3. Immediately after eating lunch
   ● 4. Between breakfast and lunch

111 Which plan for care is *most appropriate* for preventing urine and stool from soiling a hip spica cast that has been applied to an 18-month-old child?
   ○ 1. Insert cotton wadding between the cast and the skin in the perineal area.
   ● 2. Cover the perineal area of the cast with a waterproof material, such as plastic.
   ○ 3. Offer the bedpan at more frequent intervals.
   ○ 4. Place plastic pants over the perineal area.

A patient care technician is asked to assist a physician performing a lumbar puncture (spinal tap) on an 11-year-old child.

112 Which of the following indicates to the nurse that the patient care technician has positioned the client *correctly* for this procedure?
- ○ 1. The child is in the prone position with the head turned to the side.
- ○ 2. The child is in the recumbent position with the feet slightly elevated.
- ○ 3. The child is in the supine position with the head elevated 45 degrees.
- ● 4. The child is in the side-lying position with the knees drawn up and back flexed.

A nurse and a nursing assistant plan to transfer an adult client from bed to a wheelchair.

113 Which is the *best plan* for ensuring the client's safety during the transfer?
- ○ 1. Putting slippers on the client's feet
- ● 2. Locking the wheels on the wheelchair
- ○ 3. Raising the upper side rails on the bed
- ○ 4. Showing the client how to use the trapeze

114 If nurses react to a fire alarm in the following ways, which nurse is acting *most appropriately* for preventing the spread of a fire?
- ● 1. Nurse A, who closes all the inside doors
- ○ 2. Nurse B, who returns to the nursing station
- ○ 3. Nurse C, who searches for signs of smoke
- ○ 4. Nurse D, who stays with an immobile client

115 If the physician orders the irrigation of a urinary catheter but does not specify the type of solution to use, the *best choice* of solution is
- ○ 1. distilled water.
- ○ 2. warm tap water.
- ● 3. sterile normal saline.
- ○ 4. diluted hydrogen peroxide.

116 If a client has obstructive jaundice, which one of the following is the nurse *most likely* to observe?
- ● 1. Urine that is very dark brown
- ○ 2. Saliva that is tan and thick
- ○ 3. Stool that is green and watery
- ○ 4. Skin that is pale and quite dry

A nursing assistant reports that the hygiene of an African-American child has been neglected after observing a brown discoloration on the washcloth while bathing the client.

117 Which nursing explanation of the phenomenon is *most compatible* with the ethnic diversity of African-American clients?
- ○ 1. African-Americans bathe less to avoid dry skin.
- ● 2. This is a normal finding from shedding skin cells.
- ○ 3. Soap tends to remove melanin from epidermal tissue.
- ○ 4. The skin of African-Americans tends to retain oil.

When a nurse performs a mental status examination on an older adult, the previously cooperative client becomes silent when asked to spell the word "world" backwards.

118 Which is the *best nursing response* at this time?
- ○ 1. Discontinue assessing the client.
- ● 2. Go on to another mental assessment.
- ○ 3. Assume the client has early signs of dementia.
- ○ 4. Presume the client is functionally illiterate.

119 Which goal is *most appropriate* when managing the care of an older adult client who has osteoporosis?
- ○ 1. The client will consume more dairy products.
- ○ 2. The client will acquire increased bone density.
- ● 3. The client will ambulate without falling.
- ○ 4. The client will be restrained in a wheelchair.

120 Which assessment finding is *most likely* associated with the long-term effects of diabetes mellitus?
- ● 1. The client has diminished vision.
- ○ 2. The client has frequent indigestion.
- ○ 3. The client has urinary retention.
- ○ 4. The client has tremors at rest.

Correct Answers and Rationale

Part II of the Comprehensive Examination

Directions: Two numbers appear in parentheses following each rationale. The first number identifies the textbook listed in the references, page 512, and the second number identifies the page(s) in that textbook on which the correct answer can be verified. Occasionally two or more textbooks are given to verify the correct answer.

1 2. Aspirin is a known gastric irritant. It should be taken with food or milk; a buffered form would be helpful. None of the other medications are associated with gastric irritation. (18:1249)
Nursing Process—Data collection
Client Need—Physiological integrity

2 4. Getting additional rest is the best choice among the options for restoring energy during the demands of pregnancy. Although modifying the work routine to take advantage of times when energy is at its peak is beneficial, early morning rather than midafternoon is usually more of a prime energy time. It is poor advice to take more than the prescribed dose of a medication, including vitamins. Daytime napping is appropriate, even if the naps are short and frequent. (22:123)
Nursing Process—Implementation
Client Need—Health promotion/maintenance

3 2. Good sources of iron include liver, lean meats, legumes, dried fruits, green leafy vegetables, whole grain, and fortified cereals. Potatoes, oranges, and cheese are not good sources of iron. (6:208–209; 16:122)
Nursing Process—Planning
Client Need—Health promotion/maintenance

4 3. Naloxone hydrochloride (Narcan) is a narcotic antagonist that reverses the effects of opioids. Methadone hydrochloride (Dolophine) is an opiate-like drug. Both succinylcholine chloride (Anectine) and pancuronium bromide (Pavulon) are powerful neuromuscular junction blocking agents that are used as adjuncts to anesthetics. (20:195; 28:774)
Nursing Process—Implementation
Client Need—Physiological Integrity

5 1. Persons with anorexia nervosa often have *lanugo*, a growth of fine downy hair covering their body. This same condition is found among infants with low birth weights. It is thought that lanugo aids in maintaining body temperature in individuals who lack much subcutaneous body fat. The ability to manufacture blood cells may be impaired due to malnutrition. However, if bruising is noted, it is widely distributed about the body and not confined to just the upper torso. Club-shaped fingertips is a finding associated with longstanding cardiopulmonary disease. (6:374)
Nursing Process—Data collection
Client Need—Physiological integrity

6 3. A laxative is contraindicated for postpartum clients with a third- or fourth-degree laceration because this type of laceration extends into the rectal sphincter. Instead of a laxative, a stool softener is usually prescribed and clients are encouraged to increase fluid intake and ambulate to avoid constipation. Hemorrhoids, breast-feeding, and vacuum extraction are not reasons for omitting laxatives or enemas. (14:200; 16:227)
Nursing Process—Implementation
Client Need—Physiological integrity

7 2. Persons with only a few gallstones and mild symptoms experience relief by the application of shock waves that pulverize the stones. The smaller stones then move into the intestinal tract and are excreted in the stool. None of the other explanations are accurate. (4:711)
Nursing Process—Implementation
Client Need—Health promotion/maintenance

8 4. Dried beans, rice, peanut butter, peanuts, and whole grains are examples of plant proteins that are cheaper than animal proteins such as meat, chicken, fish, and dairy products. Plant proteins, taken in a sufficient amount or combined with a small amount of meat, can satisfy the protein needs of a pregnant woman. (16:121)
Nursing Process—Implementation
Client Need—Health promotion/maintenance

9 2. Postmenopausal females pick an arbitrary date and perform breast self-examination on that date each month. The time of day is not pertinent. Breasts are examined during a shower, when it is easier for the fingers to glide over the breast tissue. Breasts are examined monthly rather than once a year. (4:1022)
Nursing Process—Implementation
Client Need—Health promotion/maintenance

10 1. The presence of albumin in the urine is one of the three primary signs of preeclampsia, which is also referred to as toxemia of pregnancy and pregnancy-induced hypertension (PIH). Excreting albumin in the urine is not a sign of liver failure, amniotic embolism, or placenta previa. (14:130)

Nursing Process—Evaluation
Client Need—Physiological integrity

11 2. There is an association between infections with group A hemolytic streptococci and the development of rheumatic fever complicated by endocarditis. To prevent rheumatic heart disease and endocarditis, the American Heart Association recommends that children with streptococcal infections receive antibiotic therapy during their acute illness for at least 10 full days. Poverty and lack of insurance often deter parents from seeking medical treatment for ill children. Endocarditis is an inflammatory process that is not generally associated with birth defects, inadequate nutrition, or failure to receive immunizations for the usual childhood infectious diseases. (14:515; 16;750)

Nursing Process—Data collection
Client Need—Physiological integrity

12 2. Not all clients admitted to the labor department are given an enema, but some physicians include this as part of their routine admission orders. It is appropriate to withhold an enema for clients who are experiencing vaginal bleeding, and to collaborate with the physician. The physician and nurse collaborate on techniques for managing constipation. The nurse consults the physician before substituting a laxative for an enema. (16:163)

Nursing Process—Implementation
Client Need—Physiological integrity

13 3. The nurse's ultimate responsibility is for the safety of the patient. A change in vital signs is a sign of systemic complications such as hemorrhage and shock. Although withholding analgesic drugs may be helpful, it is not the best action to take at this time. Documenting the information, which is necessary, does not help the client improve. A Fowler's position will not raise the blood pressure. In fact, it may lower it even more. (4:453; 25:130)

Nursing Process—Implementation
Client Need—Physiological integrity

14 1. A large oral intake keeps the urine dilute and less likely to become plugged with blood clots and tissue debris. A large fluid volume does promote the excretion of toxic wastes, but that is not the best answer in this situation. The bladder capacity of a prostatectomy client is unaffected by the surgery.

Specific exercises are used to promote bladder retraining. (26:678)

Nursing Process—Implementation
Client Need—Health promotion/maintenance

15 4. The second stage of labor begins when the cervix is completely effaced and fully dilated and ends with delivery of the neonate. During the first stage of labor, the client has regular contractions that serve to dilate and thin the cervix. During the third stage of labor, the placenta is delivered. During the fourth stage of labor, the mother is monitored closely for complications such as hemorrhage. (14:186)

Nursing Process—Planning
Client Need—Health promotion/maintenance

16 2. One ounce is equal to 30 mL; therefore there are 15 mL in ½ ounce. There are approximately 5 mL per teaspoon. The equivalent of ½ ounce is 3 teaspoons. (17:35; 20:33)

Nursing Process—Implementation
Client Need—Physiological integrity

17 3. The first approach to preventing falls is to use a restraint alternative like a front-releasing harness. A restraint alternative is a protective or adaptive device that promotes safety and postural support, yet the client can release independently. Tying or locking a person in a chair is too restrictive unless previous trials with restraint alternatives have been ineffective in maintaining safety. A medical order is required before a restrictive restraint is applied. Keeping a client within sight at all times is impractical. (25:390–391)

Nursing Process—Planning
Client Need—Safe, effective care environment

18 2. The presence of a skin rash is highly suggestive of an allergic reaction common among individuals who are sensitive to penicillins. Before continuing to administer subsequent doses, the physician is consulted. The nurse uses alternative intramuscular injection sites and rotates the site of each injection when a site becomes painful. A drop in body temperature indicates that the drug is having some therapeutic effect. Constipation is not a common side effect associated with penicillin. (17:111)

Nursing Process—Data collection
Client Need—Physiological integrity

19 3. Four glasses of fluid is an inadequate volume of liquid to ensure moist stool. A healthy fluid intake from water and beverages is 1200 to 1500 mL, with an additional 700 to 1000 mL water in food sources. Eating five servings of vegetables, eating cereal with skim milk, and substituting plant protein sources for

meat are healthy dietary choices. Increasing dietary fiber promotes regular elimination of moist, bulky stools. (6:248; 25:232)
Nursing Process—Data collection
Client Need—Physiological integrity

20 3. The nurse can assume that anxiety-relieving interventions have been somewhat effective if the client says he or she is less worried. Most anxious people seem to worry unnecessarily or out of proportion to the reality of situations in which they are involved. Other data that support a reduction in anxiety include reduced heart rate and blood pressure, the ability to concentrate and remember information, restful sleep, and relaxed posture. (21:107)
Nursing Process—Evaluation
Client Need—Psychosocial integrity

21 4. The abbreviation *o.d.* indicates the right eye. The abbreviation for right ear is *a.d.,* and the abbreviation for left ear is *a.s.* The abbreviation for both eyes is *o.u.* (17:34)
Nursing Process—Implementation
Client Need—Safe, effective care environment

22 2. A Penrose and other types of open drains are placed within an operative site to help drainage escape from a surgical wound. Drains in a wound do not decrease scar formation. A drain may remove air if it is in the area of a wound, but it is not used to release intestinal gas. Nasogastric and nasointestinal tubes are used to remove air and secretions from the stomach or intestine. A drain is not used to irrigate a wound. (25:570)
Nursing Process—Implementation
Client Need—Health promotion/maintenance

23 3. Medications are never mixed with the total volume of tube feeding formula. They are instilled separately from the formula. The other steps that the client describes are safe and appropriate. (25:706)
Nursing Process—Evaluation
Client Need—Health promotion/maintenance

24 3. The solution used in a cleansing enema should be slightly higher than normal body temperature. Using temperatures higher or lower than 105° to 110°F (40° to 43°C) causes unnecessary discomfort. Solutions that are too warm or hot may burn the intestinal lining. (25:677)
Nursing Process—Implementation
Client Need—Safe, effective care environment

25 2. Coughing increases intrathoracic pressure, which facilitates raising and expelling secretions from the airways. The client's body position during postural drainage depends on which lobe(s) of the lung need draining. Lying supine does not encourage drainage from the lungs since it does not capitalize on using gravity. Selecting nutritional food is a healthy behavior, but it does not directly correlate with facilitating postural drainage. Breathing slowly may increase tidal volume, but it does not promote elimination of pulmonary secretions. (4:913)
Nursing Process—Implementation
Client Need—Physiological integrity

26 4. When introducing a nasogastric tube into a nostril, it is best to have the client, who is in a sitting position, hyperextend his or her neck. This position helps the nurse guide and direct the tip of the tube toward the pharynx. *After* the tube is in the oropharynx, the client is instructed to flex his or her neck, lower the chin to the chest, and the tube is advanced into the stomach. Circumduction and rotation of the neck do not facilitate insertion or advancement of a nasogastric tube. (25:600)
Nursing Process—Implementation
Client Need—Safe, effective care environment

27 1. Foods of an animal nature are generally involved in outbreaks of food-borne gastroenteritis. The pathogens tend to grow and reproduce when the food is not refrigerated properly or is undercooked. The appearance, flavor, and odor of contaminated food may be unaffected. The presence or absence of a fever and whether a client has previously had a food-borne infection do not necessarily reflect a diagnostic relationship to the present symptoms. (6:57)
Nursing Process—Data collection
Client Need—Physiological integrity

28 4. Care of a client receiving internal radiation therapy is best rotated among all nonpregnant members of the nursing team so that the time of any one individual's exposure to radiation is minimized. It is safe and appropriate to warn personnel and visitors of a potential hazard both verbally and using universal symbols. Radiation badges measure the amount of radiation exposure to the caregiver and, therefore, a different badge is worn by each individual involved in the client's care. (21:151–152)
Nursing Process—Evaluation
Client Need—Safe, effective care environment

29 4. Maintaining cleanliness of the perineum is essential following a perineal prostatectomy because of the high risk for wound infection from microorganisms in the stool. Straining during defecation is contraindicated; performing the Valsalva maneuver (bearing down against a closed glottis) therefore is inappropriate. A high Fowler's position can contribute to discomfort in the perineal incisional area. Laxatives generally are too harsh for prophylactically maintaining comfortable elimination of stool. (4:854; 18:1303)

Nursing Process—Planning
Client Need—Physiological integrity

30 3. An iodine-based dye is often used in diagnostic tests such as an IVP. A history of allergies is most important, especially if the client has a history of an iodine or seafood (which contains iodine) allergy. If the client is allergic to iodine, the physician is notified before the client has the IVP. (21:902)

Nursing Process—Data collection
Client Need—Physiological integrity

31 1. Of the four choices in this question, furnishing a radio or cassette tapes with recorded books or music is the most appropriate diversional activity for a newly blind client. Reading books set in Braille requires special education and time to practice the technique. The newly blind client may not be ready to interact with others as a means of diversion. Listening to the TV may create anxiety as the client can only hear and not see what is happening. (21:618)

Nursing Process—Planning
Client Need—Physiological integrity

32 4. A compound fracture is one in which the skin is impaired and the bone is exposed. Pain, impaired mobility, and crepitation may be present in closed fractures as well. (16:648)

Nursing Process—Data collection
Client Need—Physiological integrity

33 3. To determine the number of milliliters of an intravenous solution to infuse in 1 hour, the total quantity to be given (in this example, 1000 mL) is divided by the total hours of infusion (in this example, 8 hours). (25:281)

Nursing Process—Data collection
Client Need—Safe, effective care environment

34 2. An antistreptolysin O test is useful in the diagnosis of rheumatic fever. This test detects antibodies to the enzymes of the streptococcus Group A, which is thought to cause rheumatic fever, glomerulonephritis, bacterial endocarditis, scarlet fever, and other related conditions. A latex agglutination test is a nonspecific test that is elevated in many collagen diseases like lupus erythematosus. The heterophile antibody titer is performed to determine if a person has infectious mononucleosis. The fluorescent antibody test is used to diagnose syphilis. (11:357; 16:750)

Nursing Process—Data collection
Client Need—Physiological integrity

35 2. Discharge teaching for a client who has undergone a prostatectomy includes the warning to avoid heavy lifting and strenuous exercise until such activities are permitted by the physician. Constipation is avoided by eating foods high in roughage; enemas are avoided. A liberal fluid intake is encouraged. (21:878–879)

Nursing Process—Implementation
Client Need—Health promotion/maintenance

36 4. A client with expressive aphasia hears normally and understands verbal communication. However, the client has an impaired ability to provide a clear verbal response. Communication is improved in many instances if the nurse gives the client time to use motions or signs, write an answer (if able), or try to speak. Even though the speech of a client with expressive aphasia is greatly impaired, some can be understood if patience is taken when listening. It is inaccurate to assume that a client with aphasia is also compromised intellectually. (18:1107)

Nursing Process—Planning
Client Need—Physiological integrity

37 2. Continuous bubbling is abnormal in the water-seal chamber but normal in the suction-control chamber. When this finding is present in the water-seal chamber, it generally indicates that there is an air leak in the tubing between the client and the water seal chamber. The source of the air leak must be determined or the therapeutic benefit of the water-seal drainage system is compromised. (25:419)

Nursing Process—Data collection
Client Need—Safe, effective care environment

38 3. A femoral pulse is obtained by placing the fingers in the inguinal (groin) area. A popliteal pulse is felt behind the knee. The pedal pulse is felt on the dorsum of the foot. The posterior tibial pulse is felt in the lower leg. (25:149)

Nursing Process—Data collection
Client Need—Physiological integrity

39 3. During the transition phase of active labor the client may not tolerate touch, but fears being left alone. Rupture of the membranes may occur spontaneously or artificially at any point during labor. The urge to push (same feeling as urge to have a bowel movement) occurs during the second stage of labor. Shivering is a normal response that may occur during the fourth stage of labor. (16:182)

Nursing Process—Evaluation
Client Need—Health promotion/maintenance

40 1. Kegel exercises involve tightening and relaxing the pelvic floor muscles. The exercises are performed four or more times per day and 5 to 20 times each session. If performed consistently, Kegel exercises prevent or relieve stress incontinence, shorten the second stage of labor, promote healing for perineal and rectal incisions, and increase the potential for sexual orgasm. (21:941; 14:113)
    Nursing Process—Evaluation
    Client Need—Health promotion/maintenance

41 4. It is best to instill a volume of air equal to the volume that will be removed. Instilling air increases the pressure within the vial and facilitates removal of the drug. Omitting air instillation creates a vacuum in the vial once the drug has been withdrawn. Injecting more air than the amount of the drug to be withdrawn creates excessive pressure in the vial, which may force the plunger out of the syringe. It is not necessary to refrigerate a drug before withdrawing it from a vial unless refrigeration is recommended by the manufacturer. (4:420; 25:729)
    Nursing Process—Implementation
    Client Need—Physiological integrity

42 3. Recapping needles is a potentially hazardous action that can lead to needlestick injuries and possible transmission of blood-borne pathogens. Wearing gloves, swabbing the site, and depositing sharp items in a biohazard container are safe and appropriate actions. (25:728)
    Nursing Process—Evaluation
    Client Need—Safe, effective care environment

43 2. Mild to severe joint pain indicates bleeding into the joint, which can lead to joint deformities or destruction. Hemophiliacs with symptoms suggestive of bleeding need to have immediate medical attention. There is no direct connection between hemophilia and anorexia or nasal congestion. Depression may develop as a consequence of coping with a chronic illness. Depression indicates a need for additional nursing assessment for suicidal ideation and continued close observation. (18:909; 14:527)
    Nursing Process—Data collection
    Client Need—Physiological integrity

44 4. The nurse is responsible for determining that the client has sufficient information to manage his or her self-care after being discharged. Areas that are unclear, such as the medication schedule and follow-up appointments, are re-explained by the nurse and documented in the client's medical record. Questions about how the client is coping and plans for time management are thoughtful, but they are not more important that the client's ability to

manage his or her illness. It is considerate to inquire about home transportation, but the health agency is not responsible for providing transportation unless it is medically necessary. (25:88–89)
    Nursing Process—Data collection
    Client Need—Health promotion/maintenance

45 4. The use of powder is not recommended because of the risk for penumonitis secondary to aspiration of the talc. A room temperature between 72° and 75°F (22° and 24°C) is appropriate. It is also appropriate to use the elbow to assess the temperature of bath water because the elbow is most sensitive to temperature variations. Wiping the teeth with gauze is appropriate oral care for an infant; as an alternative, the mouth is cleaned by having the infant drink water. (16:540)
    Nursing Process—Evaluation
    Client Need—Safe, effective care environment

46 1. It is normal for a 4-year-old to talk to an imaginary playmate in the preschool developmental period. Preschoolers usually abandon imaginary playmates once they begin to interact more with children their own age. Since the behavior is not pathologic, it is inappropriate to look for unusual stressors, recommend the services of a child psychologist, or invoke a disciplinary timeout period. (14:373; 16:417)
    Nursing Process—Implementation
    Client Need—Health promotion/maintenance

47 1. Two abused drugs that may be injected into a vein are cocaine and heroin. Cocaine is also commonly snorted through the nose or inhaled by smoking it. Heroin is injected under the skin, a technique known as "skin popping," or directly into a vein. The other drugs are more commonly self-administered by the oral route. (20:482–483)
    Nursing Process—Data collection
    Client Need—Psychosocial integrity

48 4. An advance directive is a legal document that describes how a client wishes to be treated or not treated should the client, at some future time, be unable to make this decision independently. The client may also select a spokesperson, such as the physician or a spouse, to act on the client's behalf regarding using or withholding medical treatment. It is not necessary for *all* relatives of the client to agree or disagree on discontinuing life support. Financial cost is not considered a high priority in arriving at an ethical decision. (25:41)
    Nursing Process—Data collection
    Client Need—Safe, effective care environment

49 3. Correct treatment of poison ingestion and possibly the administration of an antidote depends on substance identification. The age of the client, who discovered the client, and the client's past medical history are relevant but of lesser importance than identifying the substance. (21:255)

Nursing Process—Data collection
Client Need—Physiological integrity

50 3. Reinforcing that easily implemented techniques can block the transmission of the virus from client to health care worker is the best information from among the choices. Being told the sources of transmission is not as reassuring as reiterating how the transmission is blocked. Even though many infected people are living longer and some receive medical benefits from insurers, that hardly gives peace of mind. (4:1171; 25:452)

Nursing Process—Implementation
Client Need—Psychosocial integrity

51 1. Immediately after the membranes have ruptured, the nurse monitors the fetal heart rate to detect fetal distress. Natural or artificial rupture of the membranes may result in prolapse of the umbilical cord, which is followed by compression of the cord and interference with fetal oxygenation. Applying pads does not take priority over assessing for fetal distress. Antibiotics are not routinely given when the amniotic membranes rupture. The physician may decide to place the client on antibiotics if the membranes have been ruptured for an extended period of time. If there is a prolapsed cord, the client is placed in the Trendelenberg position to assist with relieving umbilical cord compression. (16:181)

Nursing Process—Implementation
Client Need—Physiological integrity

52 3. Clients with slow-bleeding cerebral aneurysms are kept quiet to prevent additional or heavy bleeding. Until the physician indicates that it is safe for the client to increase activity, it is best for the nurse to position the client on a bedpan. A suppository is appropriate if the client is constipated. Clients who must avoid straining at stool, like this one, generally are given a daily stool softener to facilitate the ease of elimination. (21:559–560)

Nursing Process—Implementation
Client Need—Physiological integrity

53 2. Flaccid muscle tone is an assessment finding that is reported immediately. A healthy newborn generally is active and displays kicking of the feet and flexion of the arms. It is normal for a healthy newborn to have a pulse over 100 and display a loud, vigorous cry. The extremities may appear blue for a short time after delivery while the rest of the body

is pink. As the newborn's respirations improve and the baby is warmed, the skin color tends to become pink overall. (16:301)

Nursing Process—Data collection
Client Need—Physiological integrity

54 3. Minor burns over a small area are treated first by immersing the part in cool water. Cool compresses also may be applied. Ointments or salves are not applied to minor burns. Normally a dressing is not necessary. When a dressing is necessary, sterile gauze is first applied over the area and anchored with nonallergenic tape above and below the burn site. (4:1564)

Nursing Process—Implementation
Client Need—Physiological integrity

55 3. A therapeutic response following treatment of acute angle-closure glaucoma is a reduction or elimination of pain within the eye. Swollen eyelids are not a manifestation of acute angle-closure glaucoma. The conjunctiva is red during an acute attack of angle-closure glaucoma, but not the sclera. Loss of peripheral vision is a pathologic consequence of untreated or ineffectively treated glaucoma. (21:626)

Nursing Process—Evaluation
Client Need—Physiological integrity

56 1. Liquid and ointment otic (ear) preparations are warmed to room temperature if they have been stored in a cool or cold area. Instilling cold medication into the ear is uncomfortable. Unless the dropper is grossly covered with obvious debris, it is not necessary to clean it routinely. There is no limit on the maximum volume that is instilled within the ear. The anatomic size of the ear canal and the prescribed dose of medication are guidelines for how much drug is administered. (4:412)

Nursing Process—Implementation
Client Need—Physiological integrity

57 1. Fetal alcohol syndrome may result as a consequence of a mother consuming alcohol during a pregnancy. The syndrome leads to mental and physical retardation, structural anomalies involving the head, eyes (widely set), ears, and heart. As children with this syndrome get older, some develop attention deficit hyperactivity disorder. (9:241)

Nursing Process—Implementation
Client Need—Health promotion/maintenance

58 3. The best initial response is to assume a child is telling the truth when the subject involves sexual

abuse. Following that, nursing actions such as those in the alternative options is appropriate. (18:895)
Nursing Process—Implementation
Client Need—Psychosocial integrity

59 3. On average, signs of alcohol withdrawal are apparent in 12 to 72 hours. However, withdrawal may begin to occur as early as 4 to 6 hours among those who have a pattern of consuming large amounts of alcohol on a routine basis. Initially clients have a progressive elevation in their vital signs, tremors, and diaphoresis. If withdrawal is uncontrolled, seizures and hallucinations also occur. (9:237; 20:486)
Nursing Process—Data collection
Client Need—Psychosocial integrity

60 4. Burns around the face and neck may compromise breathing as a consequence of inhaling heated air and debris, or swelling of burned tissue. Hearing deficits and loss of hair may occur, but they do not represent as great a threat to care. Hemorrhage does not commonly occur with burns unless there has been an additional injury such as a wound or fracture. (21:1046–1047)
Nursing Process—Data collection
Client Need—Physiological integrity

61 2. Range-of-motion exercises, along with regularly changing a burned client's position, help to prevent contractures. Isometric exercises maintain muscle tone. Elevating extremities promotes venous circulation. Pressure-relieving devices maintain capillary blood flow, which is necessary for maintaining tissue integrity. (25:495)
Nursing Process—Planning
Client Need—Physiological integrity

62 3. Planned Parenthood is an organization that performs pregnancy tests, provides information on contraception and sexually transmitted diseases, supplies contraceptive devices, and assists with terminating pregnancies. Parents Anonymous provides support for abusive parents. Parents Without Partners is a social organization for divorced parents. Parent Action is a national organization that advocates for special interests affecting parents. (18:60)
Nursing Process—Implementation
Client Need—Health promotion/maintenance

63 1. A foul wound odor indicates an infection. The odor of infection is different from that of the odor associated with burn exudate. Eschar normally turns black after a period of time. An increase in urine output is unrelated to infection. Tachycardia might occur if an infection is present, but there are other physiological explanations for a rapid heart rate. (21:1051)
Nursing Process—Data collection
Client Need—Physiological integrity

64 4. When recovering from gastroenteritis, solid foods that are nonirritating to the gastrointestinal tract are added to the diet first. Foods such as bananas, rice, applesauce, toast (BRAT), tea, and yogurt (BRATTY) are provided initially. Milk products are among the last foods reintroduced to the diet. Both cereal and vanilla pudding contain milk. Salty broths, such as chicken broth, also are avoided. Furthermore, chicken broth is not a solid food. (11:195; 14:580)
Nursing Process—Implementation
Client Need—Physiological integrity

65 3. Large muscle activities that release nervous energy, such as using a treadmill, are best for clients with generalized anxiety. Playing cards, assembling models, and painting are too sedentary. (10:361)
Nursing Process—Planning
Client Need—Psychosocial integrity

66 2. Autism is characterized by unawareness of external reality, limited or no social interaction, abnormal speech patterns and conversational ability, preoccupation with repetitive behaviors, and a low range of interest in self or others. Autistic children rarely use the words "I" and "me." They do not exhibit the normal separation anxiety characteristic of the toddler. (11:250)
Nursing Process—Data collection
Client Need—Psychosocial integrity

67 3. A consistent caregiver or primary nurse facilitates development of a trusting relationship. Autistic children have a limited ability to interact with others. Restraints are not appropriate to use on a continuous basis since they increase the risk for injury; close supervision is preferred. Rocking is not appropriate because autistic children do not tolerate physical contact well. (11:250)
Nursing Process—Planning
Client Need—Psychosocial integrity

68 2. Rheumatic fever may follow a streptococcal infection. A history of a recent sore throat, which may have been due to the *Streptococcus* microorganism, is important information in the health history. Viral infections, such as measles, chickenpox, and mumps, are not known to be associated with rheumatic fever. (14:515)
Nursing Process—Data collection
Client Need—Health promotion/maintenance

69 4. Joint pain and tenderness (arthralgia) involving one or more joints is noted when assessing a client with rheumatic fever. Urticaria, hypothermia, and hypotension are not manifestations associated with rheumatic fever. (14:515)
    Nursing Process—Data collection
    Client Need—Physiological integrity

70 4. When performing a nonstress test, fetal movement must be present. For a nonstress test to be considered favorable, there also must be at least 2 fetal heart rate accelerations of at least 15 beats per minute within a 20- to 30-minute time frame. Each acceleration must last for at least 15 seconds. (16:101; 14:109).
    Nursing Process—Data collection
    Client Need—Physiological integrity

71 2. Mechanical friction further traumatizes skin that is affected by radiation. The skin is cleaned with mild soap, tepid water, and patting the area dry. The marks are never removed as they are meant to remain on the skin throughout the interim of radiation therapy. The irradiated skin is protected from direct sunlight. Clothing that covers the area of treatment should fit loosely. Powders containing metals are avoided because they absorb radiation and increase the potential for skin damage. (18:1154)
    Nursing Process—Implementation
    Client Need—Physiological integrity

72 1. Constipation is a side effect of antacids containing aluminum and calcium. Antacids containing magnesium cause a laxative effect. None of the other symptoms the client described are associated with antacid drug therapy. (17:257; 20:393)
    Nursing Process—Evaluation
    Client Need—Physiological integrity

73 2. Assessment of the temperature by the rectal route is avoided when a child has leukemia because of the danger of causing injury. Children with leukemia are maintained in protective isolation because of their compromised immune status. A sponge or gauze is appropriate to use for mouth care to prevent gums from bleeding. A sheepskin is placed under bony prominences for comfort. (18:911)
    Nursing Process—Evaluation
    Client Need—Safe, effective care environment

74 2. Sucralfate forms a protective coating similar to mucus at the site of the ulcer. This layer shields the irritated tissue from further irritation by hydrochloric acid and pepsin. Antacids neutralize gastric secretions, raising their pH. Histamine antagonists reduce gastric acid production by blocking H_2 receptors. (17:280–281)
    Nursing Process—Implementation
    Client Need—Health promotion/maintenance

75 4. The volume used to irrigate a colostomy is the same as the volume used to administer a cleansing enema. Commonly the volume for a cleansing enema and colostomy irrigation is between 500 and 1000 mL. (25:681, 689)
    Nursing Process—Planning
    Client Need—Physiological integrity

76 4. Eyedrops are instilled into the lower conjunctival sac. Before instilling eyedrops, the client is asked to look up as the lower lid margin is pulled downward by exerting downward pressure over the bony prominence of the cheek. (25:717)
    Nursing Process—Implementation
    Client Need—Physiological integrity

77 2. An IgA test is a more reliable test than the ELISA or Western blot test for determining the HIV status of infants and young children. The Western blot test and ELISA both evaluate the presence of IgG antibodies that can cross the placenta and give a false positive result if the mother is HIV-positive. IgA antibodies do not cross the placenta; thus, the presence or absence of IgA antibodies is more reliable. The rapid plasma reagin (RPR) is a serologic test used to detect syphilis. (14:522)
    Nursing Process—Data collection
    Client Need—Physiological integrity

78 1. Heroin, like morphine, causes the pupils to constrict. Although a person with a heroin overdose might be hypotensive, this finding is not as significant as finding pinpoint pupils. There may be multiple reasons as to why the client does not respond to pain. Heroin does not cause any characteristic odor to the breath as does alcohol or other medical conditions. (20:483)
    Nursing Process—Data collection
    Client Need—Psychosocial integrity

79 1. The supine position is contraindicated for a client who is receiving epidural anesthesia. The supine position causes vena caval compression and results in maternal hypotension. Hypotension reduces placental perfusion and fetal oxygenation. Semi-Fowler's and right or left side-lying positions do not cause vena caval compression. (16:211)
    Nursing Process—Implementation
    Client Need—Safe, effective care environment

80 1. The child who has attention deficit disorder needs to have an environment free of distractions to facilitate processing information. Group teaching creates

a greater potential for distraction. Rewarding desirable behavior is considered more therapeutic for effecting change than administering punishment. Having a consistent routine also proves to be more effective than varying the routine. (11:344; 14:387)
Nursing Process—Planning
Client Need—Psychosocial integrity

81 3. After the death of a spouse, it is important to eventually develop a new identity, learn new life skills, engage in new activities, and establish new relationships. Until the grief is resolved, however, it is important to delay making major changes. Rushing into decisions too soon often leads to regrets later. (3:442)
Nursing Process—Implementation
Client Need—Psychosocial integrity

82 3. Verbalization allows the bereaved to express emotions connected with their grief. Many people need to continue processing their grief over and over again, and they may not be given the opportunity by others who feel inadequate to deal with their emotional pain. Grieving is unique to each person, but it may take several years to resolve the loss of a significant person. Giving advice is nontherapeutic; clients may fear losing the support of the nurse if the advice is not taken. (3:442)
Nursing Process—Implementation
Client Need—Psychosocial integrity

83 2. Home care nurses must guard against making assumptions when their clients' environments do not reflect the nurses' values and standards. Although there are obvious health hazards in the home environment, such as its lack of cleanliness and disregard for refrigerating perishable food, the fact that there are conflicting explanations about the cause of the injuries is the most suspicious finding that suggests elder abuse. Providing a private bedroom is best, but a couch may be the only option at this time. (3:423)
Nursing Process—Data collection
Client Need—Psychosocial integrity

84 2. When a malignant breast tumor is hormone-dependent, growth is enhanced by the presence of estrogen, a hormone secreted by the ovaries. Removal of both ovaries removes the source of estrogen and thus slows metastasis and growth of any remaining tumor cells. This procedure does not enhance the action of antineoplastic drugs, prevent adverse reactions associated with the administration of antineoplastic drugs, or increase progesterone levels. (21:864)
Nursing Process—Evaluation
Client Need—Health promotion/maintenance

85 1. Symptoms similar to menopause, such as hot flashes, tend to occur when the ovaries are surgically removed. If there are no contraindications, estrogen replacement therapy can relieve many of the uncomfortable symptoms. Menstrual periods cease when the ovaries are removed. Orgasms are not affected by removal of the ovaries. Leg cramps are unrelated to the oophorectomy, but are important to report to the physician if they occur. (4:991)
Nursing Process—Planning
Client Need—Health promotion/maintenance

86 2. Involving the older adult in planning the transition reduces feelings of being powerless. Feeling that one is part of the solution is better than feeling that one is part of the problem. Obtaining factual information, consulting the physician, and reinforcing positive expected outcomes are helpful, but they are futile if the client feels a loss of control. (27:308)
Nursing Process—Planning
Client Need—Psychosocial integrity

87 2. Ambulation and movement help in preventing thrombi and hypostatic pneumonia. Early ambulation also promotes resumption of peristalsis, which facilitates oral nutrition. Although nutrition and fluids are important, the client's needs can be met temporarily with parenteral therapy. Intake and output are measures for assessing and evaluating if fluid replacement and output are adequate. The client's emotional adjustment demands nursing attention, but physical recovery is primary to the discharge goals. (26:718)
Nursing Process—Planning
Client Need—Physiological integrity

88 3. Hospice nurses are dedicated to facilitating the personal preferences of dying clients in managing how they wish to live and die. Secondarily, they are committed to supporting family members who tend to be the primary caregivers. The term "better nurses" is too subjective a statement. Hospice nurses have the same basic education and technical skills as hospital nurses. Although some dying clients live longer than expected, it is not an expected outcome of hospice care. (3:449–450)
Nursing Process—Implementation
Client Need—Psychosocial integrity

89 4. The child with attention deficit disorder has symptoms such as difficulty in concentrating, disruptive behavior, failing to complete tasks, constantly moving and fidgeting, and acting in a loud and noisy manner. The child understands, but does not follow directions well. This is attributed to the fact that

the child is easily distracted. Lack of interest in surroundings and refusal to play with others are not characteristic of this disorder. (11:344; 14:386)
Nursing Process—Data collection
Client Need—Psychosocial integrity

90 1. Infants of diabetic mothers often are hypoglycemic at birth or shortly thereafter; therefore the first nursing action is to assess the blood glucose level. If hypoglycemia is not detected and treated with either oral or intravenous glucose, the infant may develop severe, irreversible central nervous system damage and even die. Infants of diabetic mothers are often large for their gestational age, but this assessment does not take priority over determining whether or not the infant is hypoglycemic. The infant of the diabetic mother also is at risk for respiratory distress and hyperbilirubinemia. However, prior to giving oxygen or beginning phototherapy, the infant is evaluated to determine if there is a need for treatment. (11:123; 14:260)
Nursing Process—Implementation
Client Need—Physiological integrity

91 2. Signs of anticholinesterase drug therapy include muscle rigidity and spasm, salivation, and clenching of the jaw. Signs of drug underdosage are signs of the disease iteself, such as rapid fatigability, drooping of the eyelids, and difficulty breathing. (20:166)
Nursing Process—Evaluation
Client Need—Physiological integrity

92 3. Squeezing blackheads and pimples can cause spread of infection and scarring of the skin. A client with acne vulgaris can wear cosmetics, but should avoid those that are oil-based. Makeup is removed nightly with mild soap. Drying agents are avoided. (14:658)
Nursing Process—Implementation
Client Need—Health promotion/maintenance

93 1. To avoid undue strain and tension on the repaired muscle, clients who have undergone a hernia repair must avoid any activity that increases intra-abdominal pressure. Coughing, heavy lifting, sneezing, and straining to have a bowel movement can lead to an incisional hernia until the repaired area has healed. There is no reason for emptying the bladder any more frequently than to maintain comfort. There are no restrictions on turning. Ambulation is not limited unless the client develops a surgical complication. (4:694)
Nursing Process—Planning
Client Need—Physiological integrity

94 1. To facilitate movement from the stomach into the intestine, the nurse supports the tube rather than stabilizing the tube by taping it to the face. Suction is applied when the tube has reached the intestine, which may take several hours. Intestinal tubes may need to be irrigated, but that is not generally done before suction has been applied. Though the client is not allowed to drink or eat, small sips of water or ice chips may be offered after the tube is connected to suction. (21:704–706; 25:625)
Nursing Process—Implementation
Client Need—Safe, effective care environment

95 4 The most common adverse reactions with nonsteroidal anti-inflammatory drugs (NSAIDs) include nausea, vomiting, abdominal discomfort, diarrhea, constipation, and gastric or duodenal ulcers. Double vision, transient dizziness, and irregular pulse are not common side effects of NSAIDs. (20:401, 404)
Nursing Process—Evaluation
Client Need—Health promotion/maintenance

96 1. Emergency treatment of a chemical burn is directed at diluting and removing the substance as rapidly as possible by flushing the skin with large quantities of water. Water is more useful than a towel. Ointments are not applied to a burn in the initial stage of treatment. Rubbing the skin intensifies the burn injury. (18:349)
Nursing Process—Implementation
Client Need—Physiological integrity

97 3. Suctioning is performed when the client is unable to cough and raise sputum. Ineffective coughing and raising sputum, dyspnea, cyanosis, and moist breath sounds indicate suctioning is necessary. Identifying the type of cough, characteristics of sputum, and respiratory rate are important assessments, but they are not criteria for determining the necessity for suctioning a client. (18:1189–1190)
Nursing Process—Data collection
Client Need—Physiological integrity

98 3. Changes in the level of consciousness is a clinical indication of intracranial bleeding. If drowsiness or sleepiness occurs and the client cannot be easily aroused, the physician is notified. Drinking extra fluids or keeping the client in bed usually are not necessary. Although it is important to observe for signs of bleeding, the most dangerous bleeding occurs within the skull. (21:567–568)
Nursing Process—Implementation
Client Need—Health promotion/maintenance

99 2. The presence of a foul or unusual odor from within a cast indicates an infection. Blood on the cast sur-

face indicates bleeding beneath the cast. A crack or indentation in the cast does not indicate infection but compromises the integrity of the cast. (18:991)
Nursing Process—Data collection
Client Need—Physiological integrity

100 3. Studies suggest that the use of salicylates, especially aspirin, to relieve a fever or discomfort during a viral illness may lead to Reye's syndrome. Tylenol is safe for the relief of minor symptoms like fever and headache. Ibuprofen and naproxen are effective in relieving pain. (14:617)
Nursing Process—Implementation
Client Need—Health promotion/maintenance

101 3. One of the necessary criteria for maintaining the effectiveness of traction is that the weights must hang free of the floor. The legs may or may not be parallel to the bed, depending on the type of traction that is applied. Comfort is a desirable outcome of traction, but comfort is not an indication of traction effectiveness. If the feet resist the pull of traction by resting on the footboard, the traction's efficiency is reduced. (25:527)
Nursing Process—Evaluation
Client Need—Safe, effective care environment

102 2. The symptoms of pulmonary edema include sudden dyspnea, pink frothy sputum, cyanosis, bounding pulse, elevated blood pressure, severe apprehension, and moist or gurgling respirations. (21:421)
Nursing Process—Data collection
Client Need—Physiological integrity

103 3. If an actual visit to the cardiac catheterization lab cannot be arranged, then pictures of the equipment and cardiac catheterization lab facilitate the teaching process. The child should have nothing by mouth for at least 4 hours prior to the procedure. The site of catheter insertion is the femoral artery or an antecubital vessel; therefore the chest is not cleansed with an antiseptic. The child is lightly sedated, but is not unconscious. (14:507)
Nursing Process—Evaluation
Client Need—Safe, effective care environment

104 1. The first step in planning a bladder retraining program is determining the client's voiding pattern. Knowing the voiding pattern facilitates developing a voiding schedule. Limiting the fluid intake is not recommended; the client needs an adequate fluid intake to keep the urine dilute and prevent fluid deficit. Requisitioning a commode, if appropriate

for the client, is done after collecting data about the voiding pattern. (25:640)
Nursing Process—Planning
Client Need—Physiological integrity

105 4. Credé's method is performed by increasing abdominal pressure over the bladder. This technique involves using both hands to apply light pressure over the bladder. Voiding occurs without the use of a catheter. The maneuver does not include any special breathing techniques. (25:640)
Nursing Process—Evaluation
Client Need—Physiological integrity

106 3. The prone position is one in which the client is placed on his or her abdomen. If a supine position is indicated, the client is placed on his or her back. A side-lying position is a lateral position. A sitting position is referred to as a semi-Fowler's position. (18:497)
Nursing Process—Evaluation
Client Need—Safe, effective care environment

107 4. Grunting on expiration is a sign of respiratory distress. It indicates that the infant is making an extra effort to move air out of the lungs. Newborn infants normally have a respiratory rate between 30 and 60 breaths per minute. They also normally breathe abdominally and have an irregular breathing pattern. (16:290)
Nursing Process—Data collection
Client Need—Physiological integrity

108 2. Breast enlargement, also known as gynecomastia, is an expected effect of administering diethylstilbesterol, a synthetic estrogen, to a male. Other feminizing effects of diethylstilbesterol include a decrease in facial hair, a higher vocal pitch, and weight gain from fluid retention. (20:442)
Nursing Process—Data collection
Client Need—Physiological integrity

109 3. Placing a pillow on the abdomen and applying firm, light pressure reduces strain on the incision, which reduces discomfort. Flexing the knees or lying supine are not as likely to promote comfort as applying pressure. It is more advantageous to administer an analgesic shortly before a client coughs or performs other discomfort-producing activities, rather than afterward. (25:551)
Nursing Process—Planning
Client Need—Physiological integrity

110 4. Liquid nutritional supplements are best offered between meals so that the supplement is not substituted for the meal itself. A liquid supplement may not be totally consumed if it is offered with a meal or soon afterward. If it is given before a meal, the client may reduce the amount of food prepared for the meal. (1:282)

> **Nursing Process—Planning**
> **Client Need—Physiological integrity**

111 2. Covering the perineal area with waterproof material, such as plastic, helps to prevent soiling the cast. Cotton wadding is not inserted unless ordered by the physician. Offering the bedpan at more frequent intervals does not necessarily prevent soiling of the cast, especially if the child is not toilet-trained (which is unlikely for an 18-month-old child). Plastic pants are contraindicated because they hold moisture and contribute to the disintegration of the cast. (22:684)

> **Nursing Process—Planning**
> **Client Need—Physiological integrity**

112 4. When a lumbar puncture is performed, the client is placed in a side-lying position with the knees drawn up and the back flexed, or placed in a sitting position with the back flexed. Both of these positions increase the space between the vertebrae to facilitate insertion of the needle within the interspaces with minimal trauma. (16:497)

> **Nursing Process—Evaluation**
> **Client Need—Safe, effective care environment**

113 2. Locking the wheels ensures that the wheelchair remains in place during the transfer. Wearing slippers provides warmth and some protection for the client's feet, but they are not as important as locking the wheels. Raised side rails and a trapeze help the client assist in changing positions, but they are not the best safety measures during a transfer. (25:482)

> **Nursing Process—Planning**
> **Client Need—Safe, effective care environment**

114 1. Closing doors helps keep the fire confined to its location of origin and slows or prevents its spread into other areas. It is important to assemble at the nursing station to await instructions, but this activity is appropriate after the environment is secured. Searching for smoke takes valuable time that is better spent in closing doors. Staying with an immobile client is admirable, but nurses have a responsibility to ensure the protection of all clients, rather than just one who may have difficulty evacuating. (25:385)

> **Nursing Process—Evaluation**
> **Client Need—Safe, effective care environment**

115 3. Unless the physician orders otherwise, the standard for care is to use sterile, normal saline when irrigating an indwelling catheter. It is incorrect to use an unsterile solution of distilled water or tap water. Hydrogen peroxide is not commonly used when irrigating urinary catheters. (25:658)

> **Nursing Process—Planning**
> **Client Need—Physiological integrity**

116 1. A characteristic of obstructive jaundice is dark brown urine. The change in color is due to excretion of bilirubin via the kidneys rather than through the intestinal tract. The other physical assessments have no relationship to obstructive jaundice. (18:1264)

> **Nursing Process—Data collection**
> **Client Need—Physiological integrity**

117 2. All ethnic groups lose dead skin cells during bathing. In African-American clients, the dead skin cells are more obvious because they retain their pigmentation. This finding is often misinterpreted as a disregard for hygiene. There is as much ethnic variation in dryness or oiliness of skin among African-Americans as in other ethnic groups. Soap cannot physically or chemically remove pigmentation. (18:69)

> **Nursing Process—Evaluation**
> **Client Need—Safe, effective care environment**

118 2. Moving on to another area of assessment shows respect for the client; the lack of response to the assessment is documented, however. With only limited data, it is inaccurate to assume that a client who does not respond is demented or illiterate. Failure to respond to one area of assessment does not justify discontinuing further efforts to assess mental status. (1:303)

> **Nursing Process—Evaluation**
> **Client Need—Safe, effective care environment**

119 3. Preventing falls is a major goal when caring for clients with osteoporosis. Even a minor fall can result in a fracture. Consuming dairy products is a healthy behavior, but it is not likely to reverse longstanding osteoporosis. Increasing bone density may be a goal of medical therapy. Having osteoporosis does not justify restraining a client in a wheelchair. (1:191)

> **Nursing Process—Planning**
> **Client Need—Physiological integrity**

120 1. Clients with diabetes mellitus are prone to developing visual changes that may result in blindness. Other diabetic complications include renal failure, coronary artery disease, and peripheral nerve damage. Indigestion, urinary retention, and tremors are significant problems, but they are not common complications of diabetes mellitus. (1:192)

> **Nursing Process—Data collection**
> **Client Need—Physiological integrity**

11:011 — 11:44 34 min — 57 min
11:48 — 12:011 23 min

Classification of Test Items

Part II of the Comprehensive Examination

Directions: After each question the correct answer is given, as well as a classification of each test question. Compare the correct answer with your answer. If a question has been answered *incorrectly*, draw a line to the end of all the columns. When finished, add up the number of your correct answers in each column and place that number in the respective box at the end in the area identified as *Number Correct*.

To determine the percentage of questions you answered correctly and your performance in each of the test plan categories, divide the *Number Correct* in each column by the *Number Possible* in each column. Then multiply the decimal by 100. For example:

$$\frac{\text{Number Correct: } 90}{\text{Number Possible: } 120} = 0.75 \times 100 = 75\%$$

Any score that is less than 75% indicates an area where further review would be beneficial.

KEY TO ITEM CLASSIFICATION:

NURSING PROCESS

D = Data collection
P = Planning
I = Implementation
E = Evaluation

CLIENT NEEDS

S = Safe, effective care environment
P = Physiological integrity
M = Psychosocial integrity
H = Health promotion/maintenance

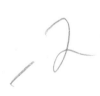

		Nursing Process				Client Needs			
Question #	Answer #	D	P	I	E	S	P	M	H
1	2	D					P		
2	4			I					H
3	2		P						H
4	3			I			P		
5	1	D					P		
6	3			I			P		
7	2			I					H
8	4			I					H
9	2			I					H
10	1				E		P		
11	2	D					P		
12	2			I			P		
13	3			I			P		
14	1			I					H
15	4		P						H

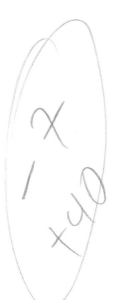

Question #	Answer #	Nursing Process				Client Needs			
		D	P	I	E	S	P	M	H
16	2			I			P		
17	3		P			S			
18	2	D					P		
19	3	D					P		
20	3				E			M	
21	4			I		S			
22	2			I					H
23	3				E				H
24	3			I		S			
25	2			I			P		
26	4			I		S			
27	1	D					P		
28	4				E	S			
29	4		P				P		
30	3	D					P		
31	1		P				P		
32	4	D					P		
33	3	D				S			
34	2	D					P		
35	2			I					H
36	4		P				P		
37	2	D				S			
38	3	D					P		
39	3				E				H
40	1				E				H
41	4			I			P		
42	3				E	S			
43	2	D					P		
44	4	D							H
45	4				E	S			
46	1			I					H
47	1	D						M	

3 | 3 | 2 | 3 | 1

		Nursing Process				Client Needs			
Question #	Answer #	D	P	I	E	S	P	M	H
48	4	D				S			
49	3	D					P		
50	3			I				M	
51	1			I			P		
52	3			I			P		
53	2	D					P		
54	3			I			P		
55	3				E		P		
56	1			I			P		
57	1			I					H
58	3			I				M	
59	3	D						M	
60	4	D					P		
61	2		P				P		
62	3			I					H
63	1	D					P		
64	4			I			P		
65	3		P					M	
66	2	D						M	
67	3		P					M	
68	2	D							H
69	4	D					P		
70	4	D					P		
71	2			I			P		
72	1				E		P		
73	2				E	S			
74	2			I					H
75	4		P				P		
76	4			I			P		
77	2	D					P		
78	1	D						M	
79	1			I		S			

	Question #	Answer #	Nursing Process				Client Needs			
			D	P	I	E	S	P	M	H
	80	1		P					M	
	81	3			I				M	
	82	3			I				M	
	83	2	D						M	
	84	2				E				H
	85	1		P						H
	86	2		P					M	
	87	2		P				P		
	88	3			I				M	
	89	4	D						M	
	90	1			I			P		
	91	2				E		P		
	92	3			I					H
	93	1		P				P		
	94	1			I		S			
	95	4				E				H
	96	1			I			P		
	97	3	D					P		
	98	3			I					H
	99	2	D					P		
	100	3			I					H
	101	3				E	S			
	102	2	D					P		
	103	3				E	S			
	104	1		P				P		
	105	4				E		P		
	106	3				E	S			
	107	4	D					P		
	108	2	D					P		
	109	3		P				P		
	110	4		P				P		
	111	2		P				P		

Question #	Answer #	Nursing Process				Client Needs			
		D	P	I	E	S	P	M	H
112	4				E	S			
113	2		P			S			
114	1				E	S			
115	3		P				P		
116	1	D					P		
117	2				E	S			
118	2				E	S			
119	3		P				P		
120	1	D					P		
Number Correct	102	29	19	34	21	18	51	11	23
Number Possible	120	36	22	40	22	21	59	16	24
Percentage Correct	85	81	86	85	95	86	86	69	96

7 3 6 1 3 8 5 1

−18
+102

REFERENCES

1. Anderson, M. A., Braun, J. V. (1995). *Caring for the elderly client*. Philadelphia: F.A. Davis.
2. Barry, P. D. (1994). *Mental health and mental illness* (5th ed.). Philadelphia: J.B. Lippincott.
3. Burke, M. M., Walsh, M. B. (1992). *Gerontologic nursing: care of the frail elderly*. St. Louis: Mosby-Year Book.
4. Christensen, B. L., Kockrow, E. O. (editors) (1995). *Foundations of nursing* (2nd ed.). St. Louis: C.V. Mosby.
5. Edmunds, M. W. (1995). *Introduction to clinical pharmacology* (2nd ed.). St. Louis: C.V. Mosby.
6. Eschleman, M. M. (1996). *Introductory nutrition and nutrition therapy* (3rd ed.). Philadelphia: J.B. Lippincott.
7. Fischbach, F. T. (1996). *A manual of laboratory and diagnostic tests* (5th ed.). Philadelphia: J.B. Lippincott.
8. Harkness, G. A., Dincher, J. R. (1996). *Medical-surgical nursing total patient care* (9th ed.). St. Louis: C.V. Mosby.
9. Kalman, N., Waughfield, C. G. (1993). *Mental health concepts* (3rd ed.). Albany: Delmar.
10. Keltner, N. L., Schwecke, L. H., Bostrom, C. E. (1995). *Psychiatric nursing* (2nd ed.). St. Louis: C.V. Mosby.
11. Marks, M. G. (1994). *Broadribb's introductory pediatric nursing* (4th ed.). Philadelphia: J.B. Lippincott.
12. Memmler, R. L., Cohen, B. J., Wood, D. L. (1996). *Structure & function of the human body* (6th ed.). Philadelphia: J.B. Lippincott.
13. Memmler, R. L., Cohen, B. J., Wood, D. L. (1996). *The human body in health and disease* (8th ed.). Philadelphia: J.B. Lippincott.
14. Neff, C., Spray, M. (1996). *Introduction to maternal and child health nursing*. Philadelphia: J.B. Lippincott.
15. Nettina, S. M. (1996). *The Lippincott manual of nursing practice* (6th ed.). Philadelphia: J.B. Lippincott.
16. Novak, J. C., Broom, B. L. (1995). *Ingall's and Salerno's maternal and child health nursing* (8th ed.). St. Louis: C.V. Mosby.
17. Reiss, B. S., Evans, M. E. (1996). *Pharmacological aspects of nursing care* (5th ed.). Albany: Delmar.
18. Rosdahl, C. B. (1995). *Textbook of basic nursing* (6th ed.). Philadelphia: J.B. Lippincott.
19. Scanlon, V. C., Sanders, T. (1991). *Essentials of anatomy and physiology* (2nd ed.). Philadelphia: F.A. Davis.
20. Scherer, J. C., Roach, S. S. (1996). *Introductory clinical pharmacology* (5th ed.). Philadelphia: J.B. Lippincott.
21. Scherer, J. C., Timby, B. K. (1995). *Introductory medical-surgical nursing* (6th ed.). Philadelphia: J.B. Lippincott.
22. Shapiro, P. J. (1995). *Basic maternal/pediatric nursing*. Albany: Delmar.
23. Shives, L. R. (1994). *Basic concepts of psychiatric-mental health nursing* (3rd ed.). Philadelphia: J.B. Lippincott.
24. Smeltzer, S. C., Bare, B. G. (1996). *Brunner and Suddarth's textbook of medical-surgical nursing* (8th ed.). Philadelphia: J.B. Lippincott.
25. Timby, B. K. (1996). *Fundamental skills and concepts in patient care* (6th ed.). Philadelphia: J.B. Lippincott.
26. Tucker, S. M., Canabbio, M. M., Paquette, E. V., Wells, M. F. (1996). *Patient care standards: collaborative practice planning guides* (6th ed.). St. Louis: C.V. Mosby.
27. Wold, G. (1993). *Basic geriatric nursing*. St. Louis: C.V. Mosby.
28. *1996 Lippincott's nursing drug guide* (1996). Philadelphia: J.B. Lippincott.

Answer Sheet

Unit I Review Test 1

With a pencil, blacken the circle below the option you have chosen for your correct answer.

	1 2 3 4		1 2 3 4		1 2 3 4		1 2 3 4
1	○○○○	22	○○○○	43	○○○○	64	○○○○
2	○○○○	23	○○○○	44	○○○○	65	○○○○
3	○○○○	24	○○○○	45	○○○○	66	○○○○
4	○○○○	25	○○○○	46	○○○○	67	○○○○
5	○○○○	26	○○○○	47	○○○○	68	○○○○
6	○○○○	27	○○○○	48	○○○○	69	○○○○
7	○○○○	28	○○○○	49	○○○○	70	○○○○
8	○○○○	29	○○○○	50	○○○○	71	○○○○
9	○○○○	30	○○○○	51	○○○○	72	○○○○
10	○○○○	31	○○○○	52	○○○○	73	○○○○
11	○○○○	32	○○○○	53	○○○○	74	○○○○
12	○○○○	33	○○○○	54	○○○○	75	○○○○
13	○○○○	34	○○○○	55	○○○○	76	○○○○
14	○○○○	35	○○○○	56	○○○○	77	○○○○
15	○○○○	36	○○○○	57	○○○○	78	○○○○
16	○○○○	37	○○○○	58	○○○○	79	○○○○
17	○○○○	38	○○○○	59	○○○○	80	○○○○
18	○○○○	39	○○○○	60	○○○○	81	○○○○
19	○○○○	40	○○○○	61	○○○○	82	○○○○
20	○○○○	41	○○○○	62	○○○○	83	○○○○
21	○○○○	42	○○○○	63	○○○○	84	○○○○

#	1 2 3 4	#	1 2 3 4	#	1 2 3 4	#	1 2 3 4
85	○ ○ ○ ○	102	○ ○ ○ ○	119	○ ○ ○ ○	136	○ ○ ○ ○
86	○ ○ ○ ○	103	○ ○ ○ ○	120	○ ○ ○ ○	137	○ ○ ○ ○
87	○ ○ ○ ○	104	○ ○ ○ ○	121	○ ○ ○ ○	138	○ ○ ○ ○
88	○ ○ ○ ○	105	○ ○ ○ ○	122	○ ○ ○ ○	139	○ ○ ○ ○
89	○ ○ ○ ○	106	○ ○ ○ ○	123	○ ○ ○ ○	140	○ ○ ○ ○
90	○ ○ ○ ○	107	○ ○ ○ ○	124	○ ○ ○ ○	141	○ ○ ○ ○
91	○ ○ ○ ○	108	○ ○ ○ ○	125	○ ○ ○ ○	142	○ ○ ○ ○
92	○ ○ ○ ○	109	○ ○ ○ ○	126	○ ○ ○ ○	143	○ ○ ○ ○
93	○ ○ ○ ○	110	○ ○ ○ ○	127	○ ○ ○ ○	144	○ ○ ○ ○
94	○ ○ ○ ○	111	○ ○ ○ ○	128	○ ○ ○ ○	145	○ ○ ○ ○
95	○ ○ ○ ○	112	○ ○ ○ ○	129	○ ○ ○ ○	146	○ ○ ○ ○
96	○ ○ ○ ○	113	○ ○ ○ ○	130	○ ○ ○ ○	147	○ ○ ○ ○
97	○ ○ ○ ○	114	○ ○ ○ ○	131	○ ○ ○ ○	148	○ ○ ○ ○
98	○ ○ ○ ○	115	○ ○ ○ ○	132	○ ○ ○ ○	149	○ ○ ○ ○
99	○ ○ ○ ○	116	○ ○ ○ ○	133	○ ○ ○ ○	150	○ ○ ○ ○
100	○ ○ ○ ○	117	○ ○ ○ ○	134	○ ○ ○ ○		
101	○ ○ ○ ○	118	○ ○ ○ ○	135	○ ○ ○ ○		

Answer Sheet

Unit **I** Review Test **2**

With a pencil, blacken the circle below the option you have chosen for your correct answer.

	1 2 3 4		1 2 3 4		1 2 3 4		1 2 3 4
1	○○○○	22	○○○○	43	○○○○	64	○○○○
2	○○○○	23	○○○○	44	○○○○	65	○○○○
3	○○○○	24	○○○○	45	○○○○	66	○○○○
4	○○○○	25	○○○○	46	○○○○	67	○○○○
5	○○○○	26	○○○○	47	○○○○	68	○○○○
6	○○○○	27	○○○○	48	○○○○	69	○○○○
7	○○○○	28	○○○○	49	○○○○	70	○○○○
8	○○○○	29	○○○○	50	○○○○	71	○○○○
9	○○○○	30	○○○○	51	○○○○	72	○○○○
10	○○○○	31	○○○○	52	○○○○	73	○○○○
11	○○○○	32	○○○○	53	○○○○	74	○○○○
12	○○○○	33	○○○○	54	○○○○	75	○○○○
13	○○○○	34	○○○○	55	○○○○	76	○○○○
14	○○○○	35	○○○○	56	○○○○	77	○○○○
15	○○○○	36	○○○○	57	○○○○	78	○○○○
16	○○○○	37	○○○○	58	○○○○	79	○○○○
17	○○○○	38	○○○○	59	○○○○	80	○○○○
18	○○○○	39	○○○○	60	○○○○	81	○○○○
19	○○○○	40	○○○○	61	○○○○	82	○○○○
20	○○○○	41	○○○○	62	○○○○	83	○○○○
21	○○○○	42	○○○○	63	○○○○	84	○○○○

	1 2 3 4		1 2 3 4		1 2 3 4		1 2 3 4
85	○○○○	94	○○○○	103	○○○○	112	○○○○
86	○○○○	95	○○○○	104	○○○○	113	○○○○
87	○○○○	96	○○○○	105	○○○○	114	○○○○
88	○○○○	97	○○○○	106	○○○○	115	○○○○
89	○○○○	98	○○○○	107	○○○○	116	○○○○
90	○○○○	99	○○○○	108	○○○○	117	○○○○
91	○○○○	100	○○○○	109	○○○○	118	○○○○
92	○○○○	101	○○○○	110	○○○○	119	○○○○
93	○○○○	102	○○○○	111	○○○○	120	○○○○

Answer Sheet

Unit I   Review Test 3

With a pencil, blacken the circle below the option you have chosen for your correct answer.

	1 2 3 4		1 2 3 4		1 2 3 4		1 2 3 4
1	○○○○	22	○○○○	43	○○○○	64	○○○○
2	○○○○	23	○○○○	44	○○○○	65	○○○○
3	○○○○	24	○○○○	45	○○○○	66	○○○○
4	○○○○	25	○○○○	46	○○○○	67	○○○○
5	○○○○	26	○○○○	47	○○○○	68	○○○○
6	○○○○	27	○○○○	48	○○○○	69	○○○○
7	○○○○	28	○○○○	49	○○○○	70	○○○○
8	○○○○	29	○○○○	50	○○○○	71	○○○○
9	○○○○	30	○○○○	51	○○○○	72	○○○○
10	○○○○	31	○○○○	52	○○○○	73	○○○○
11	○○○○	32	○○○○	53	○○○○	74	○○○○
12	○○○○	33	○○○○	54	○○○○	75	○○○○
13	○○○○	34	○○○○	55	○○○○	76	○○○○
14	○○○○	35	○○○○	56	○○○○	77	○○○○
15	○○○○	36	○○○○	57	○○○○	78	○○○○
16	○○○○	37	○○○○	58	○○○○	79	○○○○
17	○○○○	38	○○○○	59	○○○○	80	○○○○
18	○○○○	39	○○○○	60	○○○○	81	○○○○
19	○○○○	40	○○○○	61	○○○○	82	○○○○
20	○○○○	41	○○○○	62	○○○○	83	○○○○
21	○○○○	42	○○○○	63	○○○○	84	○○○○

	1 2 3 4		1 2 3 4		1 2 3 4		1 2 3 4
85	○○○○	93	○○○○	101	○○○○	109	○○○○
86	○○○○	94	○○○○	102	○○○○	110	○○○○
87	○○○○	95	○○○○	103	○○○○	111	○○○○
88	○○○○	96	○○○○	104	○○○○	112	○○○○
89	○○○○	97	○○○○	105	○○○○	113	○○○○
90	○○○○	98	○○○○	106	○○○○	114	○○○○
91	○○○○	99	○○○○	107	○○○○	115	○○○○
92	○○○○	100	○○○○	108	○○○○	116	○○○○

Answer Sheet

Unit **I** Review Test **4**

With a pencil, blacken the circle below the option you have chosen for your correct answer.

	1 2 3 4		1 2 3 4		1 2 3 4		1 2 3 4
1	○○○○	22	○○○○	43	○○○○	64	○○○○
2	○○○○	23	○○○○	44	○○○○	65	○○○○
3	○○○○	24	○○○○	45	○○○○	66	○○○○
4	○○○○	25	○○○○	46	○○○○	67	○○○○
5	○○○○	26	○○○○	47	○○○○	68	○○○○
6	○○○○	27	○○○○	48	○○○○	69	○○○○
7	○○○○	28	○○○○	49	○○○○	70	○○○○
8	○○○○	29	○○○○	50	○○○○	71	○○○○
9	○○○○	30	○○○○	51	○○○○	72	○○○○
10	○○○○	31	○○○○	52	○○○○	73	○○○○
11	○○○○	32	○○○○	53	○○○○	74	○○○○
12	○○○○	33	○○○○	54	○○○○	75	○○○○
13	○○○○	34	○○○○	55	○○○○	76	○○○○
14	○○○○	35	○○○○	56	○○○○	77	○○○○
15	○○○○	36	○○○○	57	○○○○	78	○○○○
16	○○○○	37	○○○○	58	○○○○	79	○○○○
17	○○○○	38	○○○○	59	○○○○	80	○○○○
18	○○○○	39	○○○○	60	○○○○	81	○○○○
19	○○○○	40	○○○○	61	○○○○	82	○○○○
20	○○○○	41	○○○○	62	○○○○	83	○○○○
21	○○○○	42	○○○○	63	○○○○	84	○○○○

	1 2 3 4		1 2 3 4		1 2 3 4		1 2 3 4
85	○○○○	92	○○○○	99	○○○○	106	○○○○
86	○○○○	93	○○○○	100	○○○○	107	○○○○
87	○○○○	94	○○○○	101	○○○○	108	○○○○
88	○○○○	95	○○○○	102	○○○○	109	○○○○
89	○○○○	96	○○○○	103	○○○○	110	○○○○
90	○○○○	97	○○○○	104	○○○○		
91	○○○○	98	○○○○	105	○○○○		

Answer Sheet

Unit **I**   Review Test **5**

With a pencil, blacken the circle below the option you have chosen for your correct answer.

	1 2 3 4		1 2 3 4		1 2 3 4		1 2 3 4
1	○○○○	22	○○○○	43	○○○○	64	○○○○
2	○○○○	23	○○○○	44	○○○○	65	○○○○
3	○○○○	24	○○○○	45	○○○○	66	○○○○
4	○○○○	25	○○○○	46	○○○○	67	○○○○
5	○○○○	26	○○○○	47	○○○○	68	○○○○
6	○○○○	27	○○○○	48	○○○○	69	○○○○
7	○○○○	28	○○○○	49	○○○○	70	○○○○
8	○○○○	29	○○○○	50	○○○○	71	○○○○
9	○○○○	30	○○○○	51	○○○○	72	○○○○
10	○○○○	31	○○○○	52	○○○○	73	○○○○
11	○○○○	32	○○○○	53	○○○○	74	○○○○
12	○○○○	33	○○○○	54	○○○○	75	○○○○
13	○○○○	34	○○○○	55	○○○○	76	○○○○
14	○○○○	35	○○○○	56	○○○○	77	○○○○
15	○○○○	36	○○○○	57	○○○○	78	○○○○
16	○○○○	37	○○○○	58	○○○○	79	○○○○
17	○○○○	38	○○○○	59	○○○○	80	○○○○
18	○○○○	39	○○○○	60	○○○○	81	○○○○
19	○○○○	40	○○○○	61	○○○○	82	○○○○
20	○○○○	41	○○○○	62	○○○○	83	○○○○
21	○○○○	42	○○○○	63	○○○○	84	○○○○

85　1 2 3 4　○○○○

86　1 2 3 4　○○○○

87　1 2 3 4　○○○○

88　1 2 3 4　○○○○

89　1 2 3 4　○○○○

90　1 2 3 4　○○○○

91　1 2 3 4　○○○○

92　1 2 3 4　○○○○

93　1 2 3 4　○○○○

94　1 2 3 4　○○○○

95　1 2 3 4　○○○○

96　1 2 3 4　○○○○

97　1 2 3 4　○○○○

98　1 2 3 4　○○○○

99　1 2 3 4　○○○○

100　1 2 3 4　○○○○

Answer Sheet

Unit **I**   Review Test **6**

With a pencil, blacken the circle below the option you have chosen for your correct answer.

	1 2 3 4		1 2 3 4		1 2 3 4		1 2 3 4
1	○○○○	22	○○○○	43	○○○○	64	○○○○
2	○○○○	23	○○○○	44	○○○○	65	○○○○
3	○○○○	24	○○○○	45	○○○○	66	○○○○
4	○○○○	25	○○○○	46	○○○○	67	○○○○
5	○○○○	26	○○○○	47	○○○○	68	○○○○
6	○○○○	27	○○○○	48	○○○○	69	○○○○
7	○○○○	28	○○○○	49	○○○○	70	○○○○
8	○○○○	29	○○○○	50	○○○○	71	○○○○
9	○○○○	30	○○○○	51	○○○○	72	○○○○
10	○○○○	31	○○○○	52	○○○○	73	○○○○
11	○○○○	32	○○○○	53	○○○○	74	○○○○
12	○○○○	33	○○○○	54	○○○○	75	○○○○
13	○○○○	34	○○○○	55	○○○○	76	○○○○
14	○○○○	35	○○○○	56	○○○○	77	○○○○
15	○○○○	36	○○○○	57	○○○○	78	○○○○
16	○○○○	37	○○○○	58	○○○○	79	○○○○
17	○○○○	38	○○○○	59	○○○○	80	○○○○
18	○○○○	39	○○○○	60	○○○○	81	○○○○
19	○○○○	40	○○○○	61	○○○○	82	○○○○
20	○○○○	41	○○○○	62	○○○○	83	○○○○
21	○○○○	42	○○○○	63	○○○○	84	○○○○

85 1 2 3 4 ○○○○

86 1 2 3 4 ○○○○

87 1 2 3 4 ○○○○

88 1 2 3 4 ○○○○

89 1 2 3 4 ○○○○

Answer Sheet

Unit I   Review Test 7

With a pencil, blacken the circle below the option you have chosen for your correct answer.

	1 2 3 4		1 2 3 4		1 2 3 4		1 2 3 4
1	○○○○	22	○○○○	43	○○○○	64	○○○○
2	○○○○	23	○○○○	44	○○○○	65	○○○○
3	○○○○	24	○○○○	45	○○○○	66	○○○○
4	○○○○	25	○○○○	46	○○○○	67	○○○○
5	○○○○	26	○○○○	47	○○○○	68	○○○○
6	○○○○	27	○○○○	48	○○○○	69	○○○○
7	○○○○	28	○○○○	49	○○○○	70	○○○○
8	○○○○	29	○○○○	50	○○○○	71	○○○○
9	○○○○	30	○○○○	51	○○○○	72	○○○○
10	○○○○	31	○○○○	52	○○○○	73	○○○○
11	○○○○	32	○○○○	53	○○○○	74	○○○○
12	○○○○	33	○○○○	54	○○○○	75	○○○○
13	○○○○	34	○○○○	55	○○○○	76	○○○○
14	○○○○	35	○○○○	56	○○○○	77	○○○○
15	○○○○	36	○○○○	57	○○○○	78	○○○○
16	○○○○	37	○○○○	58	○○○○	79	○○○○
17	○○○○	38	○○○○	59	○○○○	80	○○○○
18	○○○○	39	○○○○	60	○○○○	81	○○○○
19	○○○○	40	○○○○	61	○○○○	82	○○○○
20	○○○○	41	○○○○	62	○○○○	83	○○○○
21	○○○○	42	○○○○	63	○○○○	84	○○○○

	1 2 3 4		1 2 3 4		1 2 3 4		1 2 3 4
85	○○○○	91	○○○○	97	○○○○	103	○○○○
86	○○○○	92	○○○○	98	○○○○	104	○○○○
87	○○○○	93	○○○○	99	○○○○	105	○○○○
88	○○○○	94	○○○○	100	○○○○	106	○○○○
89	○○○○	95	○○○○	101	○○○○	107	○○○○
90	○○○○	96	○○○○	102	○○○○	108	○○○○

Answer Sheet

Unit **I** Review Test **8**

With a pencil, blacken the circle below the option you have chosen for your correct answer.

	1 2 3 4		1 2 3 4		1 2 3 4		1 2 3 4
1	○○○○	22	○○○○	43	○○○○	64	○○○○
2	○○○○	23	○○○○	44	○○○○	65	○○○○
3	○○○○	24	○○○○	45	○○○○	66	○○○○
4	○○○○	25	○○○○	46	○○○○	67	○○○○
5	○○○○	26	○○○○	47	○○○○	68	○○○○
6	○○○○	27	○○○○	48	○○○○	69	○○○○
7	○○○○	28	○○○○	49	○○○○	70	○○○○
8	○○○○	29	○○○○	50	○○○○	71	○○○○
9	○○○○	30	○○○○	51	○○○○	72	○○○○
10	○○○○	31	○○○○	52	○○○○	73	○○○○
11	○○○○	32	○○○○	53	○○○○	74	○○○○
12	○○○○	33	○○○○	54	○○○○	75	○○○○
13	○○○○	34	○○○○	55	○○○○	76	○○○○
14	○○○○	35	○○○○	56	○○○○	77	○○○○
15	○○○○	36	○○○○	57	○○○○	78	○○○○
16	○○○○	37	○○○○	58	○○○○	79	○○○○
17	○○○○	38	○○○○	59	○○○○	80	○○○○
18	○○○○	39	○○○○	60	○○○○	81	○○○○
19	○○○○	40	○○○○	61	○○○○	82	○○○○
20	○○○○	41	○○○○	62	○○○○		
21	○○○○	42	○○○○	63	○○○○		

Answer Sheet

Unit **I** Review Test **9**

With a pencil, blacken the circle below the option you have chosen for your correct answer.

	1 2 3 4		1 2 3 4		1 2 3 4		1 2 3 4
1	○○○○	22	○○○○	43	○○○○	64	○○○○
2	○○○○	23	○○○○	44	○○○○	65	○○○○
3	○○○○	24	○○○○	45	○○○○	66	○○○○
4	○○○○	25	○○○○	46	○○○○	67	○○○○
5	○○○○	26	○○○○	47	○○○○	68	○○○○
6	○○○○	27	○○○○	48	○○○○	69	○○○○
7	○○○○	28	○○○○	43	○○○○	70	○○○○
8	○○○○	29	○○○○	50	○○○○	71	○○○○
9	○○○○	30	○○○○	51	○○○○	72	○○○○
10	○○○○	31	○○○○	52	○○○○	73	○○○○
11	○○○○	32	○○○○	53	○○○○	74	○○○○
12	○○○○	33	○○○○	54	○○○○	75	○○○○
13	○○○○	34	○○○○	55	○○○○	76	○○○○
14	○○○○	35	○○○○	56	○○○○	77	○○○○
15	○○○○	36	○○○○	57	○○○○	78	○○○○
16	○○○○	37	○○○○	58	○○○○	79	○○○○
17	○○○○	38	○○○○	59	○○○○	80	○○○○
18	○○○○	39	○○○○	60	○○○○	81	○○○○
19	○○○○	40	○○○○	61	○○○○	82	○○○○
20	○○○○	41	○○○○	62	○○○○		
21	○○○○	42	○○○○	63	○○○○		

Answer Sheet

Unit I   Review Test **10**

With a pencil, blacken the circle below the option you have chosen for your correct answer.

	1 2 3 4		1 2 3 4		1 2 3 4		1 2 3 4
1	○○○○	22	○○○○	43	○○○○	64	○○○○
2	○○○○	23	○○○○	44	○○○○	65	○○○○
3	○○○○	24	○○○○	45	○○○○	66	○○○○
4	○○○○	25	○○○○	46	○○○○	67	○○○○
5	○○○○	26	○○○○	47	○○○○	68	○○○○
6	○○○○	27	○○○○	48	○○○○	69	○○○○
7	○○○○	28	○○○○	49	○○○○	70	○○○○
8	○○○○	29	○○○○	50	○○○○	71	○○○○
9	○○○○	30	○○○○	51	○○○○	72	○○○○
10	○○○○	31	○○○○	52	○○○○	73	○○○○
11	○○○○	32	○○○○	53	○○○○	74	○○○○
12	○○○○	33	○○○○	54	○○○○	75	○○○○
13	○○○○	34	○○○○	55	○○○○	76	○○○○
14	○○○○	35	○○○○	56	○○○○	77	○○○○
15	○○○○	36	○○○○	57	○○○○	78	○○○○
16	○○○○	37	○○○○	58	○○○○	79	○○○○
17	○○○○	38	○○○○	59	○○○○	80	○○○○
18	○○○○	39	○○○○	60	○○○○	81	○○○○
19	○○○○	40	○○○○	61	○○○○	82	○○○○
20	○○○○	41	○○○○	62	○○○○	83	○○○○
21	○○○○	42	○○○○	63	○○○○	84	○○○○

	1 2 3 4		1 2 3 4		1 2 3 4		1 2 3 4
85	○○○○	92	○○○○	99	○○○○	106	○○○○
86	○○○○	93	○○○○	100	○○○○	107	○○○○
87	○○○○	94	○○○○	101	○○○○	108	○○○○
88	○○○○	95	○○○○	102	○○○○	109	○○○○
89	○○○○	96	○○○○	103	○○○○	110	○○○○
90	○○○○	97	○○○○	104	○○○○		
91	○○○○	98	○○○○	105	○○○○		

Answer Sheet

Unit **II** Review Test **11**

With a pencil, blacken the circle below the option you have chosen for your correct answer.

	1 2 3 4		1 2 3 4		1 2 3 4		1 2 3 4
1	○○○○	22	○○○○	43	○○○○	64	○○○○
2	○○○○	23	○○○○	44	○○○○	65	○○○○
3	○○○○	24	○○○○	45	○○○○	66	○○○○
4	○○○○	25	○○○○	46	○○○○	67	○○○○
5	○○○○	26	○○○○	47	○○○○	68	○○○○
6	○○○○	27	○○○○	48	○○○○	69	○○○○
7	○○○○	28	○○○○	49	○○○○	70	○○○○
8	○○○○	29	○○○○	50	○○○○	71	○○○○
9	○○○○	30	○○○○	51	○○○○	72	○○○○
10	○○○○	31	○○○○	52	○○○○	73	○○○○
11	○○○○	32	○○○○	53	○○○○	74	○○○○
12	○○○○	33	○○○○	54	○○○○	75	○○○○
13	○○○○	34	○○○○	55	○○○○	76	○○○○
14	○○○○	35	○○○○	56	○○○○	77	○○○○
15	○○○○	36	○○○○	57	○○○○	78	○○○○
16	○○○○	37	○○○○	58	○○○○	79	○○○○
17	○○○○	38	○○○○	59	○○○○	80	○○○○
18	○○○○	39	○○○○	60	○○○○	81	○○○○
19	○○○○	40	○○○○	61	○○○○	82	○○○○
20	○○○○	41	○○○○	62	○○○○	83	○○○○
21	○○○○	42	○○○○	63	○○○○	84	○○○○

85
1 2 3 4
○○○○

86
1 2 3 4
○○○○

87
1 2 3 4
○○○○

88
1 2 3 4
○○○○

89
1 2 3 4
○○○○

90
1 2 3 4
○○○○

91
1 2 3 4
○○○○

Answer Sheet

Unit **II**   Review Test **12**

With a pencil, blacken the circle below the option you have chosen for your correct answer.

	1 2 3 4		1 2 3 4		1 2 3 4		1 2 3 4
1	○○○○	22	○○○○	43	○○○○	64	○○○○
2	○○○○	23	○○○○	44	○○○○	65	○○○○
3	○○○○	24	○○○○	45	○○○○	66	○○○○
4	○○○○	25	○○○○	46	○○○○	67	○○○○
5	○○○○	26	○○○○	47	○○○○	68	○○○○
6	○○○○	27	○○○○	48	○○○○	69	○○○○
7	○○○○	28	○○○○	49	○○○○	70	○○○○
8	○○○○	29	○○○○	50	○○○○	71	○○○○
9	○○○○	30	○○○○	51	○○○○	72	○○○○
10	○○○○	31	○○○○	52	○○○○	73	○○○○
11	○○○○	32	○○○○	53	○○○○	74	○○○○
12	○○○○	33	○○○○	54	○○○○	75	○○○○
13	○○○○	34	○○○○	55	○○○○	76	○○○○
14	○○○○	35	○○○○	56	○○○○	77	○○○○
15	○○○○	36	○○○○	57	○○○○	78	○○○○
16	○○○○	37	○○○○	58	○○○○	79	○○○○
17	○○○○	38	○○○○	59	○○○○	80	○○○○
18	○○○○	39	○○○○	60	○○○○	81	○○○○
19	○○○○	40	○○○○	61	○○○○	82	○○○○
20	○○○○	41	○○○○	62	○○○○	83	○○○○
21	○○○○	42	○○○○	63	○○○○	84	○○○○

	1 2 3 4		1 2 3 4		1 2 3 4		1 2 3 4
85	○○○○	92	○○○○	99	○○○○	106	○○○○
86	○○○○	93	○○○○	100	○○○○	107	○○○○
87	○○○○	94	○○○○	101	○○○○	108	○○○○
88	○○○○	95	○○○○	102	○○○○	109	○○○○
89	○○○○	96	○○○○	103	○○○○	110	○○○○
90	○○○○	97	○○○○	104	○○○○	111	○○○○
91	○○○○	98	○○○○	105	○○○○		

Answer Sheet

Unit **III** Review Test **13**

With a pencil, blacken the circle below the option you have chosen for your correct answer.

	1 2 3 4		1 2 3 4		1 2 3 4		1 2 3 4
1	○○○○	22	○○○○	43	○○○○	64	○○○○
2	○○○○	23	○○○○	44	○○○○	65	○○○○
3	○○○○	24	○○○○	45	○○○○	66	○○○○
4	○○○○	25	○○○○	46	○○○○	67	○○○○
5	○○○○	26	○○○○	47	○○○○	68	○○○○
6	○○○○	27	○○○○	48	○○○○	69	○○○○
7	○○○○	28	○○○○	49	○○○○	70	○○○○
8	○○○○	29	○○○○	50	○○○○	71	○○○○
9	○○○○	30	○○○○	51	○○○○	72	○○○○
10	○○○○	31	○○○○	52	○○○○	73	○○○○
11	○○○○	32	○○○○	53	○○○○	74	○○○○
12	○○○○	33	○○○○	54	○○○○	75	○○○○
13	○○○○	34	○○○○	55	○○○○	76	○○○○
14	○○○○	35	○○○○	56	○○○○	77	○○○○
15	○○○○	36	○○○○	57	○○○○	78	○○○○
16	○○○○	37	○○○○	58	○○○○	79	○○○○
17	○○○○	38	○○○○	59	○○○○	80	○○○○
18	○○○○	39	○○○○	60	○○○○	81	○○○○
19	○○○○	40	○○○○	61	○○○○	82	○○○○
20	○○○○	41	○○○○	62	○○○○	83	○○○○
21	○○○○	42	○○○○	63	○○○○	84	○○○○

	1 2 3 4		1 2 3 4		1 2 3 4		1 2 3 4
85	○○○○	93	○○○○	101	○○○○	109	○○○○
86	○○○○	94	○○○○	102	○○○○	110	○○○○
87	○○○○	95	○○○○	103	○○○○	111	○○○○
88	○○○○	96	○○○○	104	○○○○	112	○○○○
89	○○○○	97	○○○○	105	○○○○	113	○○○○
90	○○○○	98	○○○○	106	○○○○	114	○○○○
91	○○○○	99	○○○○	107	○○○○		
92	○○○○	100	○○○○	108	○○○○		

Answer Sheet

Unit **III**   Review Test **14**

With a pencil, blacken the circle below the option you have chosen for your correct answer.

	1 2 3 4		1 2 3 4		1 2 3 4		1 2 3 4
1	○○○○	22	○○○○	43	○○○○	64	○○○○
2	○○○○	23	○○○○	44	○○○○	65	○○○○
3	○○○○	24	○○○○	45	○○○○	66	○○○○
4	○○○○	25	○○○○	46	○○○○	67	○○○○
5	○○○○	26	○○○○	47	○○○○	68	○○○○
6	○○○○	27	○○○○	48	○○○○	69	○○○○
7	○○○○	28	○○○○	49	○○○○	70	○○○○
8	○○○○	29	○○○○	50	○○○○	71	○○○○
9	○○○○	30	○○○○	51	○○○○	72	○○○○
10	○○○○	31	○○○○	52	○○○○	73	○○○○
11	○○○○	32	○○○○	53	○○○○	74	○○○○
12	○○○○	33	○○○○	54	○○○○	75	○○○○
13	○○○○	34	○○○○	55	○○○○	76	○○○○
14	○○○○	35	○○○○	56	○○○○	77	○○○○
15	○○○○	36	○○○○	57	○○○○	78	○○○○
16	○○○○	37	○○○○	58	○○○○	79	○○○○
17	○○○○	38	○○○○	59	○○○○	80	○○○○
18	○○○○	39	○○○○	60	○○○○	81	○○○○
19	○○○○	40	○○○○	61	○○○○	82	○○○○
20	○○○○	41	○○○○	62	○○○○	83	○○○○
21	○○○○	42	○○○○	63	○○○○	84	○○○○

	1 2 3 4		1 2 3 4		1 2 3 4		1 2 3 4
85	○○○○	92	○○○○	99	○○○○	106	○○○○
86	○○○○	93	○○○○	100	○○○○	107	○○○○
87	○○○○	94	○○○○	101	○○○○	108	○○○○
88	○○○○	95	○○○○	102	○○○○	109	○○○○
89	○○○○	96	○○○○	103	○○○○	110	○○○○
90	○○○○	97	○○○○	104	○○○○	111	○○○○
91	○○○○	98	○○○○	105	○○○○		

Answer Sheet

Unit **IV** Review Test **15**

With a pencil, blacken the circle below the option you have chosen for your correct answer.

	1 2 3 4		1 2 3 4		1 2 3 4		1 2 3 4
1	OOOO	22	OOOO	43	OOOO	64	OOOO
2	OOOO	23	OOOO	44	OOOO	65	OOOO
3	OOOO	24	OOOO	45	OOOO	66	OOOO
4	OOOO	25	OOOO	46	OOOO	67	OOOO
5	OOOO	26	OOOO	47	OOOO	68	OOOO
6	OOOO	27	OOOO	48	OOOO	69	OOOO
7	OOOO	28	OOOO	49	OOOO	70	OOOO
8	OOOO	29	OOOO	50	OOOO	71	OOOO
9	OOOO	30	OOOO	51	OOOO	72	OOOO
10	OOOO	31	OOOO	52	OOOO	73	OOOO
11	OOOO	32	OOOO	53	OOOO	74	OOOO
12	OOOO	33	OOOO	54	OOOO	75	OOOO
13	OOOO	34	OOOO	55	OOOO	76	OOOO
14	OOOO	35	OOOO	56	OOOO	77	OOOO
15	OOOO	36	OOOO	57	OOOO	78	OOOO
16	OOOO	37	OOOO	58	OOOO	79	OOOO
17	OOOO	38	OOOO	59	OOOO	80	OOOO
18	OOOO	39	OOOO	60	OOOO	81	OOOO
19	OOOO	40	OOOO	61	OOOO	82	OOOO
20	OOOO	41	OOOO	62	OOOO	83	OOOO
21	OOOO	42	OOOO	63	OOOO	84	OOOO

	1 2 3 4		1 2 3 4		1 2 3 4		1 2 3 4
85	○○○○	89	○○○○	93	○○○○	97	○○○○
86	○○○○	90	○○○○	94	○○○○	98	○○○○
87	○○○○	91	○○○○	95	○○○○	99	○○○○
88	○○○○	92	○○○○	96	○○○○	100	○○○○

Answer Sheet

Unit **IV** Review Test **16**

With a pencil, blacken the circle below the option you have chosen for your correct answer.

	1 2 3 4		1 2 3 4		1 2 3 4		1 2 3 4
1	○○○○	22	○○○○	43	○○○○	64	○○○○
2	○○○○	23	○○○○	44	○○○○	65	○○○○
3	○○○○	24	○○○○	45	○○○○	66	○○○○
4	○○○○	25	○○○○	46	○○○○	67	○○○○
5	○○○○	26	○○○○	47	○○○○	68	○○○○
6	○○○○	27	○○○○	48	○○○○	69	○○○○
7	○○○○	28	○○○○	49	○○○○	70	○○○○
8	○○○○	29	○○○○	50	○○○○	71	○○○○
9	○○○○	30	○○○○	51	○○○○	72	○○○○
10	○○○○	31	○○○○	52	○○○○	73	○○○○
11	○○○○	32	○○○○	53	○○○○	74	○○○○
12	○○○○	33	○○○○	54	○○○○	75	○○○○
13	○○○○	34	○○○○	55	○○○○	76	○○○○
14	○○○○	35	○○○○	56	○○○○	77	○○○○
15	○○○○	36	○○○○	57	○○○○	78	○○○○
16	○○○○	37	○○○○	58	○○○○	79	○○○○
17	○○○○	38	○○○○	59	○○○○	80	○○○○
18	○○○○	39	○○○○	60	○○○○	81	○○○○
19	○○○○	40	○○○○	61	○○○○	82	○○○○
20	○○○○	41	○○○○	62	○○○○	83	○○○○
21	○○○○	42	○○○○	63	○○○○	84	○○○○

	1	2	3	4
85	○	○	○	○
86	○	○	○	○
87	○	○	○	○
88	○	○	○	○
89	○	○	○	○
90	○	○	○	○
91	○	○	○	○

	1	2	3	4
92	○	○	○	○
93	○	○	○	○
94	○	○	○	○
95	○	○	○	○
96	○	○	○	○
97	○	○	○	○
98	○	○	○	○

	1	2	3	4
99	○	○	○	○
100	○	○	○	○
101	○	○	○	○
102	○	○	○	○
103	○	○	○	○
104	○	○	○	○
105	○	○	○	○

	1	2	3	4
106	○	○	○	○
107	○	○	○	○
108	○	○	○	○
109	○	○	○	○
110	○	○	○	○

Answer Sheet

Part I Comprehensive Examination

With a pencil, blacken the circle below the option you have chosen for your correct answer.

	1 2 3 4		1 2 3 4		1 2 3 4		1 2 3 4
1	○○○○	22	○○○○	43	○○○○	64	○○○○
2	○○○○	23	○○○○	44	○○○○	65	○○○○
3	○○○○	24	○○○○	45	○○○○	66	○○○○
4	○○○○	25	○○○○	46	○○○○	67	○○○○
5	○○○○	26	○○○○	47	○○○○	68	○○○○
6	○○○○	27	○○○○	48	○○○○	69	○○○○
7	○○○○	28	○○○○	49	○○○○	70	○○○○
8	○○○○	29	○○○○	50	○○○○	71	○○○○
9	○○○○	30	○○○○	51	○○○○	72	○○○○
10	○○○○	31	○○○○	52	○○○○	73	○○○○
11	○○○○	32	○○○○	53	○○○○	74	○○○○
12	○○○○	33	○○○○	54	○○○○	75	○○○○
13	○○○○	34	○○○○	55	○○○○	76	○○○○
14	○○○○	35	○○○○	56	○○○○	77	○○○○
15	○○○○	36	○○○○	57	○○○○	78	○○○○
16	○○○○	37	○○○○	58	○○○○	79	○○○○
17	○○○○	38	○○○○	59	○○○○	80	○○○○
18	○○○○	39	○○○○	60	○○○○	81	○○○○
19	○○○○	40	○○○○	61	○○○○	82	○○○○
20	○○○○	41	○○○○	62	○○○○	83	○○○○
21	○○○○	42	○○○○	63	○○○○	84	○○○○

	1 2 3 4		1 2 3 4		1 2 3 4		1 2 3 4
85	○○○○	94	○○○○	103	○○○○	112	○○○○
86	○○○○	95	○○○○	104	○○○○	113	○○○○
87	○○○○	96	○○○○	105	○○○○	114	○○○○
88	○○○○	97	○○○○	106	○○○○	115	○○○○
89	○○○○	98	○○○○	107	○○○○	116	○○○○
90	○○○○	99	○○○○	108	○○○○	117	○○○○
91	○○○○	100	○○○○	109	○○○○	118	○○○○
92	○○○○	101	○○○○	110	○○○○	119	○○○○
93	○○○○	102	○○○○	111	○○○○	120	○○○○

Answer Sheet

Part II Comprehensive Examination

With a pencil, blacken the circle below the option you have chosen for your correct answer.

	1 2 3 4		1 2 3 4		1 2 3 4		1 2 3 4
1	○○○○	22	○○○○	43	○○○○	64	○○○○
2	○○○○	23	○○○○	44	○○○○	65	○○○○
3	○○○○	24	○○○○	45	○○○○	66	○○○○
4	○○○○	25	○○○○	46	○○○○	67	○○○○
5	○○○○	26	○○○○	47	○○○○	68	○○○○
6	○○○○	27	○○○○	48	○○○○	69	○○○○
7	○○○○	28	○○○○	49	○○○○	70	○○○○
8	○○○○	29	○○○○	50	○○○○	71	○○○○
9	○○○○	30	○○○○	51	○○○○	72	○○○○
10	○○○○	31	○○○○	52	○○○○	73	○○○○
11	○○○○	32	○○○○	53	○○○○	74	○○○○
12	○○○○	33	○○○○	54	○○○○	75	○○○○
13	○○○○	34	○○○○	55	○○○○	76	○○○○
14	○○○○	35	○○○○	56	○○○○	77	○○○○
15	○○○○	36	○○○○	57	○○○○	78	○○○○
16	○○○○	37	○○○○	58	○○○○	79	○○○○
17	○○○○	38	○○○○	59	○○○○	80	○○○○
18	○○○○	39	○○○○	60	○○○○	81	○○○○
19	○○○○	40	○○○○	61	○○○○	82	○○○○
20	○○○○	41	○○○○	62	○○○○	83	○○○○
21	○○○○	42	○○○○	63	○○○○	84	○○○○

	1 2 3 4		1 2 3 4		1 2 3 4		1 2 3 4
85	○○○○	94	○○○○	103	○○○○	112	○○○○
86	○○○○	95	○○○○	104	○○○○	113	○○○○
87	○○○○	96	○○○○	105	○○○○	114	○○○○
88	○○○○	97	○○○○	106	○○○○	115	○○○○
89	○○○○	98	○○○○	107	○○○○	116	○○○○
90	○○○○	99	○○○○	108	○○○○	117	○○○○
91	○○○○	100	○○○○	109	○○○○	118	○○○○
92	○○○○	101	○○○○	110	○○○○	119	○○○○
93	○○○○	102	○○○○	111	○○○○	120	○○○○

Lippincott's Review for NCLEX-PN,
5th Edition Disk Instructions

SYSTEM REQUIREMENTS

- A PC compatible computer with an Intel 386 or better processor
- Windows 3.1 or later
- 4 Megabytes of RAM (minimum), but recommend 8 MB RAM on Windows 3.1
- 8 Megabytes of RAM (minimum), but recommend 12 MB RAM on Windows 95.
- 3 Megabytes of available hard disk space

INSTALLING NCLEX-PN FOR WINDOWS

1. Start up Windows.
2. Insert the NCLEX-PN disk into the floppy disk drive.
3. From the Program Manager's File Menu, choose the Run command.
4. When the Run dialog box appears, type a:\setup (or b:\setup if you're using the B drive) in the Command Line box. Click OK or press the Enter button.
5. The installation process will begin. A dialog box proposing the directory "NCLEX-PN" on the drive containing Windows will appear. If the name and location are correct, click OK. If you want to change this information, type over the existing data, then click OK.
6. When the NCLEX-PN setup routine is done, a new group called "NCLEX-PN Exam Review" appears on your desktop.
7. Start the NCLEX-PN program by double clicking on its icon.

LIPPINCOTT'S REVIEW FOR NCLEX-PN, 5TH EDITION DISK PROGRAM

The NCLEX-PN disk program contains 115 questions that review the content in *Lippincott's Review for NCLEX-PN*, 5th edition.

This is not a timed test. Take your time; consider the questions and possible answers carefully.

To begin a test, click the **Start Over** button from the Main Menu screen. To continue a test that you have already begun, press the **Resume** button. To restart the exam and erase all the results from your previous session of that exam, press the **Start Over** button. To review your answers and compare them with the correct answers, press the **Results** button. When you press the **Start Over, Resume,** or **Results** button, the test and the program's Toolbar will appear.

LIPPINCOTT'S REVIEW FOR NCLEX-PN, 5TH EDITION TOOLBAR

Test Mode

The Toolbar contains a series of buttons that provide direct access to all test program functions. When you move the cursor over a button, an explanation of its function displays in the Status Bar, which is immediately above the Toolbar.

To get help at any time during the test, choose the Program Help button. Program Help reviews basic functions of the program. To close the Program Help window, click on the Program Help button again.

Answer each question by clicking on the oval to the left of an answer selection or by selecting the appropriate number on the keyboard (1, 2, 3, or 4). When an answer is selected, its oval will darken. If you change your mind about an answer, simply select that choice, by mouse or keyboard, again.

To register your answer selection and proceed to the next question, click on the Right Arrow button or press Return.

If you are unsure about an answer to a particular question, the program allows you to mark it for later review. Flag the question by clicking on the Mark Question button. To review all marked questions for a test, click on the Table of Contents button, which is immediately to the right of the Mark Question button. This will open the Table of Contents window.

The Table of Contents window lists every question included on the test and summarizes whether it has been answered, left unanswered, or marked for later review. Click on an item in the Table of Contents window and the program will move to that test question. Or, use the Arrow buttons to move to the first, previous, next, or last question.

At any time during the test or when you are finished taking the test, click on the Stop button. You may return to the session later without erasing your existing answers by selecting the Resume button on the Main Menu screen.

After taking the test, view the correct answer for each test question by using the Results button on the Main Menu. There are three different ways to review your results: Test Results, Nursing Process Report, and Client Need Report.

Study Mode

After taking the test and receiving your score, you may wish to enter the Study Mode. This mode supplies you with the test questions, the answers that you chose, and the rationale for correct and incorrect answers. To enter the Study Mode, click on the Study Mode button on the Main Menu screen. You will not be able to modify the answers that you have already given. However, you can select any of the answer choices for an explanation of that answer. You may also wish to use the Table of Contents button to show you which questions you marked for review. Each of these windows may be closed by clicking on their respective buttons.

To exit the *Lippincott's Review for NCLEX-PN* program, click the Exit button on the Main Menu.